Natural Products in Diabetes Mellitus: 2nd Edition

Natural Products in Diabetes Mellitus: 2nd Edition

Guest Editor

Ana Angélica Feregrino-Pérez

MDPI

Basel • Beijing • Wuhan • Barcelona • Belgrade • Novi Sad • Cluj • Manchester

Guest Editor
Ana Angélica Feregrino-Pérez
División de Estudios de
Posgrado, C.A. Bioingeniería
Básica y Aplicada
Universidad Autónoma de
Querétaro
Cerro de las Campanas
Mexico

Editorial Office
MDPI AG
Grosspeteranlage 5
4052 Basel, Switzerland

This is a reprint of the Special Issue, published open access by the journal *Pharmaceuticals* (ISSN 1424-8247), freely accessible at: https://www.mdpi.com/journal/pharmaceuticals/special_issues/HQ36LD85MX.

For citation purposes, cite each article independently as indicated on the article page online and as indicated below:

Lastname, A.A.; Lastname, B.B. Article Title. *Journal Name* **Year**, *Volume Number*, Page Range.

ISBN 978-3-7258-6588-8 (Hbk)
ISBN 978-3-7258-6589-5 (PDF)
https://doi.org/10.3390/books978-3-7258-6589-5

Contents

About the Editor . . . . **vii**

Preface . . . . **ix**

Ana A. Feregrino-Pérez
Natural Products in Diabetes Mellitus: 2nd Edition
Reprinted from: *Pharmaceuticals* **2025**, *18*, 1666, https://doi.org/10.3390/ph18111666 . . . . **1**

Eman B. Abbas, Asmaa M. El-Kalaawy, Noha A. Ahmed, Anwar Shams, Amal K. Khaliefa and Osama M. Ahmed
Diosmin Potentiates the Antidiabetic Effects of Linagliptin in Nicotinamide/Streptozotocin-Induced Diabetic Wistar Rats
Reprinted from: *Pharmaceuticals* **2025**, *18*, 656, https://doi.org/10.3390/ph18050656 . . . . **5**

Diana Karina Rangel-Sandoval, Lucia Guerrero-Becerra, Consuelo Lomas-Soria, Amanda Kim Rico-Chávez, José Antonio Cervantes-Chávez, Luis Antonio Reyes-Castro, et al.
Timbe (*Acaciella angustissima*) as an Alternative Source of Compounds with Biological Activity: Antidiabetic
Reprinted from: *Pharmaceuticals* **2025**, *18*, 593, https://doi.org/10.3390/ph18040593 . . . . **28**

Elena Rafailovska, Elona Xhemaili, Zorica Naumovska, Olga Gigopulu, Biljana Miova, Ljubica Suturkova and Gjoshe Stefkov
Unlocking the Antidiabetic Potential of CBD: In Vivo Preclinical Studies
Reprinted from: *Pharmaceuticals* **2025**, *18*, 446, https://doi.org/10.3390/ph18040446 . . . . **52**

Kyung-Hyun Cho, Sang Hyuk Lee, Yunki Lee, Ashutosh Bahuguna and Ji-Eun Kim
Synergistic Efficacy of Policosanol (Raydel®) and Banaba Leaf Extract to Treat Hyperglycemia and Dyslipidemia in Streptozotocin-Induced Diabetic and Hyperlipidemic Zebrafish (*Danio rerio*): Protection of Liver and Kidney with Enhanced Tissue Regeneration
Reprinted from: *Pharmaceuticals* **2025**, *18*, 362, https://doi.org/10.3390/ph18030362 . . . . **72**

Xin-Xin Zeng, Liang Wang, Ming-Yu Wang, Zhen-Ran Hu, Xiang-Ke Li, Guo-Jun Fei, et al.
BuZhong YiQi Formula Alleviates Postprandial Hyperglycemia in T2DM Rats by Inhibiting α-Amylase and α-Glucosidase In Vitro and In Vivo
Reprinted from: *Pharmaceuticals* **2025**, *18*, 201, https://doi.org/10.3390/ph18020201 . . . . **98**

Yingxiao Li, Chao-Tien Hsu, Ting-Ting Yang and Kai-Chun Cheng
Syringaldehyde Alleviates Cardiac Hypertrophy Induced by Hyperglycemia in H9c2 Cells Through GLP-1 Receptor Signals
Reprinted from: *Pharmaceuticals* **2025**, *18*, 110, https://doi.org/10.3390/ph18010110 . . . . **123**

Cristian Sandoval, Luciano Canobbi, Álvaro Orrego, Camila Reyes, Felipe Venegas, Ángeles Vera, et al.
Application of Integrated Optical Density in Evaluating Insulin Expression in the Endocrine Pancreas During Chronic Ethanol Exposure and β-Carotene Supplementation: A Novel Approach Utilizing Artificial Intelligence
Reprinted from: *Pharmaceuticals* **2024**, *17*, 1478, https://doi.org/10.3390/ph17111478 . . . . **139**

Hui-Ju Huang, Hanoch Livneh, Chieh-Tsung Yen, Ming-Chi Lu, Wei-Jen Chen and Tzung-Yi Tsai
Adjunctive Therapy with Chinese Herbal Medicine Lowers Risk of Hearing Loss in Type 2 Diabetes Patients: Results from a Cohort-Based Case-Control Study
Reprinted from: *Pharmaceuticals* **2024**, *17*, 1191, https://doi.org/10.3390/ph17091191 . . . . **153**

Felix Omoruyi, Lauren Tatina, Lizette Rios, Dewayne Stennett and Jean Sparks
Insights into the Therapeutic Use of *Kalanchoe pinnata* Supplement in Diabetes Mellitus
Reprinted from: *Pharmaceuticals* **2025**, *18*, 1518, https://doi.org/10.3390/ph18101518 . . . . **165**

Fabiola Curiel Ayala, Francisco Ignacio García Rodríguez, Sandra N. Jimenez-Garcia and Lina Garcia-Mier
Chaya Leaf: A Promising Approach for Diabetes Management
Reprinted from: *Pharmaceuticals* **2025**, *18*, 1242, https://doi.org/10.3390/ph18091242 . . . . **184**

Lucia Guerrero-Becerra, Sumiko Morimoto, Estefania Arrellano-Ordoñez, Angélica Morales-Miranda, Ramón G. Guevara-Gonzalez, Ana Angélica Feregrino-Pérez and Consuelo Lomas-Soria
Polyphenolic Compounds in Fabaceous Plants with Antidiabetic Potential
Reprinted from: *Pharmaceuticals* **2025**, *18*, 69, https://doi.org/10.3390/ph18010069 . . . . **204**

Mohammad Adi Mohammad Fadzil, Norhashimah Abu Seman and Aswir Abd Rashed
The Potential Therapeutic Use of Agarwood for Diabetes: A Scoping Review
Reprinted from: *Pharmaceuticals* **2024**, *17*, 1548, https://doi.org/10.3390/ph17111548 . . . . **224**

Xiaoyu Zhang, Jia Wang, Tingting Zhang, Shuqin Li, Junyu Liu, Mingyue Li, et al.
Updated Progress on Polysaccharides with Anti-Diabetic Effects through the Regulation of Gut Microbiota: Sources, Mechanisms, and Structure–Activity Relationships
Reprinted from: *Pharmaceuticals* **2024**, *17*, 456, https://doi.org/10.3390/ph17040456 . . . . **248**

About the Editor

Ana Angélica Feregrino-Pérez

Ana Angélica Feregrino-Pérez, Ph.D. (ORCID: 0000-0001-8001-5912), is a researcher and professor in the Universidad Autónoma de Querétaro (UAQ), Mexico. Her work integrates agricultural biotechnology, plant physiology, nanotechnology, and natural product research, with a particular focus on the metabolic and biochemical responses of plants and functional foods exposed to nanoparticles, elicitors, and abiotic stress. She specializes in the study of bioactive compounds—especially phenolics, flavonoids, and antioxidant metabolites—and their relevance to human health, including antidiabetic potential.

Dr. Feregrino-Pérez leads multidisciplinary projects involving nanotechnology in agriculture, secondary metabolite modulation, valorization of agroindustrial residues, mushroom biotechnology, and multi-omics analysis (metabolomics, transcriptomics, and proteomics). Her research group explores how nanomaterials and natural elicitors modify metabolic pathways and contribute to the sustainable production of high-value phytochemicals.

She has authored numerous scientific publications and has served as Guest Editor for Special Issues in MDPI journals, including *Pharmaceuticals*, promoting evidence-based research on natural compounds and complementary therapies for chronic diseases such as diabetes mellitus. Her academic activity also includes curriculum innovation and strengthening sustainable agroindustrial practices in semi-rural communities in central Mexico.

Dr. Feregrino-Pérez is committed to advancing integrative approaches that connect biotechnology, engineering, and public health to support sustainable food systems and the development of natural therapeutic alternatives.

Preface

The second edition of "*Natural Products in Diabetes Mellitus*" builds upon the growing body of evidence supporting the role of natural compounds as complementary approaches in the prevention and management of diabetes mellitus (DM). As the global burden of diabetes continues to rise, driven by sedentary lifestyles, dietary imbalances, and aging populations, the search for safe, effective, and sustainable therapeutic alternatives has become increasingly imperative. While conventional pharmacological treatments remain the cornerstone of clinical management, their limitations in long-term efficacy, adverse effects, and patient adherence underscore the need for integrative strategies.

This volume brings together multidisciplinary contributions that explore natural products from botanical, nutritional, and microbial origins, elucidating their mechanisms of action through molecular, cellular, and physiological pathways. The studies compiled here highlight diverse therapeutic targets, including incretin signaling, oxidative stress modulation, regulation of digestive enzymes, gut microbiota interactions, and hepatic metabolic control. The emerging evidence suggests that natural products not only possess intrinsic bioactivity but may also enhance conventional therapies through synergistic interactions, offering promising prospects for metabolic regulation and complication prevention.

Importantly, the works in this edition emphasize methodological innovation, incorporating artificial intelligence, metabolomics, and multi-omics integration to strengthen scientific rigor. Collectively, these contributions aim to inspire further translational research, promote standardization and safety assessment, and support the development of evidence-based natural interventions for diabetes management.

Ana Angélica Feregrino-Pérez
Guest Editor

pharmaceuticals

Editorial

Natural Products in Diabetes Mellitus: 2nd Edition

Ana A. Feregrino-Pérez

Posgrado en Ingeniería en Biosistemas, Facultad de Ingeniería, Universidad Autónoma de Querétaro, Carretera a Chichimequillas s/n km1, El Marques C.P. 76265, Mexico; feregrino.angge@hotmail.com

1. Introduction

Diabetes mellitus (DM) remains one of the most prevalent and challenging chronic metabolic disorders worldwide, characterized by persistent hyperglycemia due to impaired insulin secretion, insulin resistance, or both. According to recent global health reports, approximately 11.1% of adults aged 20–79 currently live with diabetes, with type 2 diabetes mellitus (T2DM) representing more than 90% of all cases [1,2]. The increasing global burden of diabetes is largely attributed to sedentary lifestyles, unbalanced diets, and aging populations, factors that collectively exacerbate the risk of cardiovascular, renal, ocular, and neurological complications [3].

Despite the diversity of pharmacological options—such as metformin, insulin analogs, DPP-4 inhibitors, GLP-1 receptor agonists, and SGLT2 inhibitors—achieving optimal glycemic control remains a significant challenge for many patients. Long-term use of these agents can lead to adverse effects, poor adherence, and increased financial burden, limiting their effectiveness in real-world settings [4]. Consequently, there is a growing scientific and clinical interest in natural compounds and complementary therapies that can provide safe, sustainable, and synergistic support to conventional pharmacotherapy.

Over the past decade, extensive research has focused on medicinal plants and bioactive phytochemicals with potential antidiabetic properties. Natural compounds have demonstrated antioxidant, anti-inflammatory, and insulin-sensitizing effects, regulating key molecular pathways involved in glucose metabolism, pancreatic β-cell protection, and glucose uptake [5–7].

Beyond phytochemicals, other natural interventions—such as those incorporating dietary fibers, probiotics, and functional foods such as apple cider vinegar—have shown promising results in improving glycemic variability, lipid metabolism, and gut microbiota composition [8,9]. The modulation of the gut–microbiota–pancreas axis appears particularly relevant, as it may enhance metabolic flexibility and reduce systemic inflammation, two hallmarks of T2DM pathogenesis.

Nevertheless, despite these encouraging findings, the safety profile and potential herb–drug interactions of natural compounds require careful assessment. To advance this field of research, future studies should prioritize integrative and multidisciplinary approaches, combining molecular, preclinical, and clinical data to elucidate mechanisms of action and optimize formulation strategies.

Collectively, the contributions presented in this Special Issue, "Natural Products in Diabetes Mellitus: 2nd Edition", of *Pharmaceuticals* highlight the importance of evidence-based natural therapies as part of a broader, sustainable strategy for diabetes prevention and management.

2. Results

The articles in this Special Issue converge on the importance of natural compounds as adjuvants to antidiabetic therapy. The contributions are listed in the backmatter of this Editorial.

In the field of phenolic metabolites, Li et al. demonstrated that syringaldehyde attenuates hyperglycemia-induced cardiac hypertrophy via GLP-1R and AMPK. Similarly, Guerrero-Becerra et al. reviewed the role of polyphenols in Fabaceae, which have antioxidant and insulinotropic potential. Other emerging botanical resources include agarwood, evaluated in a scoping review (M. Fadzil et al.), which has shown antihyperglycemic and antioxidant effects, although it has not yet been included in clinical trials.

Considering specific antioxidants, Sandoval et al. showed that β-carotene supplementation protects pancreatic β-cells against ethanol-induced damage, using artificial intelligence as an innovative histological analysis tool. Huang et al. conducted a population-based study involving over 64,000 patients, finding that adjunctive Chinese herbal medicine reduced the risk of hearing loss in T2D patients. Likewise, Zhang et al. integrated evidence on polysaccharides, highlighting their ability to modulate gut microbiota and reduce diabetic complications.

The study conducted by Curiel Ayala et al. further expanded the diversity of approaches in this domain: chaya was critically reviewed as a source of flavonoids and dietary adjuvant, with warnings about interactions with metformin. Additionally, B. Abbas et al. suggested that a diosmin–linagliptin combination showed superior efficacy compared to monocompounds in rats, restoring hepatic metabolism and pancreatic function. Omoruyi et al. reported notably antioxidant, anti-inflammatory, and antidiabetic activities in *Kalanchoe pinnata*, and Karina et al. revealed the dual antidiabetic and antimicrobial potential of timbe (*Acaciella angustissima*). Rafailovska et al. indicated that cannabidiol (CBD) lowered glucose and improved hepatic and lipid parameters in animal models, and Cho et al. clearly showed that the combination of policosanol and banaba generated synergy in glycemic control, lipid profiling, and organ protection. Finally, Zeng et al. investigated how the Buzhong Yiqi Formula (BZYQF) controls postprandial glucose by inhibiting digestive enzymes, identifying flavonoids as the primary active compounds responsible.

The presented works coincide in their insight that natural compounds act through complementary mechanisms: incretin signaling (GLP-1R, AMPK), digestive enzymes (α-amylase, α-glucosidase), hepatic metabolic regulation, oxidative stress reduction, and gut microbiota modulation. A trend toward synergy is observed, both between botanical products and in combination with conventional drugs, as in the cases of diosmin–linagliptin and policosanol–banaba. Methodological innovations such as artificial intelligence, metabolomics, and multi-omics analysis are also emphasized.

3. Research Gaps and Perspectives

The integration of natural compounds into diabetes management faces several scientific and technological challenges, notably the scarcity of controlled clinical trials, lack of standardized phytochemical characterization, and limited assessment of herb–drug interactions and long-term safety [10,11]. Establishing harmonized extraction protocols and employing advanced analytical tools such as LC–MS, metabolomics, and fingerprint profiling are essential to ensure reproducibility and safety.

To enhance translational value, integrative multi-omics analyses are required to further elucidate host–microbiota interactions [12].

Recent advances in nanotechnology have also improved the bioavailability and stability of plant-derived compounds. Nanoencapsulation of curcuminoids, polyphenols, and berberine enhances their absorption and therapeutic efficacy, paving the way toward precision nutraceuticals [13,14].

Finally, from a sustainability perspective, the valorization of regional medicinal plants promotes circular bioeconomy principles and supports the UN Sustainable Development Goals—particularly SDGs 3 and 12 [2,15]. Integrating ethnobotanical knowledge with modern biomedical approaches will be key to developing safe, effective, and sustainable phytotherapeutics for diabetes and related disorders [5,6].

4. Conclusions

This Special Issue of *Pharmaceuticals*, "Natural Products in Diabetes Mellitus: 2nd Edition", provides a broad overview of natural and complementary medicinal alternatives for diabetes management. The integrative evidence confirms the potential of phenolic compounds, polysaccharides, carotenoids, and herbal formulas, as well as the value of combined strategies. An immediate objective is progressing toward rigorous clinical trials that consolidate these options within contemporary therapeutics.

Funding: This research received no external funding.

Institutional Review Board Statement: Not applicable.

Informed Consent Statement: Not applicable.

Acknowledgments: The author would like to thank MDPI for setting up this Special Issue and anonymous editor for the support provided.

Conflicts of Interest: The author declares no conflicts of interest.

List of Contributions:

1. Li, Y.; Hsu, C.-T.; Yang, T.-T.; Cheng, K.-C. Syringaldehyde alleviates cardiac hypertrophy induced by hyperglycemia in H9c2 cells through GLP-1 receptor signals. *Pharmaceuticals* **2025**, *18*, 110. https://doi.org/10.3390/ph18010110.
2. Guerrero-Becerra, L.; Morimoto, S.; Arrellano-Ordoñez, E.; Morales-Miranda, A.; Guevara-Gonzalez, R.G.; Feregrino-Pérez, A.A.; Lomas-Soria, C. Polyphenolic compounds in fabaceous plants with antidiabetic potential. *Pharmaceuticals* **2025**, *18*, 69. https://doi.org/10.3390/ph18010069.
3. Fadzil, M.A.M.; Seman, N.A.; Rashed, A.A. The potential therapeutic use of agarwood for diabetes: A scoping review. *Pharmaceuticals* **2024**, *17*, 1548. https://doi.org/10.3390/ph17111548.
4. Sandoval, C.; Canobbi, L.; Orrego, Á.; Reyes, C.; Venegas, F.; Vera, Á.; Torrens, F.; Vásquez, B.; Godoy, K.; Zamorano, M.; et al. Application of integrated optical density in evaluating insulin expression in the endocrine pancreas during chronic ethanol exposure and β-carotene supplementation: A novel approach utilizing artificial intelligence. *Pharmaceuticals* **2024**, *17*, 1478. https://doi.org/10.3390/ph17111478.
5. Huang, H.-J.; Livneh, H.; Yen, C.-T.; Lu, M.-C.; Chen, W.-J.; Tsai, T.-Y. Adjunctive therapy with Chinese herbal medicine lowers risk of hearing loss in type 2 diabetes patients: Results from a cohort-based case-control study. *Pharmaceuticals* **2024**, *17*, 1191. https://doi.org/10.3390/ph17091191.
6. Zhang, X.; Wang, J.; Zhang, T.; Li, S.; Liu, J.; Li, M.; Lu, J.; Zhang, M.; Chen, H. Updated progress on polysaccharides with anti-diabetic effects through the regulation of gut microbiota: Sources, mechanisms, and structure–activity relationships. *Pharmaceuticals* **2024**, *17*, 456. https://doi.org/10.3390/ph17040456.
7. Ayala, F.C.; Rodríguez, F.I.G.; Jimenez-Garcia, S.N.; Garcia-Mier, L. Chaya Leaf: A Promising Approach for Diabetes Management. *Pharmaceuticals* **2025**, *18*, 1242. https://doi.org/10.3390/ph18091242.

8. Abbas, E.B.; El-Kalaawy, A.M.; Ahmed, N.A.; Shams, A.; Khaliefa, A.K.; Ahmed, O.M. Diosmin Potentiates the Antidiabetic Effects of Linagliptin in Nicotinamide/Streptozotocin-Induced Diabetic Wistar Rats. *Pharmaceuticals* **2025**, *18*, 656. https://doi.org/10.3390/ph18050656.
9. Karina, D.; Kim, A.; Antonio, J.; Antonio, L.; Angélica, A. Timbe (*Acaciella angustissima*) as an alternative source of compounds with biological activity: Antidiabetic. *Pharmaceuticals* **2025**, *18*, 593. https://doi.org/10.3390/ph18040593.
10. Rafailovska, E.; Xhemaili, E.; Naumovska, Z.; Gigopulu, O.; Miova, B.; Suturkova, L.; Stefkov, G. Unlocking the antidiabetic potential of CBD: In vivo preclinical studies. *Pharmaceuticals* **2025**, *18*, 446. https://doi.org/10.3390/ph18040446.
11. Cho, K.; Lee, S.H.; Lee, Y.; Bahuguna, A.; Kim, J. Synergistic efficacy of policosanol (Raydel®) and banaba leaf extract to treat hyperglycemia and dyslipidemia in streptozotocin-induced diabetic and hyperlipidemic zebrafish (*Danio rerio*): Protection of liver and kidney with enhanced tissue regeneration. *Pharmaceuticals* **2025**, *18*, 362. https://doi.org/10.3390/ph18030362.
12. Zeng, X.; Wang, L.; Wang, M.; Hu, Z.; Li, X.; Fei, G.; Ling, L.; Fan, Y.; Yang, Z. BuZhong YiQi formula alleviates postprandial hyperglycemia in T2DM rats by inhibiting α-amylase and α-glucosidase in vitro and in vivo. *Pharmaceuticals* **2025**, *18*, 201. https://doi.org/10.3390/ph18020201.
13. Omoruyi, F.; Tatina, L.; Rios, L.; Stennett, D.; Sparks, J. Insights into the Therapeutic Use of *Kalanchoe pinnata* Supplement in Diabetes Mellitus. *Pharmaceuticals* **2025**, *18*, 1518. https://doi.org/10.3390/ph18101518.

References

1. International Diabetes Federation. *IDF Diabetes Atlas*, 11th ed.; International Diabetes Federation: Brussels, Belgium, 2024.
2. World Health Organization. *Global Report on Diabetes 2023*; World Health Organization: Geneva, Switzerland, 2023.
3. Centers for Disease Control and Prevention. *National Diabetes Statistics Report 2024*; U.S. Department of Health and Human Services: Washington, DC, USA, 2024.
4. American Diabetes Association. Standards of medical care in diabetes—2024. *Diabetes Care* **2024**, *47* (Suppl. 1), S1–S200. [CrossRef] [PubMed]
5. Onukwuli, C.O.; Izuchukwu, E.; Paul-Chima, O. Exploring phytochemicals for diabetes management: Mechanisms, efficacy, and future directions. *Sciences* **2024**, *5*, 7–17. [CrossRef]
6. Khan, N.; Qureshi, M.A.; Shah, A. Antidiabetic effects of *Nigella sativa* and its bioactive compounds: A review. *Pharmaceuticals* **2023**, *16*, 422. [CrossRef]
7. Cheng, M.; Ding, F.; Li, L.; Dai, C.; Sun, X.; Xu, J.; Chen, F.; Li, M.; Li, X. Exploring the role of curcumin in mitigating oxidative stress to alleviate lipid metabolism disorders. *Front. Pharmacol.* **2025**, *16*, 1517174. [CrossRef] [PubMed]
8. Gómez-Ruiz, M.; Hernández-García, A.; López-Morales, J. Probiotic-based modulation of gut microbiota for glycemic control in type 2 diabetes: A systematic review. *Nutrients* **2023**, *15*, 875. [CrossRef]
9. Li, X.; Xia, Y.; Song, X.; Xiong, Z.; Ai, L.; Wang, G. Probiotics intervention for type 2 diabetes mellitus therapy: A review from proposed mechanisms to future prospects. *Crit. Rev. Food Sci. Nutr.* **2025**, *65*, 4457–4475. [CrossRef] [PubMed]
10. Suvarna, R.; Shenoy, R.P.; Hadapad, B.S.; Nayak, A.V. Effectiveness of polyherbal formulations for the treatment of type 2 Diabetes mellitus-A systematic review and meta-analysis. *J. Ayurveda Integr. Med.* **2021**, *12*, 213–222. [CrossRef] [PubMed]
11. Vijapur, L.S.; Singh, G.; Pandey, J.; Patel, B.A.; Shyamala, J.K.; Krishna, K.V.V.; Amudha, S.; Tiwari, G. Formulation standardization and quality control of polyherbal formulation for treatment of type 2 diabetes mellitus. *Nanotechnol. Percept* **2024**, *20*, 775–783.
12. Torres-Pérez, A.; García-López, C.; Martínez, D. Multi-omics approaches to understand host–microbiota interactions in metabolic disorders. *Metabolites* **2025**, *15*, 45. [CrossRef]
13. Desai, N.M. Nanotechnology Based Drug Delivery Systems of Herbal Medicine. *Biomater. Connect.* **2024**, *2*, 0009. [CrossRef]
14. Huang, L.; Luo, S.; Tong, S.; Lv, Z.; Wu, J. The development of nanocarriers for natural products. *Wiley Interdiscip. Rev. Nanomed. Nanobiotechnol.* **2024**, *16*, e1967. [CrossRef] [PubMed]
15. UNESCO. *Education for Sustainable Development Goals: Learning Objectives*; UNESCO Publishing: Paris, France, 2023.

pharmaceuticals

MDPI

Article

Diosmin Potentiates the Antidiabetic Effects of Linagliptin in Nicotinamide/Streptozotocin-Induced Diabetic Wistar Rats

Eman B. Abbas [1], Asmaa M. El-Kalaawy [2], Noha A. Ahmed [1,*], Anwar Shams [3,4,5,*], Amal K. Khaliefa [6] and Osama M. Ahmed [1]

1 Physiology Division, Department of Zoology, Faculty of Science, Beni-Suef University, P.O. Box 62521, Beni-Suef 62521, Egypt; eman_baker2002@yahoo.com (E.B.A.); osama.ahmed@science.bsu.edu.eg (O.M.A.)
2 Department of Pharmacology, Faculty of Medicine, Beni-Suef University, Beni-Suef 62521, Egypt; asmaa.hussein@med.bsu.edu.eg
3 Department of Pharmacology, College of Medicine, Taif University, P.O. Box 11099, Taif 21944, Saudi Arabia
4 Research Center for Health Sciences, Deanship of Graduate Studies and Scientific Research, Taif University, Taif 26432, Saudi Arabia
5 High Altitude Research Center, Taif University, P.O. Box 11099, Taif 21944, Saudi Arabia
6 Department of Biochemistry, Faculty of Science, Beni-Suef University, P.O. Box 62521, Beni-Suef 62521, Egypt; bio.biochemistry2011@yahoo.com
* Correspondence: drnohascience@science.bsu.edu.eg (N.A.A.); a.shams@tu.edu.sa (A.S.)

Abstract: Background/Objectives: Natural therapeutics for the treatment of diabetes mellitus represent a common challenge for many researchers. Thus, the aim of this study was to evaluate the antihyperglycemic and anti-inflammatory effects and the hepatic antioxidant activities of both diosmin and linagliptin on nicotinamide/streptozotocin-induced diabetes mellitus in rats. **Methods:** Induction of diabetes mellitus was produced by injecting an intraperitoneal dose of nicotinamide (60 mg/kg) to 16-hour-fasted rats, then after 15 min, an intraperitoneal dose of streptozotocin (60 mg/kg) was injected. The rats with diabetes were orally treated with linagliptin (1 mg/kg), diosmin (10 mg/kg), and both of them every other day for 4 weeks. **Results:** The elevated hepatic glucose-6-phosphatase and glycogen phosphorylase activities, the lowered concentrations of serum insulin, C-peptide, and hepatic glycogen, and the diminished hepatic antioxidant defense system of nicotinamide/streptozotocin-induced diabetic rats were all potentially improved by the therapies. The treatments also improved the deteriorated adiponectin and resistin mRNA expression in visceral adipose tissue of nicotinamide/streptozotocin-induced diabetic rats. In addition, the treatments induced a recovery of damaged islets of Langerhans and a regeneration of islet cells in association with the enhancement of the formation of insulin granules in β-cells and the improvement of kidney function; the combined effect was the most potent. **Conclusions:** Diosmin alone or in combination with linagliptin has potent antidiabetic effects, which were managed through their insulinotropic and insulin-improving actions. The diosmin in combination with linagliptin has the most potent antihyperglycemic effects.

Keywords: diosmin; linagliptin; nicotinamide; streptozotocin; anti-inflammatory effect; antioxidant effect; diabetic rats

1. Introduction

Diabetes mellitus (DM) is a long-term metabolic disease marked by reduced insulin action and/or absolute or relative insulin insufficiency. It is divided into three groups, also known as type 1 DM (T1DM), type 2 DM (T2DM), and other distinct forms of the disease [1].

The number of people living with DM rose from 200 million in 1990 to 830 million in 2022, and DM was the direct cause of 1.6 million deaths and 47% of all deaths in 2021 worldwide, as reported by the World Health Organization (WHO) in 2024 [2].

T1DM is a long-term inflammatory condition caused by the immune system attacking the β-cells in the pancreas that produce insulin [2]. It makes up 5–10% of DM cases, and its occurrence is increasing globally. On the other hand, T2DM accounts for 90% of the frequency of the condition and is far more common [3].

Streptozotocin (STZ) in combination with nicotinamide (NA) causes an animal model to develop a diabetes-like disease that resembles human T2DM [4]. NA is given 15 min before STZ to 2-month-old Wistar rats and causes mild and non-fasting hyperglycemia without a substantial depletion in plasma insulin concentration and a decrease in pancreatic insulin storage, making it a model of impaired insulin sensitivity [5]. STZ administered by intraperitoneal or intravenous routes enters into pancreatic islet β-cells and causes alkylation of the DNA, depletion in the NA dinucleotide, suppression in the cellular adenosine triphosphate, damage to β-cells, and insulin deficiency [6]. Thus, the antagonistic effect of NA causes only modest STZ-induced destruction to pancreatic islets' β-cells. The results and effectiveness of this two-step technique are determined by the STZ and NA dosages [7]. As a result, STZ/NA-induced animals are an appealing and effective model with pathophysiological parallels to human DM that may be used in acute and chronic research. In this model, pharmacological research of insulinotropic drugs has yielded substances that might be used to treat T2DM [7].

Gliptins, or dipeptidyl peptidase-4 (DPP-4) inhibitors, are among the most recently licensed medications for the treatment of hyperglycemia in T2DM patients. Gliptins exert their antidiabetic benefits principally by blocking the breakdown of endogenous glucagon-like peptide 1 (GLP-1) and glucose-dependent insulinotropic peptide (GIP), hence prolonging postprandial insulin production. DPP-4 inhibitors may have the ability to exhibit a broader range of valuable pleiotropic properties in the heart and vasculature, raising the level of peptides that may have vasoactive and cardioprotective properties. The DPP-4 signaling cascade has recently been shown to play a role in the pathologic characteristics of sepsis, owing to a selective cross-talk within the DPP-4 and nuclear factor-kappa B (NF-κB) signal pathways [8].

Linagliptin is an orally active dipeptidyl peptidase-4 (DPP-4) inhibitor used as T2DM therapy in many countries. This oral, highly specific DPP-4 inhibitor inhibits DPP-4 by more than 80% during a 24 h period. It has nonlinear dose-proportionate pharmacokinetic features and is virtually totally removed through the gastrointestinal system, with less than 5% detected in urine [9].

The primary characteristics of linagliptin are its high efficacy and selectivity for DPP-4 inhibition, as well as its ability to prolong the half-life of circulating hormones and enhance glucose homeostasis in preclinical investigations [9]. In a phase I trial with healthy people, it showed a true 24 h duration of effect and a safety and tolerability profile comparable to a placebo [10].

There is an increasing demand to use natural antidiabetic agents. Because herbal medicines generally have fewer side effects than conventional medications, there has been a resurgence of interest in using them to treat a variety of illnesses in recent years. The World Health Organization (WHO) has also recommended that the effectiveness of plants be evaluated in situations where safe, contemporary medications are lacking. Hence, further assessments of alternative therapies are needed [11].

Diosmin (DS) (diosmetin 7-O-rutinoside), a natural flavanone glycoside, is easily produced by dehydrogenation of hesperidin, which is rich in the pericarp of numerous citrus fruits [12]. Diosmin has anti-inflammatory effects and protects the body from free radicals and other unstable molecules [13]. It is most commonly used to treat hemorrhoids and leg sores caused by inadequate blood flow. It is also said to cure several disorders, although there is no strong evidence to support these claims [14].

Consequently, this study aims to compare the antihyperglycemic, anti-inflammatory, and hepatic antioxidant activities of diosmin and linagliptin in NA/STZ-induced diabetic rats, as well as their interactions. The study also aims to determine whether diosmin enhances linagliptin's antihyperglycemic effects in diabetic rats.

2. Results

2.1. *Effects on Oral Glucose Tolerance (OGT)*

The treatment of diabetic rats with linagliptin, diosmin, and both of them together produced a marked decrease in fasting glucose levels: 242.25 ± 65.8, 366.75 ± 76.49, and 141.25 ± 35.15 mg/dL respectively. The effect was significant ($p < 0.05$) due to treatments with linagliptin and its combination with diosmin. In the first hour of administration of glucose (3 mg/kg), the glucose levels recorded 377.50 ± 88.18, 502.00 ± 65.54, and 255.00 ± 55.6 mg/dL, respectively, reaching their peak value. Then, the glucose levels decreased in the second hour to 287.00 ± 62.09, 405.25 ± 56.05, and 169.75 ± 56.83 mg/dL, respectively. In the third hour, the glucose level recorded 319 ± 76.40 mg/dL in the diabetic rats treated with linagliptin. In the diabetic rats treated with diosmin, the glucose level decreased to 418.67 ± 87.07 mg/dL. The glucose level showed a decrease to 161.25 ± 30.99 mg/dL in the diabetic rats treated with both linagliptin and diosmin. The present data revealed that linagliptin and diosmin together are more effective than treatment with linagliptin alone or diosmin alone (Table 1).

Table 1. Effect of linagliptin and diosmin on OGT in NA/STZ-induced diabetic rats.

Groups \ Time (Min)	0 min	60 min	120 min	180 min
NC	77.125 ± 5.21 ^{a}	127.88 ± 19.75 ^{a}	111.5 ± 5.68 ^{a}	81.00 ± 7.89 ^{a}
DC	438.70± 36.21 ^{c}	598 ± 46.47 ^{d}	560 ± 80.67 ^{d}	498.00 ± 49.83 ^{c}
D + LIN	242.25 ± 65.8 ^{ab}	377.5 ± 88.18 ^{bc}	287 ± 62.09 ^{bc}	319.00 ± 76.40 ^{b}
D + DIO	366.75 ± 76.49 ^{bc}	502.25 ± 65.54 ^{cd}	405.25 ± 56.05 ^{c}	418.67 ± 87.07 ^{bc}
D + LIN + DIO	141.25 ± 35.15 ^{a}	255 ± 55.6 ^{ab}	169.75 ± 56.83 ^{ab}	161.25 ± 30.99 ^{a}

Data expressed as the means ± SE. Means which do not share the same superscript symbols (a, b, c, and d) within the same column, are significantly different at $p < 0.05$. F-probability: $p < 0.001$. NC, DC, D + LIN, D + DIO, and D + LIN + DIO refer to the normal control group, the diabetic control group, the diabetic group treated with linagliptin, the diabetic group treated with diosmin, and the diabetic group treated with linagliptin and diosmin.

2.2. *Effects on Serum Insulin and C-Peptide Levels*

Serum insulin level showed a significant depletion ($p < 0.05$) in the diabetic control (1.36 ± 0.07 ng/mL). The treatment with linagliptin, diosmin, and both of them resulted in a significant alleviation of the decreased insulin level to reach 2.41 ± 0.08, 2.67 ± 0.07, and 2.32 ± 0.07 (ng/mL), respectively; the treatment with diosmin was the most effective. Serum C-peptide levels disclosed a significant decrease ($p < 0.05$) in the diabetic rats in comparison with the normal group, reaching 3.56 ± 0.35 (ng/mL). Linagliptin, diosmin, and their combination administered to the diabetic rats recorded 8.12 ± 0.47, 7.90 ± 0.37, and 7.33 ± 0.35 (ng/mL) (Figure 1).

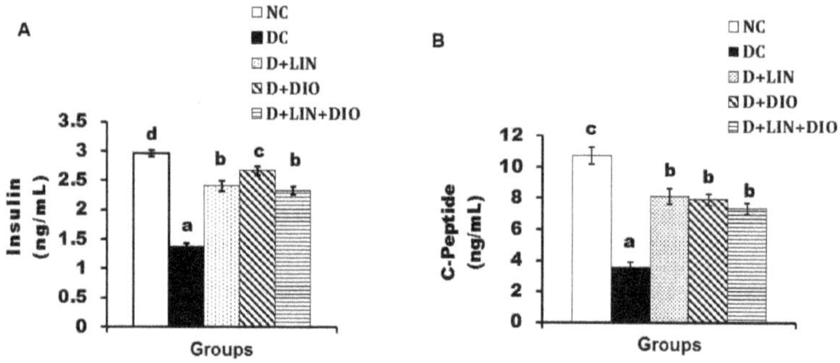

Figure 1. Effects of linagliptin, diosmin, and their combination on the serum insulin level and (**A**) the serum C-peptide level (**B**). Data expressed as the means ± SE. Means which do not share the same superscript symbols (a, b, c, and d) are significantly different at $p < 0.05$. F-probability: $p < 0.001$. NC, DC, D + LIN, D + DIO, and D + LIN + DIO refer to the normal control group, the diabetic control group, the diabetic group treated with linagliptin, the diabetic group treated with diosmin, and the diabetic group treated with linagliptin and diosmin.

2.3. *Effect on the HOMA-IR Cell Function, HOMA-IS, and HOMA-β Cell Function*

HOMA-IR manifested a significant elevation ($p < 0.05$) in the diabetic control in comparison with the healthy rats. The administration of linagliptin, diosmin, and their mixture led to a significant decrease ($p < 0.05$) of the elevated value in the diabetic rats. The HOMA-IS index expressed a significant decrease ($p < 0.05$) in the diabetic group in comparison with the healthy control. The treatment of the diabetic rats with linagliptin, diosmin, and both of them led to a significant increase. The HOMA-β cell function index showed a significant decline ($p < 0.05$) in the diabetic group as compared with the healthy group. The treatment with linagliptin, diosmin, and their mixture resulted in a significant increase ($p < 0.05$) in the diabetic rats (Figure 2).

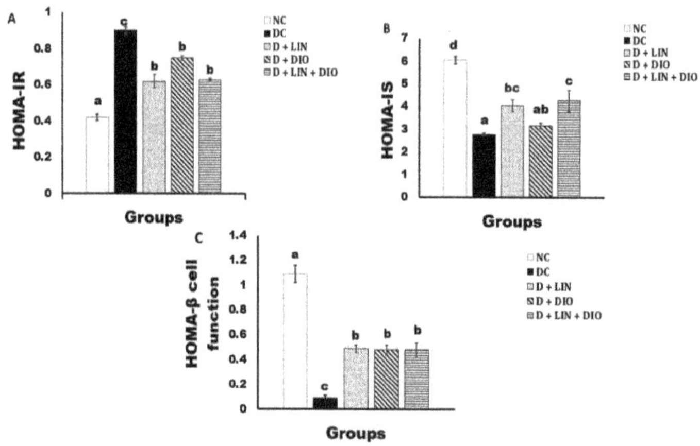

Figure 2. Effects of linagliptin and/or diosmin on the insulin resistance index (**A**), the insulin sensitivity index (**B**), and the β-cell function (**C**). Data expressed as Mean ± SE. Means, which do not share the same superscript symbols (a, b, c, and d) are significantly different at $p < 0.05$. F-probability: $p < 0.001$. NC, DC, D + LIN, D + DIO, and D + LIN + DIO refer to the normal control group, the diabetic control group, the diabetic group treated with linagliptin, the diabetic group treated with diosmin, and the diabetic group treated with linagliptin and diosmin.

2.4. *Effect on the Serum Urea and Creatinine Levels*

The serum urea level of the NA/STZ-induced diabetic rats exhibited a significant increase ($p < 0.05$) to 72.7 ± 1.81 mg/dL as compared with the normal group. The serum urea level after treatment with linagliptin recorded 38.72 ± 11.04 mg/dL, while it recorded 43.88 ± 8.06 mg/dL with treatment by diosmin. This level exhibited a significant decrease as a result of the treatment of the diabetic rats with a combination of linagliptin and diosmin together to record 35.9 ± 2.07 mg/dL (Figure 3).

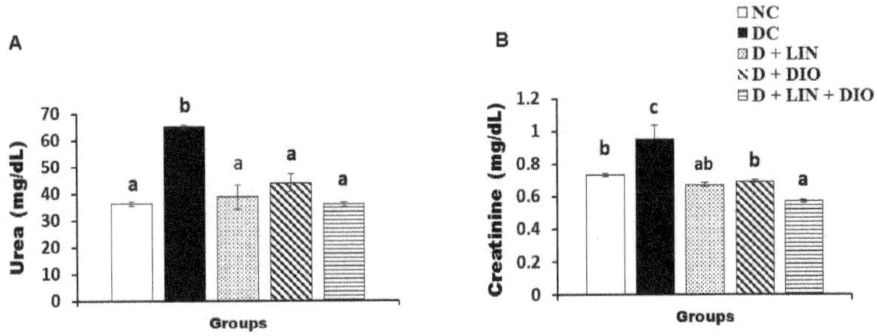

Figure 3. Effects of linagliptin and/or diosmin on the serum urea level (**A**) and creatinine level (**B**). Data expressed as the means ± SE. Means which do not share the same superscript symbols (a, b, and c) are significantly different at $p < 0.05$. F-probability: $p < 0.001$. NC, DC, D + LIN, D + DIO, and D + LIN + DIO refer to the normal control group, the diabetic control group, the diabetic group treated with linagliptin, the diabetic group treated with diosmin, and the diabetic group treated with linagliptin and diosmin.

The serum creatinine level of the NA/STZ-induced diabetic rats exhibited a significant increase ($p < 0.05$), recording 0.95 ± 0.09 mg/dl, as compared to the normal group. The serum creatinine level exhibited a significant decrease ($p < 0.05$) when treated with linagliptin, diosmin and their combination, recording 0.67 ± 0.03, 0.69 ± 0.02, and 0.57 ± 0.02 mg/dL respectively. The treatment with a combination of both linagliptin and diosmin was the more effective one (Figure 3).

2.5. *Effects on Liver Glycogen Content and Glucose-6-Phospatase and Glycogen Phosphorylase Activities*

Liver glycogen content of the diabetic rats showed a significant decrease ($p < 0.05$) when compared to the healthy group; the recorded value of the diabetic control was 6.63 ± 0.67 mg/g tissue. The treatment with linagliptin, diosmin, and a combination of them produced a highly significant alleviation ($p < 0.05$) of the liver glycogen content, recording 43.30 ± 1.47, 43.4 ± 1.11, and 27.90 ± 1.48 mg/g tissue, respectively (Figure 4A).

Liver glucose-6-phosphatase activity in the diabetic rats showed a significant elevation ($p < 0.05$) in comparison with the healthy control. The supplementation of linagliptin, diosmin, and their combination to the diabetic rats produced a significant decrease in the serum glucose-6-phosphatase activity, recording 20 ± 1.05, 22.38 ± 0.96, and 15.5 ± 0.61 mg/g tissue, respectively. Thus, the co-administration of linagliptin and diosmin was the most effective treatment (Figure 4B).

Liver glycogen phosphorylase activity in the diabetic rats showed a significant increase ($p < 0.05$) in comparison with the normal group. The treatment with linagliptin, diosmin, and their combination revealed a significant decrease in the liver glycogen phosphorylase, recording 17.62 ± 1.15, 18.07 ± 0.67, and 20.66 ± 0.33 mg/g tissue, respectively (Figure 4C).

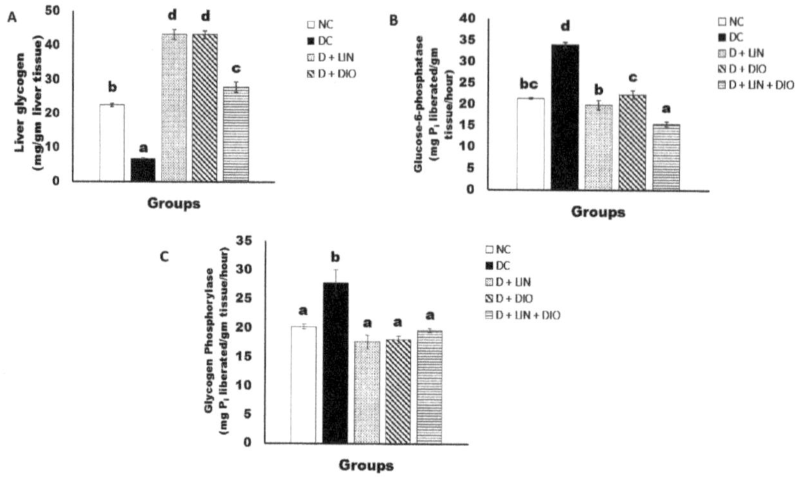

Figure 4. Effects of linagliptin and/or diosmin on the liver glycogen content (**A**), glucose-6-phosphatase activity (**B**), and glycogen phosphorylase activity (**C**). Data expressed as the means ± SE. Means which do not share the same superscript symbols (a, b, c, and d) are significantly different at $p < 0.05$. F-probability: $p < 0.001$. NC, DC, D + LIN, D + DIO, and D + LIN + DIO refer to the normal control group, the diabetic control group, the diabetic group treated with linagliptin, the diabetic group treated with diosmin, and the diabetic group treated with linagliptin and diosmin.

2.6. *Effects on the Liver Oxidative Stress and Anti-Oxidant Defense Parameters*

The data illustrating the effects of treatments with linagliptin, diosmin, and both of them are provided in Figure 5.

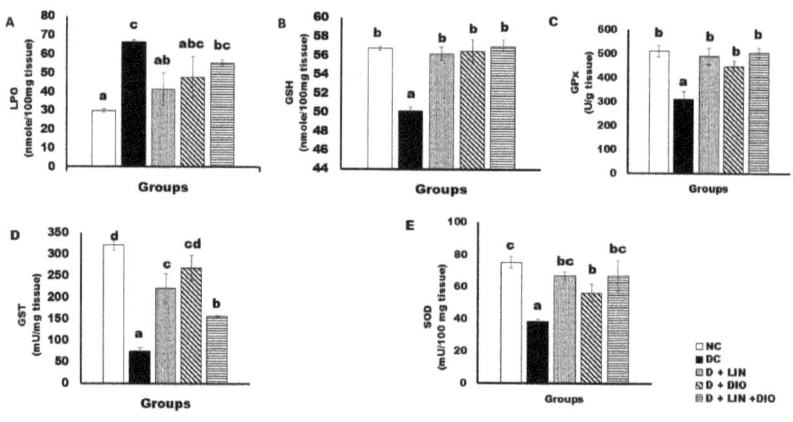

Figure 5. Effects of linagliptin and/or diosmin on LPO (**A**), GSH content (**B**), GPx activity (**C**), GST activity (**D**), and SOD activity (**E**). Data expressed as the means ± SE. Means which do not share the same superscript symbols (a, b, c, and d) are significantly different at $p < 0.05$. F-probability: $p < 0.001$. NC, DC, D + LIN, D + DIO, and D + LIN + DIO refer to the normal control group, the diabetic control group, the diabetic group treated with linagliptin, the diabetic group treated with diosmin, and the diabetic group treated with linagliptin and diosmin.

The indication of lipid peroxidation (LPO) is the formation of malondialdhyde (MDA). Its level was substantially higher ($p < 0.05$) in the rats with diabetes than in the animals without the disease. Moreover, the treatment with linagliptin resulted in a significant decrease in the MDA level, recording 41.38 ± 8.89 nmol/100 mg tissue. In addition, because of the treatment with diosmin, the MDA level exhibited a significant decrease to 47.78 ± 10.98 nmol/100 mg tissue. The co-administration of linagliptin and diosmin resulted in a decrease of LPO, recording 55.60 ± 1.42 nmol/100 mg tissue (Figure 5A).

The liver reduced glutathione (GSH) content was much lower in the rats with diabetes than in the normal group. Treatment with linagliptin resulted in a significant increase ($p < 0.05$) in the GSH content in the liver, recording 56.20 ± 0.71 nmol/100 mg tissue. Treatment with diosmin as monotherapy exhibited a significant increase in the liver GSH content, recording 56.50 ± 1.19 nmol/100 mg tissue. Under the combination therapy, the level of GSH increased significantly, recording 57.00 ± 0.71 nmol/100 mg tissue (Figure 5B).

The liver glutathione peroxidase (GPx) activity significantly decreased ($p < 0.05$) in the diabetic rats compared with normal control group; the recorded activity in the diabetic rats was 312.33 ± 29.86 U/g tissue. Treatment with linagliptin resulted in a significant increase in the GPx activity, recording 489.75 ± 33.75 U/g tissue. Diosmin treatment produced a significant increase in the GPx activity, recording 449.25 ± 23.18 U/g tissue. The most effective was the treatment with a combination of linagliptin and diosmin that resulted in an increase to 505.20 ± 20.38 U/g tissue (Figure 5C).

The liver glutathione-S-transferase (GST) activity revealed a significant decrease ($p < 0.05$) in the diabetic rats in comparison with the healthy non-diabetic rats, recording 321.40 ± 10.71 mU/mg tissue. Treatment with linagliptin led to a significant alleviation of the GST activity, recording 221.23 ± 34.73 mU/mg tissue. Moreover, treatment with diosmin produced a significant increase ($p < 0.05$) in the GST activity, recording 268.47 ± 29.38 mU/mg tissue. On treatment with a combination of linagliptin and diosmin, a significant increase in the GST activity was recorded, reaching 155.80 ± 1.9 mU/mg tissue (Figure 5D).

The superoxide dismutase (SOD) activity showed a notable reduction in the diabetic rats compared with the normal group, recording 38.50 ± 1.55 mU/100 mg tissue. On treatment with linagliptin, the SOD activity significantly increased, recording 67.00 ± 2.48 mU/100 mg tissue. Treatment with diosmin revealed a significant increase in the SOD activity, recording 56.25 ± 5.66 mU/100 mg tissue. The combination therapy of both treatments caused a significant increase in the SOD activity in the liver, recording 67.00 ± 9.23 mU/100 mg tissue (Figure 5E).

2.7. *Effect on the Interleukin 10 (IL-10) Level*

The IL-10 level is defined as an anti-inflammatory marker. It exhibited a significant decrease ($p < 0.05$) in the serum of the diabetic rats in comparison with the healthy non-diabetic rats, recording 66.87 ± 3.27 pg/mL. Linagliptin treatment effect on the IL-10 level led to a significant increase, recording 95.63 ± 4.19 pg/mL. On diosmin treatment, a significant increase in the level of IL-10 was also observed, recording 111.23 ± 1.03 pg/mL. Treatment with both linagliptin and diosmin together demonstrated a notable increase in the IL-10 level, recording 114.97 ± 2.27 pg/mL (Figure 6).

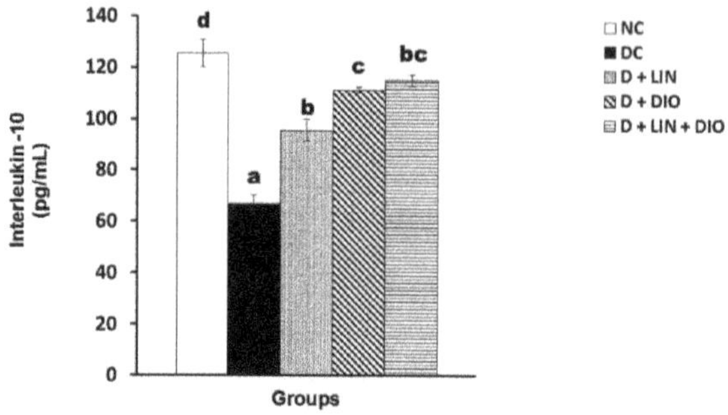

Figure 6. Effects of linagliptin and/or diosmin on the IL-10 level in the serum of the NA/STZ-induced diabetic rats. Data expressed as the means ± SE. Means which do not share the same superscript symbols (a, b, c, and d) are significantly different at $p < 0.05$. F-probability: $p < 0.001$. NC, DC, D + LIN, D + DIO, and D + LIN + DIO refer to the normal control group, the diabetic control group, the diabetic group treated with linagliptin, the diabetic group treated with diosmin, and the diabetic group treated with linagliptin and diosmin.

2.8. Effect on the mRNA Expression of Adiponectin and Resistin in Visceral Adipose Tissues

The diabetic rats showed a significant decrease ($p < 0.05$) in the mRNA expression of adiponectin in visceral adipose tissue. On the other hand, they revealed a significant elevation in the mRNA expression of resistin as compared with the healthy non-diabetic rats. The treatment of the diabetic rats with linagliptin induced a significant enhancement ($p < 0.05$) in adiponectin and a significant alleviation in the mRNA expression of resistin. On treatment with diosmin, the mRNA expression of adiponectin exhibited a significant upregulation while the expression of resistin revealed a significant downregulation. The treatment with both linagliptin and diosmin together exhibited a significant upregulation in the mRNA expression of adiponectin and a significant downregulation in the mRNA expression of resistin; the combined effect was the most potent (Figure 7).

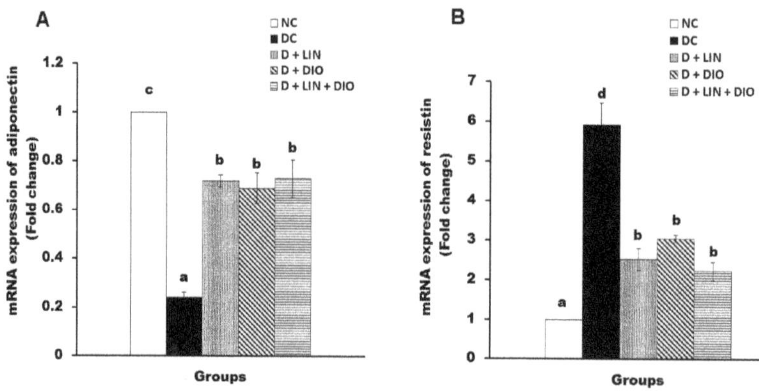

Figure 7. Effects of linagliptin and/or diosmin on the mRNA expression of adiponectin (**A**) and resistin (**B**) in visceral adipose tissue. Data expressed as the means ± SE. Means which do not share the same superscript symbols (a, b, c, and d) are significantly different at $p < 0.05$. F-probability: $p < 0.001$. NC, DC, D + LIN, D + DIO, and D + LIN + DIO refer to the normal control group, the diabetic control group, the diabetic group treated with linagliptin, the diabetic group treated with diosmin, and the diabetic group treated with linagliptin and diosmin.

2.9. *Effect on Pancreatic Histological Changes*

Figure 8 shows the pancreatic histological alterations in the diabetes control and diabetic treatment groups compared to the normal control. The pancreas is composed of an endocrine portion represented by the islets of Langerhans, which have α-cells at their periphery, β-cells in their core, and larger δ-cells. The exocrine portion is represented by pancreatic acini. The pancreases of the normal rats depicted normal architecture of pancreatic acini and islets with intact α-cells, β-cells, and δ-cells (Figure 8A). The diabetic rats, on the other hand, featured a marked decline of the islets' size and a decrease in the islet cell number in addition to fibrosis (Figure 8B). The pancreases of the diabetic rats treated with linagliptin (Figure 8C), diosmin (Figure 8D), and linagliptin and diosmin (Figure 8E) exhibited a recovery of damaged islets of Langerhans and regenerated islets. The diabetic rats treated with linagliptin revealed a moderate regeneration of islets of Langerhans. The diabetic rats treated with diosmin revealed a greater increase in the islet cells than those treated with linagliptin. The diabetic rats treated with both linagliptin and diosmin showed a nearly normal pancreatic acini and regeneration of islets of Langerhans. The combined effect seemed to be the most potent.

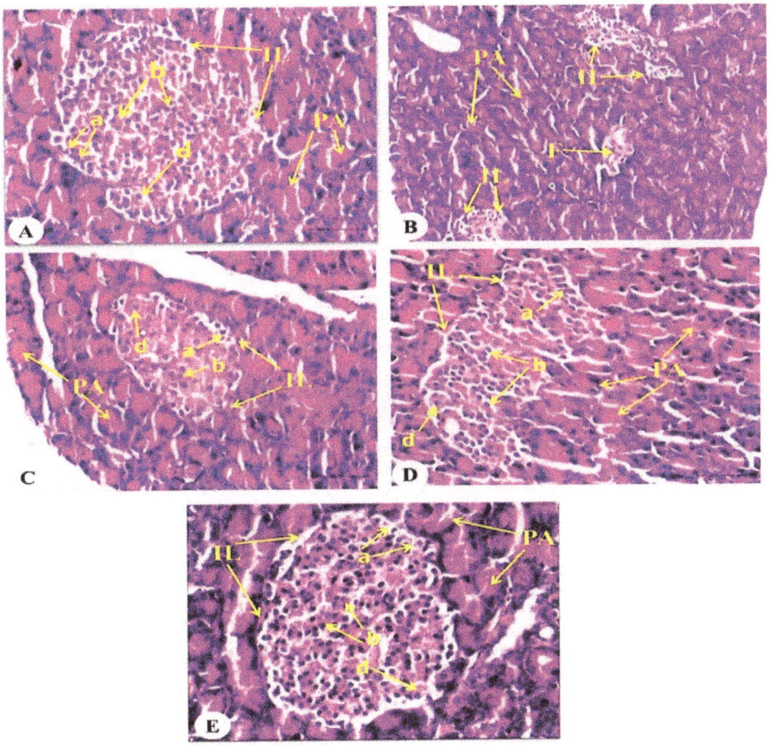

Figure 8. Photographs of H&E stained sections of the pancreas of the normal (**A**), diabetic control (**B**), and diabetic groups treated with linagliptin (**C**), diosmin (**D**), and linagliptin and diosmin (**E**). (**A**) Photograph of a pancreatic section of a healthy rat revealed normal pancreatic acini (PA) and islets of Langerhans (IL) with normal intact α-cells (a), β-cells (b), and δ-cells (d). (**B**) Photograph of a pancreatic section of a diabetic rat revealed small sizes of islets of Langerhans (IL) and fibrosis (F). The islets exhibited an enormous decrease in the islet cells. (**C**) Photograph of a pancreatic section of a diabetic rat treated with linagliptin revealed a marked improvement in the islets of Langerhans (IL) with an increased number of islet cells, including α-cells (a), β-cells (b), and δ-cells (d). (**D**) Photograph of a pancreatic section of a diabetic rat treated with diosmin revealed a

remarkable amelioration in the islets of Langerhans (IL), with an increased number of α-cells (a), β-cells (b), and δ-cells (d). (**E**) Photograph of a pancreatic section of a diabetic rat treated with linagliptin and diosmin as combination therapy showed return to normal pancreatic architecture, regenerated islets of Langerhans (IL). The islets had normal integrity, with an increased number of normal and intact α-cells (a), β-cells (b), and δ-cells (d). Magnification for photomicrographs (**A**,**C**–**E**) was 400×, while magnification for photomicrograph (**B**) was 200×.

2.10. Effect on the Expression of Insulin in Pancreatic Islets (Immunohistochemical Investigations)

The alterations in the expression of insulin in the pancreatic islets of Langerhans in different groups are depicted in Figure 9A–F. The data obtained from image analysis include density and area percentage of brown color of the immuno-stained islets represented in Figures 10A and 10B, respectively. The diabetic rats exhibited poor immunohistochemical staining (Figure 9C), reflecting a substantial decrease in the concentration of insulin granules as compared with the normal control (Figure 9A,B); the decrease was significant (Figure 10A,B). The treatments of the diabetic rats with linagliptin (Figure 9D), diosmin (Figure 9E), and linagliptin and diosmin (Figure 9F) induced a strong immunohistochemical staining of insulin granules in the pancreatic islets; the effects were significant and the combined effect was the most potent (Figure 10A,B).

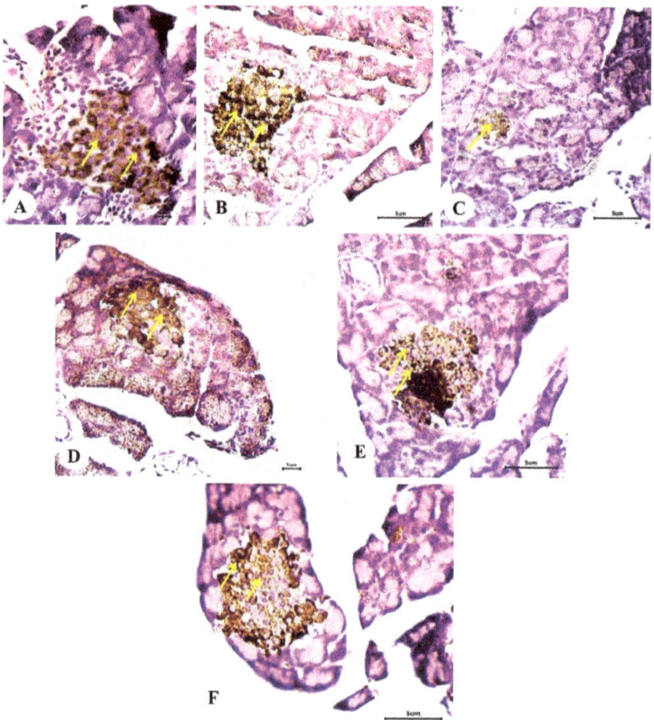

Figure 9. Photomicrographs of immunohistochemically stained sections of the pancreas showing insulin granules in the pancreatic islets of the normal (**A**,**B**), diabetic control (**C**), and diabetic groups treated with linagliptin (**D**), diosmin (**E**), and linagliptin, and diosmin (**F**). (Scale bar: 5 μm). The diabetic rats exhibited a weak expression of insulin when compared with the normal control. On the other hand, the diabetic rats treated with linagliptin and/or diosmin showed a strong expression of insulin granules; the combined effects of linagliptin and diosmin were the most potent. Arrows refer to brown color immunostaining.

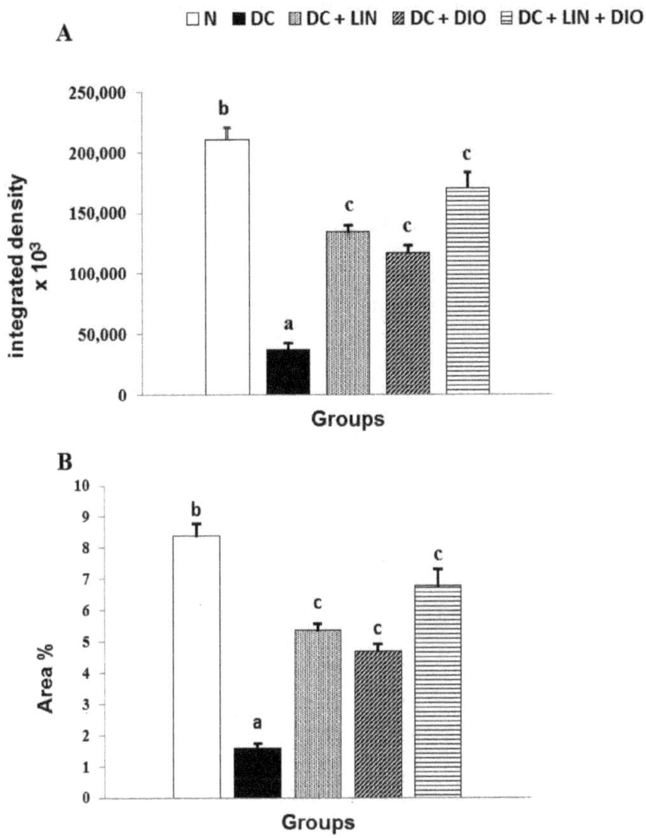

Figure 10. Effects of linagliptin and/or diosmin on the integrated density (**A**) and area percentage (**B**) of brown color produced by immunohistochemical staining of insulin granules of the pancreatic islets in the diabetic rats. Data expressed as the means ± SE. Means which do not share the same superscript symbols (a, b, and c) are significantly different at $p < 0.05$. F-probability: $p < 0.001$. NC, DC, D + LIN, D + DIO, and D + LIN + DIO refer to the normal control group, the diabetic control group, the diabetic group treated with linagliptin, the diabetic group treated with diosmin, and the diabetic group treated with linagliptin and diosmin.

3. Discussion

A large number of medicinal plants have been used in traditional medicine to treat symptoms of DM, and many of them have undergone some experimental testing for hypoglycemic and hypolipidemic activities [15]. Plant infusions and decoction fluids are widely used by populations in developing and underdeveloped countries since conventional medicines are unavailable or unaffordable. In addition, plant constituents are more preferred than crude extracts to avoid the side effects of other constituents [16,17]. Thus, this study aimed to assess the antihyperglycemic, antioxidant, and anti-inflammatory effects of one plant constituent diosmin alone and in combination with linagliptin in NA/STZ-induced diabetic rats.

STZ plus NA-induced animals with T2DM are an attractive and useful model with pathophysiological similarities to human diabetes, and it is suitable for acute and chronic studies, making it a superior model for evaluating the antihyperglycemic effects of different substances [7].

The oral glucose tolerance test (OGTT) is a valid and widely used assay for determining the antihyperglycemic effects of any hypoglycemic medication [18]. In our study, there was a significant increase in blood glucose levels in the diabetic rats as compared with the normal rats, and this agrees with the results of previous research [19–21]. The glucose levels then significantly increased to reach their peak after one hour of administration of glucose. After another hour, the level began to decline until returning to levels close to those detected before oral administration of glucose, to reach normal results in the normal groups and a high level in the diabetic ones. On the other hand, within the treatment group, the level of glucose improved and revealed normal results, especially in the case of combination treatment with both linagliptin and diosmin. This goes parallel with the antihyperglycemic effect of diosmin that was revealed by Ali et al. [22] and agrees with the results of McKeage [23] who stated that linagliptin had an improvement effect on glycemic control in diabetic patients with T2DM when used as monotherapy or in combination with other hypoglycemic agents.

C-peptide is generated during the production of insulin when the precursor molecule called proinsulin is broken down into insulin and C-peptide [24]. It has a consistent metabolic process under a variety of physiological and pathological circumstances [25]. As a result, serum C-peptide is regarded as a more accurate measure of insulin secretion and release than the serum insulin level.

Treatment of the diabetic rats with linagliptin led to a significant increase in both insulin and C-peptide secretion when compared with the diabetic animals which suffer from insulin resistance as well as damage to β-cells in the islets of Langerhans due to the effect of NA/STZ injection. The results of the present study fit with the results of Rauch et al. [26] who indicated that linagliptin was well-tolerated and significantly suppressed the plasma DPP-4 activity in T2DM patients, resulting in immediate enhancements in incretin levels, glucagon suppression, and glycemic management that lasted throughout the study.

Treatment of diabetic animals with diosmin in the present study induced glycemic control in diabetic rats by increasing the serum insulin and C-peptide levels, which may have been due to the elevated number and architecture of β-cells, as detected by histology studies. This agrees with the results of Pari and Srinivasan [27], in which diosmin promoted pancreatic β-cells, which are essential for insulin synthesis and secretion.

In our study, the combination treatment with both linagliptin and diosmin produced improvement of insulin and C-peptide secretion, showing significant glycemic control for diabetic animals by reducing the HOMA-IR and improving both HOMA-IS and HOMA-β-cell function.

In the present study, the liver glycogen content exhibited a significant increase following treatment with linagliptin when compared with the diabetic animals. In contrast with the present study, Shiraki et al. indicated that treatment with linagliptin significantly decreased the glycogen content [28]. In our study, the treatment of diabetic animals with a combination of linagliptin and diosmin revealed a significant increase in the liver glycogen content. The synthesis of hepatic glycogen content was reduced in the diabetic patients due to low insulin levels, which inactivated the glycogen synthase pathway. Thus, the liver glycogen content is a significant marker of glycemic control [28].

The rate-limiting phase in glycogen depletion is catalyzed by glycogen phosphorylase. Thus, its activity increased in the diabetic patients. According to our study, the activity of the glycogen phosphorylase enzyme declined when the diabetic animals were treated with linagliptin [29]. This occurred with treatment with diosmin as monotherapy or when it was combined with linagliptin.

The glucose-6-phosphatase activity in the current study showed a significant upregulation in the diabetic group when compared with the healthy control group. This is in agreement with the results of Mahmoud et al. [30], who demonstrated that in comparison to the normal control, there was a notable increase in the activity of the gluconeogenic enzymes fructose 1, 6-bisphosphatase and glucose-6-phosphatase, as well as of hepatic glycogen phosphorylase. The activity of glucose-6-phosphatase exhibited a significant decrease in the group of diabetic animals treated with linagliptin when compared with diabetic control.

On treatment with diosmin, the activity of glucose-6-phosphatase showed a significant decrease when compared with the diabetic control. The results fit the previous results of Pari and Srinivasan [27] and Zheng et al. [31], revealing an increase in the activity of glucose-6-phosphatase in the animals with diabetes receiving diosmin. Combination therapy with both linagliptin and diosmin revealed a significant decrease when compared to the monotherapies in this study; thus, diosmin and linagliptin might have synergistic effects on the liver glucose-6-phosphatase activity.

Insulin resistance and β-cell dysfunction have both been linked to oxidative stress [32]. Pancreatic cell damage has been linked with the development of experimental DM that was induced by STZ [33]. In this case, in addition to the damaging effects of STZ on β-cells, the subsequent hyperglycemia induces the production of free radicals, which can exhaust the antioxidant defense mechanism, resulting in oxidative damage to cell membranes and increased vulnerability to LPO [34]. In our study, oxidative stress and antioxidant defense systems were detected by measuring levels of several biomarkers in the liver.

Secondary products such as MDA are used to quantify LPO indirectly [35]. Our present exploration showed a significant increase in liver LPO levels in the diabetic rats compared with the healthy ones. The results align with the results of Mohamed et al. [36]. On treatment with linagliptin, the level of MDA exhibited a significant decrease due to the amelioration of lipids in the diabetic group treated with linagliptin and thus reflected on LPO. This result is further supported by the studies of the protective potential effect of linagliptin against hepatic encephalopathy induced by thioacetamide (TAA) in rats [37]. In the current study, the diabetic groups treated with diosmin exhibited no significant effect when compared with the untreated diabetic rats. The observed results fit the results of Ağır who studied the effect of diosmin against liver damage and detected that it had no significant effect on liver LPO represented by the level of MDA [38]. However, it contrasts with another result explained in the study of Anwer who observed that the administration of diosmin showed a significant decrease in the level of MDA in Wistar rats, which suffered from liver injury [39]. The combination of diosmin and linagliptin in our study revealed no significant effect on hepatic LPO, which suggests that the effect of linagliptin on liver LPO may be decreased by the diosmin combination, but it may have been due to the short experiment time and treatment duration.

The current study revealed modulation of the liver GSH content when treated with linagliptin because of the improvement of insulin resistance, as some results state that insulin resistance is also linked to oxidative damage. According to certain research, oxidative stress is also responsible for altering intracellular signaling pathways, which leads to insulin resistance [40]. In our research, the diabetic rats treated with diosmin showed a significant increase in hepatic GSH on comparison with the untreated group. These results are supported by the detected results of Liu in his study, which investigated the diosmin effect on the ARPE-19 human retinal pigment epithelial cells exposed to high glucose and observed the increased effect of diosmin treatment at high-glucose ARPE-19 cells on the GSH concentration level [41]. On combination therapy of the diabetic rats with linagliptin and diosmin, the level of hepatic GSH content significantly increased, indicating the improvement of hepatic oxidative stress as a diabetic complication.

The current study revealed that glutathione GPx showed a significant decrease in the diabetic rats. On the other hand, the diabetic rats treated with linagliptin and/or diosmin exhibited a significant increase in the hepatic GPx enzyme activity, indicating a potent antioxidant effect of linagliptin and diosmin.

Diabetes consequences, both microvascular and cardiovascular, are heavily influenced by oxidative stress. Diabetic metabolic problems increase mitochondrial superoxide generation. The central and significant mediator of diabetic tissue damage is increased superoxide generation [42]. SOD and GST are ROS-scavenging enzymes that decrease in the case of DM.

On the other hand, the activity of GST increased due to an increase in their production when treating the diabetic rats with linagliptin as monotherapy and in combination with diosmin. On treatment with diosmin as monotherapy, there was an improvement in the GST activity and a significant increase in comparison with the diabetic control group. This result is consistent with the results of [43], which studied the alleviative efficacy of diosmin against STZ/NA-induced oxidative stress in diabetic rats.

In our current study, the generation of SOD increased significantly in the diabetic rats treated with linagliptin as it had antioxidant effects on the diabetic rats. This significant increase in SOD was also detected with diosmin monotherapy and combination therapy with linagliptin. This approves our suggestion of the effectiveness of the combination of linagliptin with diosmin in treating DM type 2 in experimental animals. This result fits with the result of Srinivasan and Pari [43], who detected a significant increase in the recovery of SOD activity due to the treatment of diabetic animals with diosmin.

IL-10, a Th2 (T helper 2) cytokine, is considered an anti-inflammatory marker suitable for detecting inflammation in DM patients. In our present investigation, the serum level of IL-10 decreased in the diabetic rats. On the other hand, by treating the diabetic animals with linagliptin and/or diosmin, the serum IL-10 level was significantly elevated; the combined effect was the most effective, reflecting that the combination treatment has the most potent anti-inflammatory effect. These results are in accordance with those observed by Arab et al., who revealed the anti-inflammatory action of diosmin [44]. The combination therapy of linagliptin with diosmin revealed a significant increase in the serum IL-10 level compared to monotherapy with linagliptin.

Adiponectin is a peptide generated from adipocytes that has anti-inflammatory and insulin sensitivity effects [45]. A nested case–control study was undertaken to determine if baseline adiponectin concentrations in plasma are independently linked with the risk of T2DM [46]. In the presently observed results, adiponectin exhibited a significant increase in expression when linagliptin was used as monotherapy for the NA/STZ-induced diabetic rats compared with the untreated diabetic control group of animals. This observation is consistent with the results of Koyama et al. when the endothelial function in patients with T2DM and coronary artery disease was studied using linagliptin and voglibose [47]. On the other hand, the treatment with diosmin also showed a significant increase in the adiponectin expression, supporting the results of Gerges et al. who demonstrated that diosmin dramatically recovers circulating adiponectin levels [48]. In the present study, the treatment with diosmin and linagliptin produced a significant increase in the adiponectin expression, assuming the improvement of insulin sensitivity because of the increasing expression of adiponectin.

Resistin belongs to the resistin-like molecule family of tissue-specific signaling molecules. It is considered to be a proinflammatory cytokine involved in linking obesity and insulin resistance in T2DM [49]. Its levels in plasma are elevated in hyperglycemic and hyper-insulinemic rodents, as well as in T2DM patients [45,49–52]. In the present study, the resistin expression gene exhibited a significant increase in the diabetic rats when compared with the healthy non-diabetic group. By treatment with linagliptin, diosmin, and both of them, the levels of resistin expression showed a significant decrease.

The serum urea and creatinine levels were significantly elevated in the NA/STZ-induced diabetic rats; these results are in accordance with many publications [53–55]. The treatments of the diabetic rats with diosmin, linagliptin, and both of them resulted in a significant decrease in the elevated levels of urea and creatinine. The combined effect was the most potent. These changes in the serum kidney function parameters led us to suggest that diosmin, linagliptin, and both of them not only have antihyperglycemic, anti-inflammatory, and antioxidant effects, but also improve the kidney function.

In conclusion, it is clear from our data in this study that diosmin has numerous antidiabetic effects as monotherapy or in combination with linagliptin. The combined effect of diosmin with linagliptin was the most potent on OGT, hepatic glucose-6-phosphatase activity, and serum creatinine level. The antidiabetic effect was proved by the improvement that occurred in insulin resistance and the increase in insulin sensitivity in diabetic cells, as well as amelioration of the pancreatic islets' histological integrity and the insulin formation by the recovered β-cells. The recovery effect produced a decrease in the serum glucose levels, an increase in the insulin and C-peptide levels, and an improvement of the glucose homeostasis indexes. Linagliptin and diosmin improved oxidative stress parameters such as the LPO, SOD, GPx, GST activities and the GSH content in the livers of NA/STZ-induced diabetic rats. Linagliptin and diosmin exhibited a significant increase in anti-inflammatory markers such as IL-10. The current study data showed improvement in the gene expression of adiponectin and resistin in visceral adipose tissue that reveals the effective action on insulin resistance of NA/STZ-induced diabetic rats. Thus, it is speculated that diosmin in combination with linagliptin may be suggested as an efficient antihyperglycemic treatment for T2DM after approval of its efficacy and safety in humans. Further investigations for longer durations are necessary in the future to detect the effects on molecular mediators in the signaling pathways of insulin action, insulin secretion, inflammation, and antioxidant defense mechanisms.

4. Materials and Methods

4.1. Chemicals

NA and STZ were purchased from Sigma, MO, USA. The glucose kit was provided by Spinreact (Gerona, Spain). The insulin and C-peptide ELISA kit was purchased from MyBioSource (San Diego, CA, USA). Interleukin 10 was determined using a rat IL-10 Quantikine ELISA kit (R&D Systems, Inc., Minneapolis, MN, USA). Total ribonucleic acid (RNA) was extracted from the adipose tissue using a Qiagen tissue extraction kit (Qiagen, San Diego, CA, USA) based on the manufacturer's instructions. The other chemicals and reagents that were employed were all highly pure and of analytical quality.

4.2. Experimental Animals

Adult male Wistar rats weighing 120–140 g were used in the present study to perform the experiment. The experimental animals were delivered from the Animal Facilities Center of the National Research Center in Cairo, Egypt. Before the experiment started, the rats were kept under surveillance for a week in order to rule out any prior infections. The animals were housed in cages made from polypropylene and kept at controlled room temperature (25 ± 2 °C) and humidity (55 ± 5%). The animals had access to drinking water and a standard pellet diet ad libitum. All the experimental procedures were completed in accordance with the instructions and guidelines and were approved by the Animal Ethics Committee, Beni-Suef University, Egypt (Ethical Approval number 022-463). All efforts were directed towards reducing the number and suffering of animals.

4.3. Induction of DM

To induce T2DM, the groups of overnight-fasted rats were injected intraperitoneally (i.p.) with NA at a dose of 60 mg/kg (dissolved in isotonic saline) 15 min after an intraperitoneal injection of STZ (60 mg/kg; dissolved in citrate buffer, pH 4.5) [56,57]. The same volume of vehicles, citrate buffer (pH 4.5) and 0.9% saline, were administered to the corresponding normal control rats.

4.4. Experimental Design and Blood and Tissue Sampling

Blood samples were centrifuged at 3000 RPM for 15 min and the clear non-hemolyzed supernatant sera were separated into three portions for each individual animal and kept at −20 °C until used. One gram of frozen liver tissue was homogenized in 10 mL ice-cold saline (0.9% NaCl) to yield 1% homogenate (*w*/*v*) [16]. The liver homogenate was centrifuged at 3000 RPM for 15 min. The supernatants were separated and kept in a deep freezer at −20 °C until they were used in biochemical analysis. One part of organ tissues was preserved in 70% alcohol after fixation using neutral buffered formalin for 24 h to prepare for histopathological examination [58].

Five groups, each with 6 adult male Wistar rats, were utilized in this investigation:

- Normal control group (NC). These were healthy rats that were given an equivalent volume of carboxymethyl cellulose (CMC) (1% *w*/*v*) every other day for 28 days by oral gavage.
- Diabetic control group (DC). This group consisted of diabetic rats that were given the equivalent volume of CMC (1% *w*/*v*) by oral gavage every other day for 28 days.
- Diabetic group treated with linagliptin (D + LIN). This group consisted of diabetic rats, but they were treated with linagliptin at a dose of 1 mg/kg (dissolved in 1% CMC) every other day for 28 days by oral gavage [59].
- Diabetic group treated with diosmin (D + DIO). In this group, diabetic rats were treated with diosmin at a dose of 10 mg/kg (dissolved in 1% CMC) every other day for 28 days by oral gavage [60].
- Diabetic group treated with both linagliptin and diosmin (D + LIN + DIO). The rats in this group were diabetic rats that were treated with linagliptin at a dose of 1 mg/kg and diosmin at a dose of 10 mg/kg every other day for 28 days by oral gavage.

4.5. Blood Sampling and Tissue Sampling

At the end of the 4th week of the treatment period, the rats were anesthetized with ethyl ether, and from the jugular vein, blood samples were taken in Gel & Clot activator tubes. Serum was separated by centrifugation at 3000 RPM for 15 min, and clear non-hemolyzed supernatant sera were separated and kept at −20 °C until used. After decapitation and dissection, organ tissue specimens, liver, and pancreas were excised for histological and biochemical analyses.

4.6. Biochemical Analysis

To assess the antihyperglycemic effects, OGTT was performed. OGTT was performed by measuring the blood glucose of the rats at time intervals of 0, 60, 120 and 180 min after oral uptake of the glucose dose (3 g/kg) according to Ibrahim et al. [61] (using a glucometer and Gluco Dr.auto strips (All Medicus, Co., Ltd., Anyang-si, Republic of Korea)). The day before the sacrifice, blood samples were obtained by puncturing the lateral tail vein following a 10–12 h fast.

To assess the effect on insulin formation and insulin secretory response of β-cells, serum insulin and C-peptide levels were detected. Using an ELISA kit from MyBioSource

(San Diego, CA, USA), serum insulin and C-peptide concentrations were measured in accordance with the manufacturer's instructions.

Hepatic glycogen content, which is another glycemic indicator, was determined according to Seifter et al. [62]. To assess the effects on hepatic glucose output, hepatic glucose-6-phosphatase and glycogen phosphorylase activities were determined. Hepatic glucose-6-phosphatase activity was estimated based on the procedure of Kabir and Begum [63]. Hepatic glycogen phosphorylase activity was detected based on the method of Stalmans and Hers [64] using reagents prepared in the laboratory.

The homeostasis model assessment (HOMA) indices were evaluated to scrutinize the effects on insulin action and β-cell function. HOMA-insulin resistance (HOMA-IR), HOMA-insulin sensitivity (HOMA-IS), and HOMA-β-cell function (HOMA-β) were calculated according to the following equations [65–67]:

$$\text{HOMA-IR} = (\text{fasting insulin } [\mu\text{IU/mL}] \times \text{fasting glucose } [\text{mg/dL}])/405$$

$$\text{HOMA-IS} = 10{,}000/(\text{fasting insulin } [\mu\text{IU/mL}] \times \text{fasting glucose } [\text{mg/dL}])$$

$$\text{HOMA-}\beta \text{ cell function} = (20 \times \text{fasting insulin } [\mu\text{IU/mL}])/(\text{fasting glucose } [\text{mg/dL}] - 3.5)$$

Serum urea and creatinine were detected to assess the effects on the kidney function. Serum urea was determined by a method using kits obtained from Randox Laboratories Company (Crumlin, UK) according to Patton and Crouch [68]. The serum creatinine level was determined by a method using kits obtained from Randox Laboratories Company (UK) according to Bartels and Bohmer [69].

IL-10, which is an anti-inflammatory cytokine, was determined using a rat ELISA kit according to the guidelines and instructions of the manufacturer (Bio-Techne, Minneapolis, MN, USA). This assay depends on the quantitative sandwich enzyme-linked immunoassay technique.

4.7. RNA Isolation and Quantitative Real-Time Polymerase Chain Reaction (qRT-PCR)

Total RNA was extracted from the adipose tissue using a Qiagen tissue extraction kit in accordance with the manufacturer's instructions (Qiagen, Germantown, MD, USA). Quantitative real-time polymerase chain reaction (qRT-PCR) amplification and analysis were performed using an Applied Biosystem running software version 3.1. (Applied Biosystems, Waltham, MA, USA).

Complementary DNA (cDNA) was synthesized according to the manufacturer's protocol (Thermo Fisher Scientific, Waltham, MA, USA). A 2 μg of cDNA template, SYBR®-Green Master Mix (Thermo Fisher Scientific, Waltham, MA, USA), and the appropriate primers were used to conduct qRT-PCR analyses, which were conducted in triplicate. The $2^{-\Delta\Delta Ct}$ method [70] was used for calculating the relative gene expression levels. The β-actin gene was amplified as an internal control. The primer sequences used included the following: for adiponectin F: 5′-AATCCTGCCCAGTCATGAAG-3′ and R: 5′-CATCTCCTGGGTCACCCTTA-3′ [71]; for resistin F: 5′-GGGAGTTGTGCCCTGCT-3′; R: 5′-CAGCACTCGGAGGGCAA-3′ [72].

4.8. Determination of Oxidative Stress and Anti-Oxidant Defense Parameters

The technique of Marklund and Marklund [73] was applied to measure the liver SOD enzyme activity. In short, pyrogallol quickly underwent auto-oxidation in an aqueous solution to generate a yellow color that was detectable at 430 nm. A 0.1 mL of Tris buffer (pH 8) was added to one mL of homogenate supernatant. Then, 0.05 mL of pyrogallol were added. The initial absorbance was read immediately and read again 10 min after adding pyrogallol. The control consisted of 0.1 mL Tris buffer and one mL distilled water; then, 0.05 mL of pyrogallol were added. The enzyme activity and the inhibition of the yellow color that emerged at 430 nm were computed. An enzyme unit was defined as the quantity of the enzyme that resulted in a 50% suppression of the extinction changes in 1 min as compared to the control.

Formation of thiobarbituric acid-reacting substances (TBARS), low-molecular-weight end products (mainly MDA) that are formed during the decomposition of lipid peroxidation products, estimates the amount of lipid peroxidation (LPO). MDA was assayed based on the procedure described by Preuss et al. [74]. The protein was precipitated by mixing 1 mL of the liver homogenate with 0.15 mL of 76% trichloroacetic acid (TCA). Then, as a color-developing agent, 0.35 mL of thiobarbituric acid (TBA) were added to the separated supernatant. After being incubated for 30 min at 80 °C in a water bath, the formed faint pink color was detected at 532 nm. MDA, also known as 1,1,3,3-tetramethoxypropane, was employed as the standard.

The amount of GSH was measured using the technique of Beutler [75]. In brief, Ellman's reagent (as a color-developing agent), 0.5 mL DTNB [5,5′-dithiobis (2-nitrobenzoic acid)], and phosphate buffer solution (pH 7) were added to the supernatant following protein precipitation in order to quantify GSH. The sample and standard's produced yellow color was measured at 412 nm in comparison to the blank, and the GSH concentration in the sample was calculated.

The activity of GPx was estimated using the suggested method of Matkovics et al. [76]. In this method, the residual GSH after a certain time from the known concentration of GSH added to the sample was measured photometrically at 412 nm by reacting with DTNB. Then, the reduced form of GSH was converted to the oxidized form (GSSG), and the total amount was calculated. Briefly, 350 µL Tris buffer (pH 7.6), 50 µL GSH solution (2 mM), and 50 µL H_2O_2 (3.38 mM) were placed in a Wasserman tube, and 50 µL homogenate supernatant was added. Following ten minutes of incubation, the previously described method [75] for determining GSH at 430 nm was used to measure the residual GSH content. The blank test was made by adding 100 µL of distilled water in place of 50 µL of the sample and 50 µL of the GSH solution, and the standard test was performed by adding 50 µL of distilled water in place of 50 µL of the sample. Following the identification of the sample's residual GSH content, the GSH converted to the oxidized form (GSSG), and the enzyme activity can be computed.

GST activity was determined based on the chemical method described in a previous publication [77]. In brief, 250 µL of 4 mM 1-chloro-2,4-dinitrobenzene (CDNB) was introduced into a Wasserman tube that had 250 µL of the sample, 250 µL of the GSH solution (4 mM), and 250 µL of phosphate buffer (pH 7.3). After 10 min of incubation at 25 °C, the developed color was measured.

4.9. Histological and Immunohistochemical Investigations

The pancreas was quickly removed after dissection, chopped into tiny three mm^3 pieces, and then preserved for 24 h in 10% neutral buffered formalin. The tissues were washed and dehydrated in two changes of 100% ethyl alcohol for 30 min each after the excess fixative removed. This was followed by 45 min each of increasing grades of ethyl alcohol: 70%, 80%, 90%, and 95%. After that, two changes of xylene were used to clear the tissues for thirty minutes each. After being impregnated with paraplast plus (three changes) for three hours at 60 degrees Celsius, the tissues were implanted in paraplast plus. Sections 4 to 5 µm thick were created using a microtome, and for histological examination, they were then stained with hematoxylin and eosin [78].

For immunohistochemical investigation, sections 5–6 µm thick that were mounted on positive slides and stained using the streptavidin–biotin–peroxidase staining method were used for anti-insulin immunolocalization [17,79]. To enable comparison of the immunostaining outcomes across the different experimental groups, each section was incubated with the same quantity of primary and secondary antibodies for the same length of time and under the same circumstances [16]. Following immunohistochemical staining, light microscopy was used to examine the stained sections. A positive reaction was shown by a brown hue. Insulin granules' integrated density and area percentage as indicated by brown color were evaluated using the ImageJ (1.54d version) (http://imagej.org, accessed on 13 September 2023; Wayne Rasband and Contributors, National Institutes of Health, Bethesda, MD, USA).

4.10. Statistical Analysis

The average ± standard deviation (SD) was used to express the data. SPSS version 20 statistical analysis was used to analyze the data using one-way analysis of variance (ANOVA) followed by Tukey's test to compare various groups with each other. Significant differences were found for values of $p < 0.05$.

Author Contributions: Conceptualization, A.K.K. and O.M.A.; project administration, A.K.K., N.A.A., A.S. and O.M.A.; supervision, A.K.K. and O.M.A.; funding acquisition, E.B.A., A.S. and A.K.K.; methodology, E.B.A., N.A.A. and O.M.A.; data curation, E.B.A., N.A.A., A.K.K. and O.M.A.; statistical analysis, E.B.A., N.A.A. and O.M.A.; software, E.B.A.; validation and visualization, E.B.A., A.M.E.-K., N.A.A., A.S., A.K.K. and O.M.A.; formal analysis, E.B.A. and O.M.A.; writing—original draft preparation, E.B.A.; writing—revision and editing, E.B.A., A.M.E.-K., N.A.A., A.S., A.K.K. and O.M.A. All authors have read and agreed to the published version of the manuscript.

Funding: This research was funded by Taif University, Taif, Saudi Arabia, project No. TU-DSPP-2024-288.

Institutional Review Board Statement: The animal experiments were approved by the Experimental Animal Ethics Committee, Faculty of Science, Beni-Suef University, Egypt (Ethical Approval Number 022-463; date: 22 October 2023).

Informed Consent Statement: Not applicable.

Data Availability Statement: All data are available from the corresponding author upon reasonable request.

Acknowledgments: The authors extend their appreciation to Taif University, Saudi Arabia, for supporting this work through project number TU-DSPP-2024-288.

Conflicts of Interest: The authors declare no conflict of interest.

Abbreviations

DM: diabetes mellitus; DS: diosmin; DPP4: dipeptidyl peptidase-4;WHO: World Health Organization; CMC: carboxy methyl cellulose; ELISA: sandwich enzyme-linked immunosorbent assay; GPx: glutathione peroxidase; GST: glutathione-S-transferase; IL: islet of Langerhans; H&E: hematoxylin and eosin; HOMA-IR: homeostatic model assessment-insulin resistance; HOMA-IS: homeostatic model assessment-insulin sensitivity; HOMA-β cell function: homeostatic model assessment-β cell function; GSH: reduced glutathione; i.p.: intraperitoneal; IR: insulin resistance; IS: insulin sensitivity; LPO: lipid peroxidation; MDA: malondialdehyde; mRNA: messenger RNA; OGTT: oral glucose tolerance test; RNA: ribonucleic acid; qRT-PCR: quantitative real-time polymerase chain reaction; SOD: superoxide dismutase; STZ: streptozotocin; T2DM: type 2 DM; DTNB: 5,5′dithiobis-2-nitrobenzoic acid; CDNB: 1-choloro-2,4-dinitrobenzene; IL-10: interleukin 10; SE: standard error.

References

1. ADA Classification and diagnosis of diabetes: Standards of Medical Care in Diabetes-2020. *Diabetes Care* **2020**, *43*, S14–S31. [CrossRef]
2. Jalili, R.B.; Moeen Rezakhanlou, A.; Hosseini-Tabatabaei, A.; Ao, Z.; Warnock, G.L.; Ghahary, A. Fibroblast populated collagen matrix promotes islet survival and reduces the number of islets required for diabetes reversal. *J. Cell. Physiol.* **2011**, *226*, 1813–1819. [CrossRef]
3. Petersmann, A.; Müller-Wieland, D.; Müller, U.A.; Landgraf, R.; Nauck, M.; Freckmann, G.; Heinemann, L.; Schleicher, E. Definition, Classification and Diagnosis. *Exp. Clin. Endocrinol. Diabetes* **2019**, *127*, S1–S7. [CrossRef] [PubMed]
4. Masiello, P.; Broca, C.; Gross, R.; Roye, M.; Manteghetti, M.; Hillaire-Buys, D.; Novelli, M.; Ribes, G. Experimental NIDDM: Development of a new model in adult rats administered streptozotocin and nicotinamide. *Diabetes* **1998**, *47*, 224–229. [CrossRef] [PubMed]
5. Bolzán, A.D.; Bianchi, M.S. Genotoxicity of Streptozotocin. *Mutat. Res. Mutat. Res.* **2002**, *512*, 121–134. [CrossRef] [PubMed]
6. Dhuria, R.S.; Singh, G.; Kaur, A.; Kaur, R.; Kaur, T. Current status and patent prospective of animal models in diabetic research. *Adv. Biomed. Res.* **2015**, *4*, 117.
7. Asrafuzzaman, M.; Cao, Y.; Afroz, R.; Kamato, D.; Gray, S.; Little, P.J. Animal models for assessing the impact of natural products on the aetiology and metabolic pathophysiology of Type 2 diabetes. *Biomed. Pharmacother.* **2017**, *89*, 1242–1251. [CrossRef]
8. Klemann, C.; Wagner, L.; Stephan, M.; von Hörsten, S. Cut to the chase: A review of CD26/dipeptidyl peptidase-4's (DPP4) entanglement in the immune system. *Clin. Exp. Immunol.* **2016**, *185*, 1–21. [CrossRef]
9. Del Prato, S.; Barnett, A.H.; Huisman, H.; Neubacher, D.; Woerle, H.J.; Dugi, K.A. Effect of linagliptin monotherapy on glycaemic control and markers of β-cell function in patients with inadequately controlled type 2 diabetes: A randomized controlled trial. *Diabetes Obes. Metab.* **2011**, *13*, 258–267. [CrossRef]

10. Heise, T.; Graefe-Mody, E.U.; Hüttner, S.; Ring, S.; Trommeshauser, D.; Dugi, K.A. Pharmacokinetics, pharmacodynamics and tolerability of multiple oral doses of linagliptin, a dipeptidyl peptidase-4 inhibitor in male type 2 diabetes patients. *Diabetes Obes Metab.* **2009**, *11*, 786–794. [CrossRef]
11. World Health Organization. *WHO Guidelines on Safety Monitoring of Herbal Medicines in Pharmacovigilance Systems*; World Health Organization: Geneva, Switzerland, 2004; Available online: https://iris.who.int/bitstream/handle/10665/43034/9241592214_eng.pdf (accessed on 5 June 2004).
12. Campanero, M.A.; Escolar, M.; Garcia-Quetglas, E.P.; Sadaba, B.; Azanza, J.R. Simultaneous determination of diosmin and diosmetin in human plasma by ion trap liquid chromatography-atmospheric pressure chemical ionization tandem mass spectrometry. *J. Pharm. Biomed. Anal.* **2010**, *51*, 875–881. [CrossRef] [PubMed]
13. Bogucka-Kockaa, A.; Wozniaka, M.; Feldob, M.; Kockic, J.; Szewczyk, K. Diosmin -isolation techniques, determination in plant material and pharmaceutical formulations, and clinical use. *Nat. Prod. Commun.* **2013**, *8*, 545–550. [CrossRef]
14. Thanapongsathorn, W.; Vajrabukka, T. Clinical trial of oral diosmin (Daflon®) in the treatment of hemorrhoids. *Dis. Colon. Rectum.* **1992**, *35*, 1085–1088. [CrossRef]
15. AbouZid, S.F.; Ahmed, O.M.; Ahmed, R.R.; Mahmoud, A.; Abdella, E.; Ashour, M.B. Antihyperglycemic Effect of Crude Extracts of Some Egyptian Plants and Algae. *J. Med. Food* **2014**, *17*, 400–406. [CrossRef] [PubMed]
16. Sayed, H.M.; Awaad, A.S.; Abdel Rahman, F.E.Z.S.; Al-Dossari, M.; Abd El-Gawaad, N.S.; Ahmed, O.M. Combinatory Effect and Modes of Action of Chrysin and Bone Marrow-Derived Mesenchymal Stem Cells on Streptozotocin/Nicotinamide-Induced Diabetic Rats. *Pharmaceuticals* **2023**, *16*, 34. [CrossRef] [PubMed]
17. Ahmed, O.M.; Saleh, A.S.; Ahmed, E.A.; Ghoneim, M.M.; Ebrahim, H.A.; Abdelgawad, M.A.; Abdel-Gabbar, M. Efficiency of Bone Marrow-Derived Mesenchymal Stem Cells and Hesperetin in the Treatment of Streptozotocin-Induced Type 1 Diabetes in Wistar Rats. *Pharmaceuticals* **2023**, *16*, 859. [CrossRef]
18. Ali, A.M.; Gabbar, M.A.; Abdel-Twab, S.M.; Fahmy, E.M.; Ebaid, H.; Alhazza, I.M.; Ahmed, O.M. Antidiabetic Potency, Antioxidant Effects, and Mode of Actions of Citrus reticulata Fruit Peel Hydroethanolic Extract, Hesperidin, and Quercetin in Nicotinamide/Streptozotocin-Induced Wistar Diabetic Rats. *Oxid. Med. Cell. Longev.* **2020**, *2020*, 1730492. [CrossRef] [PubMed] [PubMed Central]
19. Akhani, S.P.; Vishwakarma, S.L.; Goyal, R.K. Anti-diabetic activity of Zingiber officinale in streptozotocin-induced type I diabetic rats. *J. Pharm. Pharmacol.* **2004**, *56*, 101–105. [CrossRef]
20. Ahmed, O.; Abdel Moneim, A.; Yazid, I.; Mahmoud, A. Antihyperglycemic, antihyperlipidemic and antioxidant effects and the probable mechanisms of action of Ruta graveolens infusion and rutin in nicotinamide-streptozotocin-induced diabetic rats. *Diabetol. Croat.* **2010**, *39*, 15–35.
21. Schaalan, M.; El-Abhar, H.S.; Barakat, M.; El-Denshary, E.S. Westernized-like-diet-fed rats: Effect on glucose homeostasis, lipid profile, and adipocyte hormones and their modulation by rosiglitazone and glimepiride. *J. Diabetes Complicat.* **2009**, *23*, 199–208. [CrossRef]
22. Ali, T.M.; Abo-Salem, O.M.; El Esawy, B.H.; El Askary, A. The Potential Protective Effects of Diosmin on Streptozotocin-Induced Diabetic Cardiomyopathy in Rats. *Am. J. Med. Sci.* **2020**, *359*, 32–41. [CrossRef]
23. McKeage, K. Linagliptin: An update of its use in patients with type 2 diabetes mellitus. *Drugs* **2014**, *74*, 1927–1946. [CrossRef] [PubMed]
24. Wahren, J.; Ekberg, K.; Samnegård, B.; Johansson, B.L. C-peptide: A new potential in the treatment of diabetic nephropathy. *Curr. Diab. Rep.* **2001**, *1*, 261–266. [CrossRef]
25. Steiner, D.F. The Proinsulin C-peptide—A Multirole Model. *J. Diabetes Res.* **2004**, *5*, 7–14. [CrossRef] [PubMed]
26. Rauch, T.; Graefe-Mody, U.; Deacon, C.F.; Ring, A.; Holst, J.J.; Woerle, H.J.; Dugi, K.A.; Heise, T. Linagliptin increases incretin levels, lowers glucagon, and improves glycemic control in type 2 diabetes mellitus. *Diabetes Ther.* **2012**, *3*, 1–14. [CrossRef] [PubMed]
27. Pari, L.; Srinivasan, S. Antihyperglycemic effect of diosmin on hepatic key enzymes of carbohydrate metabolism in streptozotocin-nicotinamide-induced diabetic rats. *Biomed. Pharmacother.* **2010**, *64*, 477–481. [CrossRef]
28. Shiraki, A.; Oyama, J.; Shimizu, T.; Node, N. The DPP4 inhibitor linagliptin exacerbated heart failure due to energy deficiency via downregulation of glucose absorption and utilization in mice. *Eur. Heart J.* **2022**, *43*, ehac544-2682. [CrossRef]
29. Enes, P.; Panserat, S.; Kaushik, S.; Oliva-Teles, A. Nutritional regulation of hepatic glucose metabolism in fish. *Fish. Physiol. Biochem.* **2009**, *35*, 519–539. [CrossRef]
30. Mahmoud, A.M.; Ahmed, O.M.; Ashour, M.B.; Abdel-Moneim, A. In vivo and in vitro antidiabetic effects of citrus flavonoids; a study on the mechanism of action. *Int. J. Diabetes Dev. Ctries.* **2015**, *35*, 250–263. [CrossRef]
31. Zheng, Y.; Zhang, R.; Shi, W.; Li, L.; Liu, H.; Chen, Z.; Wu, L. Metabolism and pharmacological activities of the natural health-benefiting compound diosmin. *Food Funct.* **2020**, *11*, 8472–8492. [CrossRef]
32. Vetrivel Venkatasamy, V.; Pericherla, S.; Manthuruthil, S.; Mishra, S.; Hanno, R. Effect of Physical activity on Insulin Resistance, Inflammation and Oxidative Stress in Diabetes Mellitus. *J. Clin. Diagn. Res.* **2013**, *7*, 1764. [PubMed] [PubMed Central]

33. Coskun, O.; Kanter, M.; Korkmaz, A.; Oter, S. Quercetin, a flavonoid antioxidant, prevents and protects streptozotocin-induced oxidative stress and β-cell damage in rat pancreas. *Pharmacol. Res.* **2005**, *51*, 117–123. [CrossRef]
34. Son, S.M.; Whalin, M.K.; Harrison, D.G.; Taylor, W.R.; Griendling, K.K. Oxidative stress and diabetic vascular complications. *Curr. Diab. Rep.* **2004**, *4*, 247–252. [CrossRef]
35. Anoopkumar-Dukie, S.; Walker, R.B.; Daya, S. A sensitive and reliable method for the detection of lipid peroxidation in biological tissues. *J. Pharm. Pharmacol.* **2010**, *53*, 263–266. [CrossRef]
36. Mohamed, N.A.; Hussein, M.M.; Ahmed, O.M.; Al-Jameel, S.S.; Al-Muzafar, H.M.; Amin, K.A.; Abdou, H.M. Oleuropein ameliorates hyperlipidemia, oxidative stress, inflammatory and liver dysfunction biomarkers, in streptozotocin-induced diabetic rats. *J. Appl. Pharm. Sci.* **2024**, *14*, 227–234. [CrossRef]
37. Hussien, Y.A.; Mansour, D.F.; Nada, S.A.; Abd El-Rahman, S.S.; Abdelsalam, R.M.; Attia, A.S.; El-Tanbouly, D.M. Linagliptin attenuates thioacetamide-induced hepatic encephalopathy in rats: Modulation of C/EBP-β and CX3CL1/Fractalkine, neuro-inflammation, oxidative stress and behavioral defects. *Life Sci.* **2022**, *295*, 120378. [CrossRef] [PubMed]
38. Ağır, M.S.; Eraslan, G. The effect of diosmin against liver damage caused by cadmium in rats. *J. Food Biochem.* **2019**, *43*, e12966. [CrossRef]
39. Anwer, T.; Alruwaili, M.N.; Alshahrani, S.; Alqahtani, S.S.; Jali, A.; Ahmed, R.A.; Alam, M.F.; Moni, S.S. Hepatoprotective potential of diosmin against hepatotoxic effect of isoniazid and rifampin in wistar rats. *Hum. Exp. Toxicol.* **2023**, *42*, 09603271221149199. [CrossRef]
40. Dong, K.; Ni, H.; Wu, M.; Tang, Z.; Halim, M.; Shi, D. ROS-mediated glucose metabolic reprogram induces insulin resistance in type 2 diabetes. *Biochem. Biophys. Res. Commun.* **2016**, *476*, 204–211. [CrossRef]
41. Liu, W.Y.; Liou, S.S.; Hong, T.Y.; Liu, I.M. The benefits of the citrus flavonoid diosmin on human retinal pigment epithelial cells under high-glucose conditions. *Molecules* **2017**, *22*, 2251. [CrossRef]
42. Giacco, F.; Brownlee, M. Oxidative stress and diabetic complications. *Circ. Res.* **2010**, *107*, 1058–1070. [CrossRef] [PubMed]
43. Srinivasan, S.; Pari, L. Ameliorative effect of diosmin, a citrus flavonoid against streptozotocin-nicotinamide generated oxidative stress induced diabetic rats. *Chem. Biol. Interact.* **2012**, *195*, 43–51. [CrossRef]
44. Arab, H.H.; Salama, S.A.; Omar, H.A.; Arafa, E.S.A.; Maghrabi, I.A. Diosmin Protects against Ethanol-Induced Gastric Injury in Rats: Novel Anti-Ulcer Actions. *PLoS ONE* **2015**, *10*, e0122417. [CrossRef] [PubMed]
45. El Husseny, M.W.A.; Mamdouh, M.; Shaban, S.; Ibrahim Abushouk, A.; Zaki, M.M.M.; Ahmed, O.M.; Abdel-Daim, M.M. Adipokines: Potential Therapeutic Targets for Vascular Dysfunction in Type II Diabetes Mellitus and Obesity. *J. Diabetes Res.* **2017**, *2017*, 8095926. [CrossRef]
46. Ferris, H.A.; Kahn, C.R. New mechanisms of glucocorticoid-induced insulin resistance: Make no bones about it. *J. Clin. Investig.* **2012**, *122*, 3854–3857. [CrossRef] [PubMed]
47. Koyama, T.; Tanaka, A.; Yoshida, H.; Oyama, J.-I.; Toyoda, S.; Sakuma, M.; Inoue, T.; Otsuka, Y.; Node, K. Comparison of the effects of linagliptin and voglibose on endothelial function in patients with type 2 diabetes and coronary artery disease: A prospective, randomized, pilot study (EFFORT). *Heart Vessels* **2018**, *33*, 958–964. [CrossRef]
48. Gerges, S.H.; Wahdan, S.A.; Elsherbiny, D.A.; El-Demerdash, E. Diosmin ameliorates inflammation, insulin resistance, and fibrosis in an experimental model of non-alcoholic steatohepatitis in rats. *Toxicol. Appl. Pharmacol.* **2020**, *401*, 115101. [CrossRef]
49. Rajala, M.W.; Qi, Y.; Patel, H.R.; Takahashi, N.; Banerjee, R.; Pajvani, U.B.; Sinha, M.K.; Gingerich, R.L.; Scherer, P.E.; Ahima, R.S. Regulation of Resistin Expression and Circulating Levels in Obesity, Diabetes, and Fasting. *Diabetes* **2004**, *53*, 1671–1679. [CrossRef]
50. Stofkova, A. Resistin and visfatin: Regulators of insulin sensitivity, inflammation and immunity. *Endocr. Regul.* **2010**, *44*, 25–36. [CrossRef]
51. Lazar, M.A. Resistin- and obesity-associated metabolic diseases. *Horm. Metab. Res.* **2007**, *39*, 710–716. [CrossRef]
52. Hartman, H.B.; Hu, X.; Tyler, K.X.; Dalal, C.K.; Lazar, M.A. Mechanisms regulating adipocyte expression of resistin. *J. Biol. Chem.* **2002**, *277*, 19754–19761. [CrossRef] [PubMed]
53. Ahmed, O.M.; Ali, T.M.; Abdel Gaid, M.A.; Elberry, A.A. Effects of enalapril and paricalcitol treatment on diabetic nephropathy and renal expressions of TNF-α, p53, caspase-3 and Bcl-2 in STZ-induced diabetic rats. *PLoS ONE* **2019**, *14*, e0214349. [CrossRef] [PubMed] [PubMed Central]
54. Ahmed, O.M.; Mosa, N.M.; Abou-Seif, H.S. Therapeutic role of Arabic gum against nicotinamide/streptozotocin-induced diabetes and nephropathy in Wistar rats. *Egypt. Pharm. J.* **2024**, *23*, 643–653. [CrossRef]
55. Yan, L.J. The Nicotinamide/Streptozotocin Rodent Model of Type 2 Diabetes: Renal Pathophysiology and Redox Imbalance Features. *Biomolecules* **2022**, *12*, 1225. [CrossRef] [PubMed] [PubMed Central]
56. Ahmed, O.M.; Abdel Fattah, A.A.; Abdul-Hamid, M.; Abdel-Aziz, A.M.; Sakr, H.I.; Damanhory, A.A.; Abdel-Kawi, S.H.; Ghaboura, N.; Awad, M.M.Y. Antidiabetic and liver histological and ultrastructural effects of Cynara scolymus leaf and flower head hydroethanolic extracts in nicotinamide/streptozotocin-induced diabetic rats. *Evid.-Based Complement. Altern. Med.* **2023**, *2023*, 4223026. [CrossRef]

57. Zaky, A.S.; Kandeil, M.; Abdel-Gabbar, M.; Fahmy, E.M.; Almehmadi, M.M.; Ali, T.M.; Ahmed, O.M. The Antidiabetic Effects and Modes of Action of the Balanites aegyptiaca Fruit and Seed Aqueous Extracts in NA/STZ-Induced Diabetic Rats. *Pharmaceutics* **2022**, *14*, 263. [CrossRef]
58. Mahmoud, A.M.; Mohamed, B.M.; Ibraheem, I.B.M.; Soliman, H.A.; Ahmed, O.M. Characterization of *Ulva fasciata* ethanolic extract-mediated biosynthesized silver nanoparticles and evaluation of their nephrocadiopreventive effects in doxorubicin-injected wistar rats. *Adv. Anim. Vet. Sci.* **2020**, *8* (Suppl. S2), 98–111. [CrossRef]
59. Jones, R.B.; Vickers, S.B.; Cheetham, S.C.; Headland, K.R.; Mark, M.; Klein, T. Effect of linagliptin, alone and in combination with voglibose or exendin-4, on glucose control in male ZDF rats. *Eur. J. Pharmacol.* **2014**, *729*, 59–66. [CrossRef]
60. Mohamed, K.; Abuelsaad, A.; Abdelaziz, M.; Sakr, H.; Abdel-Aziz, A.; Ahmed, O. The preventive effects of diosmin alone or combined with irinotecan on 1,2-dimethylhydrazine-induced colon cancer in rats. *Eur. Rev. Med. Pharmacol. Sci.* **2024**, *28*, 4003–4021. [CrossRef] [PubMed]
61. Ibrahim, G.M.; Ahmed, O.M.; Abbas, N.H.; El Fateh, M.M. Evaluation of the anti-diabetic effects of epicatechin and/or gallic acid in STZ/NA- induced diabetic Wister rats. *Res. J. Appl. Biotechnol.* **2018**, *4*, 87–104. [CrossRef]
62. Seifter, S.; Dayton, S.; Novic, B.; Muntwyler, E. The estimation of glycogen with the anthrone reagent. *Arch. Biochem.* **1950**, *25*, 191–200. [PubMed]
63. Kabir, S.M.H.; Begum, R. Toxicity of three organophosphorus insecticides to shinghi fish, Heteropneustes fossilis (Block). *Dacca Univ. Stud. (Bangladesh) Part B* **1978**, *26*, 115–122.
64. Stalmans, W.; Hers, H.-G. The stimulation of liver phosphorylase b by AMP, fluoride and sulfate. A technical note on the specific determination of the a and b forms of liver glycogen phosphorylase. *Eur. J. Biochem.* **1975**, *54*, 341–350. [CrossRef]
65. Hsing, A.W.; Gao, Y.-T.; Chua, S.; Deng, J.; Stanczyk, F.Z. Insulin Resistance and Prostate Cancer Risk. *JNCI J. Natl. Cancer Inst.* **2003**, *95*, 67–71. [CrossRef]
66. Aref, A.B.M.; Ahmed, O.M.; Ali, L.A.; Semmler, M. Maternal rat diabetes mellitus deleteriously affects insulin sensitivity and beta-cell function in the offspring. *J. Diabetes Res.* **2013**, *2013*, 429154. [CrossRef]
67. Park, J.M.; Bong, H.Y.; Jeong, H.I.; Kim, Y.K.; Kim, J.Y.; Kwon, O. Postprandial hypoglycemic effect of mulberry leaf in Goto-Kakizaki rats and counterpart control Wistar rats. *Nutr. Res. Pract.* **2009**, *3*, 272–278. [CrossRef]
68. Patton, C.J.; Crouch, S.R. Spectrophotometric and Kinetics Investigation of the Berthelot Reaction for the Determination of Ammonia. *Anal. Chem.* **1977**, *49*, 464–469. [CrossRef]
69. Bartels, H.; Böhmer, M.; Heierli, C. Serum creatinine determination without protein precipitation. *Clin. Chim. Acta* **1972**, *37*, 193–197. [CrossRef]
70. Livak, K.J.; Schmittgen, T.D. Analysis of relative gene expression data using realtime quantitative PCR and the $2^{-\Delta\Delta C_T}$ method. *Methods* **2001**, *25*, 402–408. [CrossRef]
71. Caminos, J.E.; Nogueiras, R.; Gallego, R.; Bravo, S.; Tovar, S.; García-Caballero, T.; Casanueva, F.F.; Diéguez, C. Expression and Regulation of Adiponectin and Receptor in Human and Rat Placenta. *J. Clin. Endocrinol. Metab.* **2005**, *90*, 4276–4286. [CrossRef]
72. Levy, J.R.; Davenport, B.; Clore, J.N.; Stevens, W. Lipid metabolism and resistin gene expression in insulin-resistant Fischer 344 rats. *Am. J. Physiol.-Endocrinol. Metab.* **2002**, *282*, E626–E633. [CrossRef] [PubMed]
73. Marklund, S.; Marklund, G. Involvement of the Superoxide Anion Radical in the Autoxidation of Pyrogallol and a Convenient Assay for Superoxide Dismutase. *Eur. J. Biochem.* **1974**, *47*, 469–474. [CrossRef] [PubMed]
74. Preuss, H.G.; Jarrell, S.T.; Scheckenbach, R.; Lieberman, S.; Anderson, R.A. Comparative Effects of Chromium, Vanadium and Gymnema Sylvestre on Sugar-Induced Blood Pressure Elevations in SHR. *J. Am. Coll. Nutr.* **1998**, *17*, 116–123. [CrossRef] [PubMed]
75. Beutler, E.; Duron, O.; Kelly, B.M. Improved method for the determination of blood glutathione. *J. Lab. Clin. Med.* **1963**, *61*, 882–888. [PubMed]
76. Matkovics, B.; Kotorman, M.; Sz Varga, I.; Quy Hai, D.; Varga, C. Oxidative stress in experimental diabetes induced by streptozotocin. *Acta Physiol. Hung.* **1997**, *85*, 29–38. [PubMed]
77. Ahmed, O.M.; Abd El-Twab, S.M.; Al-Muzafar, H.M.; Adel Amin, K.; Abdel Aziz, S.M.; Abdel-Gabbar, M. *Musa paradisiaca* L. leaf and fruit peel hydroethanolic extracts improved the lipid profile, glycemic index and oxidative stress in nicotinamide/streptozotocin-induced diabetic rats. *Vet. Med. Sci.* **2021**, *7*, 500–511. [CrossRef] [PubMed] [PubMed Central]

78. Bancroft, J.D.; Gamble, M. Theory and Practice of Histological Techniques, 6th Edition. *J. Neuropathol. Exp. Neurol.* **2008**, *67*, 633. [CrossRef]
79. Ramadan, H.; Moustafa, N.; Ahmed, R.R.; El-Shahawy, A.A.G.; Eldin, Z.E.; Al-Jameel, S.S.; Amin, K.A.; Ahmed, O.M.; Abdul-Hamid, M. Therapeutic effect of oral insulin-chitosan nanobeads pectin-dextrin shell on streptozotocin-diabetic male albino rats. *Heliyon* **2024**, *10*, e35636. [CrossRef] [PubMed] [PubMed Central]

pharmaceuticals

MDPI

Article

Timbe (*Acaciella angustissima*) as an Alternative Source of Compounds with Biological Activity: Antidiabetic

Diana Karina Rangel-Sandoval [1,†], Lucia Guerrero-Becerra [2,†], Consuelo Lomas-Soria [3], Amanda Kim Rico-Chávez [4], José Antonio Cervantes-Chávez [1], Luis Antonio Reyes-Castro [3], Angélica Morales-Miranda [3] and Ana Angélica Feregrino-Pérez [2,*]

1 Facultad de Ciencias Naturales, Universidad Autónoma de Querétaro, Campus Aeropuerto, Carretera a Chichimequillas s/n, Anillo Vial Fray Junípero Serra, Km 8, Querétaro 76000, Mexico; drangel11@alumnos.uaq.mx (D.K.R.-S.); jose.antonio.cervantes@uaq.mx (J.A.C.-C.)

2 Facultad de Ingeniería, Universidad Autónoma de Querétaro, Campus Amazcala, Carretera a Chichimequillas Km 1 s/n, Amazcala, El Marqués 76265, Mexico; gubel28@gmail.com

3 Departamento de Biología de la Reproducción, Instituto Nacional de Ciencias Médicas y Nutrición Salvador Zubirán, Mexico City 14080, Mexico; consuelo.lomass@incmnsz.mx (C.L.-S.); luis.reyesc@incmnsz.mx (L.A.R.-C.); angelica.moralesm@incmnsz.mx (A.M.-M.)

4 Facultad de Química, Universidad Autónoma de Querétaro, Campus Centro Universitario, Cerro de las Campanas s/n, Querétaro 76010, Mexico

* Correspondence: feregrino.angge@hotmail.com; Tel.: +52-01-442-192-12-00 (ext. 6016)

† These authors contributed equally to this work.

Abstract: Background/Objectives: Timbe (*Acaciella angustissima*) is a legume recognized for its environmental benefits, such as soil restoration, wildlife nutrition, and the presence of biologically active compounds. This study investigates the antioxidant, pharmacological, and antimicrobial properties of Timbe. **Methods:** The total phenolic content, flavonoids, and condensed tannins from Timbe flowers, seeds, and pods were quantified, and their antioxidant activity was evaluated using the DPPH and ABTS assays. Enzymatic activities were assessed through α-amylase, α-glucosidase, and ACE-I inhibition, and antimicrobial properties were tested against various bacterial strains. **Results:** The pods and flowers exhibited higher antioxidant capacities compared to seeds, effectively neutralizing free radicals. Flavonoids and condensed tannins showed positive correlations with antioxidant activity and the inhibition of α-amylase and α-glucosidase, suggesting the potential benefits of these metabolites in blood glucose control. Timbe also demonstrated ACE-I inhibition, particularly the flowers. Regarding antimicrobial activity, the pods displayed moderate inhibition against *E. coli*, *K. pneumoniae*, and *S. aureus*. **Conclusions:** The results indicate that different parts of Timbe (flowers, seeds, and pods) possess significant therapeutic potential for preventing and treating metabolic disorders and bacterial infections.

Keywords: antimicrobial activity; antioxidant activity; diabetes mellitus; hypertensive; legume; phenolic compounds

1. Introduction

Traditional medicine encompasses knowledge and practices transmitted from generation to generation based on the experiences and beliefs of diverse cultures. It is essential in maintaining health and preventing diseases and is especially accessible in rural and remote areas [1]. Traditional medicine is based on the use of plants (seeds, roots, stems, leaves, flowers, and fruits) that contain bioactive compounds, such as secondary metabolites, which can also serve as precursors for designing new drugs, especially for chronic and degenerative diseases [2–4]. On the other hand, interest in medicinal herbs has grown in recent years because they usually cause fewer side effects than conventional drugs. The increase in the search for medicinal alternatives is valuable, particularly where modern and safe drugs do not exist, which is why the World Health Organization (WHO) recommends evaluating the effectiveness of plants in treating diseases [5–7]. Among bioactive plant metabolites, phenolic compounds are prominent because they are widely distributed in plants and have health-promoting effects [3,8]. The phenolic compounds found in many plant foods have a wide range of biological properties, including antioxidant, anti-inflammatory, and enzyme activity-modulating effects [9,10]. Although several processes through which phenolic compounds contribute to preventing metabolic diseases have been identified, the exact mechanisms by which they exert these effects are still under investigation [9]. However, growing evidence suggests that regular consumption may be an effective strategy for improving metabolic health and preventing the onset of diseases like diabetes mellitus (DM) [11,12].

DM is a chronic and complex metabolic disease characterized by elevated blood glucose levels and is common worldwide [13]. People with DM develop infections more frequently than the general population, and these tend to be more severe, increasing the risk of death, especially in low-income countries [14,15]. Infections, and in some cases, the treatments applied to them, can alter the balance of glucose in the body, affecting insulin production and effectiveness and increasing the risk of developing diabetes [14]. Additionally, modifying the diversity of the gut microbiota and gut-related metabolites is associated with beneficial effects that help combat diabetes [13,16]. The human gut microbiota, composed of trillions of bacteria from over 1000 species and other microorganisms such as archaea, viruses, fungi, and protists, plays a crucial role in health. Its imbalance or alteration can contribute to the development of various diseases, such as obesity, type 2 diabetes, nonalcoholic hepatic steatosis, hypertension, and osteoporosis. Due to the increasing prevalence of DM and its complications, natural plant-based treatments, such as legumes, are being investigated. Thanks to their bioactive compounds, they can regulate glucose levels and prevent metabolic complications [17].

Timbe (*Acaciella angustissima*) is a legume with a distribution ranging from the southern United States to Costa Rica, and it is adapted to dry and semi-arid ecosystems in Mexico. Its resistance to drought and ability to improve soil quality make it a key species for bioremediation and ecosystem restoration. Its morphological characteristics include taproot, compound leaves, white flowers, and pod-shaped fruits, and it is used to produce firewood, wood, fodder, and traditional medicinal products [18,19]. Timbe is valuable for its high protein content and ability to regrow, which makes it helpful as fodder in dry seasons. In addition, it has outstanding biological properties, such as antioxidant, antimicrobial, and antimutagenic activity, which gives it the potential for pharmacological and cosmetic applications [19–21]. The roots and bark are used in traditional medicine to relieve toothache, arthritis, gastritis, rheumatic disorders, and skin lesions and even to treat digestive problems and diarrhea [18,20]. Its effect on diseases such as diabetes and its ability to produce bioactive compounds give Timbe a promising biotechnological potential in the health sector. However, despite these benefits, Timbe has been threatened by deforestation, leading to the advent of reforestation and conservation initiatives [22,23]. Given its agroforestry importance, a deeper understanding of its value, including its bioactive potential, could strengthen sustainable utilization strategies. Therefore, this research aimed to identify and analyze the bioactive compounds present in the flowers, seeds, and pods of the Timbe (*Acaciella angustissima*) plant, not only to explore underexploited therapeutic applications but also to support conservation by highlighting its multifunctional role. This study focuses on the antioxidant, pharmacological (antidiabetic), and antimicrobial properties of the Timbe tree with a pioneering approach to exploring its bioactive compounds in the context of new therapeutic alternatives.

2. Results

2.1. Phenolic Compounds and Antioxidant Capacity

The analysis presented in Table 1 reveals significant differences in the content of bioactive compounds and antioxidant capacity between the flowers, seeds, and pods. The pods showed the highest concentration of total phenols (7.151 ± 0.04 mg GAE/g), with a statistically significant difference compared to the flowers and seeds, the latter having the lowest concentration. Regarding the flavonoid content, the flowers stood out with the highest value (4.052 ± 0.26 mg RE/g), while the seeds had the lowest concentration of these compounds. In the case of condensed tannins, the pods again stood out with the highest concentration (6.213 ± 0.64 mg CE/g), significantly surpassing the flowers and seeds, between which no significant differences were found. Regarding antioxidant capacity, the pods showed the highest value in the DPPH assay, followed by the flowers and, finally, the seeds, with the lowest activity. On the other hand, in the ABTS assay, the flowers and the pods showed significantly higher antioxidant activity than that observed for the seeds.

Table 1. Content of phenolic compounds and antioxidant capacity of flowers, seeds, and pods of *Acacciella angustissima*.

Analysis	Flowers	Seeds	Pods
Total Phenols (mg GAE/g)	6.281 ± 0.07 [b]	4.810 ± 0.05 [c]	7.151 ± 0.04 [a]
Flavonoids (mg RE/g)	4.052 ± 0.26 [a]	0.121 ± 0.02 [c]	2.235 ± 0.20 [b]
Condensed Tannins (mg CE/g)	2.714 ± 0.36 [b]	1.677 ± 0.36 [b]	6.213 ± 0.64 [a]
DPPH (mg Trolox/g)	7.160 ± 0.02 [b]	3.979 ± 0.09 [c]	9.745 ± 0.07 [a]
ABTS (mg Trolox/g)	8.261 ± 0.08 [a]	5.989 ± 0.37 [b]	7.931 ± 0.08 [a]

Data are expressed as Mean ± SD; $p < 0.05$. A one-way ANOVA followed by Tukey's test was performed to determine differences among tissues (flowers, seeds, and pods) for each analysis. Different letters indicate significant statistical differences ($p < 0.05$) among the flowers, seeds, and pods for each phenolic compound and antioxidant capacity. mg GAE/g: mg eq. gallic acid/g of sample; mg RE/g: mg eq. rutin/g of sample; mg CE/g: mg eq. (+) catechin/g of sample; mg Trolox/g: mg eq. Trolox/g of dry sample.

The antioxidant capacity of the samples (Table 1) was expressed in terms of the Trolox concentration that generates a similar decrease in absorbance compared to the reference sample. In the DPPH (2,2-diphenyl-1-picrylhydrazyl) assay, the pods showed the highest efficiency in neutralizing free radicals, with a value of 9.745 ± 0.07 mg Trolox/g, while the seeds presented the lowest antioxidant capacity, with a value of 3.979 ± 0.09 mg Trolox/g. In the ABTS (2,2′-azino-bis-3-ethylbenzothiazoline-6-sulfonic acid) assay, the flowers and pods showed higher antioxidant activity (8.261 ± 0.08 and 7.931 ± 0.08 mg Trolox/g, respectively) compared to the seeds, whose activity was significantly lower, reaching 5.989 ± 0.37 mg Trolox/g.

Comparing the antioxidant activity from the ABTS and DPPH assays of the three samples, it can be observed that for the flowers, the ABTS method reaches almost 100% inhibition, while DPPH shows a value of 53.09%. In the seeds, both methods presented lower inhibition percentages than the flowers and pods, with DPPH being the lowest, with a value of 14.43%. Both methods show high inhibition percentages in the pods, reaching 96.36% and 84.52% (ABTS and DPPH, respectively), with ABTS slightly higher (Figure 1).

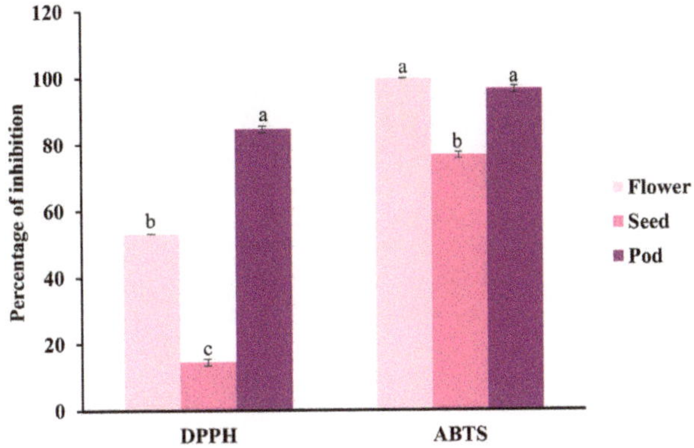

Figure 1. Percentage of inhibition of the antioxidant capacity of the flowers, seeds, and pods of *Acaciella angustissima*. Data are expressed as Mean ± SD; $p < 0.05$. A one-way ANOVA using Tukey's test was performed to determine differences among tissues (flowers, seeds, pods) for each analysis. Different letters indicate statistical differences ($p < 0.05$).

2.2. Metabolic Composition and Fatty Acid Content

The most relevant components of the metabolic profile of the flowers, seeds, and pods of *A. angustissima* were identified (Table 2) as the main metabolites in these parts of the plant, and their biotechnological potential was highlighted. D-pinitol and stigmasterol occur in the pods, seeds, and flowers (see footnote Table 2), while β-amyrin was predominantly in the flowers and pods; these compounds stand out for their potential biological properties.

Table 2. Metabolic profile of *Acaciella angustissima* flowers, seeds, and pods obtained by gas chromatography coupled with mass spectrometry (GC-MS).

Sample	Retention Time (min)	Name	Area (%)	Associated Biological Activity
Flowers	7.200	L-Proline	2.724	Precursor to the synthesis of compounds with antioxidant and antidiabetic potential [24,25].
	12.491	L-Threonic acid	1.607	In the form of magnesium salt, it could have beneficial neurofunctional effects in the treatment of Attention-deficit hyperactivity disorder [26].
	17.489	D-Pinitol	5.528	It has been found in other fabaceous, such as soybeans and tamarind, and is credited with antidiabetic, anti-inflammatory, antioxidant, and immunosuppressive properties [27–29].
	39.682	Stigmasterol	6.905	It has anticancer, anti-inflammatory, antioxidant, neuroprotective, antidiabetic, and antiparasitic effects, as well as anti-osteoarthritis, immunomodulatory, antifungal, and antibacterial properties [30–32].
	40.441	β-Amyrin	11.324	It has antioxidant potential, anti-inflammatory effects, antimicrobial activity, and antidiabetic properties [33,34].
Seeds		Amino acid		Amino acids can act as precursors in the synthesis of antibacterial and anticancer agents, while non-essential amino acids can modulate and enhance antitumor function [35–37].
	5.759	L-Valine	0.694	
	6.741	L-Leucine	0.126	
	7.202	L-Proline	0.187	
	8.456	Serine	0.107	
	8.987	L-Threonine	0.115	
	9.595	L-Aspartic acid	0.216	
	19.652	D-pinitol	0.502	It is the same compound as in flowers.
	21.697	Myo-Inositol	1.289	It shows protective effects against oxidative damage in proteins and lipids, improving vascular function and blood coagulation [38].
	39.678	Stigmasterol	0.247	It is the same compound as in flowers.

Table 2. *Cont.*

Sample	Retention Time (min)	Name	Area (%)	Associated Biological Activity
Pods	11.515	Picolinic acid	2.565	Picolinic acid derivatives have demonstrated antitumor, antiangiogenic, and antimicrobial effects [39,40].
		D-pinitol	8.083	It is the same compound as in flowers.
	19.367	2-Ketoglutaric acid	1.953	It acts as a prebiotic that reduces inflammation, improves the function of the intestinal barrier, and restores the balance of the intestinal microbiota [41].
	39.678	Stigmasterol	13.063	It is the same compound as in flowers.
	40.438	β-Amyrin	3.282	It is the same compound as in flowers.

Note: Only compounds whose presence or concentration are directly related to the activities analyzed in this study are reported. Other compounds present in the sample were not included in the table.

The fatty acid profile (Table 3) revealed that most of the acids present in the samples are unsaturated fatty acids, predominantly in the seeds. However, it only contains two unsaturated fatty acids (oleic acid and linoleic acid), and their concentration is higher compared to the pods, which contain three unsaturated acids (6-Octadecenoic acid, linoleic acid, and 1,3,14,16-Nonadecatetraene). On the other hand, the flowers have the lowest concentration, with only linolenic acid present. The flowers stood out for their higher concentration of hexadecanoic acid. At the same time, the Timbe seeds contain a higher total amount of fatty acids, the most prominent being linoleic acid and oleic acid. Both were unsaturated acids, with the first being an essential fatty acid (omega 6) and the second an omega 9. The pods presented a great diversity of short-chain fatty acids, but the most abundant was 6-octadecenoic acid, although linoleic and palmitic acids were also present.

Table 3. Fatty acid profile of *Acaciella angustissima* flowers, seeds, and pods obtained by gas chromatography coupled with mass spectrometry (GC-MS).

Sample	Retention Time (min)	Name	Area (%)	Concentration (μg/g Sample)
Flowers	14.011	Hexadecanoic acid	58.54	334.329
	16.711	Stearic acid	13.69	125.154
	20.451	Linolenic acid	25.99	215.076
	22.739	Popenoic acid	1.78	NQ
Seeds	14.017	Palmitic acid	23.07	843.249
	16.676	Stearic acid	4.02	237.454
	17.408	Oleic acid	17.10	2424.105
	18.700	Linoleic acid	55.31	3404.042
	20.490	Eicosanoic acid	0.48	50.888
Pods	8.858	Ethanedioic acid	0.76	NQ
	9.439	Propanedioic acid	0.32	NQ
	10.194	Butanedioic acid	0.54	NQ
	12.130	Tetradecanoate acid	1.67	ND
	13.997	Palmitic acid	37.87	498.944
	14.436	Butanoic acid	0.64	NQ
	15.712	Nonanedioic acid	0.60	ND
	16.640	Stearic acid	12.05	260.789
	17.313	6-Octadecenoic acid	20.17	1033.730
	18.667	Linoleic acid	23.06	511.773
	20.532	1,3,14,16-Nonadecatetraene	2.29	42.122

NQ: not quantified; ND: not detected (concentrations were under the detection limit).

2.3. *α-glucosidase, α-amylase, and ACE-I Inhibitory Activities*

α-amylase, α-glucosidase, and ACE-I inhibition assays were carried out to determine the potential of Timbe flowers, pods, and seeds (concentration: 10 mg/mL) against diabetes and hypertension-related enzymes. The Timbe pods had a remarkable potential against enzyme activity related to diabetes and hypertension. In particular, they showed the most significant inhibitory activity for α-amylase, with 74.77%, compared to the flowers and seeds. However, regarding α-glucosidase inhibition, the pods showed the lowest inhibition, with 15.92%. On the other hand, the seeds presented the highest percentage of α-glucosidase inhibition, with 48.12%, followed closely by the flowers, with 47.72%. Notably, regarding ACE-I inhibition, lisinopril (reference standard) showed inhibition of 91.46 ± 4%, underscoring the importance of continuing to investigate the therapeutic potential of Timbe extracts for treating diabetes and hypertension to achieve the same percentages of inhibition as lisinopril, for example. The structure with the highest inhibitory activity was the flowers, whose extract showed 69.14% more inhibition than the pods and seeds (Table 4).

Table 4. Evaluation of enzymatic activity: α-amylase, α-glucosidase, and ACE-I.

	% Inhibition		
Assay	Flowers	Seeds	Pods
α-amylase	25.31 ± 3 [b]	31.01 ± 4 [b]	74.77 ± 3 [a]
α-glucosidase	47.72 ± 6 [a]	48.12 ± 2 [a]	15.92 ± 1 [b]
ACE-I	69.14 ± 3 [a]	19.95 ± 2 [b]	28.39 ± 7 [b]

Data are expressed as Mean ± SD; $p < 0.05$. A one-way ANOVA followed by Tukey's test was performed to determine differences among tissues (flowers, seeds, and pods) for each analysis. Different letters indicate significant statistical differences ($p < 0.05$) among the flowers, seeds, and pods. ACE-I: angiotensin I-converting enzyme inhibition.

A correlation analysis was carried out between the percentages of inhibition of the α-amylase, α-glucosidase, and ACE-I enzymes and the total phenolic content (Figure 2). The pods demonstrated both a high content of phenolic compounds and inhibitory activity, especially with α-amylase. Even though the seeds have the lowest phenolic content, they showed the highest percentage of inhibition for α-glucosidase. Nevertheless, the inhibition percentages of the flowers and seeds were not significantly different, which led to both having the highest inhibitory activity for α-glucosidase. The ACE-I inhibitory activity is the lowest in all the parts tested. In addition, the phenol levels follow a similar trend to enzyme inhibition, with higher values in the flowers and pods and lower values in the seeds.

The correlation matrix between three types of bioactive compounds (total phenols, flavonoids, and tannins) and five biological activities (ABTS, DPPH, ACE-I, α-amylase, and α-glucosidase) is shown in Figure 3. Each graph presented a linear regression with its corresponding Pearson correlation value (r), which allowed the evaluation of the relationship between each pair of variables. Overall, the total phenols and tannins had strong positive correlations with the antioxidant activity (ABTS and DPPH), especially between phenols and DPPH ($r = 0.99$), suggesting a high antioxidant potential for these compounds. Furthermore, tannins showed significant negative correlations with α-glucosidase inhibition ($r = -0.93$) and positive correlations with α-amylase ($r = 0.91$), indicating a possible effect on enzyme modulation. On the other hand, flavonoids correlated well with ABTS and ACE-I but showed no clear relationship with digestive enzymes. Together, these results showed that certain phenolic compounds may have played a relevant role in antioxidant activity and the inhibition of enzymes associated with metabolic diseases, with additional details provided in Supplementary Material (Table S1).

2.4. Antimicrobial Activity

In this study, the MIC (minimum inhibitory concentration) values of the Timbe flowers, pods, and seeds against *Listeria monocytogenes*, *Staphylococcus aureus*, *Escherichia coli*, *Pseudomonas aeruginosa*, *Salmonella typhimurium*, and *Klebsiella pneumoniae* were determined by the microdilution method (Table 5). The extract dilutions considered were 20, 10, 5, 2.5, 1.25, 0.625, 0.312, 0.156, 0.078, and 0.039 mg/mL. The Timbe structures with the most prominent inhibitory activity were the pods against *S. aureus* and *K. pneumoniae*, showing the lowest MIC value at 0.625 mg/mL. These were followed by the seeds (MIC 1.25 mg/mL) and pods (MIC 1.25 mg/mL) against *S. aureus* and *E. coli*, respectively. Overall, the seeds showed the lowest performance regarding inhibitory effects against most of the bacteria tested, as the MIC obtained for most cases was ≥20 mg/mL, the highest concentration tested. The flowers presented a diverse spectrum of inhibition, ranging from MIC 2.5 mg/mL (against *S. aureus*) to MIC > 20 mg/mL (against *E. coli*).

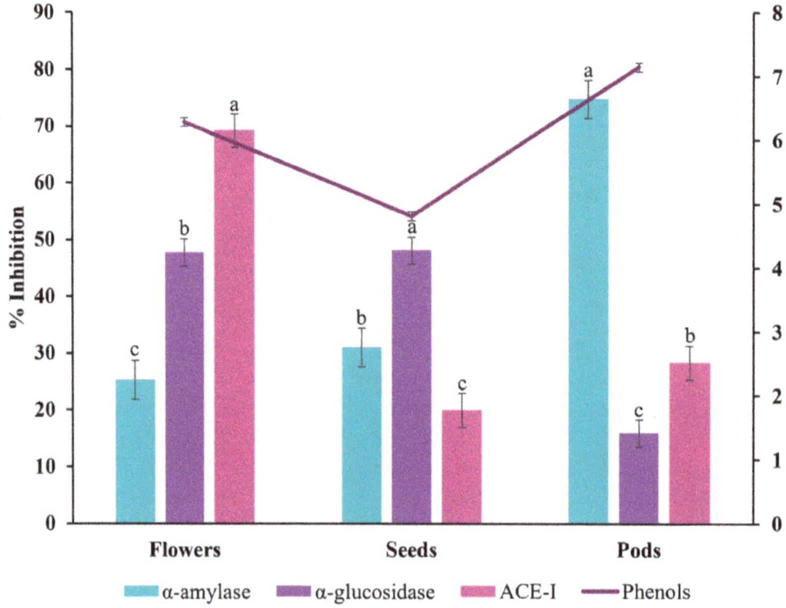

Figure 2. Comparison of the total phenolic content with the inhibitory activity of α-amylase, α-glucosidase, and ACE-I. Data are expressed as Mean ± SD. A one-way ANOVA followed by Tukey's test was performed to determine differences among tissues (flowers, seeds, and pods) for each analysis. Different letters indicate statistical differences ($p < 0.05$). ACE-I: angiotensin I-converting enzyme inhibition; mg GAE/g: mg eq. gallic acid/g of sample.

Table 5. Minimum inhibitory concentration (MIC) of *Acaciella angustissima* flowers, seeds, and pods.

Bacteria	Minimum Inhibitory Concentration (mg/mL)			
	Gentamicin	Flowers	Seeds	Pods
S. typhimurium	0.039	5	>20	5
E. coli	20	>20	>20	1.25
P. aeruginosa	0.039	5	20	5
S. aureus	0.039	2.5	1.25	0.625
K. pneumoniae	0.039	10	>20	0.625
L. monocytogenes	0.039	5	>20	5

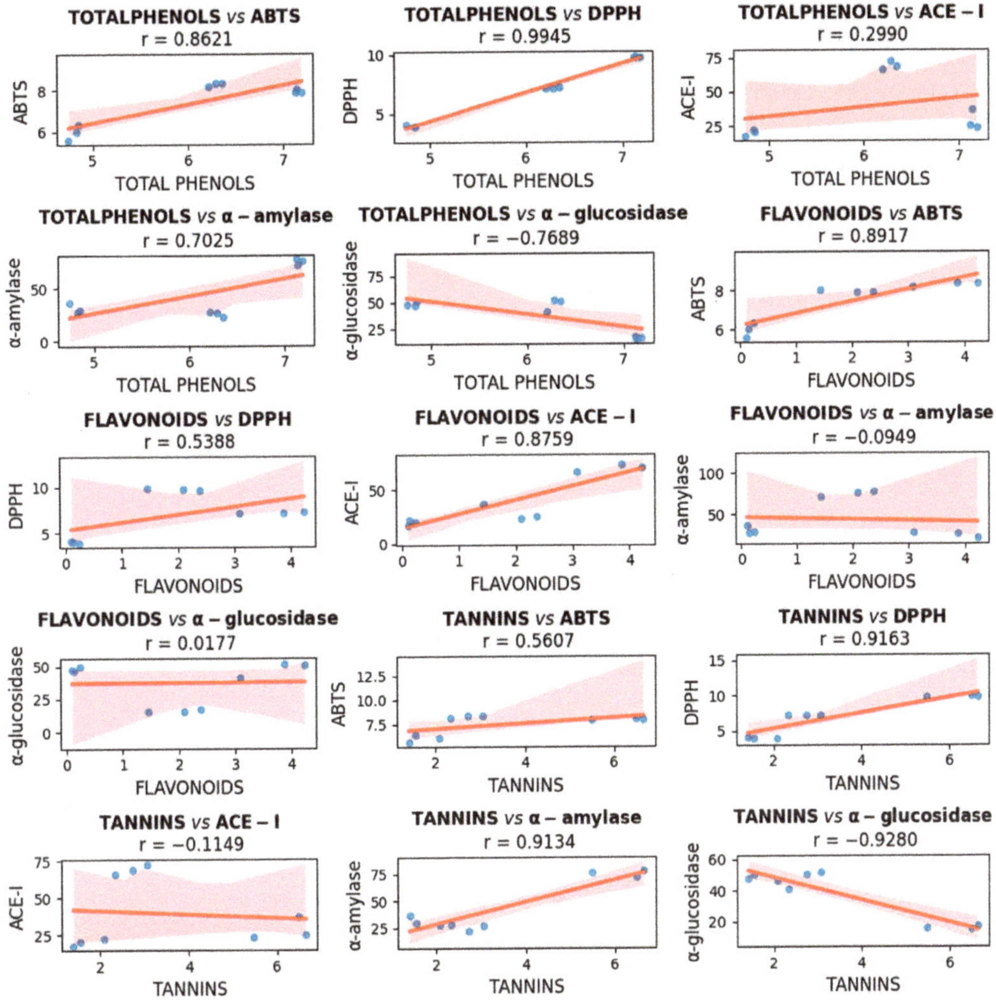

Figure 3. Correlation between total phenols, flavonoids, and tannins with DPPH, ABTS, α-amylase, α-glucosidase, and ACE-I (p-value < 0.05). Total phenols: mg eq. gallic acid/g of sample; flavonoids: mg eq. rutin/g of sample; condensed tannins: mg eq. (+) catechin/g of sample; DPPH, ABTS, α-amylase, α-glucosidase, and ACE-I: percentage of inhibition.

3. Discussion

3.1. Antioxidant Capacity by Phenolic Compounds

A. angustissima is characterized by its remarkable resistance to extreme heat and drought conditions, which makes it an ecological and sustainable option in arid regions. In addition, these conditions favor the development of secondary metabolites (phenolic compounds, nitrogen compounds, sulfur compounds, and terpenes) that the plant produces as a defense mechanism. These compounds are relevant in both the chemical and pharmaceutical fields [19]. In the results presented, significant differences were observed in the concentrations of phenolic compounds between the different parts of the plant (flowers, seeds, and pods). These compounds were extracted using methanol from methanolic extracts using the technique employed in this study, which has proven to be more efficient compared to water extraction, as reported by Rodríguez-Méndez in 2018 [22]. The pods presented the highest concentration of phenolic compounds, with an average value of 7.151 $\pm$ 0.04 mg GAE/g, suggesting that this part of the plant could play a fundamental role in the storage or accumulation of these compounds as a strategy to protect the seeds [42,43]. The data obtained were lower than those that Rodriguez-Méndez et al. reported in a Timbe pod methanolic extract [22]. These variations could be attributed to the specific conditions in which the plant is found at the time of harvest since the threats faced by the plant can induce a greater production of secondary metabolites, particularly phenolic ones, which play a protective role [42–44].

On the other hand, the flowers showed the highest concentration of flavonoids, which contribute to the protection of the flowers from damage by pathogens and even from ultraviolet light. In addition, flavonoids give color to the flowers and attract pollinators, thus ensuring the perpetuation of the species and its continuity in the ecosystem [45]. Furthermore, the Timbe seeds presented the lowest amount of phenolic compounds, which agrees with that reported by Alonso-Herrera et al., who compared the seeds and the flowers [19]. These results could be explained by the distribution of the plant's defense compounds, which are mainly concentrated in the parts most exposed to adverse environmental factors, such as the flowers and the pods, which protect the seeds from possible damage before germination [46].

Differences in the concentration of phenolic compounds between plant organs may be related to defense mechanisms optimized for their survival. Given its role in antioxidant capacity, this variation could help specifically counteract oxidative stress. Oxidative stress, caused by an imbalance between free radicals and antioxidants, is linked to chronic diseases. Genetic or environmental variations can influence antioxidant production, allowing some people to neutralize cellular damage more efficiently. Thus, these individual differences could offer more effective protection against the effects of oxidative stress. Dietary antioxidants, especially plant-derived polyphenols, help restore this balance by neutralizing free radicals by transferring a hydrogen atom, thus reducing cell damage [47,48]. A higher antioxidant capacity in a sample indicates a better ability to neutralize these free radicals, protecting cell health and preventing potential damage [49].

Among the parts of *A. angustissima* analyzed by ABTS, the flowers presented the highest concentration of Trolox equivalents, reaching almost 100% inhibition, suggesting a high efficacy against free radicals. In contrast, the seeds showed the lowest antioxidant capacity, reflected in the lowest percentage of inhibition. The results suggest that the antioxidant compounds present in the flowers react more efficiently with the ABTS radical than with DPPH. Both methods show the lowest inhibition percentages in the seeds, with DPPH showing the lowest value. This could be due to a lower concentration or effectiveness of antioxidant compounds in this part of the plant. In contrast, the highest inhibition values are observed in the pods for both methods, with ABTS showing a slightly higher percentage than DPPH. This behavior could be due to the presence of antioxidant compounds that are highly reactive against both radicals, although with a greater affinity towards ABTS, since a positive correlation has been seen between antioxidant activity with ABTS and DPPH, being more sensitive [50–52]. The relationship between antioxidant capacity and diabetes is that diabetic patients have greater oxidative stress due to high blood glucose levels, which can damage cells and tissues, contributing to complications such as cardiovascular problems, kidney damage, and neuropathy. Increasing antioxidant capacity helps neutralize free radicals generated by excess glucose, protecting cells and reducing the risk of complications [53–55].

Tannins act as effective electron and hydrogen donors, enabling them to neutralize free radicals and exhibit antioxidant activity. Their antioxidant potential depends on factors such as chemical structure and the oxidizing agent involved, with higher molecular mass generally enhancing activity. However, studies suggest that their effectiveness against DPPH radicals is primarily determined by the accessibility of hydroxyl groups [56]. On the other hand, there is a strong positive correlation between the concentration of flavonoids and their antioxidant capacity measured by ABTS. That is, the higher the content of flavonoids in a plant extract, the more significant the reduction in the ABTS radical and, therefore, the greater the measured antioxidant capacity [57,58]. A negative correlation between certain compounds, such as phenolics with α-glucosidase, flavonoids with α-amylase, and tannins with ACE-I and α-glucosidase, suggests that as the concentration of these compounds increases, their inhibitory capacity decreases. This could be due to competition with inhibitors at the enzyme's active site or the activation of compensatory mechanisms that counteract the inhibition. Hyperglycemia favors oxidative stress since the autooxidation of glucose generates free radicals. Antioxidant capacity is crucial since hyperglycemia reduces this capacity, affecting various tissues and contributing to microvascular complications associated with diabetes. Improving erythrocytes' antioxidant capacity and structure could prevent and treat such complications [59,60]. Polyphenols from plant sources have been associated with a lower incidence of metabolic diseases such as obesity, diabetes, and hypertension, which are related to insulin resistance [61]. These compounds improve insulin sensitivity, which is essential for people with diabetes. Furthermore, by reducing oxidative stress, polyphenols can prevent diabetes complications, such as blood glucose spikes and cardiovascular diseases, so their inclusion in the diet has positive effects [62–64]. Polyphenols may influence the activity of enzymes and hormones in the body, such as stimulating the release of GLP-1 (glucagon-like peptide-1), a hormone important for regulating blood sugar. GLP-1 and PYY (peptide tyrosine-tyrosine) reduce the risk of diabetes and obesity. They also modify the intestinal microbiota and may inhibit the enzyme DPP-IV (dipeptidyl peptidase-IV), which favors glucose control [65]. On the other hand, reactive oxygen species (ROS) are essential for regulating vascular and cardiac function. However, when their levels are elevated, they can cause cellular damage and contribute to the development of vascular disease, especially in conditions such as hypertension [66,67], which is a common complication of diabetes [68]. The flowers, seeds, and pods of *A. angustissima* presented a relevant antioxidant capacity attributed to their phenolic compounds. Phenolic compounds are known for their antioxidant properties, which help neutralize free radicals and prevent cellular damage, which could explain their ability to protect against mutations. This antioxidant activity is particularly relevant since, as Vargas-Hernández et al. point out, an extract with high phenolic content could protect DNA and minimize cellular damage [21]. However, although they show antimutagenic potential, evaluating their cytotoxicity is crucial to ensure that, at effective concentrations, they do not cause cellular damage.

3.2. Metabolic Profile and Fatty Acid Profile

The metabolic profiles of the flowers, seeds, and pods of *A. angustissima* were obtained by gas chromatography–mass spectrometry (GC-MS), revealing compounds with diverse biological activities. Three major compounds were identified in the flowers: D-pinitol (a sugar alcohol), stigmasterol (a sterol), and β-amyrin (a triterpene). Although only D-pinitol exhibits hydroxyl groups reminiscent of phenolics, all three are associated with antioxidant, anti-inflammatory, antidiabetic, anticancer, and immunomodulatory properties [27–34]. Moreover, phytosterols and triterpenes are known for modulating cellular processes and combating oxidative stress. Essential and non-essential amino acids, as well as myoinositol, were identified in the seeds, which are compounds with protective and regulatory effects on metabolic functions [35–38]. From the pods, picolinic acid and 2-ketoglutaric acid are reported to exhibit anti-inflammatory, antimicrobial, and prebiotic properties [41]. The presence of essential amino acids, phytonutrients, and antioxidant compounds, such as β-amyrin and picolinic acid, indicates that this plant may have protective properties, making it interesting from a pharmacological and nutritional perspective. The promising results suggest that the flowers, seeds, and pods contain a combination of bioactive metabolites that could benefit both the plant and humans.

Furthermore, the fatty acid profile found for the different parts of *A. angustissima* revealed a composition rich in compounds of nutritional and therapeutic relevance. The presence of saturated fatty acids, such as palmitic and stearic, along with unsaturated fatty acids, such as oleic, linoleic, and linolenic, suggested that this plant could play a beneficial role in human health, particularly in regulating cholesterol and cardiovascular function and modulating inflammatory processes. Polyunsaturated fatty acids, such as linoleic and linolenic, are essential, as the human body cannot synthesize them and must obtain them from the diet. They also play a key role in neuronal development, immune response, and the prevention of chronic diseases. The high concentration of these compounds in the pods, especially 6-octadecenoic acid, highlighted its potential as an alternative source of functional lipids. A comparison of the fatty acid profile of red lentil seeds shows similar results to those of Timbe seeds. Its main fatty acid is linoleic acid (46.81%), followed by oleic acid (23.27%) and palmitic acid (14.41%) [69,70], which shows a comparable trend to the content of the Timbe seeds, which presents values of 48.91%, 34.83%, and 12.12%, respectively. On the other hand, soy, another seed widely consumed for its nutritional value and health benefits [71–73], shows the same trend with higher concentrations of linoleic acid (52.8%), oleic acid (19%), and palmitic acid (13.1%) [74]. A moderate amount of linoleic acid in the diet may help lower total blood cholesterol levels and low-density lipoprotein cholesterol (known as "bad" cholesterol) [75].

The unique phytochemical profile of *A. angustissima*, featuring phenolic metabolites, sterols, and triterpenoids, positions it as a prime candidate for drug development and functional foods. Further research on the pharmacokinetics and structure–activity relationships of these compounds is warranted to unlock their full therapeutic potential.

3.3. *α-glucosidase, α-amylase and ACE-I Inhibitory Activities*

Type 2 diabetes is characterized by a rapid rise in blood glucose levels due to the breakdown of starch by pancreatic α-amylase and glucose absorption in the small intestine by α-glucosidase. This condition may be managed by inhibiting the enzymes involved in carbohydrate digestion. The consumption of natural inhibitors from dietary components could effectively control postprandial hyperglycemia with minimal side effects, unlike traditional drug treatments such as acarbose [76].

The effects of Timbe on enzymes associated with diabetes and hypertension have not been thoroughly investigated. However, it has been reported that in rats with streptozotocin-induced diabetes, Timbe (pods) significantly reduced blood glucose levels, increased serum insulin concentrations, decreased lipid levels, and improved indicators of kidney damage [22]. The present work assessed the inhibitory activity of α-glucosidase and α-amylase. The *A. angustissima* pod extract demonstrated the highest content of phenolic compounds and inhibitory activity of the α-amylase enzyme. In contrast, the seeds and flowers showed the most prominent inhibitory effect of the α-glucosidase enzyme. Therefore, all the studied structures of *A. angustissima* have potential as an alternative diabetes treatment. However, further studies are still required since none of the extracts evaluated achieved the percentage of inhibition reported in the standard, such as acarbose, which is 93% [77].

In addition, hypertension is one of the major macrovascular complications of diabetes and is a significant risk factor for many cardiovascular diseases. Hypertension is twice as common in people with diabetes as in those without. People with hypertension often have insulin resistance and are more likely to develop diabetes than people with normal blood pressure [78]. ACE-I plays a crucial role in the regulation of vascular tone. ACE-I converts angiotensin I into angiotensin II, a potent vasoconstrictor stimulating aldosterone secretion from the adrenal glands. ACE-I inhibition is an effective therapeutic approach for the treatment of hypertension in both diabetic and non-diabetic patients [79].

In this study, the inhibitory activity of ACE-I was evaluated. The flowers showed the best performance for ACE-I inhibition, making them the best candidate for treating hypertension of all the *A. angustissima* structures studied. Although the seeds and pods did not show as pronounced an inhibitory effect as the flowers, their activity on α-glucosidase and α-amylase was greater, making all structures relevant to the possible treatment and prevention of diabetes and hypertension. Plant extracts have been used worldwide as complementary or alternative treatments for patients with diabetes and hypertension. Their efficacy is largely attributed to the presence of polyphenolic compounds in various plants and foods, whose antioxidant activity helps neutralize free radicals and, consequently, prevent diabetes [80]. In addition, the hypoglycemic effects of these plants are also linked to the presence of compounds such as alkaloids, terpenes, flavonoids, and saponins, among others, which are thought to have insulin-mimetic activity. However, their exact mechanism of action remains unclear [22].

The correlation analysis showed that total phenols, flavonoids, and tannins exhibited varying degrees of association with the biological activities evaluated. These findings reinforce the importance of phenolic compounds as bioactive agents with multiple functional effects, especially in oxidative stress and metabolic diseases such as diabetes and hypertension.

3.4. Antimicrobial Testing

People with diabetes are more susceptible to new infections and relapses due to weakened immune defenses and complications of the disease. Rare, life-threatening infections are more common in people with diabetes than in those without diabetes [15].

Hyperglycemia, a key symptom of poorly controlled diabetes, plays a crucial role in exacerbating bacterial infections by providing an optimal environment for pathogen growth [14]. People with inadequate glycemic control have higher glucose levels in various tissues and organs throughout the body, which many bacterial pathogens, including staphylococci, streptococci, and enterococci, use as their primary carbon source to support their growth and enhance their virulence [81].

Plant-derived antimicrobials have immense potential for treating bacterial, fungal, protozoal, and viral infections without known adverse effects due to secondary metabolites, which include phenolic compounds such as flavones, flavanols, flavonoids, quinones, and tannins [82]. These are commonly found in medicinal plants and are widely used against pathogenic bacteria. *A. angustissima* is rich in phenolic compounds, which are effective in preventing a wide variety of diseases as they possess antidiabetic, antioxidant, anticancer, antimicrobial, and anti-inflammatory biological activities [18,83]. Timbe is also rich in flavonoids, which are particularly recognized for their antiviral, anti-inflammatory, and antimicrobial effects. Moreover, flavonoids exhibit promising activity against *E. coli*, *P. aeruginosa*, *K. pneumoniae*, and *Mycobacterium tuberculosis* [84,85]. Tannins have also been shown to inhibit the growth of several Gram-positive and Gram-negative bacteria and are known to have the ability to disrupt biofilms [86].

The antimicrobial activity of *A. angustissima* has been studied. Ethanolic extracts of this plant have shown a complete inhibition of growth on *Bacillus subtilis*, *Klebsiella pneumoniae*, and *Staphylococcus aureus* [87]. Methanolic extracts of pods have displayed antifungal activity against *Fusarium oxysporum, Rhizoctonia solani,* and *Phytophtora capsica,* as well as against the human pathogen *Candida albicans* [21]. In addition, methanolic extracts of pods have also demonstrated antifungal activity against *Sclerotium cepivorum* Berk in garlic cultivation [88]. Currently, there are many pharmacological treatment options for diabetic patients, but the associated side effects, such as gastrointestinal symptoms, heart failure, weight gain, edema, impaired renal function, pancreatitis, genital infections, etc., become an additional burden for patients [89]. Treatments with fewer side effects are needed, and plant extracts could be an effective therapeutic intervention.

The literature regarding the antimicrobial activity of *Acaciella angustissima*, or Acaciella as a genus, is limited, which makes interpreting results challenging. Nevertheless, several studies have been conducted concerning the Fabaceae family and reported the resulting minimal inhibitory concentration (MIC) and the different thresholds considered to classify the results. The MIC ranges considered to classify the antimicrobial activity of Fabaceae can vary vastly; in a study by Bussmann et al. [90] strong antimicrobial activity was defined as an MIC of less than 5 mg/mL, while other authors like Nielsen et al. [91], Dalmarco et al. [92], Tamokou et al. [93], and Wamba et al. [94] considered significant, excellent, or highly active when MIC < 0.1 mg/mL.

The difference in the thresholds used to classify the antimicrobial activity could be explained when looking at the MIC values obtained from plants from the Fabaceae family, as these also vary greatly. In the study by Bussmann et al. [90] it was shown that against *S. aureus*, *Caesalpinia paipai* and *Cassia fistula* showed an MIC value of 1 mg/mL; *Senna monilifera* and *Spartium junceum* of 4 mg/mL; *Caesalpinia spinosa* of 16 mg/mL; and *Senna bicapsularis* of 256 mg/mL. On the other hand, the MIC values for *E. coli* were 0.016 mg/mL for *Senna bicapsularis*, and 64 mg/mL for *Caesalpinia spinosa* and *Medicago sativa*. The MIC attained stand out for their high values, which might explain why strong antimicrobial activity was considered when MIC < 5 mg/mL.

Nielsen et al. [91] evaluated the antibacterial activities of the leaves and stems of *A. karroo*, obtaining an MIC value of 0.15625 mg/mL against βL+EC (β-lactamase-positive *Escherichia coli*) and CRPA (Carbenicillin-resistant *Pseudomonas aeruginosa*) for both leaf and stem extracts. In addition, the MIC values against MRSA (Methicillin-resistant *Staphylococcus aureus*) and ARKP (Ampicillin-resistant *Klebsiella pneumoniae*) were 0.15625 mg/mL and 0.07812 mg/mL in the case of leaves and stem, respectively. The activity was considered to be significant if the MIC values were below 0.100 mg/mL and moderate when 0.100 < MIC < 0.625 mg/mL.

The antimicrobial activity and MIC values of seeds and leaves of *Albizia masikororum* (Fabaceae) were analyzed in a study by Razafindrakoto et al. [95]. The MIC value against *S. aureus* was determined to be 0.19531 mg/mL and 0.78125 mg/mL for seeds and leaves, respectively. The MIC interpretation standards followed those established by Dalmarco et al. [92], where an MIC below 0.1 mg/mL was regarded as excellent, between 0.1 mg/mL and 0.5 mg/mL as moderate, between 0.5 mg/mL and 1 mg/mL as weak, and above 1 mg/mL as inactive.

A study by Mahamat Djamalladine et al. [96] analyzed the antimicrobial activity of the aerial parts of *Abrus canescens* (Fabaceae), which demonstrated notable antibacterial effects against *P. aeruginosa, E. coli, E. faecalis,* and *S. aureus,* with MIC values between 0.256 and 0.512 mg/mL. Another study by Álvarez-Martínez et al. [97] reviewed the antimicrobial activity of compounds derived from plants and their mechanisms of action in which some Fabaceae plants were assessed. The flowers of *Bauhinia kockiana* presented an MIC of 0.0625 mg/mL against Methicillin-resistant *S. aureus* (MRSA), and the leaves of *Phaseolus vulgaris* against *E. coli* had an MIC of 0.256 mg/mL. In both articles, the threshold values proposed by Tamokou et al. [93] were considered: highly active (MIC below 0.100 mg/mL), significantly active (0.100 ≤ MIC ≤ 0.512 mg/mL), moderately active (0.512 < MIC ≤ 2.048 mg/mL), low activity (MIC > 2.048 mg/mL), and not active (MIC > 10 mg/mL).

An experiment conducted by Mpude et al. [98] showed that the leaves of *Acacia sieberiana* were most active against Methicillin-susceptible *Staphylococcus aureus* (MSSA) A1 with an MIC of 0.032 mg/mL and against Methicillin-resistant *Staphylococcus aureus* (MRSA) A4 with an MIC of 0.128 mg/mL. The thresholds considered were significant activity (MIC < 0.1 mg/mL), moderate (0.1 mg/mL < MIC ≤ 0.625 mg/mL), and low or negligible (MIC > 0.625 mg/mL). Nevertheless, in this study is remarked the updated and rationally defined cutoff points of antibacterial botanicals obtained from Wamba et al. [94]: outstanding activity—minimal inhibitory concentration (MIC) ≤ 0.008 mg/mL; excellent activity—0.008 < MIC ≤ 0.04 mg/mL; very good activity—0.04 < MIC ≤ 0.128 mg/mL; good activity—0.128 < MIC ≤ 0.32 mg/mL; average activity—0.32 < MIC ≤ 0.625 mg/mL; weak activity—0.625 < MIC ≤ 1.024 mg/mL; not active—MIC values > 1.024 mg/mL.

Overall, the similarity between the threshold values for MIC proposed by Tamokou et al. [93] (considered by Mahamat Djamalladine et al. [96] and Álvarez-Martínez et al. [97]) and the ones proposed by Wamba et al. [94] (contemplated by Mpude et al. [98]) and by Dalmarco et al. [92] (considered by Razafindrakoto et al. [95]) creates a more solid and well-founded classification of the results for plants from the Fabaceae family.

Considering those ranges, the most prominent results obtained for *A. angustissima* come from the pods, with a weak or moderate antimicrobial activity against *S. aureus* (MIC 0.625 mg/mL) and *K. pneumoniae* (MIC 0.625 mg/mL). Both bacterial strains are relevant to common diabetes infections: *S. aureus* is recurrent in infections like pneumonia and bronchopneumonia, infections in skin lesions, necrotizing fasciitis, diabetic foot, osteomyelitis, septic arthritis, and bacteremia [15,99]; *K. pneumoniae* has been linked to endophthalmitis, pneumonia, bronchopneumonia, and hepatic and intra-abdominal abscesses in people with diabetes [15]. *K. pneumoniae* is also known to cause urinary tract infections in diabetic patients, which often become more severe due to immunosuppression [100,101].

The inhibition of *E. coli* due to the pods (MIC 1.25 mg/mL), as well as the inhibition caused by the seeds against *S. aureus* (MIC 1.25 mg/mL), can also be classified as moderately active if just the classification by Tamokou et al. [93] is considered. Although the pods did not show the best inhibitory effect of this experiment, it stands out from the rest as its inhibition towards *E. coli* (MIC 1.25 mg/mL) surpassed that of gentamicin (MIC 20 mg/mL). *E. coli* is also a microorganism responsible for common infections in people with diabetes, such as endophthalmitis, bacteremia, sepsis, and urinary tract infections (UTIs) like cystitis, urethritis, and pyelonephritis [15].

The inhibition of the rest of the tested bacteria caused by the seeds and pods was not enough to classify them in an excellent, strong, high, or even a moderate category, receiving a lower classification just like for the flowers, which are classified as inactive, low activity, or negligible as none of the concentrations against any of the tested bacteria reached an MIC value low enough (lowest MIC = 2.5 mg/mL against *S. aureus*). Even though the antimicrobial activity against the rest of the tested bacteria was not as prominent as the ones already described, their potential should not be ignored as other common infections in people with diabetes are caused by *Salmonella* spp. (necrotizing fasciitis [15]), *P. aeruginosa* (malignant otitis externa, bacteremia, sepsis [15], and tissue damage in diabetic foot ulcers [102]), and *L. monocytogenes* (the combination of incomplete Freund's adjuvant (IFA) and *L. monocytogenes* treatment effectively delays type I diabetes in non-obese diabetes (NOD) mice [103]).

4. Materials and Methods

4.1. Collection of Plant Material

In 2022, the flowers and mature pods were collected from *Acaciella angustissima* trees at the Autonomous University of Querétaro, Amazcala Campus, in El Marqués, Querétaro. The flowers were collected in July, and after selection, they were frozen for subsequent freeze-drying. The pods collected in February were left to dry at room temperature for 72 h; then, the seeds were separated from the pods for later handling. The samples were ground and sifted.

4.2. Content of Total Phenols, Flavonoids, and Condensed Tannins

To determine phenolic content, methanolic extracts were prepared following the methodology of Cardador-Martínez et al. [104] with some modifications. A total of 200 mg of the sample was weighed, and 10 mL of methanol was added. The mixture was subjected to sonication for 30 min at room temperature, and then centrifuged at 8000 rpm for 20 min at 4 °C. The supernatant obtained was recovered and stored at −20 °C until further use.

The total content of phenolic compounds was determined by the Folin–Ciocalteu method reported by Oomah et al. [105], one of the most used techniques for quantifying phenolic compounds due to its high sensitivity and reproducibility. For the standard curve, gallic acid was used (points between 0 and 0.032 mg/mL). The methodology proposed by Oomah et al. [68] was also followed to determine the flavonoid content, with a routine standard curve with points ranging from 2 to 200 mg/mL. Regarding the analysis of condensed tannins, the vanillin-HCl method was used according to the procedure described by Deshpande and Cheryan [106], with a Catechin standard curve within a 0 to 1 mg/mL concentration.

4.3. Antioxidant Capacity: DPPH Y ABTS

4.3.1. DPPH

The DPPH (2,2-diphenyl-1-picrylhydrazyl) radical scavenging capacity was evaluated using the methodology described by Brand-Williams et al. [107], with some modifications. A total of 20 µL of the sample (methanolic extract described in Section 4.2) and 200 µL of a methanolic solution (80%) of DPPH (0.06 mg/mL) were added. The mixture was allowed to stand at room temperature for 30 min in the dark. Methanol was used instead of the DPPH solution for the blank, and deionized water was used instead of the sample for the control. The absorbance was measured at 515 nm. The free radical scavenging capacity was calculated using Equation (1).

$$\%\text{Free radical scavenging} = [1 - (A_{\text{sample}} - (A_{blank}/A_{control}))] * 100 \quad (1)$$

Several points with concentrations ranging from 0 to 0.250 mg/mL of Trolox were used for the standard curve.

4.3.2. ABTS

The ABTS (2,2′-azinobis-(3-ethylbenzothiazoline-6-sulfonic acid)) radical scavenging capacity was determined following the methodology described by Re et al. [108] with some modifications. A solution of ABTS radical (3.84 g/mL) was prepared with potassium persulfate (2.45 mmol/L), and it was left in the dark at room temperature for 12 h. A total of 20 µL of the sample (methanolic extract described in Section 4.2) and 230 µL of ABTS solution were added. For the blank, 20 µL of methanol plus 230 µL of ethanol were used, and for the control, only methanol was used. The absorbance was measured at 734 nm. The free radical scavenging capacity was calculated using Equation (2).

$$\%\text{Free radical scavenging} = [1 - (\text{A}_{\text{sample}}/A_{control})] * 100 \quad (2)$$

The standard curve was constructed using different points ranging from 0 to 0.250 mg/ml Trolox concentrations.

4.4. Analysis by Gas Chromatography–Mass Spectrometry (GC-MS)

4.4.1. Fatty Acid Profile

To determine fatty acids, 50 mg of the sample (ground and sieved) was weighed and 400 µL of NaOH (1.5 M, prepared in methanol) was added, following the methodology of Gómez-Velázquez et al. [109]. The mixture was vortexed for 1 min and then sonicated at 40 kHz for 5 min. Then, 400 µL of H_2SO_4 (1.75 M, prepared in methanol) was added, vortexed again for 1 min, and sonicated for 5 more minutes. A total of 800 µL of hexane was added to each sample, vortexed for 30 s, and centrifuged at 10,000× *g* for 5 min to recover the supernatant. This was filtered and injected into the gas chromatograph.

4.4.2. Metabolic Profile

The metabolic profile of the *A. angustissima* flowers, seeds, and pods was determined using 50 mg samples (ground and sieved), following the methodology of Rico-Chávez et al. [110]. Each sample was added with 1 mL of methanol, sonicated for 15 min, and then vortexed for 30 s. They were kept under constant agitation at 200 rpm in an orbital shaker for 3 h. The samples were centrifuged at 12,000 RCF for 10 min at 4 °C. A 250 µL aliquot was taken from the supernatant and dried in a SpeedVac at room temperature. For the derivatization of the samples, 100 µL of derivatizing agent (BSTFA + 1% TMS) was added, sonicated for 3 min, and centrifuged at 10,000× *g* for 5 min to recover the supernatant, which was then filtered to be injected into the gas chromatograph.

4.5. Evaluation of Enzymatic Activity

4.5.1. Extract Preparation

The flower, pod, and seed extracts of *A. angustissima* were prepared using different solvents. For the α-amylase and α-glucosidase assays, distilled water was used at concentrations of 50 mg/mL and 20 mg/mL, respectively [79]. Methanol was used as the solvent at 1 mg/mL per extract for the ACE-I assay [111]. The samples were mixed and stirred at 160 rpm for 24 h in the dark at room temperature [112]. The homogenates were then centrifuged at 10,000 rpm at 4 °C for 20 min, and the supernatant obtained was used as the extract [113].

4.5.2. α-amylase Inhibition Assay

A modified version of the assay described in the Worthington Enzyme Manual was used to evaluate the α-amylase inhibitory activity [79,114,115]. A 0.02 M sodium phosphate buffer (pH 6.9 with 0.006 M NaCl) was prepared to suspend the α-amylase solution (0.5 mg/mL) and a 1% starch solution. In total, 500 µL of each extract and the α-amylase solution were mixed and incubated at 25 °C for 10 min. Then, 500 µL of the 1% starch solution was added and incubated at 25 °C for another 10 min. The reaction was stopped by adding 1.0 mL of DNS dye reagent, and the tubes were boiled for 5 min, cooled, and diluted with 15 mL of distilled water. The absorbance was measured at 540 nm, and the blank and control values were recorded. The percentage inhibition was calculated using Equation (3) [113].

$$\%\text{Inhibition} = [(A_{control} - A_{sample})/(A_{control})] * 100 \quad (3)$$

4.5.3. α-glucosidase Inhibition Assay

For α-glucosidase inhibitory activity, a modified version of the assay described in the Worthington Enzyme Manual [79,115,116] was used. A total of 50 µL of the sample extract, diluted with 50 μL of 0.1 M potassium phosphate buffer (pH 6.9), and 100 μL of 0.1 M potassium phosphate buffer (pH 6.9) were incubated with α-glucosidase solution (1.0 U/mL) at 25 °C for 10 min. Then, 50 μL of a 5 mM solution of *p*-nitrophenyl-α-D-glucopyranoside in 0.1 M potassium phosphate buffer (pH 6.9) was added and incubated at 25 °C for 5 min. A control with 50 μL buffer solution was included instead of the extract (A405 control). Absorbance readings were taken at 405 nm, and the percentage inhibition was calculated using Equation (3) [113].

4.5.4. ACE-I Assay

The inhibition of angiotensin I-converting enzyme (ACE-I) activity was evaluated using the method established by Hou and collaborators [117], with modification [111]. All the tests were performed in triplicate. A Tris-HCl solution (50 mM, NaCl 0.3 M, pH = 7.5) was prepared as a solvent for an N-[3(2-furyl)acryloyl]-phe-gly-gly solution. First, 200 μL of this solution was mixed with 250 μL of the extract and 30 μL of Tris-HCl buffer. The enzymatic reaction was started by adding 20 μL of the ACE-I solution derived from rabbit lungs (1 U/mL) and later monitored for 5 min at 345 nm using a UV-Vis spectrophotometer. A blank containing no substrate was used as a control, while Lisinopril (2 mg/mL) was the positive inhibition control. For inhibition calculations, the enzyme activity without extract was considered to be 100%.

4.6. Assessment Antimicrobial Activity

4.6.1. Extract Preparation

Methanol was used as a solvent to extract bioactive compounds from Timbe flowers, pods, and seeds. A total of 5 g of each Timbe structure was weighed and mixed separately with 500 mL of methanol. The mixtures were shaken in an orbital shaker at 160 rpm for 24 h at room temperature in the dark. After extraction, the methanol was evaporated using a rotary evaporator [118]. The resulting powder was dissolved in Mueller–Hinton Broth to obtain a 20 mg/mL concentration.

4.6.2. Microorganisms and Growing Conditions

Six types of microorganisms were obtained from the collection of the Molecular Microbiology Laboratory from the Basic and Applied Microbiology Unit, Natural Sciences Faculty of the Autonomous University of Queretaro for the evaluation of the antibacterial activities of the Timbe flower, pod, and seed extracts. *Listeria monocytogenes* ATCC 19115, *Staphylococcus aureus* ATCC 25923, *Escherichia coli* ATCC 25922, *Pseudomonas aeruginosa* ATCC27853, *Salmonella typhimurium* ATCC 14028, and *Klebsiella pneumoniae* ATCC 13883 were standardized to a concentration of 10^8 CFU/mL for the antibacterial susceptibility test.

4.6.3. Broth Microdilution Method

To evaluate the antimicrobial activity, a microdilution assay was performed to determine the minimum inhibitory concentrations (MICs) following the Clinical and Laboratory Standards Institute (CLSI) guidelines [119].

Serial dilutions of gentamicin (80 mg/2 mL) and the extracts at different concentrations (20, 10, 5, 2.5, 1.25, 0.625, 0.312, 0.156, 0.078, and 0.039 mg/mL) prepared in Mueller–Hinton Broth (MHB) and 50 μL of each dilution was transferred into a 96-well microtiter plate. The inoculants were standardized to 10^8 CFU/mL and diluted to 10^6 CFU/mL. A total of 50 μL of the diluted bacterial suspension was added to each well, resulting in a final concentration of 5 × 10^5 CFU/mL [120]. Positive controls (inoculants) and sterility controls (culture media) were considered [121]. The microplates were then incubated at 37 °C, and the wells were examined for turbidity 24 h later by optical density readings at 600 nm and by the direct observation of turbidity. At least three repetitions were run for each assay [122]. The lowest concentration of each extract that inhibited each bacteria's growth was considered the MIC.

4.7. Statistical Analysis

All the tests were performed in triplicate, and the results were analyzed using a one-way ANOVA analysis followed by Tukey's test. Significant differences between treatments were considered when the p-value < 0.05. All the statistical analyses were performed using the JMP Pro-16.2.0 software. To explore possible correlations between variables (total phenols, flavonoids, condensed tannins, ABTS, DPPH, ACE-I, α-amylase, and α-glucosidase), Python 3.13.2 was used together with the Pingouin library 0.5.5. This tool allowed for calculating pairwise correlations between variables using the Pearson method.

5. Conclusions and Perspectives

Acaciella angustissima is a promising alternative in biotechnology and health due to its bioactive properties. The flowers, pods, and seeds exhibit distinct phenolic compound content, correlating to their antioxidant, antidiabetic, and antihypertensive potential. The pods stood out for their high phenolic compound content, tannin content, and antioxidant capacity in the DPPH assay. At the same time, the flowers, the main source of flavonoids, showed the highest antioxidant activity in ABTS. In contrast, the seeds showed the lowest values in all the analyses, indicating a lower antioxidant potential. These results underline the therapeutic value of the plant, particularly in the regulation of blood glucose levels through the inhibition of alpha-amylase (with the pods being the most effective) and alpha-glucosidase (with the flowers and seeds being the most effective), in addition to its antihypertensive action through ACE-I inhibition (with the flowers having the greatest inhibition). These effects make *Acaciella angustissima* an attractive option for developing natural therapeutic products. Regarding antimicrobial activity, the pods showed the greatest inhibitory effect on bacteria, such as *Escherichia coli*, *Klebsiella pneumoniae*, and *Staphylococcus aureus*, suggesting their potential as natural agents for controlling bacterial infections. These results open the door for future research to explore their application in developing new antimicrobial treatments.

However, despite the promising results, further research is needed to explore the full therapeutic potential of the plant. Future studies should focus on understanding the specific mechanisms by which the bioactive compounds exert their effects, assessing the bioavailability and safety of the active constituents, and conducting clinical trials to confirm their efficacy in humans. In addition, research into the synergistic effects of their compounds could lead to more effective formulations for treating diseases such as diabetes and hypertension. A key area of future research will be to evaluate how these compounds affect the body's homeostasis, particularly in the regulation of insulin secretion, which could offer new approaches to the treatment of metabolic disorders. Exploring sustainable extraction methods and expanding their applications in pharmaceuticals and nutraceuticals could also enhance their commercial potential and consolidate them as a valuable resource in natural medicine.

Supplementary Materials: The following supporting information can be downloaded at: https://www.mdpi.com/article/10.3390/ph18040593/s1, Table S1. Person correlation for total phenols, flavonoids, tannins, DPPH, ABTS, α-amylase, α-glucosidase, and ACE-I (p-value < 0.05).

Author Contributions: Conceptualization, D.K.R.-S., L.G.-B., C.L.-S., A.K.R.-C. and A.A.F.-P.; original draft preparation, D.K.R.-S. and L.G.-B.; methodology, D.K.R.-S., L.G.-B. and A.K.R.-C.; investigation, D.K.R.-S., L.G.-B., C.L.-S., A.K.R.-C. and A.A.F.-P.; writing, D.K.R.-S. and L.G.-B.; supervision, C.L.-S. and A.A.F.-P.; editor, D.K.R.-S., L.G.-B., C.L.-S., A.K.R.-C., J.A.C.-C., L.A.R.-C., A.M.-M. and A.A.F.-P. All authors have read and agreed to the published version of the manuscript.

Funding: This work was supported by the CONAHCyT grant (Ciencia de Fronteras G-1176) and the UAQ grant (CA141UAQ).

Institutional Review Board Statement: Not applicable.

Informed Consent Statement: Not applicable.

Data Availability Statement: The original contributions presented in this study are included in the article/Supplementary Material. Further inquiries can be directed to the corresponding author.

Acknowledgments: The authors want to thank CONAHCyT for the PhD scholarship to the student L.G.-B. We would also like to thank L.G.-B. for creating the graphical abstract with BioRender.com, access: 20 February 2025.

Conflicts of Interest: The authors declare no conflicts of interest.

References

1. WHO. Traditional, Complementary and Integrative Medicine. Available online: https://www.who.int/ (accessed on 17 January 2025).
2. Madariaga-Mazón, A.; Naveja, J.J.; Medina-Franco, J.L.; Noriega-Colima, K.O.; Martinez-Mayorga, K. DiaNat-DB: A Molecular Database of Antidiabetic Compounds from Medicinal Plants. *RSC Adv.* **2021**, *11*, 5172–5178. [CrossRef] [PubMed]
3. Sun, W.; Shahrajabian, M.H. Therapeutic Potential of Phenolic Compounds in Medicinal Plants—Natural Health Products for Human Health. *Molecules* **2023**, *28*, 1845. [CrossRef] [PubMed]
4. Alqahtani, A.S.; Ullah, R.; Shahat, A.A. Bioactive Constituents and Toxicological Evaluation of Selected Antidiabetic Medicinal Plants of Saudi Arabia. *eCAM* **2022**, *2022*, 7123521. [CrossRef]
5. Ali, A.M.; Gabbar, M.A.; Abdel-Twab, S.M.; Fahmy, E.M.; Ebaid, H.; Alhazza, I.M.; Ahmed, O.M. Antidiabetic Potency, Antioxidant Effects, and Mode of Actions of *Citrus reticulata* Fruit Peel Hydroethanolic Extract, Hesperidin, and Quercetin in Nicotinamide/Streptozotocin-Induced Wistar Diabetic Rats. *Oxid. Med. Cell. Longev.* **2020**, *2020*, 1730492. [CrossRef] [PubMed]
6. Mohamed, N.A.; Hussein, M.M.; Ahmed, O.M.; Al-Jameel, S.S.; Al-Muzafar, H.M.; Amin, K.A.; Abdou, H.M. Oleuropein Ameliorates Hyperlipidemia, Oxidative Stress, Inflammatory and Liver Dysfunction Biomarkers, in Streptozotocin-Induced Diabetic Rats. *J. Appl. Pharm. Sci.* **2024**, *14*, 227–234. [CrossRef]
7. Ahmed, O.M.; Abd El-Twab, S.M.; Al-Muzafar, H.M.; Adel Amin, K.; Abdel Aziz, S.M.; Abdel-Gabbar, M. *Musa paradisiaca* L. Leaf and Fruit Peel Hydroethanolic Extracts Improved the Lipid Profile, Glycemic Index and Oxidative Stress in Nicotinamide/Streptozotocin-Induced Diabetic Rats. *Vet. Med. Sci.* **2021**, *7*, 500–511. [CrossRef]
8. Przeor, M. Some Common Medicinal Plants with Antidiabetic Activity, Known and Available in Europe (A Mini-Review). *Pharmaceuticals* **2022**, *15*, 65. [CrossRef]
9. Zeb, A. Concept, Mechanism, and Applications of Phenolic Antioxidants in Foods. *J. Food Biochem.* **2020**, *44*, e13394. [CrossRef]
10. Zhang, Y.; Cai, P.; Cheng, G.; Zhang, Y. A Brief Review of Phenolic Compounds Identified from Plants: Their Extraction, Analysis, and Biological Activity. *Nat. Prod. Commun.* **2022**, *17*, 1934578X211069721. [CrossRef]
11. Rahman, M.M.; Rahaman, M.S.; Islam, M.R.; Rahman, F.; Mithi, F.M.; Alqahtani, T.; Almikhlafi, M.A.; Alghamdi, S.Q.; Alruwaili, A.S.; Hossain, M.S.; et al. Role of Phenolic Compounds in Human Disease: Current Knowledge and Future Prospects. *Molecules* **2021**, *27*, 233. [CrossRef]
12. Lv, Q.; Long, J.; Gong, Z.; Nong, K.; Liang, X.; Qin, T.; Huang, W.; Yang, L. Current State of Knowledge on the Antioxidant Effects and Mechanisms of Action of Polyphenolic Compounds. *Nat. Prod. Commun.* **2021**, *16*, 1934578X211027745. [CrossRef]
13. Zhang, X.; Wang, J.; Zhang, T.; Li, S.; Liu, J.; Li, M.; Lu, J.; Zhang, M.; Chen, H. Updated Progress on Polysaccharides with Anti-Diabetic Effects through the Regulation of Gut Microbiota: Sources, Mechanisms, and Structure–Activity Relationships. *Pharmaceuticals* **2024**, *17*, 456. [CrossRef]
14. Holt, R.I.G.; Cockram, C.S.; Ma, R.C.W.; Luk, A.O.Y. Diabetes and Infection: Review of the Epidemiology, Mechanisms and Principles of Treatment. *Diabetologia* **2024**, *67*, 1168–1180. [CrossRef] [PubMed]
15. Toniolo, A.; Cassani, G.; Puggioni, A.; Rossi, A.; Colombo, A.; Onodera, T.; Ferrannini, E. The Diabetes Pandemic and Associated Infections: Suggestions for Clinical Microbiology. *Rev. Res. Med. Microbiol.* **2019**, *30*, 1–17. [CrossRef]
16. Iatcu, C.O.; Steen, A.; Covasa, M. Gut Microbiota and Complications of Type-2 Diabetes. *Nutrients* **2022**, *14*, 166. [CrossRef]

17. Singhal, P.; Kaushik, G.; Mathur, P. Antidiabetic Potential of Commonly Consumed Legumes: A Review. *Crit. Rev. Food Sci. Nutr.* **2014**, *54*, 655–672. [CrossRef]
18. Musara, C.; Bosede Aladejana, E. *Acaciella angustissima* (Mill.) Brit. & Rose: Botanical Features, Distribution, Medicinal and Pharmacological Properties. *J. Pharm. Nutr. Sci.* **2020**, *10*, 325–330. [CrossRef]
19. Alonso-Herrada, J.; Rico-Reséndiz, F.; Campos-Guillén, J.; Guevara-González, R.G.; Torres-Pacheco, I.; Cruz-Hernández, A. Establishment of in Vitro Regeneration System for *Acaciella angustissima* (Timbe) a Shrubby Plant Endemic of México for the Production of Phenolic Compounds. *Ind. Crops Prod.* **2016**, *86*, 49–57. [CrossRef]
20. Rico Arce, M.d.L.; Bachman, S. A Taxonomic Revision of Acaciella (Leguminosae, Mimosoideae). *An. Jardín Botánico Madrid* **2006**, *63*, 189–244. [CrossRef]
21. Vargas-Hernández, M.; Munguía-Fragozo, P.V.; Cruz-Hernández, A.; Guerrero, B.Z.; Gonzalez-Chavira, M.M.; Feregrino-Pérez, A.A.; Mendoza-Díaz, S.O.; Loarca-Piña, G.; Torres-Pacheco, I.; Hernández-Salazar, M.; et al. Bioactivity and Gene Expression Studies of an Arbustive Mexican Specie *Acaciella angustissima* (Timbe). *Ind. Crops Prod.* **2014**, *52*, 649–655. [CrossRef]
22. Rodríguez-Méndez, A.J.; Carmen-Sandoval, W.; Lomas-Soria, C.; Guevara-González, R.G.; Reynoso-Camacho, R.; Villagran-Herrera, M.E.; Salazar-Olivo, L.; Torres-Pacheco, I.; Feregrino-Pérez, A.A. Timbe (*Acaciella angustissima*) Pods Extracts Reduce the Levels of Glucose, Insulin and Improved Physiological Parameters, Hypolipidemic Effect, Oxidative Stress and Renal Damage in Streptozotocin-Induced Diabetic Rats. *Molecules* **2018**, *23*, 2812. [CrossRef] [PubMed]
23. Odenyo, A.A.; Osuji, P.O.; Reed, J.D.; Smith, A.H.; Mackie, R.I.; Mcsweeney, C.S.; Hanson, J. *Acacia angustissima*: Its Anti-Nutrients Constituents, Toxicity and Possible Mechanisms to Alleviate the Toxicity-a Short Review. *Agrofor. Syst.* **2003**, *5*, 141–147. [CrossRef]
24. Gomha, S.M.; Abolibda, T.Z.; Alruwaili, A.H.; Farag, B.; Boraie, W.E.; Al-Hussain, S.A.; Zaki, M.E.A.; Hussein, A.M. Efficient Green Synthesis of Hydrazide Derivatives Using L-Proline: Structural Characterization, Anticancer Activity, and Molecular Docking Studies. *Catalysts* **2024**, *14*, 489. [CrossRef]
25. Vettore, L.A.; Westbrook, R.L.; Tennant, D.A. Proline Metabolism and Redox; Maintaining a Balance in Health and Disease. *Amino Acids* **2021**, *53*, 1779–1788. [CrossRef] [PubMed]
26. Lange, K.W.; Lange, K.M.; Nakamura, Y.; Reissmann, A. Nutrition in the Management of ADHD: A Review of Recent Research. *Curr. Nutr. Rep.* **2023**, *12*, 383–394. [CrossRef]
27. Poongothai, G.; Sripathi, S.K. A Review on Insulinomimetic Pinitol from Plants. *Int. J. Pharm. Bio. Sci.* **2013**, *4*, 992–1009.
28. Azab, A. D-Pinitol—Active Natural Product from Carob with Notable Insulin Regulation. *Nutrients* **2022**, *14*, 1453. [CrossRef]
29. Pandi, A.; Kalappan, V.M.; Chandrashekar, N. Effects of D-Pinitol on Diabetes Mellitus: An Updated Review. *Bull. Natl. Res. Cent.* **2022**, *46*, 130. [CrossRef]
30. Zhang, X.; Wang, J.; Zhu, L.; Wang, X.; Meng, F.; Xia, L.; Zhang, H. Advances in Stigmasterol on Its Anti-Tumor Effect and Mechanism of Action. *Front. Oncol.* **2022**, *12*, 1101289. [CrossRef]
31. Bakrim, S.; Benkhaira, N.; Bourais, I.; Benali, T.; Lee, L.H.; El Omari, N.; Sheikh, R.A.; Goh, K.W.; Ming, L.C.; Bouyahya, A. Health Benefits and Pharmacological Properties of Stigmasterol. *Antioxidants* **2022**, *11*, 1912. [CrossRef]
32. Valitova, J.; Renkova, A.; Beckett, R.; Minibayeva, F. Stigmasterol: An Enigmatic Plant Stress Sterol with Versatile Functions. *Int. J. Mol. Sci.* **2024**, *25*, 8122. [CrossRef] [PubMed]
33. Ngenge Tamfu, A.; Mfifen Munvera, A.; Veronica Dediu Botezatu, A.; Talla, E.; Ceylan, O.; Tagatsing Fotsing, M.; Tanyi Mbafor, J.; Shaheen, F.; Mihaela Dinica, R. Synthesis of Benzoyl Esters of β-Amyrin and Lupeol and Evaluation of Their Antibiofilm and Antidiabetic Activities. *Results Chem.* **2022**, *4*, 100322. [CrossRef]
34. Viet, T.D.; Xuan, T.D.; Anh, L.H. α-Amyrin and β-Amyrin Isolated from *Celastrus hindsii* Leaves and Their Antioxidant, Anti-Xanthine Oxidase, and Anti-Tyrosinase Potentials. *Molecules* **2021**, *26*, 7248. [CrossRef]
35. Li, H.; Fu, S.; Wang, Y.; Yuan, X.; Liu, L.; Dong, H.; Wang, Q.; Zhang, Z. Antimicrobial and Antitumor Activity of Peptidomimetics Synthesized from Amino Acids. *Bioorg. Chem.* **2021**, *106*, 104506. [CrossRef] [PubMed]
36. Umumararungu, T.; Gahamanyi, N.; Mukiza, J.; Habarurema, G.; Katandula, J.; Rugamba, A.; Kagisha, V. Proline, a Unique Amino Acid Whose Polymer, Polyproline II Helix, and Its Analogues Are Involved in Many Biological Processes: A Review. *Amino Acids* **2024**, *56*, 50. [CrossRef] [PubMed]
37. Hope, H.C.; Salmond, R.J. The Role of Non-Essential Amino Acids in T Cell Function and Anti-Tumour Immunity. *Arch. Immunol. Ther. Exp.* **2021**, *69*, 29. [CrossRef]
38. Rolnik, A.; Olas, B.; Szablińska-Piernik, J.; Lahuta, L.B.; Gromadziński, L.; Majewski, M.S. Antioxidant and Anticoagulant Properties of Myo-Inositol Determined in an Ex Vivo Studies and Gas Chromatography Analysis. *Sci. Rep.* **2024**, *14*, 25633. [CrossRef]
39. Abbas, A.H.; Mahmood, A.A.R.; Tahtamouni, L.H.; Al-Mazaydeh, Z.A.; Rammaha, M.S.; Alsoubani, F.; Al-Bayati, R.I. A Novel Derivative of Picolinic Acid Induces Endoplasmic Reticulum Stress-Mediated Apoptosis in Human Non-Small Cell Lung Cancer Cells: Synthesis, Docking Study, and Anticancer Activity. *Pharmacia* **2021**, *68*, 679–692. [CrossRef]

40. Borawska, M.H.; Czechowska, S.K.; Markiewicz, R.; Pałka, J.; Świsłocka, R.; Lewandowski, W. Antimicrobial Activity and Cytotoxicity of Picolinic Acid and Selected Picolinates as New Potential Food Preservatives. *Pol. J. Food Nutr. Sci.* **2008**, *58*, 415–418.
41. Kim, S.; Jang, S.H.; Kim, M.J.; Lee, J.J.; Kim, K.M.; Kim, Y.H.; Lee, J.H.; Jung, S.K. Hybrid Nutraceutical of 2-Ketoglutaric Acid in Improving Inflammatory Bowel Disease: Role of Prebiotics and TAK1 Inhibitor. *Biomed. Pharmacother.* **2024**, *171*, 116126. [CrossRef]
42. Divekar, P.A.; Narayana, S.; Divekar, B.A.; Kumar, R.; Gadratagi, B.G.; Ray, A.; Singh, A.K.; Rani, V.; Singh, V.; Singh, A.K.; et al. Plant Secondary Metabolites as Defense Tools against Herbivores for Sustainable Crop Protection. *Int. J. Mol. Sci.* **2022**, *23*, 2690. [CrossRef]
43. Li, Y.; Kong, D.; Fu, Y.; Sussman, M.R.; Wu, H. The Effect of Developmental and Environmental Factors on Secondary Metabolites in Medicinal Plants. *Plant Physiol. Biochem.* **2020**, *148*, 80–89. [CrossRef]
44. Twaij, B.M.; Hasan, M.N. Bioactive Secondary Metabolites from Plant Sources: Types, Synthesis, and Their Therapeutic Uses. *Int. J. Plant Bioly.* **2022**, *13*, 4–14. [CrossRef]
45. Stavenga, D.G.; Leertouwer, H.L.; Dudek, B.; van der Kooi, C.J. Coloration of Flowers by Flavonoids and Consequences of PH Dependent Absorption. *Front. Plant Sci.* **2021**, *11*, 600124. [CrossRef]
46. Elshafie, H.S.; Camele, I.; Mohamed, A.A. A Comprehensive Review on the Biological, Agricultural and Pharmaceutical Properties of Secondary Metabolites Based-Plant Origin. *Int. J. Mol. Sci.* **2023**, *24*, 3266. [CrossRef] [PubMed]
47. Garcés-Rimón, M.; Morales, D.; Miguel-Castro, M. Potential Role of Bioactive Proteins and Peptides Derived from Legumes towards Metabolic Syndrome. *Nutrients* **2022**, *14*, 5271. [CrossRef] [PubMed]
48. Bešlo, D.; Golubić, N.; Rastija, V.; Agić, D.; Karnaš, M.; Šubarić, D.; Lučić, B. Antioxidant Activity, Metabolism, and Bioavailability of Polyphenols in the Diet of Animals. *Antioxidants* **2023**, *12*, 1141. [CrossRef]
49. Sadowska-Bartosz, I.; Bartosz, G. Evaluation of The Antioxidant Capacity of Food Products: Methods, Applications and Limitations. *Processes* **2022**, *10*, 2031. [CrossRef]
50. Rumpf, J.; Burger, R.; Schulze, M. Statistical Evaluation of DPPH, ABTS, FRAP, and Folin-Ciocalteu Assays to Assess the Antioxidant Capacity of Lignins. *Int. J. Biol. Macromol.* **2023**, *233*, 123470. [CrossRef]
51. Gaber, N.B.; El-Dahy, S.I.; Shalaby, E.A. Comparison of ABTS, DPPH, Permanganate, and Methylene Blue Assays for Determining Antioxidant Potential of Successive Extracts from Pomegranate and Guava Residues. *Biomass. Convers. Biorefin.* **2023**, *13*, 4011–4020. [CrossRef]
52. Wołosiak, R.; Drużyńska, B.; Derewiaka, D.; Piecyk, M.; Majewska, E.; Ciecierska, M.; Worobiej, E.; Pakosz, P. Verification of the Conditions for Determination of Antioxidant Activity by Abts and Dpph Assays—A Practical Approach. *Molecules* **2022**, *27*, 50. [CrossRef] [PubMed]
53. Tan, Y.; Chang, S.K.C.; Zhang, Y. Comparison of α-Amylase, α-Glucosidase and Lipase Inhibitory Activity of the Phenolic Substances in Two Black Legumes of Different Genera. *Food Chem.* **2017**, *214*, 259–268. [CrossRef]
54. Park, S.; Park, S.-Y. Can Antioxidants Be Effective Therapeutics for Type 2 Diabetes? *Yeungnam Univ. J. Med.* **2021**, *38*, 83–94. [CrossRef]
55. Leh, H.E.; Lee, L.K. Lycopene: A Potent Antioxidant for the Amelioration of Type II Diabetes Mellitus. *Molecules* **2022**, *27*, 2335. [CrossRef]
56. Sekowski, S.; Veiko, A.; Olchowik-Grabarek, E.; Dubis, A.; Wilczewska, A.Z.; Markiewicz, K.H.; Zavodnik, I.B.; Lapshina, E.; Dobrzynska, I.; Abdulladjanova, N.; et al. Hydrolysable Tannins Change Physicochemical Parameters of Lipid Nano-Vesicles and Reduce DPPH Radical—Experimental Studies and Quantum Chemical Analysis. *Biochim. Biophys. Acta Biomembr.* **2022**, *1864*, 183778. [CrossRef] [PubMed]
57. Barreca, D.; Bellocco, E.; Leuzzi, U.; Gattuso, G. First Evidence of C- and O-Glycosyl Flavone in Blood Orange (*Citrus sinensis* (L.) Osbeck) Juice and Their Influence on Antioxidant Properties. *Food Chem.* **2014**, *149*, 244–252. [CrossRef]
58. Papoutsis, K.; Pristijono, P.; Golding, J.B.; Stathopoulos, C.E.; Bowyer, M.C.; Scarlett, C.J.; Vuong, Q.V. Optimisation of Aqueous Extraction Conditions for the Recovery of Phenolic Compounds and Antioxidants from Lemon Pomace. *Int. J. Food Sci. Technol.* **2016**, *51*, 2009–2018. [CrossRef]
59. Wang, Y.; Yang, P.; Yan, Z.; Liu, Z.; Ma, Q.; Zhang, Z.; Wang, Y.; Su, Y. The Relationship between Erythrocytes and Diabetes Mellitus. *J. Diabetes Res.* **2021**, *2021*, 6656062. [CrossRef]
60. Wang, W.; Wang, X.; Cao, S.; Duan, Y.; Xu, C.; Gan, D.; He, W. Dietary Antioxidant Indices in Relation to All-Cause and Cause-Specific Mortality Among Adults with Diabetes: A Prospective Cohort Study. *Front. Nutr.* **2022**, *9*, 849727. [CrossRef]
61. Da Porto, A.; Cavarape, A.; Colussi, G.; Casarsa, V.; Catena, C.; Sechi, L.A. Polyphenols Rich Diets and Risk of Type 2 Diabetes. *Nutrients* **2021**, *13*, 1445. [CrossRef]
62. Naz, R.; Saqib, F.; Awadallah, S.; Wahid, M.; Latif, M.F.; Iqbal, I.; Mubarak, M.S. Food Polyphenols and Type II Diabetes Mellitus: Pharmacology and Mechanisms. *Molecules* **2023**, *28*, 3996. [CrossRef] [PubMed]

63. Fernandes, I.; Oliveira, J.; Pinho, A.; Carvalho, E. The Role of Nutraceutical Containing Polyphenols in Diabetes Prevention. *Metabolites* **2022**, *12*, 184. [CrossRef]
64. Aryaeian, N.; Sedehi, S.K.; Arablou, T. Polyphenols and Their Effects on Diabetes Management: A Review. *Med. J. Islam. Repub. Iran* **2017**, *31*, 886–892. [CrossRef]
65. Wang, Y.; Alkhalidy, H.; Liu, D. The Emerging Role of Polyphenols in the Management of Type 2 Diabetes. *Molecules* **2021**, *26*, 703. [CrossRef] [PubMed]
66. Amponsah-Offeh, M.; Diaba-Nuhoho, P.; Speier, S.; Morawietz, H. Oxidative Stress, Antioxidants and Hypertension. *Antioxidants* **2023**, *12*, 281. [CrossRef]
67. Gać, P.; Poręba, M.; Januszewska, L.; Prokopowicz, A.; Martynowicz, H.; Mazur, G.; Poręba, R. The Total Antioxidant Status, Serum Selenium Concentrations and the Ultrasound Assessment Carotid Intima Media Thickness in Patients with Arterial Hypertension. *Antioxidants* **2021**, *10*, 63. [CrossRef] [PubMed]
68. Serina, J.J.C.; Castilho, P.C.M.F. Using Polyphenols as a Relevant Therapy to Diabetes and Its Complications, a Review. *Crit. Rev. Food Sci. Nutr.* **2022**, *62*, 8355–8387. [CrossRef]
69. Taghi-Gharibzahedi, S.M.; Mousavi, S.M.; Jafari, M.S.; Faraji, K. Proximate Composition, Mineral Content, and Fatty Acids Profile of Two Varieties of Lentil Seeds Cultivated in Iran. *Chem. Nat. Compd.* **2012**, *47*, 976–978. [CrossRef]
70. Lastras, C.; Revilla, I.; González-Martín, M.I.; Vivar-Quintana, A.M. Prediction of Fatty Acid and Mineral Composition of Lentils Using near Infrared Spectroscopy. *J. Food Compos. Anal.* **2021**, *102*, 104023. [CrossRef]
71. Chandra, S.; Saklani, S.; Mathur, A. Study on Nutritional and Phytochemical Profile of Seven Edible Food Supplements of Uttarakhand (*Garhwal himalaya*). *Vegetos* **2021**, *34*, 678–683. [CrossRef]
72. Lin, Y.; Wu, S. Vegetable Soybean (*Glycine max* (L.) Merr.) Leaf Extracts: Functional Components and Antioxidant and Anti-Inflammatory Activities. *J. Food Sci.* **2021**, *86*, 2468–2480. [CrossRef] [PubMed]
73. Khosravi, A.; Razavi, S.H. Therapeutic Effects of Polyphenols in Fermented Soybean and Black Soybean Products. *J. Funct. Foods* **2021**, *81*, 104467. [CrossRef]
74. Szpunar-Krok, E.; Wondołowska-Grabowska, A.; Bobrecka-Jamro, D.; Jańczak-Pieniążek, M.; Kotecki, A.; Kozak, M. Effect of Nitrogen Fertilisation and Inoculation with Bradyrhizobium Japonicum on the Fatty Acid Profile of Soybean (*Glycine max* (L.) Merrill) Seeds. *Agronomy* **2021**, *11*, 941. [CrossRef]
75. Rodríguez Madrera, R.; Campa Negrillo, A.; Ferreira Fernández, J.J. Fatty Acids in Dry Beans (*Phaseolus vulgaris* L.): A Contribution to Their Analysis and the Characterization of a Diversity Panel. *Foods* **2024**, *13*, 2023. [CrossRef] [PubMed]
76. Kwon, Y.-I.I.; Vattem, D.A.; Shetty, K. Evaluation of Clonal Herbs of Lamiaceae Species for Management of Diabetes and Hypertension. *Asia Pac. J. Clin. Nutr.* **2006**, *15*, 107–118.
77. Sevilla-Asencio, A.; Dublán-García, O.; Gómez-Oliván, L.M.; López-Martínez, L.X. Actividad α-glucosidasa y α-amilasa de extractos acuosos de algunas especias en la mexicana. *Ciencia UAT* **2013**, *8*, 42–47. [CrossRef]
78. Petrie, J.R.; Guzik, T.J.; Touyz, R.M. Diabetes, Hypertension, and Cardiovascular Disease: Clinical Insights and Vascular Mechanisms. *Can. J. Cardiol.* **2018**, *34*, 575–584. [CrossRef]
79. Ranilla, L.G.; Kwon, Y.I.; Apostolidis, E.; Shetty, K. Phenolic Compounds, Antioxidant Activity and in Vitro Inhibitory Potential against Key Enzymes Relevant for Hyperglycemia and Hypertension of Commonly Used Medicinal Plants, Herbs and Spices in Latin America. *Bioresour. Technol.* **2010**, *101*, 4676–4689. [CrossRef]
80. Loarca-Piña, G.; Mendoza, S.; Ramos-Gómez, M.; Reynoso, R. Antioxidant, Antimutagenic, and Antidiabetic Activities of Edible Leaves from *Cnidoscolus chayamansa* Mc. Vaugh. *J. Food Sci.* **2010**, *75*, H68–H72. [CrossRef]
81. Darwitz, B.P.; Genito, C.J.; Thurlow, L.R. Triple Threat: How Diabetes Results in Worsened Bacterial Infections. *Infect. Immun.* **2024**, *92*, e00509-23. [CrossRef]
82. Chandra, H.; Bishnoi, P.; Yadav, A.; Patni, B.; Mishra, A.P.; Nautiyal, A.R. Antimicrobial Resistance and the Alternative Resources with Special Emphasis on Plant-Based Antimicrobials—A Review. *Plants* **2017**, *6*, 457–462. [CrossRef] [PubMed]
83. Feregrino-Pérez, A.A.; Torres-Pacheco, I.; Vargas-Hernández, M.; Munguía-Fragozo, P.V.; Loarca-Piña, G.F.; Mendoza-Díaz, S.O.; Ocampo-Velázquez, R.V.; Rico-García, E.; Guevara-Gónzalez, R.G. Antioxidant and Antimutagenic Activities of Acacia Pennatula Pods. *J. Sci. Ind. Res.* **2011**, *70*, 859–864.
84. Vaou, N.; Stavropoulou, E.; Voidarou, C.; Tsigalou, C.; Bezirtzoglou, E. Towards Advances in Medicinal Plant Antimicrobial Activity: A Review Study on Challenges and Future Perspectives. *Microorganisms* **2021**, *9*, 2041. [CrossRef]
85. Araújo, M.G.D.F.; Hilário, F.; Nogueira, L.G.; Vilegas, W.; Dos Santos, L.C.; Bauab, T.M. Chemical Constituents of the Methanolic Extract of Leaves of Leiothrix Spiralis Ruhland and Their Antimicrobial Activity. *Molecules* **2011**, *16*, 10479–10490. [CrossRef] [PubMed]
86. Villanueva, X.; Zhen, L.; Ares, J.N.; Vackier, T.; Lange, H.; Crestini, C.; Steenackers, H.P. Effect of Chemical Modifications of Tannins on Their Antimicrobial and Antibiofilm Effect against Gram-Negative and Gram-Positive Bacteria. *Front. Microbiol.* **2023**, *13*, 987164. [CrossRef]

87. Hoffman, J.J.; Timmermann, B.N.; Mclaughlin, S.P.; Punnapayak, H. Potential Antimicrobial Activity of Plants from the Southwest-Ern United States. *Int. J. Pharmacog* **1993**, *31*, 101–115. [CrossRef]
88. Martínez Sánchez, A.K. Evaluación de Actividad Antimicrobiana de Extractos Metanólicos de Timbe (Acaciella Mill.), En Ajo Contra Sclerotium Cepivorum Berk. Bachelor's Thesis, UAQ, Querétaro, México, 2013.
89. Lee, J.; Noh, S.; Lim, S.; Kim, B. Plant Extracts for Type 2 Diabetes: From Traditional Medicine to Modern Drug Discovery. *Antioxidants* **2021**, *10*, 81. [CrossRef]
90. Bussmann, R.W.; Malca-García, G.; Glenn, A.; Sharon, D.; Chait, G.; Díaz, D.; Pourmand, K.; Jonat, B.; Somogy, S.; Guardado, G.; et al. Minimum Inhibitory Concentrations of Medicinal Plants Used in Northern Peru as Antibacterial Remedies. *J. Ethnopharmacol.* **2010**, *132*, 101–108. [CrossRef]
91. Nielsen, T.R.H.; Kuete, V.; Jäger, A.K.; Meyer, J.J.M.; Lall, N. Antimicrobial Activity of Selected South African Medicinal Plants. *BMC Complement. Altern. Med.* **2012**, *12*, 74. [CrossRef]
92. Dalmarco, J.; Dalmarco, E.; Koelzer, J.; Pizzolatti, M.; Fröde, T. Isolation and Identification of Bioactive Compounds Responsible for the Anti-Bacterial Efficacy of Lotus Corniculatus Var. So Gabriel. *Int. J. Green Pharm.* **2010**, *4*, 108–114. [CrossRef]
93. Tamokou, J.d.D.; Mbaveng, A.T.; Kuete, V. Antimicrobial Activities of African Medicinal Spices and Vegetables. In *Medicinal Spices and Vegetables from Africa: Therapeutic Potential Against Metabolic, Inflammatory, Infectious and Systemic Diseases*; Elsevier Inc.: Amsterdam, The Netherlands, 2017; pp. 207–237. [CrossRef]
94. Wamba, B.E.N.; Mbaveng, A.T.; Kuete, V. Fighting Gram-Positive Bacteria with African Medicinal Plants: Cut-off Values for the Classification of the Activity of Natural Products. *Adv. Bot. Res.* **2023**, *106*, 413–522. [CrossRef]
95. Razafindrakoto, R.; Lovarintsoa, J.R.; Eliane, R.V.; Hanitra, R.R.; Danielle, A.D.R.; Victor, L.J. Antimicrobial Activity of the Extracts of Albizia Masikororum R.Vig., a Fabaceae from Madagascar. *Afr. J. Microbiol. Res.* **2018**, *12*, 464–469. [CrossRef]
96. Mahamat Djamalladine, D.; Mabou, F.D.; Feugap Tsamo, D.L.; Tamokou, J.D.D.; Voutquenne-Nazabadioko, L.; Tsopmo, A.; Ngnokam, D. New Triterpenoid Saponin from the Aerial Part of *Abrus canescens* Welw Ex. Bak. (Fabaceae) and Their Antibacterial Activities. *Nat. Prod. Res.* **2025**, *39*, 362–373. [CrossRef] [PubMed]
97. Álvarez-Martínez, F.J.; Barrajón-Catalán, E.; Herranz-López, M.; Micol, V. Antibacterial Plant Compounds, Extracts and Essential Oils: An Updated Review on Their Effects and Putative Mechanisms of Action. *Phytomedicine* **2021**, *90*, 153626. [CrossRef]
98. Mpude, L.; Yendze, A.W.B.; Assonfack, D.J.; Cadet, E.; Matieta, V.Y.; Megaptche, J.F.; Mbaveng, A.T.; Kuete, V. Antibacterial Activity of *Sarcocephalus latifolius* and *Acacia sieberiana*, and the Effect of Their Association with Antibiotics against Multidrug-Resistant Staphylococcus Aureus. *Investig. Med. Chem. Pharmacol.* **2024**, *7*, 96. [CrossRef]
99. Morton, K.E.; Coghill, S.H. Staphylococcus Aureus Is the Predominant Pathogen in Hospitalised Patients with Diabetes-Related Foot Infections: An Australian Perspective. *Antibiotics* **2024**, *13*, 594. [CrossRef]
100. Sonkoue Lambou, J.C.; Noubom, M.; Djoumsie Gomseu, B.E.; Takougoum Marbou, W.J.; Tamokou, J.D.D.; Gatsing, D. Multidrug-Resistant Escherichia Coli Causing Urinary Tract Infections among Controlled and Uncontrolled Type 2 Diabetic Patients at Laquintinie Hospital in Douala, Cameroon. *Genet. Res.* **2022**, *2022*, 1250264. [CrossRef]
101. Thapliyal, S.; Dandriyal, A. A Literature Review on Urinary Tract Infection Due to Diabetes Mellitus and Development of Antimicrobial Resistance. *Int. J. Sci. Res.* **2023**, *12*, 2461–2465. [CrossRef]
102. Arfaoui, A.; Rojo-Bezares, B.; Fethi, M.; López, M.; Toledano, P.; Sayem, N.; Ben Khelifa Melki, S.; Ouzari, H.-I.; Klibi, N.; Sáenz, Y. Molecular Characterization of *Pseudomonas aeruginosa* from Diabetic Foot Infections in Tunisia. *J. Med. Microbiol.* **2024**, *73*, 001851. [CrossRef]
103. Wang, H.P.; He, Z.G. Treatment with Incomplete Freund's Adjuvant and Listeria Monocytogenes Delays Diabetes via an Interleukin-17-Secretion-Independent Pathway. *Exp. Ther. Med.* **2015**, *9*, 1934–1938. [CrossRef]
104. Cardador-Martínez, A.; Castaño-Tostado, E.; Loarca-Piña, G. Antimutagenic Activity of Natural Phenolic Compounds Present in the Common Bean (*Phaseolus vulgaris*) against Aflatoxin B1. *Food Addit. Contam.* **2002**, *19*, 62–69. [CrossRef] [PubMed]
105. Oomah, B.D.; Cardador-Martínez, A.; Loarca-Piña, G. Phenolics and Antioxidative Activities in Common Beans (*Phaseolus vulgaris* L.). *J. Sci. Food Agric.* **2005**, *85*, 935–942. [CrossRef]
106. Deshpande, S.S.; Cheryan, M. Determination of Phenolic Compounds of Dry Beans Using Vanillin, Redox and Precipitation Assays. *J. Food Sci.* **1987**, *52*, 332–334. [CrossRef]
107. Brand-Williams, W.; Cuvelier, M.E.; Berset, C. Use of a Free Radical Method to Evaluate Antioxidant Activity. *LWT—Food Sci. Technol.* **1995**, *28*, 25–30. [CrossRef]
108. Re, R.; Pellegrini, N.; Proteggente, A.; Pannala, A.; Yang, M.; Rice-Evans, C. Antioxidant Activity Applying an Improved ABTS Radical Cation Decolorization Assay. *Free Radic. Biol. Med.* **1999**, *26*, 1231–1237. [CrossRef] [PubMed]
109. Gómez-Velázquez, H.D.J.; Aparicio-Fernández, X.; Escobar-Ortiz, A.; Feregrino-Pérez, A.A.; Reynoso-Camacho, R.; Pérez-Ramírez, I.F. Phytochemical Fingerprint of Chia Sprouts Grown Under Chemical Elicitation with Salicylic Acid and Hydrogen Peroxide. *Plant Foods Hum. Nutr.* **2024**, *79*, 127–136. [CrossRef]

110. Rico-Chávez, A.K.; Pérez-Ramírez, I.F.; Escobar-Ortíz, A.; Feregrino-Pérez, A.A.; Torres-Pacheco, I.; Guevara-González, R.G. Hormetic Elicitation of Phthalides in Celery Seeds (*Apium graveolens* L. Var Dulce) and Its Effect on Seedling Development. *Ind. Crops Prod.* **2023**, *202*, 117022. [CrossRef]
111. Salazar-Aranda, R.; de la Torre-Rodríguez, Y.C.; Alicia Alanís-Garza, B.; Alejandro Pérez-López, L.; Waksman-de-Torres, N. Evaluación de La Actividad Biológica de Productos Herbolarios Comerciales. *Med. Univ.* **2009**, *11*, 156–164.
112. Aguirre-Becerra, H.; Pineda-Nieto, S.A.; García-Trejo, J.F.; Guevara-González, R.G.; Feregrino-Pérez, A.A.; Álvarez-Mayorga, B.L.; Rivera Pastrana, D.M. Jacaranda Flower (*Jacaranda mimosifolia*) as an Alternative for Antioxidant and Antimicrobial Use. *Heliyon* **2020**, *6*, e05802. [CrossRef]
113. Mccue, P.; Kwon, Y.-I.; Shetty, K. All Rights Reserved. 278 Blackwell Science, LtdOxford. *J. Food Biochem.* **2005**, *29*, 278–294. [CrossRef]
114. Worthington Biochemical Corp (a). Alpha amylase. In *Worthington Enzyme Manual*; Worthington, V., Ed.; Worthington Biochemical Corp.: Lakewood, NJ, USA, 1993; pp. 36–41.
115. Abdulmunem, O.; Makky, E.A.; Tawfiq, A.A.; Mahendran, K.; Zamri, N. Evaluating the Effect of Combined Plant Extracts on α-Amylase and α-Glucosidase Inhibition Activity as Antidiabetic Agents. *Pakistan J. Biol. Sci.* **2020**, *23*, 287–294. [CrossRef]
116. Worthington Biochemical Corp (b). Maltase-α-glucosidase. In *Worthington Enzyme Manual*; Worthington, V., Ed.; Worthington Biochemical Corp.: Lakewood, NJ, USA, 1993; p. 261.
117. Hou, W.C.; Lee, M.H.; Hsu, F.L.; Lin, Y.H. Inhibitory Activities of Semicarbazide-Sensitive Amine Oxidase and Angiotensin Converting Enzyme of Pectin Hydroxamic Acid. *J. Agric. Food Chem.* **2003**, *51*, 6362–6366. [CrossRef]
118. Bennour, N.; Mighri, H.; Eljani, H.; Zammouri, T.; Akrout, A. Effect of Solvent Evaporation Method on Phenolic Compounds and the Antioxidant Activity of Moringa Oleifera Cultivated in Southern Tunisia. *S. Afr. J. Bot.* **2020**, *129*, 181–190. [CrossRef]
119. Clinical and Laboratory Standards Institute (CLSI). *M100: Performance Standards for Antimicrobial Susceptibility Testing*, 33rd ed.; CLSI: Malvern, PA, USA, 2023.
120. Swebocki, T.; Barras, A.; Maria Kocot, A. Minimum Inhibitory Concentration (MIC) and Minimum Bactericidal Concentration (MBC) Assays Using Broth Microdilution Method. *JUN* **2023**, *23*.
121. Vanegas, D.; Novillo, A.A.; Khachatryan, A.; Jerves Andrade, L.; Peñaherrera, E.; Cuzco, N.; Wilches, I.; Calle, J.; León-Tamariz, F. Validation of a Method of Broth Microdilution for the Determination of Antibacterial Activity of Essential Oils. *BMC Res. Notes* **2021**, *14*, 439. [CrossRef]
122. Panpaliya, N.P.; Dahake, P.T.; Kale, Y.J.; Dadpe, M.V.; Kendre, S.B.; Siddiqi, A.G.; Maggavi, U.R. In Vitro Evaluation of Antimicrobial Property of Silver Nanoparticles and Chlorhexidine against Five Different Oral Pathogenic Bacteria. *Saudi Dent. J.* **2019**, *31*, 76–83. [CrossRef]

pharmaceuticals

MDPI

Article

Unlocking the Antidiabetic Potential of CBD: In Vivo Preclinical Studies

Elena Rafailovska [1], Elona Xhemaili [2], Zorica Naumovska [3], Olga Gigopulu [3], Biljana Miova [1], Ljubica Suturkova [3] and Gjoshe Stefkov [3,*]

[1] Institute of Biology, Faculty of Natural Sciences and Mathematics, Ss. Cyril and Methodius University in Skopje, Arhimedova 3, 1000 Skopje, North Macedonia; elena.rafailovska@pmf.ukim.mk (E.R.); bmiova@pmf.ukim.mk (B.M.)

[2] Department of Pharmacy, Faculty of Medical Sciences, University of Tetovo, Ilinden bb, 1200 Tetovo, North Macedonia; xhemailielona@gmail.com

[3] Faculty of Pharmacy, Ss. Cyril and Methodius University in Skopje, Majka Tereza 47, 1000 Skopje, North Macedonia; zose@ff.ukim.edu.mk (Z.N.); olga.gigopulu@ff.ukim.edu.mk (O.G.); ljubica.suturkova@ff.ukim.edu.mk (L.S.)

* Correspondence: gost@ff.ukim.edu.mk

Abstract: Background/Objectives: Diabetes mellitus is a growing global health concern, driving the exploration of new therapies like cannabidiol (CBD), which shows potential in improving insulin sensitivity and glycemic control, though its effects on glucose metabolism remain unclear. This study evaluates CBD's dose-dependent effects on glycemia, insulin, and hepatic carbohydrate metabolism in diabetic rats. **Methods**: The Oral Glucose Tolerance Test (OGTT) was performed in healthy rats to compare intragastric vs. intraperitoneal CBD (0.5, 5, 50 mg/kg). Diabetic rats were treated with intragastric CBD (25, 50, 100 mg/kg) or metformin (70 mg/kg) for 8 days. Blood glucose, insulin, lipid profiles, and key carbohydrate-metabolizing enzymes were analyzed. **Results**: In the OGTT, intragastric CBD reduced glycemic AUC, with 50 mg/kg showing the strongest effect, while intraperitoneal CBD had no impact. In diabetic rats, metformin and 25 mg/kg CBD lowered blood glucose, but only CBD increased insulin. The 50 mg/kg dose caused the greatest glucose reduction and moderate insulin rise, while 100 mg/kg had no effect. At 25 mg/kg, CBD inhibited glucose-6-phosphatase and increased glucose-6-phosphate. The 50 mg/kg dose further suppressed gluconeogenic enzymes, reduced glycogen phosphorylase and liver glucose, and enhanced glucose-6-phosphate, showing the strongest metabolic effects. The 100 mg/kg dose increased hexokinase but had weaker metabolic effects. Metformin improved glucose utilization and glycogen storage. CBD at 25 and 50 mg/kg reduced triacylglycerols and increased HDL, while 100 mg/kg had no effect. **Conclusions:** This study provides strong evidence of CBD's antidiabetic potential, especially at 50 mg/kg, particularly through its modulation of glucose metabolism and tendency to regulate insulin levels.

Keywords: cannabidiol; diabetes mellitus; insulin sensitivity; hepatic carbohydrate metabolism; laboratory animals; OGTT

1. Introduction

Cannabis sativa has garnered significant attention over the past 50 years due to its pharmacological properties and potential therapeutic applications [1]. The plant contains approximately 750 compounds, including the major phytocannabinoids tetrahydrocannabinol (THC) and cannabidiol (CBD) [2]. While Δ9-THC is well known for its psychoactive effects [3,4], CBD, which is primarily derived from the flowers and leaves of *C. sativa* and also present in smaller amounts in other Cannabis species [2], lacks such properties and has gained widespread use in medical contexts, including therapeutic applications and clinical trials in Europe [5].

Several medical applications of *C. sativa* are supported by reliable clinical data, including its use in managing chronic pain, multiple sclerosis, refractory epilepsy, chemotherapy-induced nausea and vomiting, appetite and weight loss associated with anxiety and sleep disorders, PTSD, and schizophrenia [6,7]. Beyond these well-documented effects, both *C. sativa* extracts and its active compounds, such as CBD and THC, have shown additional therapeutic benefits in in vitro and in vivo studies, including reductions in blood pressure, triglycerides, and cholesterol, along with antioxidant properties [6]. Notably, recent research has expanded to explore the role of CBD in metabolic disorders, particularly diabetes mellitus (DM) [8]. DM is a major global health concern, with its prevalence steadily increasing. According to the International Diabetes Federation (IDF), approximately 537 million adults were living with diabetes in 2021, a number projected to rise to 783 million by 2045 [9]. Moreover, the World Health Organization (WHO) estimates that DM-related mortality will increase by 50% by 2030, further underscoring the urgent need for effective treatment strategies [10]. Given these alarming statistics, there is a growing interest in exploring alternative therapies that may complement conventional diabetes treatments.

CBD has emerged as a potential adjunct therapy for diabetes management due to its anti-inflammatory, antioxidant, and insulin-sensitizing properties. Even though clinical trials on CBD are still limited, a Phase I study investigating the efficacy of a sublingual CBD/THC regimen (10:1) in type 2 diabetes patients found significant improvements in fasting blood sugar, HbA1c, and 2 h Oral Glucose Tolerance Test (OGTT) values, along with reduced insulin secretion and HOMA2-IR values, suggesting that CBD may enhance insulin sensitivity and glycemic control [11]. Moreover, unlike some antidiabetic treatments, CBD does not appear to be associated with an increased prevalence of liver enzyme elevation indicative of hepatic damage [12]. Preclinical studies indicate that CBD improves insulin sensitivity in both in vitro [13] and in vivo models, primarily by reducing inflammation, which plays a key role in insulin resistance [5]. In diabetic animal models, CBD has been shown to enhance glycemic control, and its effects appear to be mediated via CB2 receptor signaling [14]. Some research suggests that CBD lowers fasting and postprandial blood glucose [14] and inhibits α-glucosidase, an enzyme involved in carbohydrate digestion [15]. Furthermore, CBD may protect pancreatic β-cells from autoimmune destruction in Type 1 diabetes models, leading to improved glucose homeostasis [16]. Studies also suggest that CBD treatment ameliorates metabolic dysfunctions such as hyperglycemia and increases insulin levels in diabetic rats [14]. While these findings are promising, the precise mechanisms by which CBD modulates endogenous glucose metabolism remain unclear.

Dysregulation of hepatic glucose metabolism is a hallmark of diabetes, affecting processes such as gluconeogenesis, glycogenolysis, and glycolysis [17,18]. The liver plays a central role in maintaining glucose homeostasis, and alterations in key carbohydrate-metabolizing enzymes contribute to diabetic pathophysiology [18]. CBD has been shown to decrease the expression of genes responsible for glucose metabolism, glycolysis, and gluconeogenesis in vitro [19]. However, limited studies have investigated CBD's direct effects on enzyme activity in hepatic carbohydrate metabolism.

Moreover, several in vivo studies have shown mixed effects on glycemic measures [20–23], or found no improvement in blood glucose levels at all [24,25]. These inconsistencies are mainly due to the different routes of administration of CBD (intraperitoneal or oral) and the different doses used in the studies (ranging from 10 mg/kg to 60 mg/kg body weight) [20,21,23].

Thus, there is a need to establish the most favorable route of administration and assess the dose-dependent effects of CBD.

The present study aims to examine the route of administration and evaluate the dose-dependent effects of CBD on glycemia. Furthermore, it assesses alterations in glucose and insulin levels to determine the potential regulatory role of CBD in maintaining glucose homeostasis. In addition, the study investigates the impact of CBD on hepatic carbohydrate metabolism in diabetic rats, focusing on its dose-dependent effects on key metabolic pathways, including gluconeogenesis, glycolysis, and glycogen metabolism, through its effects on enzyme activities and substrate concentrations.

2. Results

2.1. Oral Glucose Tolerance Test (OGTT)—Intragastric vs. Intraperitoneal Application of CBD

During the OGTT measurements in healthy rats receiving CBD treatment intragastically (Figure 1A), glucose levels peaked at similar levels across all three groups 15 min after glucose administration. Notably, the 50 mg/kg CBD group exhibited a lesser glucose increasement compared to controls and metformin-treated groups during this period. At 60 min post-administration, the 0.5 mg/kg and 50 mg/kg i.g. CBD groups, akin to the metformin-treated group, reached glucose levels comparable to controls. However, the 5 mg/kg CBD group took 90 min to reach control values. The AUC analysis of the OGTT in rats receiving CBD intragastrically (Figure 1B) revealed that the 50 mg/kg CBD treatment resulted in a significantly lower glycemic AUC compared to the other groups. Specifically, the AUC in the 50 mg/kg CBD group was approximately 10% lower than in the metformin-treated group (Met:CBD 50, $p < 0.05$), and it was also 10% and 15% lower than the AUC values in the 0.5 mg/kg and 5 mg/kg CBD groups (CBD 0.5:CBD 50, $p < 0.05$; CBD 5:CBD 50, $p < 0.05$), respectively.

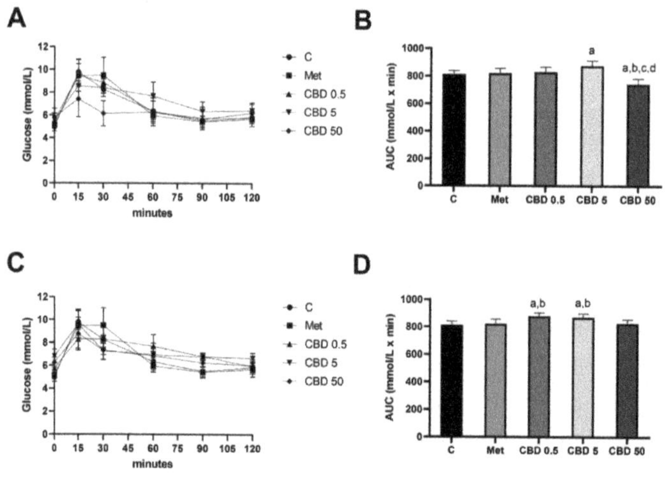

Figure 1. Blood glucose levels (**A**,**C**) and area under the curve (AUC) of blood glucose levels (**B**,**D**) measured during the Oral Glucose Tolerance Test (OGTT) in healthy rats treated with cannabidiol (CBD). CBD was administered in doses of 0.5 mg/kg, 5 mg/kg, and 50 mg/kg body weight either intragastrically (**A**,**B**) or intraperitoneally (**C**,**D**). Treatment groups included a control group (C), a metformin-treated group (Met, 70 mg/kg), and CBD-treated groups receiving 0.5 mg/kg (CBD 0.5), 5 mg/kg (CBD 5), or 50 mg/kg (CBD 50). Data are presented as mean ± SD. Significant differences ($p < 0.05$) are indicated as follows: a—compared to C; b—compared to Met; c—compared to CBD 0.5; d—compared to CBD 5.

The results of the OGTT performed on healthy rats receiving CBD treatment intraperitoneally (Figure 1C) showed that both metformin- and CBD-treated groups have similar dynamics regarding blood glucose levels during 120 min measurement. Namely, glucose levels in all groups peaked at similar levels 15 min after glucose administration. Similar to the metformin-treated group, the CBD-treated groups with the doses 0.5 mg/kg and 50 mg/kg reached the values of control rats 60 min after the glucose administration, while the rats treated with 5 mg/kg CBD reached control values 90 min after the glucose administration. The AUC analysis of the OGTT following intraperitoneal CBD administration (Figure 1D) revealed that treatment with 0.5 mg/kg and 5 mg/kg CBD resulted in significantly higher AUC values, compared to the control (C:CBD 0.5, $p < 0.05$; C:CBD5, $p < 0.05$) and metformin-treated group (Met:CBD 0.5, $p < 0.05$; Met:CBD5, $p < 0.05$). However, no significant differences were observed between the different CBD doses.

2.2. Daily Glucose Regulation During Multiple-Dose Study

The results of blood glucose levels (A) and the area under the curve (AUC) of blood glucose levels (B), measured daily during the multiple-dose study in streptozotocin-induced diabetic rats, are shown in Figure 2. The AUC results indicate that the untreated diabetic group consistently exhibited significantly higher blood glucose levels compared to the control group (C:D, $p < 0.05$). Notably, both the metformin-treated group and the CBD-treated group receiving 25 mg/kg body weight showed similar effects, significantly reducing the AUC by approximately 10% compared to the diabetic group (D:Met, $p < 0.05$; D:CBD25, $p < 0.05$; Met:CBD25, ns). Administration of CBD at a dose of 50 mg/kg body weight resulted in the most pronounced reduction, lowering the AUC by 20% (D:CBD50, $p < 0.05$). This dose also yielded a significantly lower AUC compared to the metformin-treated group (Met:CBD50, $p < 0.05$). In contrast, treatment with CBD at a dose of 100 mg/kg body weight did not produce a significant change in the AUC compared to the diabetic group (D:CBD100, ns). This treatment also showed significantly higher AUC values compared to the Met, CBD25, and CBD50 groups, respectively.

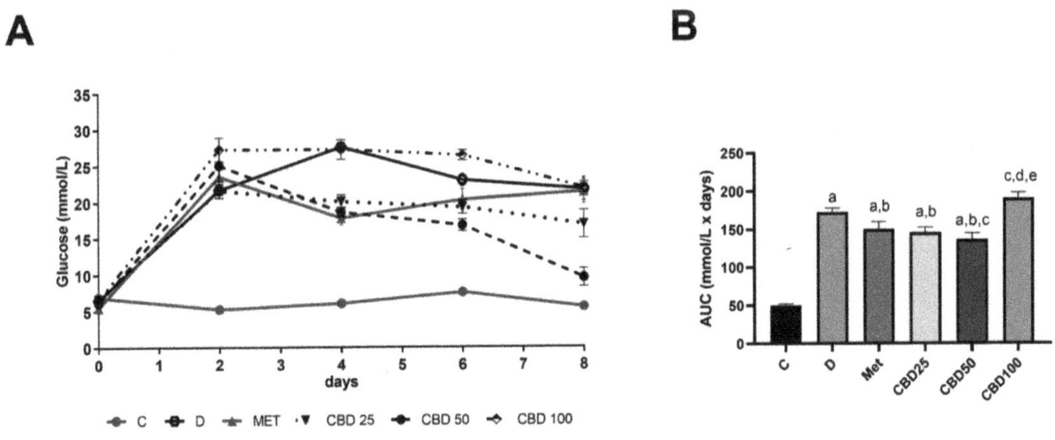

Figure 2. Blood glucose levels (**A**) monitored daily and area under the curve (AUC) of blood glucose levels (**B**) measured daily during the multiple-dose study in streptozotocin-induced diabetic rats. Treatment groups included a control group (C), a diabetic control group (D), a metformin-treated group (Met, 70 mg/kg), and cannabidiol (CBD) treatment groups receiving 25 mg/kg (CBD25), 50 mg/kg (CBD50), or 100 mg/kg (CBD100). Data are presented as mean ± SD. Significant differences ($p < 0.05$) are indicated as follows: a—compared to C; b—compared to D; c—compared to Met; d—compared to CBD25; e—compared to CBD50.

2.3. *Hourly Profile of Blood Glucose Levels During Multiple-Dose Study on Days 2 and 6*

Figure 3 depicts the hourly change in blood glucose concentration (Figure 3A,C) and area under the curve of blood glucose (Figure 3B,D) monitored on the second and sixth day of the multiple-dose study in streptozotocin-induced diabetic rats, respectively.

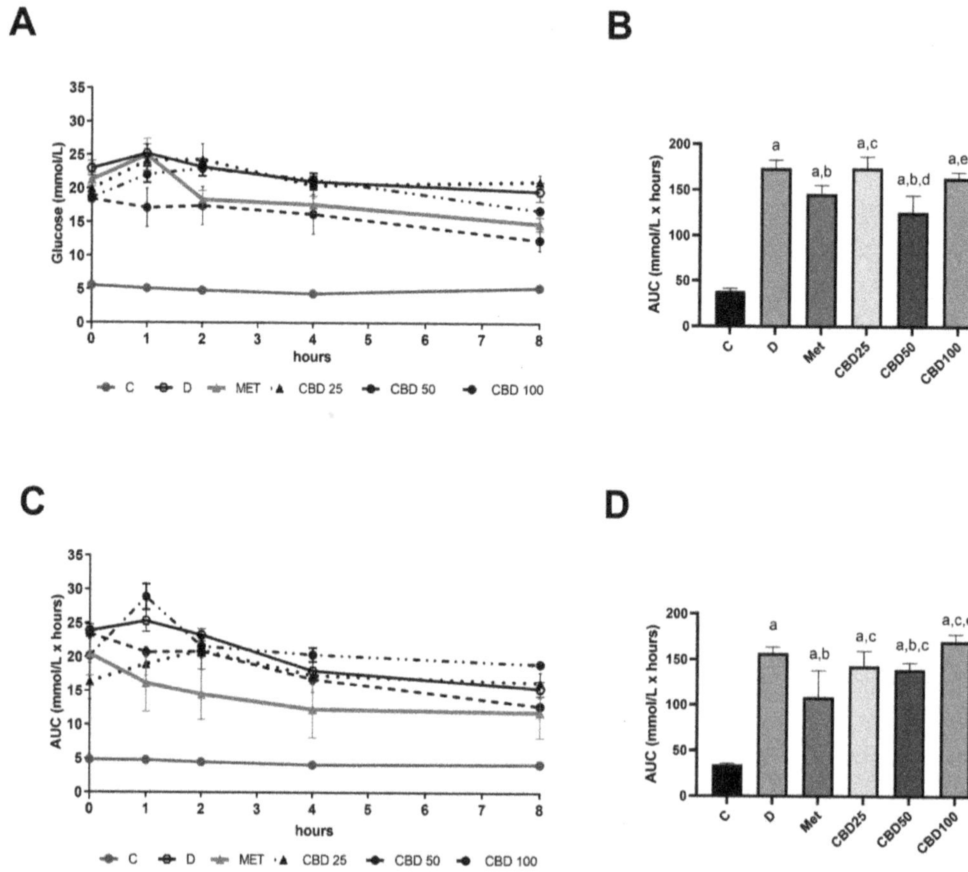

Figure 3. Blood glucose levels (**A**) monitored hourly, and the corresponding area under the curve (AUC) values (**B**) measured on the 2nd day; blood glucose levels (**C**) monitored hourly and the corresponding area under the curve (AUC) values (**D**) measured on the 6th day of the multiple-dose study in streptozotocin-induced diabetic rats. Treatment groups included a control group (C), a diabetic control group (D), a metformin-treated group (Met, 70 mg/kg), and cannabidiol (CBD) treatment groups receiving 25 mg/kg (CBD25), 50 mg/kg (CBD50), or 100 mg/kg (CBD100). Data are presented as mean ± SD. Significant differences ($p < 0.05$) are indicated as follows: a—compared to C; b—compared to D; c—compared to Met; d—compared to CBD25; e—compared to CBD50.

The AUC results showed that untreated diabetic rats consistently exhibited higher blood glucose levels on days 2 and 6 compared to the control group (Figure 3B, C:D, $p < 0.05$; Figure 3D, C:D, $p < 0.05$). On the second day, the CBD50 group demonstrated the most pronounced reduction in glycemic AUC values, with a 27.6% decrease in the first 8 h (D:CBD50, $p < 0.05$) (Figure 3B). Although this reduction was greater than that observed in the metformin group (−16.9%), the difference between the two treatments was not statistically significant (Met:CBD50, ns) (Figure 3B). In contrast, the glycemic AUC values in the CBD25 and CBD100 groups did not differ significantly from those of the untreated diabetic group (D:CBD25, D:CBD100, ns). By the sixth day, metformin exhibited a more substantial effect, reducing the glycemic AUC value by 31.2% (D:Met, $p < 0.05$), while the CBD50 group showed a more modest reduction of 12.1% (D:CBD50, $p < 0.05$) (Figure 3D). The effect of metformin on the 6th day compared to CBD50 was significantly more pronounced (Met:CBD50, $p < 0.05$). Meanwhile, the glycemic AUC values in the CBD25 and CBD100 groups remained unchanged compared to the untreated diabetic group (D:CBD25, D:CBD100, ns).

2.4. Blood Glucose and Insulin Concentration

Figure 4 illustrates the alterations in blood glucose (A) and insulin concentration (B) observed in both healthy and diabetic rats following treatment with three different concentrations of CBD oil and metformin during the multiple-dose study in streptozotocin-induced diabetic rats. A notable reduction in insulin concentration and high blood glucose levels were evident in the untreated diabetic group (C:D, $p < 0.05$). Metformin administration in diabetic rats did not yield significant changes compared to the diabetic control group (D:Met, ns). Treatment with CBD oil at a dose of 25 mg/kg resulted in a slight yet significant reduction in blood glucose levels (D:CBD25,−21%, $p < 0.05$), alongside a noteworthy increase in insulin concentration by 45% compared to diabetic rats (D:CBD25, $p < 0.05$). Most notably, a substantial 67% decrease in blood glucose levels (D:CBD50, $p < 0.05$) and a significant 20% increase in insulin levels were observed in the CBD50 group. Contrariwise, the treatment with a dosage of 100 mg/kg b.w. CBD did not lead to significant alterations in blood glucose nor insulin concentration compared to the diabetic control group.

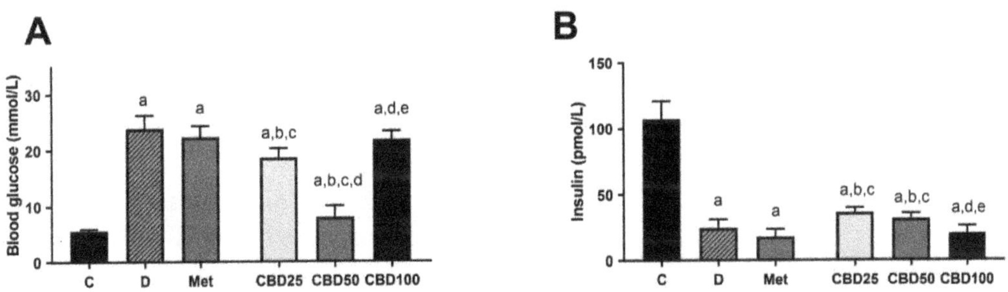

Figure 4. Blood glucose (**A**) and plasma insulin concentration (**B**) in healthy and STZ-induced diabetic rats treated with CBD oil at three different doses and metformin, measured at the end of the multiple-dose study. Treatment groups included a control group (C), a diabetic control group (D), a metformin-treated group (Met, 70 mg/kg), and cannabidiol (CBD) treatment groups receiving 25 mg/kg (CBD25), 50 mg/kg (CBD50), or 100 mg/kg (CBD100). Data are presented as mean ± SD. Significant differences ($p < 0.05$) are indicated as follows: a—compared to C; b—compared to D; c—compared to Met; d—compared to CBD25; e—compared to CBD50.

2.5. Carbohydrate Metabolism in the Liver

Figure 5 depicts the changes in enzyme activities and substrate concentrations of carbohydrate metabolism in the liver of healthy and diabetic rats following treatment with three different doses of CBD oil and metformin during the multiple-dose study in streptozotocin-induced diabetic rats.

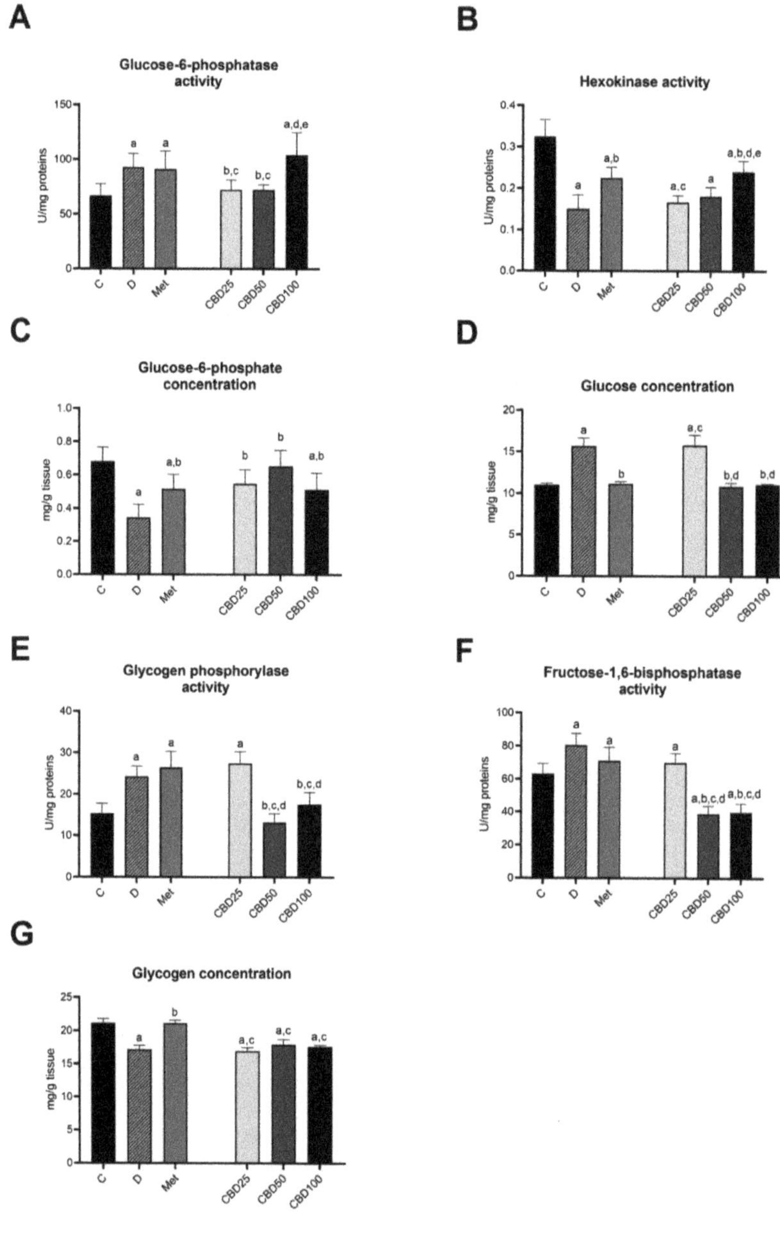

Figure 5. Activity of glucose-6-phosphatase (**A**), hexokinase (**B**), glucose-6-phosphate concentration (**C**), glucose concentration (**D**), glycogen phosphorylase activity (**E**), fructose-1,6-bisphosphatase activity (**F**), and glycogen concentration (**G**) in the liver of healthy and STZ-induced diabetic rats treated with CBD extracts and metformin in the multiple-dose study. Treatment groups included a control group (C), a diabetic control group (D), a metformin-treated group (Met, 70 mg/kg), and cannabidiol (CBD) treatment groups receiving 25 mg/kg (CBD25), 50 mg/kg (CBD50), or 100 mg/kg (CBD100). Data are presented as mean ± SD. Significant differences ($p < 0.05$) are indicated as follows: a—compared to C; b—compared to D; c—compared to Met; d—compared to CBD25; e—compared to CBD50.

Compared to control animals, experimental diabetes resulted in significant increases in glucose-6-phosphatase activity (Figure 5A), alongside significant decreases in hexokinase activity (Figure 5B) and glucose-6-phosphate concentration (Figure 5C). Moreover, there were significant rises in glucose concentration (Figure 5D) and the activities of glycogen phosphorylase (Figure 5E) and fructose-1,6-bisphosphatase (Figure 5F), coupled with notable decreases in glycogen content (Figure 5G).

Metformin treatment did not induce significant changes in the activity of glucose-6-phosphatase (Figure 5A), glycogen phosphorylase (Figure 5E), or fructose-1,6-bisphosphatase (Figure 5F). However, it significantly increased hexokinase activity (Figure 5B), glucose-6-phosphate concentration (Figure 5C), and glycogen concentration (Figure 5G), while also significantly decreasing liver glucose levels (Figure 5D) compared to diabetic rats.

CBD treatment at a dose of 25 mg/kg led to a significant decrease in glucose-6-phosphatase activity (Figure 5A), with no noticeable effect on hexokinase activity (Figure 5B). It resulted in an increase in glucose-6-phosphate concentration (Figure 5C) but did not significantly affect liver glucose concentration (Figure 5D), glycogen phosphorylase activity (Figure 5E), fructose-1,6-bisphosphatase activity (Figure 5F), or glycogen concentration (Figure 5G) compared to diabetic rats.

Compared to diabetic rats, CBD treatment at a dose of 50 mg/kg resulted in a significant decrease in glucose-6-phosphatase activity (Figure 5A) while having no noticeable effect on hexokinase activity (Figure 5B). Additionally, it significantly increased glucose-6-phosphate concentration (Figure 5C) and led to a significant decrease in liver glucose concentration (Figure 5D), glycogen phosphorylase activity (Figure 5E), and fructose-1,6-bisphosphatase activity (Figure 5F), though it did not alter liver glycogen concentration (Figure 5G). The activities of glycogen phosphorylase and fructose-1,6-bisphosphatase, as well as hepatic glucose concentration in diabetic rats treated with CBD at a dose of 50 mg/kg, were significantly lower compared to diabetic rats treated with CBD at a dose of 25 mg/kg (Figure 5D,G).

Compared to diabetic rats, treatment with CBD at a dose of 100 mg/kg did not alter glucose-6-phosphatase activity (Figure 5A) or glycogen content (Figure 5G). However, it notably increased hexokinase activity (Figure 5B) and glucose-6-phosphate concentration (Figure 5C), while significantly reducing liver glucose concentration (Figure 5D), glycogen phosphorylase activity (Figure 5E), and fructose-1,6-bisphosphatase activity (Figure 5F). Additionally, glucose concentration, glycogen phosphorylase activity, and fructose-1,6-bisphosphatase activity in the CBD100 group were significantly lower compared to the CBD25 group, whereas the activities of glucose-6-phosphatase and hexokinase in the CBD100 group were significantly higher compared to both the CBD25 and CBD50 groups.

2.6. Blood Lipid Parameters

Figure 6 illustrates the changes in triacylglycerol, total cholesterol, and HDL levels in the blood of healthy and diabetic rats following treatment with three different doses of CBD oil (25 mg/kg, 50 mg/kg, and 100 mg/kg) and metformin during the multiple-dose study in streptozotocin-induced diabetic rats.

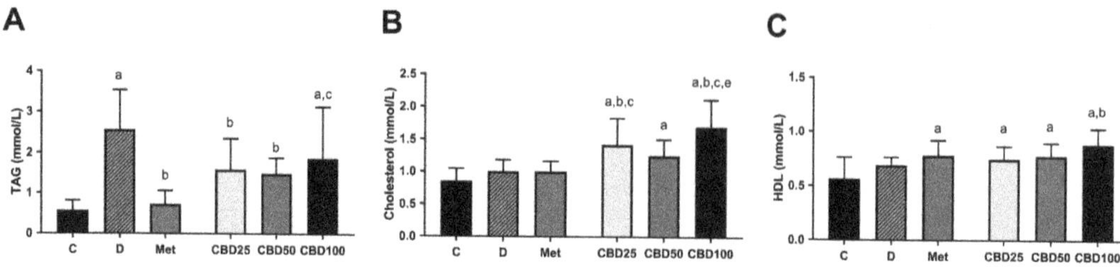

Figure 6. Triacylglycerol (TAG) (**A**), total cholesterol (**B**), and HDL cholesterol (**C**) levels, measured at the end of the multiple-dose study in streptozotocin-induced diabetic rats. Treatment groups included a control group (C), a diabetic control group (D), a metformin-treated group (Met, 70 mg/kg), and cannabidiol (CBD) treatment groups receiving 25 mg/kg (CBD25), 50 mg/kg (CBD50), or 100 mg/kg (CBD100). Data are presented as mean ± SD. Significant differences ($p < 0.05$) are indicated as follows: a—compared to C; b—compared to D; c—compared to Met; d—compared to CBD25; e—compared to CBD50.

Diabetic rats exhibited a marked increase in triacylglycerol (TAG) levels compared to controls (C:D, $p < 0.05$), while total cholesterol and HDL levels remained unchanged (C:D, ns). Compared to diabetic rats, metformin treatment led to a significant decrease in TAG levels (D:Met, $p < 0.05$), without affecting total cholesterol and HDL levels (D:Met, ns). However, HDL levels in metformin-treated rats were significantly higher compared to healthy controls (C:Met, $p < 0.05$).

CBD treatment at a dose of 25 mg/kg led to a significant decrease in TAG levels, alongside a significant increase in total cholesterol levels compared to diabetic rats (D:CBD25, $p < 0.05$). Additionally, total cholesterol and HDL levels in the CBD25 group were significantly higher compared to healthy controls (C:CBD25, $p < 0.05$). Similarly, treatment with 50 mg/kg CBD significantly lowered TAG levels compared to diabetic rats (D:CBD50, $p < 0.05$). Total cholesterol and HDL concentrations in the CBD50 group significantly exceeded control values (C:CBD50, $p < 0.05$). In contrast, treatment with 100 mg/kg CBD had no significant effect on TAG levels (D:CBD100, ns), but significantly increased total cholesterol and HDL levels compared to diabetic rats (D:CBD100, $p < 0.05$).

3. Discussion

In addition to its known pharmacological properties and potential therapeutic benefits in managing metabolic syndrome and diabetes, this study provides compelling evidence supporting the antihyperglycemic and antidiabetic effects of cannabidiol (CBD) and provides insights into its mechanisms of action. Our results demonstrate the strong antidiabetic potential of CBD in diabetic animal models, particularly through its modulation of blood glucose and insulin levels as well as hepatic enzymes involved in carbohydrate metabolism.

The results from the Oral Glucose Tolerance Test (OGTT) in this study highlight the importance of optimizing CBD administration methods to enhance its efficacy in glucose regulation. The doses (0.5 mg/kg, 5 mg/kg, and 50 mg/kg) were selected based on previous studies showing glucose-lowering effects within the 5–30 mg/kg range [26–28]. Our findings demonstrate that intragastrically administered CBD at the highest dose (50 mg/kg) significantly improved glucose regulation, while lower doses (0.5 mg/kg and 5 mg/kg) did not produce similar effects, indicating a dose-dependent response. In contrast, intraperitoneal CBD administration did not result in significant differences in the glycemic area under the curve (AUC) across doses, suggesting that the route of administration plays a key role in CBD's bioavailability and efficacy. This lack of effect with intraperitoneal administration aligns with findings from other studies [23]. One explanation for the better outcomes with intragastrically administered CBD is its lipophilic nature, which allows for more efficient absorption through the gastrointestinal (GI) tract and accumulation in highly vascularized tissues like the liver, essential for glucose metabolism [29,30]. Despite low oral bioavailability (around 6%) [31,32], the absorption via the GI tract, combined with CBD's protein-binding capacity and long half-life, may enhance its therapeutic effects when administered at appropriate doses [33,34].

Based on the results of the OGTT, we selected intragastric administration for the STZ-induced diabetes experiment. The doses of 25 mg/kg, 50 mg/kg, and 100 mg/kg were chosen based on previous studies demonstrating the beneficial effects of CBD in diabetic and insulin resistance models. Namely, studies using doses between 10 mg/kg and 30 mg/kg have shown improvements in glycemic control and insulin sensitivity [1,27,35,36]. The inclusion of higher doses aimed to explore potential enhanced therapeutic effects and assess whether increasing concentrations would yield stronger metabolic benefits or reveal a saturation threshold.

Throughout the 8-day treatment period, the administration of 50 mg/kg CBD consistently showed the most significant reduction in daily blood glucose levels among diabetic rats, lowering blood glucose by approximately 20%. Notably, this effect was more pronounced than that observed with metformin, a standard antidiabetic treatment. Interestingly, the 100 mg/kg dose did not provide additional benefits and was less effective than the lower doses. This inverted-U dose–response relationship aligns with previous research on cannabinoids, where biphasic effects have been reported for different pathologies [37,38]. At higher doses, CBD's efficacy may be reduced due to receptor saturation or receptor desensitization. Chronic activation of CB1 receptors, which play a key role in energy homeostasis [39], can trigger feedback processes that counteract initial receptor activity [40], potentially explaining the diminished therapeutic effects observed at increased CBD dosages. Additionally, CBD interacts with multiple receptors, including transient receptor potential (TRP) channels, particularly TRPV1 [41], which is involved in glucose homeostasis [42]. Activation of TRPV1 can initially enhance signaling but may subsequently lead to a prolonged refractory state, commonly referred to as desensitization [43]. This desensitization could contribute to the reduced efficacy observed at higher CBD doses.

Hourly glycemic profiling further supported the efficacy of the 50 mg/kg dose, which reduced blood glucose levels by 27.6% within 8 h on the second day of treatment, comparable to the effect of metformin. However, by the sixth day of treatment, metformin exhibited superior glycemic control (31.2% reduction) compared to CBD50 (12.1% reduction). These findings suggest that while CBD is effective in providing short-term glycemic control, metformin offers more sustained benefits over longer treatment periods. Metformin's prolonged efficacy could be attributed to its well-established mechanisms of action, including the cumulative reduction in hepatic glucose production [44], activation of AMP-activated protein kinase (AMPK), and modulation of cellular redox balance [45], all of which collectively contribute to stable blood sugar levels over time. In contrast, the transient nature of CBD's efficacy raises the possibility of combination therapies to leverage the rapid effects of CBD alongside metformin's sustained benefits.

This study also highlights the dose-dependent impact of CBD on glycemic control and insulin levels, with significant changes observed at lower doses (25 and 50 mg/kg), while the highest dose (100 mg/kg) exhibited minimal effects. Previous studies have demonstrated CBD's potential in modulating glucose homeostasis [14,26,36,46], and the dose-dependent effects observed here underscore the complexity of its action. In vivo studies have shown that CBD reduces hyperglycemia and increases plasma insulin levels at doses ranging from 5 mg/kg to 30 mg/kg [28,46]. However, starting at 60 mg/kg, no improvement in glycemic measures was observed in male Wistar rats [23], and similarly, no changes in blood glucose or serum insulin were noted in humans after 13 weeks of daily oral administration of 200 mg CBD [20]. This lack of effect at higher doses may suggest a saturation point beyond which CBD fails to enhance glycemic control. As previously speculated, at higher doses, CBD may lose its efficacy in glycemic control due to receptor desensitization, activation of counter-regulatory mechanisms, and non-specific interactions. Moreover, CBD at higher doses may interact with alternative molecular targets, leading to metabolic outcomes that counteract its glucose-lowering effects [47]. While we focused on glycemic control and insulin levels, future studies on insulin sensitivity using the Homeostatic Model Assessment of Insulin Resistance (HOMA-IR) could enhance the translational value of these findings.

The findings of this study further emphasize the liver's pivotal role in mediating CBD's antidiabetic effects, given its centrality in glucose metabolism. CBD's influence on hepatic gluconeogenesis, glycogenolysis, and glycolysis may account for the observed improvements in glycemic control. In this sense, experimental diabetes significantly altered the activities of enzymes and substrates involved in carbohydrate metabolism. Our findings indicate that experimental diabetes increased gluconeogenesis, as evidenced by the elevated activities of glucose-6-phosphatase and fructose-1,6-bisphosphatase, likely due to decreased insulin levels in diabetic rats. Since insulin directly suppresses gluconeogenic enzymes [48], its deficiency contributes to this upregulation. Simultaneously, the lack of insulin suppresses the activity of enzymes associated with glucose metabolism [49], such as hexokinase (HK), as demonstrated in our results. The reduced activity of hexokinase in diabetic rats accounts for the decrease in glucose-6-phosphate (G6P) concentration, as HK is responsible for glucose phosphorylation and subsequent G6P production [50]. The diabetic state also lowered the glycogen content in the liver, probably due to diminished glucose uptake in hepatocytes [51] and reduced activity in glycogen synthetase in response to decreased insulin levels [52]. Additionally, we observed lower activity of glycogen phosphorylase in the liver of diabetic animals, likely due to reduced glycogen stores, as phosphorylase is inactivated when glycogen levels are low to minimize glycogenolysis [53].

The treatment of diabetic animals with CBD at a dose of 25 mg/kg selectively modulated certain aspects of carbohydrate metabolism, particularly by lowering the activity of the gluconeogenic enzyme glucose-6-phosphatase. The increase in glucose-6-phosphate concentration is consistent with the decreased activity of glucose-6-phosphatase. Since less glucose-6-phosphate is being converted back to glucose, its intracellular concentration rises [54]. These changes support the slight glycemic control observed in this experimental group.

The treatment with CBD at dose of 50 mg/kg exerts a stronger inhibitory effect on gluconeogenesis and glycogenolysis compared to the lower dose. Treatment with this concentration leads to a notable decrease in glucose-6-phosphatase and fructose-1,6-bisphosphatase activities, reflecting a robust inhibition of gluconeogenesis [55]. This effect is further supported by the significant reduction in liver glucose concentration, indicating that 50 mg/kg CBD effectively reduces hepatic glucose production [56]. These findings align with previous literature demonstrating that fructose-1,6-bisphosphatase and glucose-6-phosphatase activities are suppressed in vitro, in a dose-dependent manner, when incubated with cannabidiol. Specifically, doses ranging from 120 to 240 μg/mL of CBD have been shown to inhibit these key gluconeogenic enzymes [57]. Additionally, CBD has been reported to decrease the expression of genes involved in gluconeogenesis in vitro [19], further supporting our observed suppression of glucose-6-phosphatase at 25 mg/kg and the stronger inhibition at 50 mg/kg. The observed decrease in gluconeogenesis and glycogenolysis might be due to the modulation of gene expression by CBD; however, further studies are needed to clarify its precise mechanism of action. Additionally, the treatment at a dose of 50 mg/kg reduces glycogen phosphorylase activity, indicating a suppression of glycogenolysis, which helps to preserve glycogen stores. This is consistent with reports that cannabidiol suppresses glycogen phosphorylase activity in a dose-dependent manner [57]. Despite this suppression, in our results, liver glycogen concentration remains unchanged, suggesting that while glycogen breakdown is inhibited, glycogen synthesis may still be impaired [58]. Furthermore, we observed non-significant changes in hexokinase activity, despite the significant increase in glucose-6-phosphate concentration, which might be explained by feedback inhibition of hexokinase by high levels of glucose-6-phosphate [59]. Interestingly, the literature indicates that CBD significantly upregulates mRNA expression of hexokinases [60], suggesting that CBD's effects on hexokinase may involve regulatory mechanisms at the transcriptional level, which may not immediately translate into changes in enzyme activity.

The effects of CBD treatment at a dose of 100 mg/kg present a distinct pattern compared to the 25 mg/kg and 50 mg/kg doses, revealing different impacts on hepatic carbohydrate metabolism in diabetic rats. The 100 mg/kg CBD dose did not reduce glucose-6-phosphatase activity, indicating that gluconeogenesis continues [55], which contributes to persistent hyperglycemia. Despite increased hexokinase activity and glucose-6-phosphate levels, liver glucose concentrations are lower, likely because glucose is being released into the bloodstream. Although glycogen phosphorylase activity is reduced, glycogen levels remain low, suggesting that glycogen synthesis is still impaired [58], similar to the effects observed at 50 mg/kg. Consistent with our earlier observations, this dose of CBD did not result in effective glycemic control.

The results from metformin treatment in this study showed that it did not induce significant changes in the activity of key enzymes involved in gluconeogenesis (glucose-6-phosphatase, fructose-1,6-bisphosphatase) or glycogenolysis (glycogen phosphorylase). However, metformin significantly increased hexokinase activity, glucose-6-phosphate levels, and glycogen concentration, while reducing liver glucose levels compared to diabetic rats. These findings suggest that during the 8-day treatment, metformin's action likely focuses on improving glucose metabolism by increasing the efficiency of glucose utilization, rather than directly inhibiting glucose production [61]. The increase in hexokinase activity indicates enhanced glucose phosphorylation, facilitating glucose storage and utilization within liver cells [62]. The elevated glucose-6-phosphate concentration further supports this, as glucose-6-phosphate is a key intermediate in both glycolysis and glycogen synthesis [54]. The increased levels of glucose-6-phosphate together with lowered liver glucose levels could also indicate enhanced glucose utilization in the liver by storing glucose as glycogen [63], which subsequently results in increased glycogen levels in the liver. This pattern of results aligns with the known mechanisms of action of metformin, where it promotes glucose utilization [64]. Overall, CBD at 50 mg/kg reduces liver glucose production by inhibiting gluconeogenesis and glycogenolysis, while metformin enhances glucose utilization and storage. Notably, CBD exhibits metabolic effects similar to other natural compounds, such as berberine, curcumin, and resveratrol, which enhance glucose metabolism by reducing hepatic glucose production [65] or promoting glucose uptake [66]. However, future research is needed to address the underlying molecular mechanisms of action or long-term effects of CBD treatment, and to better compare the efficacy of CBD with metformin, which is known for its long-term benefits in glucose metabolism and insulin sensitivity [64].

CBD oil at doses of 25, 50, and 100 mg/kg significantly reduced triglyceride (TAG) levels in diabetic rats, although its efficacy in restoring TAG levels to control values was lower than that of metformin. This effect is consistent with previous findings, where CBD at doses of 10 and 30 mg/kg was shown to lower plasma triglycerides in Wistar rats [25].

The observed reduction in TAG levels may be attributed to CBD's ability to modulate lipid metabolism through PPARγ activation, which has been implicated in improving lipid profiles in diabetic conditions [25].

Interestingly, the highest CBD dose (100 mg/kg) resulted in increased total cholesterol and HDL levels, a finding that aligns with previous studies [27,67]. This increase in HDL may suggest a potential cardioprotective role of CBD, as elevated HDL levels are typically associated with improved lipid transport and reduced cardiovascular risk [67]. Human trials have provided additional insights into the lipid-modulating effects of CBD, with CBD-rich treatments in type 2 diabetic patients leading to reductions in both plasma triglycerides and total cholesterol [11]. However, the concurrent rise in total cholesterol warrants further investigation, as it could indicate a shift in lipid metabolism rather than an overall improvement in lipid homeostasis.

This study demonstrates that orally administered CBD reduces blood glucose levels in diabetic rats by inhibiting hepatic glucose production, showing effects comparable to but shorter-lasting than metformin. These findings suggest potential therapeutic benefits for humans. CBD oil could offer advantages as an antidiabetic treatment due to its excellent safety profile and lack of liver toxicity, with human trials indicating that doses up to 1500 mg per day are well tolerated [12,68]. However, individual responses to CBD may vary, potentially leading to inconsistent effects [69].

A significant drawback of CBD is its interaction with liver enzymes, particularly those in the cytochrome P450 system, which plays a key role in drug metabolism [70]. CBD inhibits CYP2C9 and CYP3A4, enzymes responsible for metabolizing many drugs, including antidiabetic medications such as sulfonylureas and metformin [68,71]. While CBD oil shows promise as an adjunct therapy for diabetes [8], further research is needed to evaluate the effects of chronic CBD use and the potential for drug interactions before it can be widely recommended for diabetic patients.

4. Materials and Methods

4.1. Animals and Tissue Procedures

For the experimental purposes, male Wistar rats (3–4 months old with a body weight of 250–300 g) were used. The animals were fed with standard laboratory chow and given water ad libitum. A total of 112 rats were used, consisting of 64 rats for the OGTT experiment (8 rats per group across 8 groups) and 48 rats for the multiple-dose experiment in the streptozotocin-induced diabetes experiment (8 rats per group across 6 groups).

During the whole experimental period, they were housed under a 12-hour light regime (6 a.m.–6 p.m. light). The animals were always sacrificed at the same time of the day (9–10 a.m.), with a standard laparotomic procedure, after induction of anesthesia with Na-thiopental narcosis (45 mg/kg), given by the guide of the EC Directive 86/609/EEC.

All experiments were performed in accordance with the current ethical norms approved by the Animal Ethics Committee of the University "Ss. Cyril and Methodius", Skopje, R. North Macedonia (License number 10-409/6 from 10-03-2024), following the Directive 2010/63/EU for the protection of animals used for scientific purposes of the European Commission.

4.2. Treatment of Animals

A commercially available 20% CBD oil, suspended in olive oil (Replek Farm Ltd., Skopje, North Macedonia), was purchased from a local pharmacy and used in this study. As a reference antidiabetic agent (positive control), metformin hydrochloride was used in the form of a secondary reference standard with a molecular weight of 165.62 g/mol and a purity of 99.89% (Alkaloid AD, Skopje, North Macedonia). Metformin was dissolved in distilled water and administered at a dose of 70 mg/kg body weight [72].

4.3. Oral Glucose Tolerance Test (OGTT)

To evaluate the hypoglycemic effect of CBD oil, an experiment was conducted using healthy male and female rats. The CBD oil used in the study was suspended in olive oil and administered in three doses: 0.5 mg/kg, 5 mg/kg, and 50 mg/kg. CBD oil treatments were applied using two different administration routes, intragastric (i.g.) and intraperitoneal (i.p.), to determine the more effective method of delivery.

The experiment aimed to assess glycemic regulation following a single administration of metformin or CBD oil at three different concentrations (0.5 mg/kg, 5 mg/kg, and 50 mg/kg). The rats were divided into eight experimental groups, 8 rats per group (n = 64), which are presented in Table 1.

Table 1. Groups of healthy rats included in the Oral Glucose Tolerance Test (OGTT) study divided according to the treatment regime.

Code	Treatment	Dose
C	Water	1 mL/100 g body weight
Met	Metformin	70 mg/kg body weight
CBD 0.5 i.g.	CBD oil extract	0.5 mg/kg
CBD 5 i.g.	CBD oil extract	5 mg/kg
CBD 50 i.g.	CBD oil extract	50 mg/kg
CBD 0.5 i.p.	CBD oil extract	0.5 mg/kg
CBD 5 i.p.	CBD oil extract	5 mg/kg
CBD 50 i.p.	CBD oil extract	50 mg/kg

Glycemia was measured in all experimental groups using a glucometer, with blood samples collected from the tail vein immediately before CBD oil administration. Thirty minutes after treatment, all animals received a glucose solution (2 g/kg body weight) via an intragastric tube [73,74]. Blood glucose levels were subsequently measured at 0, 15, 30, 60, 90, and 120 min after glucose administration in the same animals at each time-point. Blood samples were taken from the tail with great care to minimize stress and ensure accuracy in glucose readings. Six hours prior to treatment, food was withheld from all experimental groups, and animals remained fasted throughout the measurement period, while water was available ad libitum [75].

4.4. Multiple-Dose Study in Streptozotocin-Induced Diabetic Rats

Streptozotocin (STZ)-induced diabetes was established by a single intraperitoneal injection of STZ (45 mg/kg body weight), freshly dissolved in 0.1 M citrate buffer (pH 4.5) [75]. For experimental purposes, only animals that exhibited clear diabetic symptoms (fasting blood glucose levels above 15 mmol/L) 24–48 h after diabetes induction were included in the study [14,75].

To investigate the effect of an 8-day treatment with different doses of CBD, the rats were randomly divided into the following groups, with 8 rats per group (n = 48), as presented in Table 2.

Table 2. Groups of rats included in the multiple-dose study divided according to the treatment regime.

Code	Type of Rats	Treatment	Dose
C	Normal control	Water	1 mL/100 g body weight
D	Diabetic control	Olive oil	1 mL/100 g body weight
Met	Diabetic rats	Metformin	70 mg/kg body weight
CBD25	Diabetic rats	CBD oil extract	25 mg/kg body weight
CBD50	Diabetic rats	CBD oil extract	50 mg/kg body weight
CBD100	Diabetic rats	CBD oil extract	100 mg/kg body weight

All treatments were administered once daily to 8 h fasted rats (with water available ad libitum). After treatment, the rats were given free access to food and water. Fasting blood glucose was measured before treatment initiation using a glucometer, with blood samples collected from the tail vein. During the 8-day treatment period, blood glucose levels were also assessed on days 2 and 6 of the experiment at 0h (baseline) and at 1, 2, 4, and 8 h post-administration. At the end of the experiment, the rats were sacrificed, and blood samples were collected from the dorsal vein into serum and plasma separation tubes. After centrifugation, the resulting supernatant, designated as serum or plasma, was transferred into clean polypropylene tubes and stored at 2–8 °C until further analysis. The rats' livers were isolated, washed with a cold saline solution, and immediately immersed in liquid nitrogen. Tissue powder was prepared at liquid nitrogen temperature, and portions were kept at −80 °C. Before analysis, the tissue powder was homogenized with an ultrasonic homogenizer (Cole-Parmer Instrument-4710, USA/Illionis) for 7–10 s, maintaining a temperature of 0–4 °C (on ice) throughout the process.

4.5. Biochemical Analysis

Blood glucose was measured using the GOD method with a colorimetric kit (Human, Weisbaden, Germany). Plasma insulin levels were assessed using a commercially available enzyme-linked immunosorbent assay (ELISA) kit (Mercodia AB, Uppsala, Sweden). Additionally, serum levels of triglycerides (TAGs), total cholesterol (TC), and high-density lipoprotein (HDL) were evaluated using commercial enzymatic tests (Human, Germany).

4.6. Enzymes Activities and Substrates Concentration

All the enzymes' activities and substrates concentrations were measured in liver homogenates, prepared in appropriate homogenization media. Liver glycogen, glucose, and glucose-6-phosphate concentrations [76] were determined in perchlorate homogenates, neutralized with 5M K_2CO_3, by production of NADPH at 340 nm. The substrate concentration was expressed as µmol/g tissue. Glucose-6-phosphatase (E.C. 3.1.3.9) was assayed by the method of Hers [77], while the fructose-1,6-bisphosphatase (E.C. 3.1.3.11) activity was assayed using the method by Freedland and Harper [78]. The activity of liver glycogen phosphorylase *a* (E.C. 2.4.1.1) was determined by Stalmans et al. [79]. For determination of hexokinase (EC 2.7.1.1) activity [80], we measured the production of NADH at 340 nm. For the interpretation of enzyme activity as specific enzyme activity in the tissue extracts, the total quantity of the proteins was determined by Lowry et al. [81], by using bovine serum albumin as a standard. Enzyme activity was expressed as nmol Pi/min/mg protein. The amount of released inorganic phosphate was determined by Fiske and Subbarow [82].

4.7. Statistics

Results are presented as means ± SD. Normality of the data was assessed using the Shapiro–Wilk test. Since the data met the assumption of normality, one-way ANOVA with Tukey's post hoc test was used for comparisons between groups. Statistical analysis was performed using GraphPad Prism 9. A *p*-value of <0.05 was considered statistically significant.

5. Conclusions

This study provides promising evidence for the potential antihyperglycemic and antidiabetic effects of cannabidiol (CBD), highlighting its ability to modulate blood glucose and insulin levels in diabetic animal models. The findings suggest that CBD's efficacy may be dose-dependent and influenced by the route of administration, with intragastric administration at 50 mg/kg producing the most notable glucose-lowering effects. Interestingly, at this dose, CBD demonstrated greater short-term glycemic control compared to metformin; however, its effects appeared transient, whereas metformin maintained prolonged benefits. Mechanistically, CBD at 50 mg/kg was associated with the suppression of gluconeogenesis and glycogenolysis, likely through the inhibition of key enzymes such as glucose-6-phosphatase and fructose-1,6-bisphosphatase, leading to reduced hepatic glucose production. Nevertheless, higher doses (100 mg/kg) did not further enhance these metabolic effects.

While these findings provide valuable insights into CBD's metabolic effects, further research is required to fully elucidate its long-term efficacy and mechanisms of action, particularly in chronic treatment models. Future studies should also explore potential molecular targets and signaling pathways to better understand the role of CBD in glucose homeostasis.

Author Contributions: Conceptualization, E.R. and B.M.; methodology, E.R., B.M. and G.S.; formal analysis, E.X.; investigation, E.R. and E.X.; resources, G.S. and L.S.; data curation, Z.N.; writing—original draft preparation, E.R., E.X., Z.N., O.G., B.M., L.S. and G.S.; writing—review and editing, E.R. and B.M.; visualization, O.G.; supervision, L.S.; project administration, G.S. and B.M. All authors have read and agreed to the published version of the manuscript.

Funding: This research received no external funding.

Institutional Review Board Statement: The animal study protocol was approved by the Institutional Animal Ethics Committee of the University "Ss. Cyril and Methodius", Skopje, R. North Macedonia (License number 10-409/6 from 10-03-2024), following the Directive 2010/63/EU for the protection of animals used for scientific purposes of the European Commission.

Informed Consent Statement: Not applicable.

Data Availability Statement: The original contributions presented in this study are included in the article. Further inquiries can be directed to the corresponding author.

Acknowledgments: The authors wish to thank Elena Mirova for her assistance with English proofreading and her technical support during the manuscript preparation process.

Conflicts of Interest: The authors declare no conflicts of interest.

References

1. Bielawiec, P.; Harasim-Symbor, E.; Chabowski, A. Phytocannabinoids: Useful Drugs for the Treatment of Obesity? Special Focus on Cannabidiol. *Front. Endocrinol.* **2020**, *11*, 114. [CrossRef] [PubMed]
2. Pertwee, R.G. Cannabinoid Pharmacology: The First 66 Years. *Br. J. Pharmacol.* **2006**, *147*, S163–S171. [CrossRef] [PubMed]
3. Montoya-Alatriste, C.A.; Alarcón-Aguilar, F.J. Cannabis and Cannabinoids as an Alternative Remedy in Metabolic Syndrome. *Braz. J. Pharm. Sci.* **2022**, *58*, e20161. [CrossRef]
4. Devsi, A.; Kiyota, B.; Ouellette, T.; Hegle, A.P.; Rivera-Acevedo, R.E.; Wong, J.; Dong, Y.; Pugsley, M.K.; Fung, T. A Pharmacological Characterization of *Cannabis sativa* Chemovar Extracts. *J. Cannabis Res.* **2020**, *2*, 17. [CrossRef]
5. Wiciński, M.; Fajkiel-Madajczyk, A.; Kurant, Z.; Gryczka, K.; Kurant, D.; Szambelan, M.; Malinowski, B.; Falkowski, M.; Zabrzyński, J.; Słupski, M. The Use of Cannabidiol in Metabolic Syndrome—An Opportunity to Improve the Patient's Health or Much Ado about Nothing? *J. Clin. Med.* **2023**, *12*, 4620. [CrossRef]

6. Bilbao, A.; Spanagel, R. Medical Cannabinoids: A Pharmacology-Based Systematic Review and Meta-Analysis for All Relevant Medical Indications. *BMC Med.* **2022**, *20*, 259. [CrossRef]
7. National Academies of Sciences, Engineering, and Medicine. *The Health Effects of Cannabis and Cannabinoids: The Current State of Evidence and Recommendations for Research*; The National Academies Press: Washington, DC, USA, 2017.
8. Zhang, J.S.; Lin, C.; Jiang, S.; Wang, H.; Wang, Y.; Du, X.; Hutchinson, M.R.; Zhao, H.; Fang, L.; Wang, X. The Pharmacology and Therapeutic Role of Cannabidiol in Diabetes. *Exploration* **2023**, *3*, 20230047. [CrossRef]
9. CBD & Diabetes | American Diabetes Association. Available online: https://diabetes.org/health-wellness/cbd-and-diabetes (accessed on 6 April 2024).
10. Vieira, R.; Souto, S.B.; Sánchez-López, E.; Machado, A.L.; Severino, P.; Jose, S.; Santini, A.; Fortuna, A.; García, M.L.; Silva, A.M.; et al. Sugar-Lowering Drugs for Type 2 Diabetes Mellitus and Metabolic Syndrome—Review of Classical and New Compounds: Part-I. *Pharmaceuticals* **2019**, *12*, 152. [CrossRef]
11. Afshar, S.; Khalili, S.; Amin, G.; Abbasinazari, M. A Phase I Randomized, Double-Blind, Placebo-Controlled Study on Efficacy and Safety Profile of a Sublingually Administered Cannabidiol /Delta 9-Tetrahydrocannabidiol (10: 1) Regimen in Diabetes Type 2 Patients. *Iran. J. Pharm. Res.* **2023**, *21*, e132647. [CrossRef]
12. Kaufmann, R.; Aqua, K.; Lombardo, J.; Lee, M. Observed Impact of Long-Term Consumption of Oral Cannabidiol on Liver Function in Healthy Adults. *Cannabis Cannabinoid Res.* **2023**, *8*, 148–154. [CrossRef]
13. Silvestri, C.; Paris, D.; Martella, A.; Melck, D.; Guadagnino, I.; Cawthorne, M.; Motta, A.; Di Marzo, V. Two Non-Psychoactive Cannabinoids Reduce Intracellular Lipid Levels and Inhibit Hepatosteatosis. *J. Hepatol.* **2015**, *62*, 1382–1390. [CrossRef] [PubMed]
14. Chaves, Y.C.; Genaro, K.; Crippa, J.A.; da Cunha, J.M.; Zanoveli, J.M. Cannabidiol Induces Antidepressant and Anxiolytic-like Effects in Experimental Type-1 Diabetic Animals by Multiple Sites of Action. *Metab. Brain Dis.* **2021**, *36*, 639–652. [CrossRef] [PubMed]
15. Ma, H.; Li, H.; Liu, C.; Seeram, N.P. Evaluation of Cannabidiol's Inhibitory Effect on Alpha-Glucosidase and Its Stability in Simulated Gastric and Intestinal Fluids. *J. Cannabis Res.* **2021**, *3*, 20. [CrossRef]
16. Weiss, L.; Zeira, M.; Reich, S.; Har-Noy, M.; Mechoulam, R.; Slavin, S.; Gallily, R. Cannabidiol Lowers Incidence of Diabetes in Non-Obese Diabetic Mice. *Autoimmunity* **2006**, *39*, 143–151. [CrossRef]
17. Molehin, O.R.; Fakayode, A.E.; Olaoye, A.B.; Teibo, J.O.; Adeola, O.A. Biochemical Pathways Involved in Diabetes Mellitus. In *Biochemical Immunology of Diabetes and Associated Complications*; Tripathi, P., Tripathi, R.P., Kaushik, M.P., Eds.; Academic Press: New York, NY, USA, 2024.
18. Raddatz, D.; Ramadori, G. Carbohydrate Metabolism and the Liver: Actual Aspects from Physiology and Disease. *Z. Gastroenterol.* **2007**, *45*, 51–62. [CrossRef]
19. Cherkasova, V.; Ilnytskyy, Y.; Kovalchuk, O.; Kovalchuk, I. Transcriptome Analysis of Cisplatin, Cannabidiol, and Intermittent Serum Starvation Alone and in Various Combinations on Colorectal Cancer Cells. *Int. J. Mol. Sci.* **2023**, *24*, 14743. [CrossRef] [PubMed]
20. Jadoon, K.A.; Ratcliffe, S.H.; Barrett, D.A.; Thomas, E.L.; Stott, C.; Bell, J.D.; O'Sullivan, S.E.; Tan, G.D. Efficacy and Safety of Cannabidiol and Tetrahydrocannabivarin on Glycemic and Lipid Parameters in Patients with Type 2 Diabetes: A Randomized, Double-Blind, Placebo-Controlled, Parallel Group Pilot Study. *Diabetes Care* **2016**, *39*, 1777–1786. [CrossRef]
21. Kajero, J.A.; Seedat, S.; Ohaeri, J.; Akindele, A.; Aina, O. Investigation of the Effects of Cannabidiol on Vacuous Chewing Movements, Locomotion, Oxidative Stress and Blood Glucose in Rats Treated with Oral Haloperidol. *World J. Biol. Psychiatry* **2020**, *21*, 612–626. [CrossRef]
22. Kajero, J.A.; Seedat, S.; Ohaeri, J.U.; Akindele, A.J.; Aina, O. Effects of Cannabidiol on Vacuous Chewing Movements, Plasma Glucose and Oxidative Stress Indices in Rats Administered High Dose Risperidone. *Sci. Rep.* **2022**, *12*, 19718. [CrossRef]
23. de Morais, H.; Chaves, Y.C.; Waltrick, A.P.F.; Jesus, C.H.A.; Genaro, K.; Crippa, J.A.; da Cunha, J.M.; Zanoveli, J.M. Sub-Chronic Treatment with Cannabidiol but Not with URB597 Induced a Mild Antidepressant-like Effect in Diabetic Rats. *Neurosci. Lett.* **2018**, *682*, 62–68. [CrossRef]
24. Ten Ham, M.; De Yong, Y. Effects of Δ9 Tetrahydrocannabinol and Cannabidiol on Blood Glucose Concentrations in Rabbits and Rats. *Pharm. Weekbl.* **1975**, *110*, 1157–1161.
25. Reyes-Cuapio, E.; Coronado-Álvarez, A.; Quiroga, C.; Alcaraz-Silva, J.; Ruíz-Ruíz, J.C.; Imperatori, C.; Murillo-Rodríguez, E. Juvenile Cannabidiol Chronic Treatments Produce Robust Changes in Metabolic Markers in Adult Male Wistar Rats. *Eur. J. Pharmacol.* **2021**, *910*, 174463. [CrossRef] [PubMed]
26. Santiago, A.N.; Mori, M.A.; Guimarães, F.S.; Milani, H.; Weffort, M. Effects of Cannabidiol on Diabetes Outcomes and Chronic Cerebral Hypoperfusion Comorbidities in Middle-Aged Rats. *Neurotox. Res.* **2019**, *35*, 463–474. [CrossRef] [PubMed]
27. Zorzenon, M.R.T.; Santiago, A.N.; Mori, M.A.; Piovan, S.; Jansen, C.A.; Perina Padilha, M.E.; Ciotta, S.R.; Cezar de Freitas Mathias, P.; Guimarães, F.S.; Weffort de Oliveira, R.M.; et al. Cannabidiol Improves Metabolic Dysfunction in Middle-Aged Diabetic Rats Submitted to a Chronic Cerebral Hypoperfusion. *Chem. Biol. Interact.* **2019**, *312*, 108819. [CrossRef]

28. Chaves, Y.C.; Genaro, K.; Stern, C.A.; de Oliveira Guaita, G.; de Souza Crippa, J.A.; da Cunha, J.M.; Zanoveli, J.M. Two-Weeks Treatment with Cannabidiol Improves Biophysical and Behavioral Deficits Associated with Experimental Type-1 Diabetes. *Neurosci. Lett.* **2020**, *729*, 135020. [CrossRef]
29. Lucas, C.J.; Galettis, P.; Schneider, J. The Pharmacokinetics and the Pharmacodynamics of Cannabinoids. *Br. J. Clin. Pharmacol.* **2018**, *84*, 2477–2482. [CrossRef]
30. Bardhi, K.; Coates, S.; Watson, C.J.W.; Lazarus, P. Cannabinoids and Drug Metabolizing Enzymes: Potential for Drug-Drug Interactions and Implications for Drug Safety and Efficacy. *Expert Rev. Clin. Pharmacol.* **2022**, *15*, 1443–1460. [CrossRef]
31. Ahmed, S.A.; Ross, S.A.; Slade, D.; Radwan, M.M.; Khan, I.A.; ElSohly, M.A. Minor Oxygenated Cannabinoids from High Potency *Cannabis sativa* L. *Phytochemistry* **2015**, *117*, 194–199. [CrossRef]
32. Rock, E.M.; Parker, L.A. Constituents of *Cannabis sativa*. In *Cannabinoids and Neuropsychiatric Disorders*; Murillo-Rodriguez, E., Pandi-Perumal, S.R., Monti, J.M., Eds.; Springer International Publishing: Cham, Switzerland, 2021; pp. 1–13.
33. Jones, P.G.; Falvello, L.; Kennard, O.; Sheldrick, G.M.; Mechoulam, R. Cannabidiol. *Acta Crystallogr. Sect. B* **1977**, *33*, 3211–3214. [CrossRef]
34. Taylor, L.; Gidal, B.; Blakey, G.; Tayo, B.; Morrison, G. A Phase I, Randomized, Double-Blind, Placebo-Controlled, Single Ascending Dose, Multiple Dose, and Food Effect Trial of the Safety, Tolerability and Pharmacokinetics of Highly Purified Cannabidiol in Healthy Subjects. *CNS Drugs* **2018**, *32*, 1053–1067. [CrossRef]
35. Charytoniuk, T.; Sztolsztener, K.; Harasim-Symbor, E.; Berk, K.; Chabowski, A.; Konstantynowicz-Nowicka, K. Cannabidiol—A Phytocannabinoid That Widely Affects Sphingolipid Metabolism under Conditions of Brain Insulin Resistance. *Biomed. Pharmacother.* **2021**, *142*, 112057. [CrossRef] [PubMed]
36. Berk, K.; Konstantynowicz-Nowicka, K.; Charytoniuk, T.; Harasim-Symbor, E.; Chabowski, A. Distinct Effects of Cannabidiol on Sphingolipid Metabolism in Subcutaneous and Visceral Adipose Tissues Derived from High-Fat-Diet-Fed Male Wistar Rats. *Int. J. Mol. Sci.* **2022**, *23*, 5382. [CrossRef] [PubMed]
37. Linares, I.M.; Zuardi, A.W.; Pereira, L.C.; Queiroz, R.H.; Mechoulam, R.; Guimarães, F.S.; Crippa, J.A. Cannabidiol Presents an Inverted U-Shaped Dose-Response Curve in a Simulated Public Speaking Test. *Braz. J. Psychiatry* **2019**, *41*, 9–14. [CrossRef] [PubMed]
38. Deiana, S.; Watanabe, A.; Yamasaki, Y.; Amada, N.; Arthur, M.; Fleming, S.; Woodcock, H.; Dorward, P.; Pigliacampo, B.; Close, S.; et al. Plasma and Brain Pharmacokinetic Profile of Cannabidiol (CBD), Cannabidivarine (CBDV), Δ9-Tetrahydrocannabivarin (THCV) and Cannabigerol (CBG) in Rats and Mice Following Oral and Intraperitoneal Administration and CBD Action on Obsessive–Compulsive Behaviour. *Psychopharmacology* **2011**, *219*, 859–873.
39. Cinar, R.; Iyer, M.R.; Kunos, G. The Therapeutic Potential of Second and Third Generation CB1R Antagonists. *Pharmacol. Ther.* **2020**, *208*, 107477. [CrossRef]
40. Laprairie, R.B.; Bagher, A.M.; Kelly, M.E.M.; Denovan-Wright, E.M. Cannabidiol Is a Negative Allosteric Modulator of the Cannabinoid CB1Receptor. *Br. J. Pharmacol.* **2015**, *172*, 4790–4805. [CrossRef]
41. De Petrocellis, L.; Ligresti, A.; Moriello, A.S.; Allarà, M.; Bisogno, T.; Petrosino, S.; Stott, C.G.; Di Marzo, V. Effects of Cannabinoids and Cannabinoid-EnrichedCannabisextracts on TRP Channels and Endocannabinoid Metabolic Enzymes. *Br. J. Pharmacol.* **2011**, *163*, 1479–1494. [CrossRef]
42. Colsoul, B.; Nilius, B.; Vennekens, R. Transient Receptor Potential (TRP) Cation Channels in Diabetes. *Curr. Top. Med. Chem.* **2013**, *13*, 258–269. [CrossRef]
43. Szallasi, A.; Di Marzo, V. New Perspectives on Enigmatic Vanilloid Receptors. *Trends Neurosci.* **2000**, *23*, 491–497. [CrossRef]
44. Viollet, B.; Guigas, B.; Garcia, N.S.; Leclerc, J.; Foretz, M.; Andreelli, F. Cellular and Molecular Mechanisms of Metformin: An Overview. *Clin. Sci.* **2011**, *122*, 253–270. [CrossRef]
45. Zhu, H.; Jia, Z.; Li, Y.R.; Danelisen, I. Molecular Mechanisms of Action of Metformin: Latest Advances and Therapeutic Implications. *Clin. Exp. Med.* **2023**, *23*, 2941–2951. [CrossRef] [PubMed]
46. Ehud, Z.; Lola, W.; Itamar, R.; Natan, P.; Zhanna, Y.; Ruth, G. Islet Protection and Amelioration of Diabetes Type 2 in Psammomys Obesus by Treatment with Cannabidiol. *J. Diabetes Mellit.* **2012**, *2*, 27–34. [CrossRef]
47. McGrath, S.; Bartner, L.R.; Rao, S.; Packer, R.A.; Gustafson, D.L. Randomized Blinded Controlled Clinical Trial to Assess the Effect of Oral Cannabidiol Administration in Addition to Conventional Antiepileptic Treatment on Seizure Frequency in Dogs with Intractable Idiopathic Epilepsy. *J. Am. Vet. Med. Assoc.* **2019**, *254*, 1301–1308. [CrossRef]
48. Jiang, S.; Young, J.; Wang, K.; Qian, Y.; Cai, L. Diabetic-Induced Alterations in Hepatic Glucose and Lipid Metabolism: The Role of Type 1 and Type 2 Diabetes Mellitus (Review). *Mol. Med. Rep.* **2020**, *22*, 603–611. [CrossRef]
49. Agius, L. Glucokinase and Molecular Aspects of Liver Glycogen Metabolism. *Biochem. J.* **2008**, *414*, 1–18. [CrossRef]
50. Rines, A.K.; Sharabi, K.; Tavares, C.D.J.; Puigserver, P. Targeting Hepatic Glucose Output in the Treatment of Type 2 Diabetes. *Nat. Rev. Drug Discov.* **2016**, *15*, 786–804. [CrossRef]
51. Sharabi, K.; Tavares, C.D.J.; Rines, A.K.; Puigserver, P. Molecular Pathophysiology of Hepatic Glucose Production. *Mol. Asp. Med.* **2015**, *46*, 21–33. [CrossRef]

52. Halse, R.; Bonavaud, S.M.; Armstrong, J.L.; McCormack, J.G.; Yeaman, S.J. Control of Glycogen Synthesis by Glucose, Glycogen, and Insulin in Cultured Human Muscle Cells. *Diabetes* **2001**, *50*, 720–726. [CrossRef]
53. Agius, L. Role of Glycogen Phosphorylase in Liver Glycogen Metabolism. *Mol. Asp. Med.* **2015**, *46*, 34–45. [CrossRef]
54. Rajas, F.; Gautier-Stein, A.; Mithieux, G. Glucose-6 Phosphate, a Central Hub for Liver Carbohydrate Metabolism. *Metabolites* **2019**, *9*, 282. [CrossRef]
55. Wajngot, A.; Chandramouli, V.; Schumann, W.C.; Ekberg, K.; Jones, P.K.; Efendic, S.; Landau, B.R. Quantitative Contributions of Gluconeogenesis to Glucose Production during Fasting in Type 2 Diabetes Mellitus. *Metabolism* **2001**, *50*, 47–52. [CrossRef] [PubMed]
56. Roden, M.; Bernroider, E. Hepatic Glucose Metabolism in Humans—Its Role in Health and Disease. *Best Pract. Res. Clin. Endocrinol. Metab.* **2003**, *17*, 365–383. [CrossRef] [PubMed]
57. Erukainure, O.L.; Matsabisa, M.G.; Salau, V.F.; Olofinsan, K.A.; Oyedemi, S.O.; Chukwuma, C.I.; Nde, A.L.; Islam, M.S. Cannabidiol Improves Glucose Utilization and Modulates Glucose-Induced Dysmetabolic Activities in Isolated Rats' Peripheral Adipose Tissues. *Biomed. Pharmacother.* **2022**, *149*, 112863. [CrossRef]
58. Sargsyan, A.; Herman, M.A. Regulation of Glucose Production in the Pathogenesis of Type 2 Diabetes. *Curr. Diabetes Rep.* **2019**, *19*, 22. [CrossRef] [PubMed]
59. Pastorino, J.G.; Hoek, J.B. Hexokinase II: The Integration of Energy Metabolism and Control of Apoptosis. *Curr. Med. Chem.* **2003**, *10*, 1535–1551. [CrossRef]
60. Mahmoud, A.M.; Kostrzewa, M.K.; Marolda, V.; Cerasuolo, M.; Maccarinelli, F.; Coltrini, D.; Rezzola, S.; Giacomini, A.; Mollica, M.P.; Motta, A.; et al. Cannabidiol Alters Mitochondrial Bioenergetics via VDAC1 and Triggers Cell Death in Hormone-Refractory Prostate Cancer. *Pharmacol. Res.* **2023**, *189*, 106683. [CrossRef]
61. Minassian, C.; Tarpin, S.; Mithieux, G. Role of Glucose-6 Phosphatase, Glucokinase, and Glucose-6 Phosphate in Liver Insulin Resistance and Its Correction by Metformin. *Biochem. Pharmacol.* **1998**, *55*, 1213–1219. [CrossRef]
62. Rabbani, N.; Xue, M.; Thornalley, P.J. Hexokinase-2-Linked Glycolytic Overload and Unscheduled Glycolysis—Driver of Insulin Resistance and Development of Vascular Complications of Diabetes. *Int. J. Mol. Sci.* **2022**, *23*, 2165. [CrossRef]
63. Villar-Palasí, C.; Guinovart, J.J. The Role of Glucose 6-Phosphate in the Control of Glycogen Synthase. *FASEB J.* **1997**, *11*, 544–558. [CrossRef]
64. Rena, G.; Hardie, D.G.; Pearson, E.R. The Mechanisms of Action of Metformin. *Diabetologia* **2017**, *60*, 1577–1585. [CrossRef]
65. Zhang, D.; Fu, M.; Gao, S.-H.; Liu, J.-L. Curcumin and Diabetes: A Systematic Review. *Evid.-Based Complement. Altern. Med.* **2013**, *2013*, 636053. [CrossRef] [PubMed]
66. Xie, W.; Su, F.; Wang, G.; Peng, Z.; Xu, Y.; Zhang, Y.; Xu, N.; Hou, K.; Hu, Z.; Chen, Y.; et al. Glucose-Lowering Effect of Berberine on Type 2 Diabetes: A Systematic Review and Meta-Analysis. *Front. Pharmacol.* **2022**, *13*, 1015045. [CrossRef] [PubMed]
67. Stanley, C.P.; Wheal, A.J.; Randall, M.D.; O'Sullivan, S.E. Cannabinoids Alter Endothelial Function in the Zucker Rat Model of Type 2 Diabetes. *Eur. J. Pharmacol.* **2013**, *720*, 376–382. [CrossRef] [PubMed]
68. Grotenhermen, F.; Müller-Vahl, K. Cannabis Und Cannabinoide in Der Medizin: Fakten Und Ausblick. *Suchttherapie* **2016**, *17*, 71–76. [CrossRef]
69. Iffland, K.; Grotenhermen, F. An Update on Safety and Side Effects of Cannabidiol: A Review of Clinical Data and Relevant Animal Studies. *Cannabis Cannabinoid Res.* **2017**, *2*, 139–154. [CrossRef]
70. Pelkonen, O.; Turpeinen, M.; Hakkola, J.; Honkakoski, P.; Hukkanen, J.; Raunio, H. Inhibition and Induction of Human Cytochrome P450 Enzymes: Current Status. *Arch. Toxicol.* **2008**, *82*, 667–715. [CrossRef]
71. Ujváry, I.; Hanuš, L. Human Metabolites of Cannabidiol: A Review on Their Formation, Biological Activity, and Relevance in Therapy. *Cannabis Cannabinoid Res.* **2016**, *1*, 90–101. [CrossRef]
72. Zhang, Y.; Zhou, F.; Guan, J.; Zhou, L.; Chen, B. Action Mechanism of Metformin and Its Application in Hematological Malignancy Treatments: A Review. *Biomolecules* **2023**, *13*, 250. [CrossRef]
73. Nakakaawa, L.; Gbala, I.D.; Bargul, J.L.; Cheseto, X.; Wesonga, J.M. Therapeutic Potential of Brassica Carinata Microgreens Extract in Alleviating Symptoms of Type 2 Diabetes in Wistar Rats. *Food Sci. Nutr.* **2025**, *13*, e4635. [CrossRef]
74. Igbayilola, Y.D.; Gujja, M.G. Alpha-Amylase and Alpha-Glucosidase Upregulated Glucose Homeostasis in High-Fat Fed Wistar Rats Supplemented with Cocoa Flavonoid-Rich Aqueous. *Food Biosci.* **2024**, *59*, 104070. [CrossRef]
75. Furman, B.L. Streptozotocin-Induced Diabetic Models in Mice and Rats. *Curr. Protoc.* **2021**, *1*, e78. [CrossRef] [PubMed]
76. Keppler, D.; Decker, K. Glycogen Determination with Amyloglucosidase. In *Methods of Enzymatic Analysis*; Academic Press: New York, NY, USA, 1974; pp. 1127–1131.
77. Hers, H.G. Glycogen Storage Disease. In *Advances in Metabolic Disorders*; Levine, R., Luft, R., Eds.; Academic Press: New York, NY, USA, 1959; pp. 36–85.
78. Freedland, R.A.; Harper, A.E. Metabolic Adaptations in Higher Animals. The Study of Metabolic Pathways by Means of Metabolic Adaptations. *J. Biol. Chem.* **1959**, *234*, 1350–1354. [CrossRef] [PubMed]

79. Stalmans, W.; Wulf, H.D.; Hue, L.; Hers, H.-G. The Sequential Inactivation of Glycogen Phosphorylase and Activation of Glycogen Synthetase in Liver after the Administration of Glucose to Mice and Rats. *Eur. J. Biochem.* **1974**, *41*, 127–134. [CrossRef] [PubMed]
80. Bontemps, F.; Hue, L.; Hers, H.-G. Phosphorylation of Glucose in Isolated Rat Hepatocytes. Sigmoidal Kinetics Explained by the Activity of Glucokinase Alone. *Biochem. J.* **1978**, *174*, 603–611. [CrossRef]
81. Lowry, O.H.; Rosenbrough, N.J.; Farr, A.L.; Randall, R.J. Protein Measurement with the Folin Phenol Reagent. *J. Biol. Chem.* **1951**, *193*, 265–275. [CrossRef]
82. Fiske, C.H.; Subbarow, Y. The Colorimetric Determination of Phosphorus. *J. Biol. Chem.* **1978**, *66*, 357–400. [CrossRef]

pharmaceuticals

MDPI

Article

Synergistic Efficacy of Policosanol (Raydel®) and Banaba Leaf Extract to Treat Hyperglycemia and Dyslipidemia in Streptozotocin-Induced Diabetic and Hyperlipidemic Zebrafish (*Danio rerio*): Protection of Liver and Kidney with Enhanced Tissue Regeneration

Kyung-Hyun Cho *, Sang Hyuk Lee, Yunki Lee, Ashutosh Bahuguna and Ji-Eun Kim

Raydel Research Institute, Medical Innovation Complex, Daegu 41061, Republic of Korea
* Correspondence: chok@raydel.co.kr; Tel.: +82-53-964-1990; Fax: +82-53-965-1992

Abstract: Background: The efficacy of banaba leaf extract was tested against carboxymethyllysine (CML)-induced toxicity in embryos and adult zebrafish. Additionally, the individual and combined effects of banaba (BNB) and policosanol (PCO) were analyzed to alleviate dyslipidemia, hyperglycemia, and associated effects in streptozotocin (STZ)-induced hyperlipidemic diabetic zebrafish. **Methodology:** The high cholesterol diet (HCD, final 4%, w/w)-fed zebrafish were injected with STZ to develop diabetes and were subsequently fed with either HCD or HCD+BNB (final 0.1% w/w) or HCD+PCO (final 0.1% w/w) or HCD+BNB+PCO (each final 0.1%, w/w) each for 14 days. The zebrafish tail fin was amputated to assess tissue regeneration, while the organs and blood were collected for histological and biochemical analysis. **Results:** Severely compromised embryo survivability and developmental defects were noticed in the CML-injected group that significantly improved following BNB exposure. Similarly, CML-induced acute paralysis and mortality of adult zebrafish were effectively mitigated by the treatment with BNB. In the hyperlipidemic diabetic zebrafish, both BNB and PCO supplementation displayed the hypoglycemic effect; however, a remarkable reduction ($p < 0.05$) in blood glucose levels was observed in the BNB+PCO group, around 14% and 16% less than the BNB group and PCO group, respectively. Likewise, higher tail fin regeneration was noticed in response to BNB+PCO supplementation. Both BNB and PCO have a substantial counter-effect against HCD+STZ-induced dyslipidemia. However, the combined supplementation (BNB+PCO) displayed a significantly better effect than that of BNB and PCO alone to alleviate total cholesterol (TC), triglycerides (TGs), and low-density lipoprotein cholesterol (LDL-C). The most impressive impact of BNB+PCO was noticed in the elevation of high-density lipoprotein cholesterol (HDL-C), which was ~1.5 times higher than the HDL-C level in response to BNB and PCO. Also, BNB+PCO effectively reduced the malondialdehyde (MDA) and elevated the plasma sulfhydryl content, paraoxonase (PON), and ferric ion reduction (FRA) activity. Histological analyses revealed a significant effect of BNB+PCO in preventing inflammatory infiltration, fatty liver changes, and interleukin-6 production. Similarly, a notably better effect of BNB+PCO compared to their individual effect was noticed in preventing kidney damage and mitigation of ROS generation, apoptosis, and cellular senescence. **Conclusions:** The finding establishes the substantial effect of BNB and PCO in countering hyperglycemia, dyslipidemia, and associated disorders, which synergistically improved following the combined supplementation with BNB+PCO.

Keywords: banaba; diabetes; policosanol; hyperglycemia; fatty liver; oxidative stress; inflammation; senescence; tissue regeneration

1. Introduction

Diabetes is a metabolic disease characterized by hyperglycemia which is spreading across the globe, with the alarming rate reflected by 463 million diabetic patients in 2019, predicted to reach over 700 million by 2045 [1,2]. The sedentary lifestyle, poor nutrition, obesity, smoking, and aging are among the important factors contributing to the onset of diabetes [3,4]. Type 2 diabetes is the most predominant form of diabetes, arising from the combination of insulin resistance and impaired insulin secretion due to the dysfunction of pancreatic β-cells [5]. Diabetes has a detrimental effect on multiple organs, leading to a morbid state like retinopathy, vasculopathy, neuropathy, nephropathy, and cardiovascular diseases [6]. Patients with diabetes are prone to coronary artery disease, myocardial infarction, and cardiovascular diseases compared to non-diabetic individuals [7]. It has been reported that about 12% of diabetic individuals present with diabetic cardiomyopathy attributed to myocardial fibrosis and myocellular hypertrophy and are at a higher risk of heart failure [7,8]. In addition, a substantial adverse effect of diabetes has been noticed with respect to the induction of fatty liver disease, liver fibrosis, and cirrhosis [6].

The hyperglycemic environment exacerbates hepatocyte damage in fatty liver disease and, consequently, augments the morbidity and mortality of diabetic patients [6,9]. Furthermore, diabetes adversely affects the normal tissue regeneration process, leading to varied complications such as diabetic foot ulcers [10]. The elevated glycemic condition also leads to the production of a variety of advanced glycation end-products (AGE) [11] such as carboxymethyllysine (CML) (chronic wound+CML). The elevated AGE upregulates the receptor for advanced glycation end-product (RAGE) expression in the pancreatic β-cells and the AGE-RAGE interaction induces nuclear factor-kB (NF-kB) signaling, leading to the intense inflammation and programmed cell death that ultimately affect the pancreatic β-cells [11].

Insulin resistance and hyperglycemia substantially elevate blood pressure and provoke dyslipidemia [2], highlighted by elevated blood total cholesterol (TC), triglycerides (TGs), low-density lipoproteins (LDL-C), and decreased high-density lipoproteins (HDL-C) levels, thereby amplifying the risk of cardiovascular complications associated with diabetes [7]. There are many synthetic drugs of different classes used to prevent diabetes and dyslipidemia. However, the toxicity associated with their long-term consumption is always a matter of concern [12] and highlights the significance of natural compounds in therapeutic applications [12]. Natural compounds and alternative therapies are gaining attention owing to their affordability and safety over conventional pharmaceutical treatments [12]. Furthermore, when used in combination with established therapies, natural compounds have demonstrated substantial potential in effectively managing the advanced stage of type 2 diabetes [12,13]. Several natural compounds and extracts have been explored as an alternative therapy to mitigate diabetes [12] and dyslipidemia [14].

Among the natural compounds, policosanol, which is a typical mixture of long-chain aliphatic alcohols (LCAA), has gained huge attention due to its diverse functionality including antiglycation and tissue regeneration activity [15,16]. However, the prominent effect of policosanol has been observed to counter dyslipidemia [17] and hypertension [18]. Several preclinical and clinical studies have documented the impactful role of policosanol in reducing TC, TGs, and LDL-C levels as well as augmenting HDL-C levels [17,19] via the inhibitory impact on the cholesterylester transfer protein (CETP) [16,20]. Also, policosanol prevents LDL oxidation, augments the cholesterol efflux ability, and boosts the HDL-C functionality through the activity enhancement of HDL-associated paraoxonase (PON)-1 [21]. In a comparative study, policosanol displayed a better effect than lovastatin (a conventional statin drug) on the elevation of HDL-C levels and reduced the LDL/HDL ratio in human subjects of type 2 diabetes and hypercholesterolemia [22]. The effect of policosanol in preventing CML (an important AGE)-induced toxicity has been described [18], indicating that policosanol may ameliorate the hyperglycemic-induced events.

Banaba (*Lagerstroemia speciosa*), a perennial medicinal plant from the Lythraceae family, is widely cultivated across South Asian countries and has long been utilized in traditional medicine for its therapeutic properties [23]. The reports highlight the analgesic, antimicrobial, anti-obesity, antioxidant, anti-inflammatory, antifibrotic, and antihypertensive properties of banaba leaves [24]. However, banaba leaves and their important phytoconstituents, e.g., corosolic acid [23], have been extensively studied for antidiabetic properties by improving glucose metabolism, insulin secretion, insulin sensitization/resistance, and inhibition of enzymes like α-amylase and α-glucosidase [23,25]. Several studies have observed the impactful role of banaba and corosolic acid in decreasing the blood glucose levels in genetically diabetic and chemically induced diabetic animals [23]. Corosolic acid exerts its antidiabetic effects by regulating insulin receptor substrate-1 (IRS-1), protein kinase B (Akt), and liver kinase B1 (LkB1), thereby mitigating adenosine monophosphate-activated protein kinase (AMPK) activation to alleviate insulin resistance [26]. Also, IRS-1 modulates phosphoinositide 3-kinase (PI3K), facilitating Akt/mTOR pathway activation, which influences the translocation of glucose transporter type 4 (GLUT4) and leads to the absorption of glucose [26]. Furthermore, corosolic acid reduces cyclic adenosine 3′,5′-monophosphate (cAMP) levels and inhibits protein kinase A activity, leading to decreased fructose-2,6 diphosphate and suppression of gluconeogenesis [23,26]. Despite several beneficial effects, the banaba has not been probed for diabetic tissue regeneration and AGE-triggered toxicity.

Given banaba substantial antidiabetic properties and the established efficacy of policosanol in managing dyslipidemia, we hypothesize that their combination might effectively mitigate the chronic complications of diabetes and hyperlipidemia. Concerning this, the present study investigates the effect of banaba on CML-induced toxicity in embryos and adult zebrafish (*Danio rerio*). Additionally, the comparative tissue regeneration effect of banaba and policosanol alone or in combination (banaba+policosanol) is assessed on streptozotocin (STZ) and high cholesterol diet (HCD)-induced diabetic and hyperlipidemic zebrafish. Furthermore, the effect of these treatments on the blood oxidative and antioxidant variables, lipid profiles, and liver and kidney functionality of diabetic hyperlipidemic zebrafish are evaluated.

2. Results

2.1. Zebrafish Embryo Protective Effect of Banaba

Figure 1A illustrates that survivability was significantly influenced by time ($F = 2130.1$, $p < 0.001$), treatment type ($F = 3237.9$, $p < 0.001$), and their interaction ($F = 292.6$, $p < 0.001$), indicating the influence of both factors on survivability. The survivability of zebrafish embryos was severely compromised in the CML-injected group. A periodic sharp decline in the survivability of embryos was observed in the CML-injected group, starting from 57% 5 h post injection, reaching 12% 24 h post injection, and, finally, ending with a mere 4% survivability 72 h post injection (Figure 1A). In contrast, banaba co-injection at both concentrations (5 ng and 10 ng) effectively protected the embryos from the CML-triggered mortality. The 5 ng and 10 ng banaba-treated groups showed a 61% and a 65% embryo survivability 72 h post injection, a level which was 15.2 ($p < 0.001$) and 16.2 ($p < 0.001$) times higher than the survivability of embryos observed in the CML-injected group.

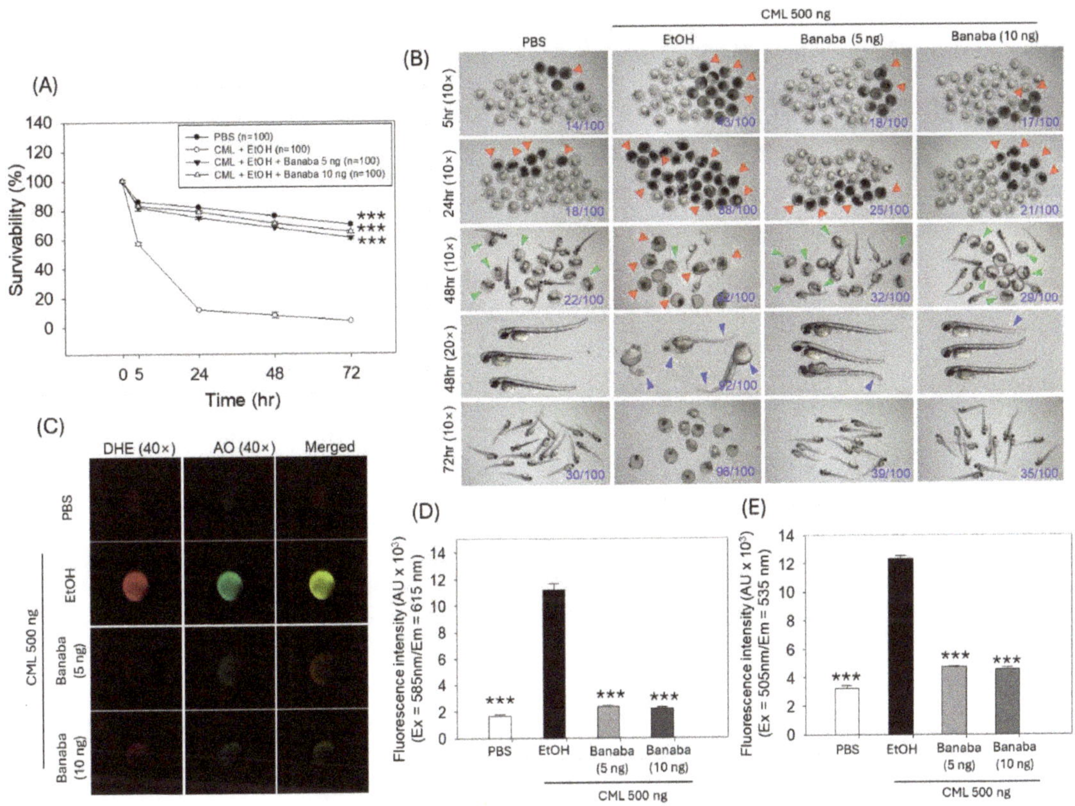

Figure 1. Effect of banaba leaf extract against carboxymethyllysine (CML)-induced toxicity in zebrafish embryos (n = 100). (**A**) The embryo survivability kinetics at two different concentrations (5 ng or 10 ng banaba/embryo). The symbol *** ($p < 0.001$) indicates the statistical significance of the difference between groups vs. EtOH+CML-injected group as determined by a two-way ANOVA, followed by Tukey's post-hoc analysis. (**B**) Pictorial representation of zebrafish embryos among the different groups 5 h to 72 h post injection. Blue numerical values inside the images represent the number of dead embryos/total embryos (n = 100). The red arrowhead highlights the dead embryos, the green arrowhead represents the unhatched embryos 48 h post injection, and the blue arrowhead underscores the developmental deformities. (**C**) Dihydroethidium (DHE) and acridine orange (AO) fluorescent imaging of the embryos. (**D**,**E**) Quantification of DHE and AO fluorescence intensity using the Image J software. Abbreviations: PBS (phosphate buffered saline), EtOH (ethanol), CML (carboxymethyllysine). The symbol *** signifies the statistical difference at $p < 0.001$ vs. EtOH+CML-injected group.

The morphological analysis revealed severe developmental defects (indicated by the blue arrow) and delayed embryo hatching (indicated by the green arrow) in response to CML injection (Figure 1B). At 48 h post injection, only 10% hatching was observed among the embryos who survived in the CML-injected group, such a percentage increasing to 23.3% and 30% when CML was co-injected with 5 ng and 10 ng of banaba extract, respectively. Notably, most of the surviving embryos appeared to have severe developmental deformities (indicated by the blue arrow) concerning the tail fin curvature, the yolk sac, and the pericardial edema in the CML-injected group. In contrast, CML-induced developmental defects were prevented by the injection of banaba. However, the occasional tail fin curvature and yolk sac edema were noticed in the banaba-treated groups.

DHE and AO staining revealed massive ROS production and apoptosis in the embryos exposed to CML. The CML-induced ROS and apoptosis in the embryos were significantly protected by the co-injection of 5 ng and 10 ng of banaba extract. As depicted in Figure 1C–E, a ~five-fold ($p < 0.001$) and ~2.5-fold ($p < 0.001$) decrease in DHE and AO fluorescence intensity was quantified in the banaba extract (5 ng and 10 ng) group compared to the CML-injected groups, attesting a substantial effect of the banaba extract to ameliorate the CML-induced toxicity promoted by ROS-mediated apoptotic embryo death.

2.2. Banaba Mitigates CML-Induced Paralysis and Mortality in Adult Zebrafish

The statistical outcomes derived from the two-way ANOVA, as depicted in Figure 2A,B, demonstrate that treatment type (F = 202.9, $p < 0.001$ and F = 533.1, $p < 0.001$), time (F = 68.8, $p < 0.001$ and F = 135.4, $p < 0.001$), and their interactions (F = 19.9, $p < 0.001$ and F = 38.2, $p < 0.001$) significantly influenced zebrafish survivability and swimming recovery. These findings highlight the impact of both treatment conditions and time in determining zebrafish survivability and swimming recovery. In the PBS-injected group, a 96.7% survivability was observed 90 min post injection. In contrast, the severe impact of the CML injection on zebrafish survivability was noticed (Figure 2A), where survivability declined to 43.3% 30 min post injection and eventually reached 23.4% 90 min post injection. Contrary to this, the co-injection of banaba effectively prevented CML-induced mortality, reflected by a 63.3% and 56.7% survivability 60 and 90 min post injection that was ~2.4 times ($p < 0.001$) higher than the survivability observed in the CML-injected group at the respective time.

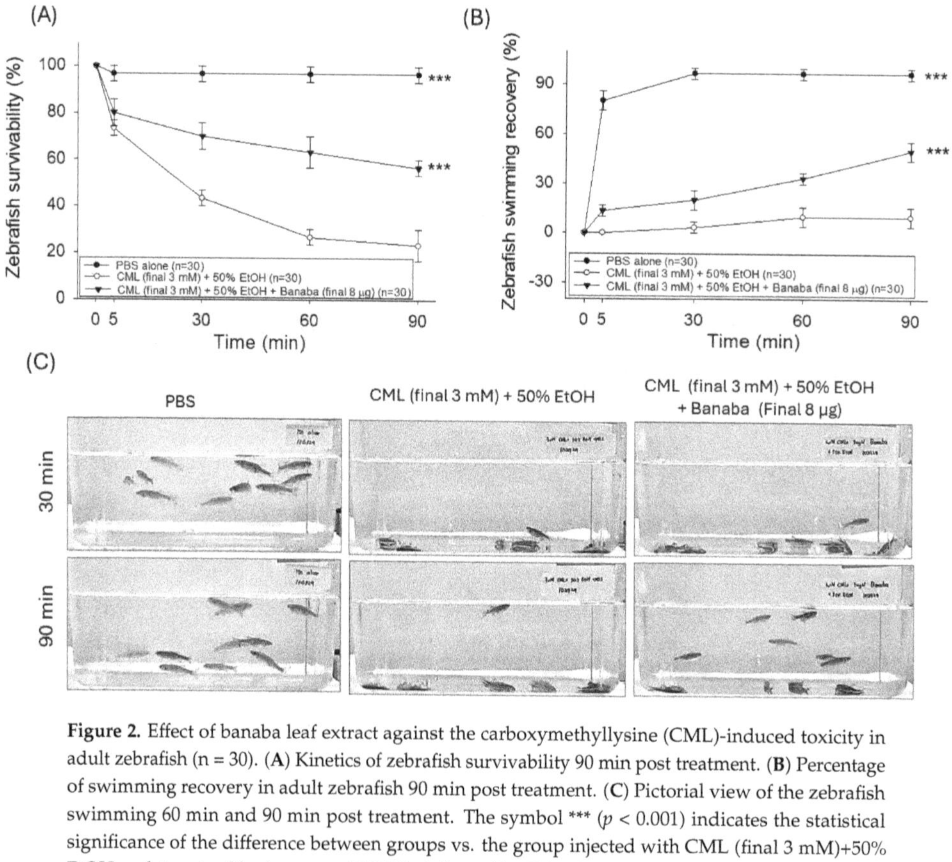

Figure 2. Effect of banaba leaf extract against the carboxymethyllysine (CML)-induced toxicity in adult zebrafish (n = 30). (**A**) Kinetics of zebrafish survivability 90 min post treatment. (**B**) Percentage of swimming recovery in adult zebrafish 90 min post treatment. (**C**) Pictorial view of the zebrafish swimming 60 min and 90 min post treatment. The symbol *** ($p < 0.001$) indicates the statistical significance of the difference between groups vs. the group injected with CML (final 3 mM)+50% EtOH as determined by two-way ANOVA, followed by Tukey's post-hoc analysis.

A severe paralytic effect of the CML injection was noticed in the zebrafish. As reflected in Figure 2B,C, all the zebrafish were lying at the bottom of the tanks without any sign of movement 30 min post injection in the CML-injected group, contrary to 96.7% of the zebrafish swimming in the PBS-injected group. With the progression of time (at 90 min), a slight recovery was observed, with 10.0% of the zebrafish swimming in the CML-injected groups. In contrast, the banaba extract effectively reverted the CML-provoked paralysis, as reflected by the 20% and 50% restoration of zebrafish swimming behavior, values that are approximately three times and five times ($p < 0.001$) higher than the zebrafish swimming activity noticed in the CML-injected group 30 and 90 min post injection.

2.3. Banaba Extract Augmented CML-Impaired Plasma Antioxidant Variables

An elevated MDA level was quantified in the plasma of the CML-injected group which was 2.2 times ($p < 0.01$) higher than the basal level detected in the PBS-injected group (Figure 3A). In response to the injection of banaba, a significant 32.8% ($p < 0.05$) reduction in the MDA level was observed compared to the CML-injected group.

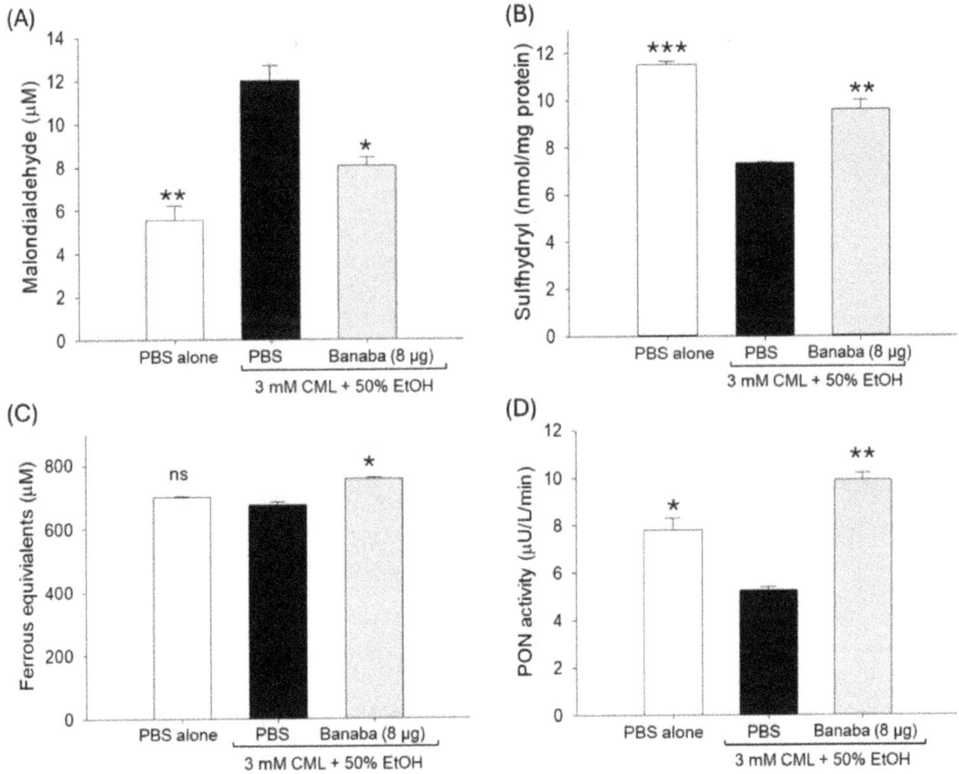

Figure 3. The plasma antioxidant status of adult zebrafish injected with carboxymethyllysine (CML) with or without the banaba leaf extract. (**A**) Quantification of the lipid peroxidation assessed by thiobarbituric acid reactive substance (TBARS) assay using malondialdehyde (MDA) as the standard. (**B**) Ferric ion reduction assay (FRA). (**C**) Sulfhydryl content quantification. (**D**) Paraoxonase (PON) activity assay. Each analysis was performed using triplicate experiments with duplicate samples, resulting in a total of six replicates (n = 6). * ($p < 0.01$), ** ($p < 0.01$), and *** ($p < 0.001$) displayed the statistical difference between the groups with respect to the group injected with 3 mM CML+50% EtOH; ns represents a non-significant ($p > 0.05$) difference.

The plasma sulfhydryl content was significantly reduced, by a factor of 1.6, in the CML-injected group compared to the basal level as detected in the PBS group (Figure 3B). The CML-diminished sulfhydryl content experienced a significant increase of 31.1% ($p < 0.01$) following the injection of banaba, attesting to the positive effect of the banaba extract on the plasma sulfhydryl content. Likewise, reduced plasma ferric ion reduction ability (FRA) (Figure 3C) and paraoxonase (PON) activity (Figure 3D) were noticed in the CML-injected group, such a decrease turning into a significant increase of 12.4% ($p < 0.05$) and 78.1% ($p < 0.01$), respectively, in the banaba-injected group. The combined results underline the effective role of the banaba extract in improving plasma oxidative and antioxidant variables.

2.4. Banaba and Policosanol Improved STZ-Impaired Tail Fin Regeneration

The amputated tail fin regenerative effect of banaba and policosanol alone or in combination was assessed in a time-dependent manner under the influence of diabetic hyperlipidemic conditions induced by HCD+STZ (Figure 4A,B). The statistical outcomes (two-way ANOVA), as depicted in Figure 4B, reveal that time ($F = 122.7$, $p < 0.001$), treatments ($F = 268.8$, $p < 0.001$), and their interactions ($F = 13.7$, $p < 0.001$) had a significant effect on the amputated tail fin generation, attesting the importance of both time and treatments on tail fin regeneration. The smallest degree of tail fin regeneration (9.5 ± 0.3 mm^2) was observed in the HCD+STZ group, with values 1.8 times ($p < 0.001$) lower than the tissue regenerative area (16.6 ± 0.8 mm^2) observed in the HCD group after 14 days, underscoring the adverse effect of STZ on the tail fin regeneration. The consumption of banaba and policosanol had a substantial curative impact on the STZ-impaired tissue regeneration, reflected by a 40.1% (13.3 ± 0.4 mm^2, $p < 0.001$) and 34.2% (12.7 ± 0.3 mm^2, $p < 0.001$) higher regenerated tissue area compared to that in the HCD+STZ group (9.5 ± 0.3 mm^2) after 14 days. The combined effect of banaba and policosanol (BNB+PCO) showed the most promising outcome, evident through a significant 54.6% (14.7 ± 0.3 mm^2, $p < 0.001$) higher tissue regeneration compared to that in the HCD+STZ group and a significant 15% and 10% increase in tail fin regeneration compared to the effect observed in the banaba only and policosanol only groups, respectively. Notably, the frequent presence of tissue fissures (Figure 4A, indicated by the blue arrows) was observed in the regenerated tail fin of the HCD+STZ group, such fissures completely disappearing in the banaba, policosanol, and banaba+policosanol groups, strengthening the significant tissue regenerative effect of banaba and policosanol alone or in combination against the STZ-posed adversity.

2.5. Banaba and Policosanol Displayed a Hypoglycemic Effect

An elevated blood glucose level (81.8 ± 3.6 mg/dL) was observed in the STZ-injected group which was 1.7 times ($p < 0.001$) higher than the basal glucose level (48.7 ± 2.0 mg/dL) detected in the HCD group (Figure 4C). The STZ-induced elevated blood glucose level was significantly reduced to 21.0% and 18.8% following the consumption of banaba (64.8 ± 1.6 mg/dL, $p < 0.01$) and policosanol (66.4 ± 2.5 mg/dL, $p < 0.01$). The combination of banaba+policosanol emerged with the lowest glucose level (56.1 ± 1.9 mg/dL) that was, notably, 32% ($p < 0.001$) lower than the glucose level quantified in the STZ-injected group and 14% ($p < 0.05$) and 16% ($p < 0.05$) lower than the individual effect of banana and policosanol, respectively.

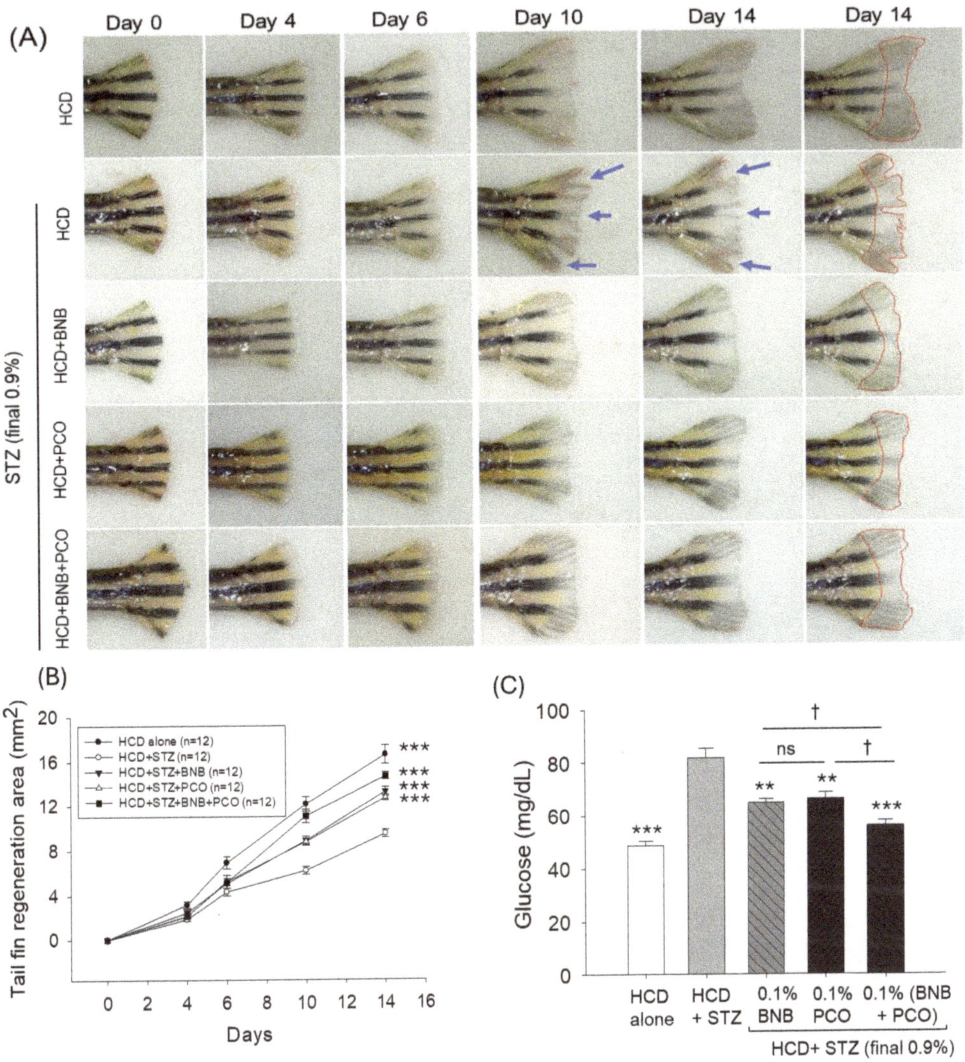

Figure 4. Effect of banaba leaf extract and policosanol (alone or in combination) supplementation on the tail fin regeneration and blood glucose level of the hyperlipidemic zebrafish injected with streptozotocin (n = 12). (**A**) Pictorial view of amputated tail fin regeneration (tissue regeneration) after 14 days. The blue arrow indicates the tail fissure, while the red line depicts the regenerated tail fin area after 14 days. (**B**) A time-dependent (0–14 days) tail fin regenerated area was observed among the different treatment groups. The symbol *** ($p < 0.001$) indicates the statistical significance of the difference between groups vs the group injected with EtOH+CML, as determined by the two-way ANOVA, followed by Tukey's post-hoc analysis. (**C**) The blood glucose level was examined after 14 days. Abbreviations: HCD (high cholesterol diet), STZ (streptozotocin), BNB (banaba), and PCO (policosanol). The symbols **, and *** underline the statistical significance at $p < 0.01$, and 0.001, respectively, vs. the HCD+STZ group. † indicate statistical significance at $p < 0.05$ in relation to the BNB+PCO group; ns represents a non-significant ($p > 0.05$) difference.

2.6. Blood Lipid Profile

The total cholesterol (TC, 272.2 ± 18.4 mg/dL), triglyceride (TG, 49.2 ± 7.2 mg/dL), high-density lipoprotein cholesterol (HDL-C, 19.2 ± 5.0 mg/dL), and low-density lipoprotein cholesterol (LDL-C, 243.3 ± 16.9 mg/dL) levels in the STZ-injected group non-significantly ($p > 0.05$) changed compared to the only HCD-consuming group (Figure 5A–D). The consumption of banaba and policosanol significantly diminished the HCD+STZ elevated blood TC, TG, and LDL-C levels. In contrast, banaba, in combination with policosanol (BNP+PCO), displayed a much stronger effect on the reduction of HCD+STZ-altered TC, TG, and LDL-C levels. Significantly lower levels of TC, by 34.2% (179.2 ± 12.6 mg/dL, $p < 0.01$), TGs, by 59.1% (20.1 ± 3.2 mg/dL, $p < 0.05$), and LDL-C, by 67.9% (77.9 ± 15.9 mg/dL, $p < 0.05$) were quantified in the BNB+PCO-consuming group compared to the HCD+STZ group. Both policosanol and banaba increased the HDL-C level by a factor of three ($p < 0.001$) compared to the HCD+STZ groups. However, the most notable effect of a 5.1-fold ($p < 0.001$) augmentation in the HDL-C level was observed as a result of the combination of banaba and policosanol compared to the HCD+STZ groups. Compared to policosanol and banaba supplementation, ~1.5 times ($p < 0.01$) higher HDL-C levels were observed in the BNP+PCO-consuming group.

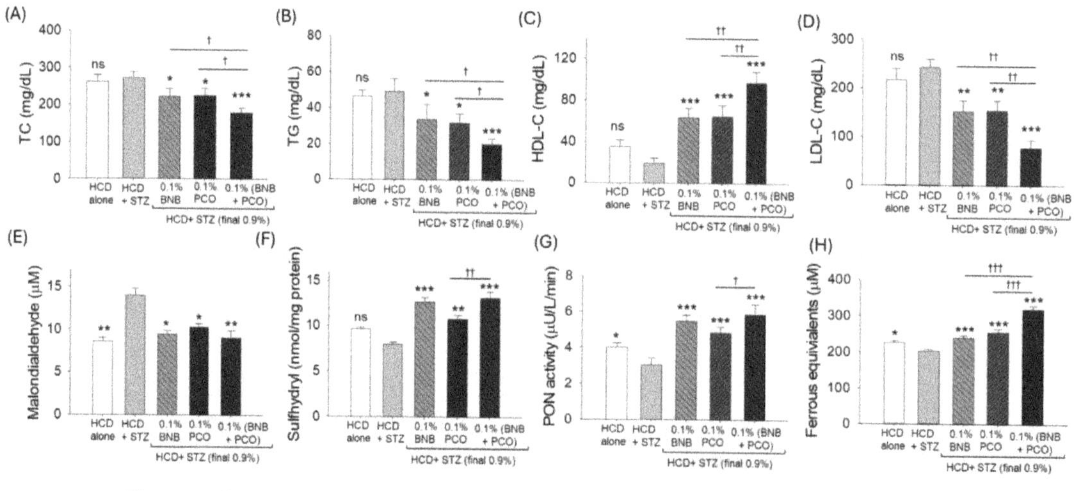

Figure 5. Effect of banaba leaf extract and policosanol (alone or in combination) on the lipoprotein profile and oxidative and antioxidant variables of plasma from the hyperlipidemic zebrafish treated with streptozotocin (n = 12). (**A**) Total cholesterol (TC), (**B**) triglycerides (TGs), (**C**) high-density lipoprotein cholesterol (HDL-C), (**D**) low-density lipoprotein cholesterol (LDL-C), (**E**) malondialdehyde (MDA), (**F**) sulfhydryl content, (**G**) paraoxonase (PON), and (**H**) ferric ion reduction (FRA) ability. Each analysis was performed using triplicate experiments with duplicate samples, resulting in a total of six replicates (n = 6). Abbreviations: HCD (high cholesterol diet), STZ (streptozotocin), BNB (banaba), and PCO (policosanol). The symbols *, **, and *** underline the statistical significance at $p < 0.05$, $p < 0.01$, and $p < 0.001$, respectively, vs. the HCD+STZ group. †, ††, and ††† indicate statistical significance at $p < 0.05$, $p < 0.01$, and 0.001 vs. the BNB+PCO group; ns represents a non-significant ($p > 0.05$) difference vs. the HCD+STZ group.

2.7. Effect of Banaba and Policosanol Consumption on Blood Antioxidant Status

A significant 1.6-fold increase in the MDA level was detected in the blood of individuals in the HCD+STZ group compared to the only HCD-consuming group, indicating the adverse effect of STZ on the plasma lipid peroxidation (Figure 5E). Consumption of policosanol and banaba alone or in combination significantly reduced HCD+STZ-induced MDA levels by 32.8% ($p < 0.05$), 26.7% ($p < 0.05$), and 35.7% ($p < 0.01$), respectively.

The HCD+STZ treatment substantially diminished the plasma sulfhydryl content, which was ~1.6 times ($p < 0.001$), 1.4 times ($p < 0.01$), and 1.6 times ($p < 0.001$) higher in response to the consumption of policosanol, banaba, and the combination of banaba and policosanol, respectively (Figure 5F).

A significant 10.5% reduction in FRA activity was observed in the blood of the HCD+STZ group compared to the HCD only group (Figure 5G). PON activity in the HCD+STZ group was increased by 18.6%, 24.4%, and 55.5% following the consumption of policosanol, banaba, and the combination of policosanol with banaba, respectively. Similarly to FRA activity, ~1.8 ($p < 0.05$), 1.5 ($p < 0.05$), and 1.8 times ($p < 0.001$) higher PON activity was observed in the plasma obtained from the groups consuming policosanol, banaba, and banaba+policosanol, respectively, compared to the HCD+STZ groups (Figure 5H).

The combined results reflect the fact that banaba and policosanol supplementation have a substantial protective effect against the HCD+STZ-induced oxidative effect and the restoration of plasma antioxidant status.

2.8. Hepatic Histology and Inflammation

The histology outcomes, as exemplified in Figure 6, display substantial hepatic degeneration and neutrophil infiltration in the HCD+STZ group. The HCD+STZ-induced hepatic changes were significantly prevented by the consumption of banaba and policosanol, as indicated by ~two-fold ($p < 0.05$) decrease in neutrophil counts compared to the HCD+STZ group. Compared to the individual supplementation with banaba or policosanol, the combination of both showed a significantly better hepatoprotective effect marked by a 3.7-fold ($p < 0.01$) and 1.6-fold ($p < 0.05$) decrease in neutrophil counts compared to that detected in the HCD+STZ group and in the policosanol- and banaba-consuming groups, respectively.

The IHC staining reflects the higher IL-6 production rate in the HCD+STZ group which accounts for 11.5% of the IL-6-stained area (Figure 6 C,D,G). In contrast to this, a reduced IL-6-stained area in the hepatic section of banaba- (6.5%) and policosanol-supplemented (6.3%) individuals was noticed that accounted for a ~1.8-fold ($p < 0.001$) reduction in the IL-6-stained area compared to that of the HCD+STZ group, indicating a substantial antiinflammatory effect of banaba and policosanol. Compared to the individual supplementation, the combined supplementation with banaba and policosanol displayed a higher reduction of IL-6 production, reflected by a 4.4% IL-6-stained area that was 2.6 times ($p < 0.001$) lower than the IL-6 production observed in the HCD+STZ group and ~1.5 times ($p < 0.001$) lower than the IL-6-stained area observed in the banaba- and policosanol-consuming groups.

The ORO staining revealed fatty liver changes indicated by a high lipid accumulation in the HCD+STZ-consuming group which was, notably, 1.4 times ($p < 0.001$) higher than the ORO-stained area of the only HCD-consuming group (Figure 6E,H). The HCD+STZ-provoked fatty liver changes were effectively curtailed by the consumption of banaba and policosanol, evident by a two-fold ($p < 0.001$) and a 1.8-fold ($p < 0.001$) decrease in lipid accumulation compared to the HCD+STZ group. However, the combined supplementation with banaba+policosanol showed a much stronger protective effect, reflected by a ~two-fold ($p < 0.001$) decrease in the ORO-stained area compared to the policosanol- and banaba-supplemented groups and a 3.6-fold ($p < 0.05$) decrease in the ORO-stained relative to the HCD+STZ group.

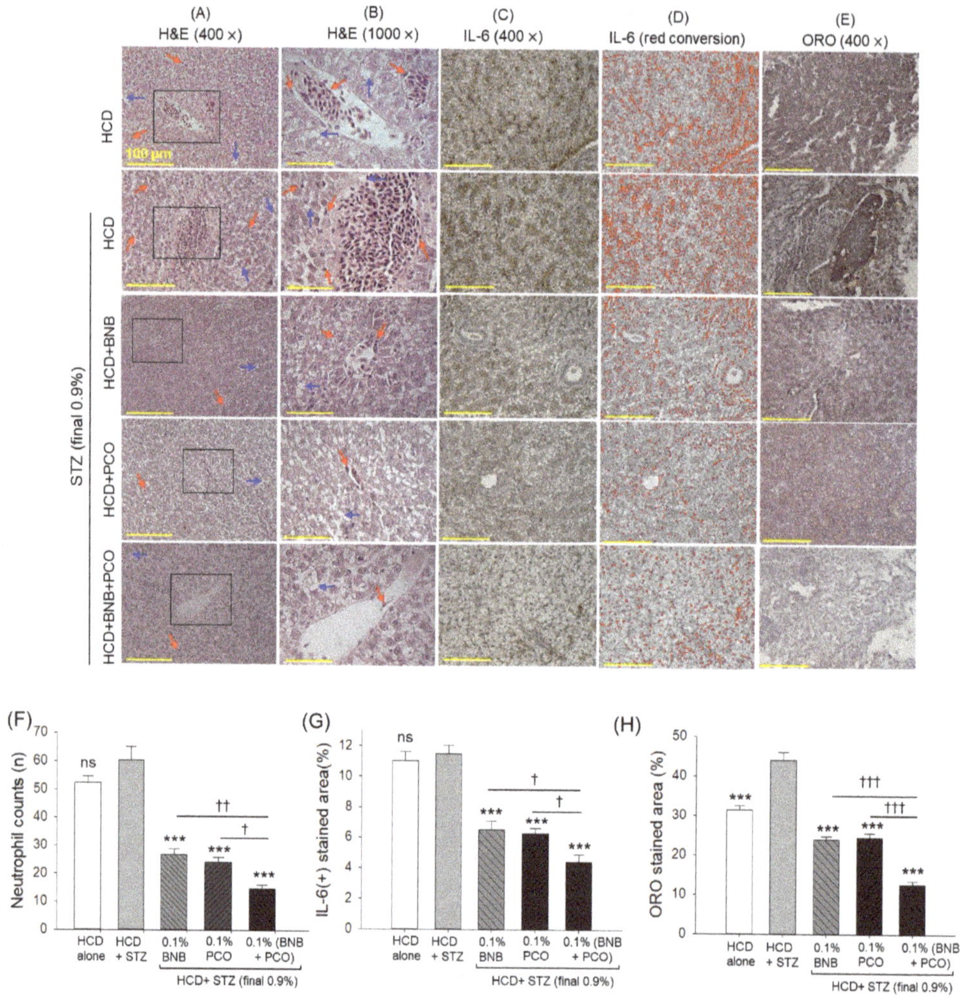

Figure 6. A comparative effect of banaba leaf extract and policosanol (alone or in combination) on the hepatic histology of the streptozotocin-treated hyperlipidemic zebrafish (n = 3). (**A**) Hematoxylin and eosin (H&E) staining (400× magnified): blue and red arrows highlight the infiltration of neutrophils and lipid droplets, respectively [100 μm, scale bar]. The H&E area in the black box is 1000× magnified and images (**B**) represent this magnified view. (**C**) Oil red O (ORO) staining. (**D**) Immunohistochemical (IHC) staining for the detection of interleukin (IL)-6. (**E**) Red conversion of the IL-6-stained area (brown color) using the Image J software with a brown color threshold value of 20–120; the red conversion was performed to improve the intensity of the IL-6-stained area. (**F**) Percentage neutrophil counts. A semiquantitative evaluation of neutrophils (stained with a dark purple color) was conducted through a microscopic analysis of a predefined region (1.23 mm^2) across three independent sections, with five distinct areas assessed per section. (**G**,**H**) illustrate the quantification of ORO and IL-6-stained areas, respectively. Abbreviations: HCD (high cholesterol diet), STZ (streptozotocin), BNB (banaba), and PCO (policosanol). The symbols *** underline the statistical significance at $p < 0.001$vs the HCD+STZ group. †, †† and ††† indicate statistical significance at $p < 0.05$, $p < 0.01$ and $p < 0.001$ vs. the BNB+PCO group; ns represents a non-significant ($p > 0.05$) difference.

2.9. ROS Production, Apoptosis, Senescence, and Hepatic Function Biomarkers

DHE staining revealed severe ROS production in the HCD+STZ group that was effectively reduced by a factor of 1.6 ($p < 0.001$) and 1.5 ($p < 0.001$) following the supplementation with banaba and policosanol (Figure 7A,D). Furthermore, a more beneficial effect with respect to the inhibition of ROS generation was observed in response to the combined supplementation with banaba and policosanol, evidenced by a significant 23.3% ($p < 0.01$) and 31.4% ($p < 0.01$) decrease in DHE fluorescence intensity compared to the banaba- and policosanol-supplemented groups, respectively.

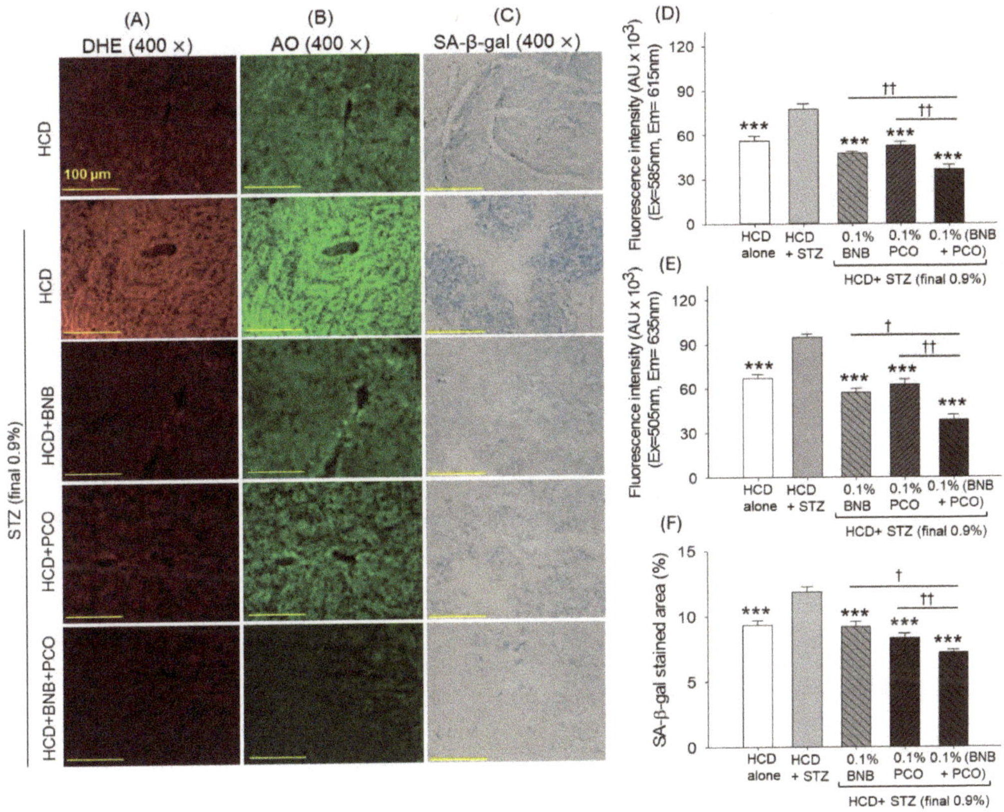

Figure 7. Effect of banaba leaf extract and policosanol (alone or in combination) on the reactive oxygen species (ROS), apoptosis, and senescence in the liver of the streptozotocin-treated hyperlipidemic zebrafish (n = 3). (**A**,**B**) dihydroethidium (DHE) and acridine orange (AO) fluorescent staining to determine ROS and apoptosis, respectively. (**C**) Senescence-associated β-galactosidase (SA-β-gal) staining. (**D**,**E**) Quantification of DHE and AO fluorescence intensity. (**F**) Percentage quantification of the SA-β-gal-positive area. Abbreviations: HCD (high cholesterol diet), STZ (streptozotocin), BNB (banaba), and PCO (policosanol). The symbol *** underlines the statistical significance at $p < 0.001$ vs. the HCD+STZ group. † and †† indicate statistical significance at $p < 0.05$ and $p < 0.01$ vs. the BNB+PCO group.

A similar trend was observed for apoptosis, where the HCD+STZ treatment induced a higher AO fluorescence intensity, which was effectively reduced by a factor of 1.6 ($p < 0.001$), 1.5 ($p < 0.001$), and 2.4 ($p < 0.001$) following the supplementation with policosanol, banaba, and the combination of banaba+policosanol, respectively (Figure 7B,E). Compared with the effect of banaba and policosanol alone, a 32.2% and a 37.7% decrease in AO fluorescence intensity was observed relative to the banaba+policosanol-supplemented group.

The SA-β-gal staining showed a higher abundance of senescent positive cells (%) in the HCD+STZ group that significantly ($p < 0.001$) decreased to 22.8%, 29.8%, and 38.9% following supplementation with banaba, policosanol, and the combination of banaba+policosanol, respectively (Figure 7C,F). By comparing policosanol, banaba, and their combination, the banaba+policosanol-supplemented group demonstrated a 21.7% and a 14.0% reduction in SA-β-gal-positive cells compared to the banaba and policosanol groups, respectively.

The STZ-induced increase in the blood hepatic function biomarkers AST and ALT substantially decreased following supplementation with banaba, policosanol, and their combination. A 17% and a 19% reduction in AST and a 27% and a 30% reduction in ALT levels were observed in the banaba- and policosanol-supplemented groups, respectively (Figure 8). Contrary to the individual supplementation, the combined supplementation with banaba+policosanol displayed the greatest reduction of AST and ALT levels, amounting to a 35% and a 44% reduction compared to the STZ-injected group.

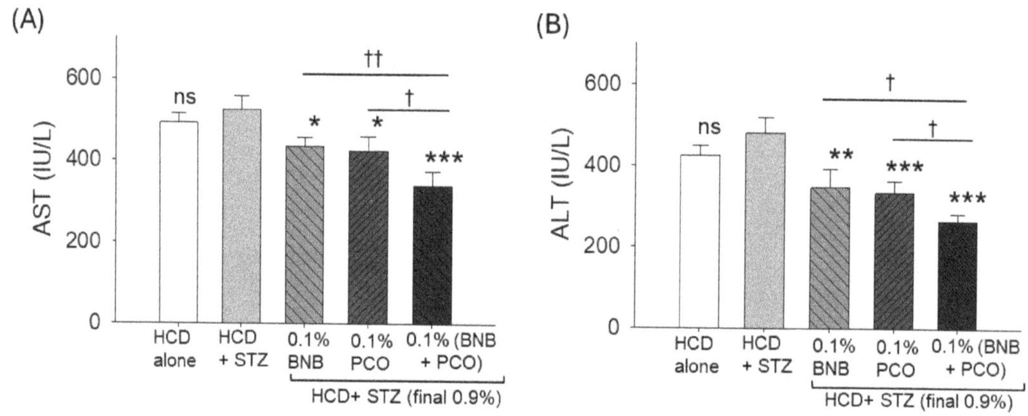

Figure 8. Effect of banaba leaf extract and policosanol (alone or in combination) on the blood hepatic function biomarkers in streptozotocin-treated hyperlipidemia zebrafish (n = 12). (**A**) Aspartate amino transferase (AST) and (**B**) alanine amino transferase (ALT). Each analysis was performed using triplicate experiments with duplicate samples, resulting in a total of six replicates (n = 6). Abbreviations: HCD (high cholesterol diet), STZ (streptozotocin), BNB (banaba), and PCO (policosanol). The symbols *, ** and *** underline the statistical significance at $p < 0.05$, $p < 0.01$ and $p < 0.001$, respectively, vs. the HCD+STZ group. † and †† indicate statistical significance at $p < 0.05$ and $p < 0.01$ vs. the BNB+PCO group; ns represents a non-significant ($p > 0.05$) difference.

2.10. Histological Analysis of the Kidney

As exemplified in Figure 9A, highly disorganized distal and proximal tubules with the frequent appearance of enlarged tubular lumen and luminal debris were noticed in the kidney section of the HCD+STZ group. The supplementation with banaba and policosanol effectively prevented the HCD+STZ-induced nephrotoxicity and restored the disturbed distal and proximal tubular arrangement; however, the occasional presence of increased luminal tubules with tubular debris was noticed. Conversely, the combined effect of banaba+policosanol supplementation prevented the HCD+STZ-triggered kidney damage, as shown by the regular distribution of proximal and distal tubules, which were mostly free from the cellular debris in the tubular cast.

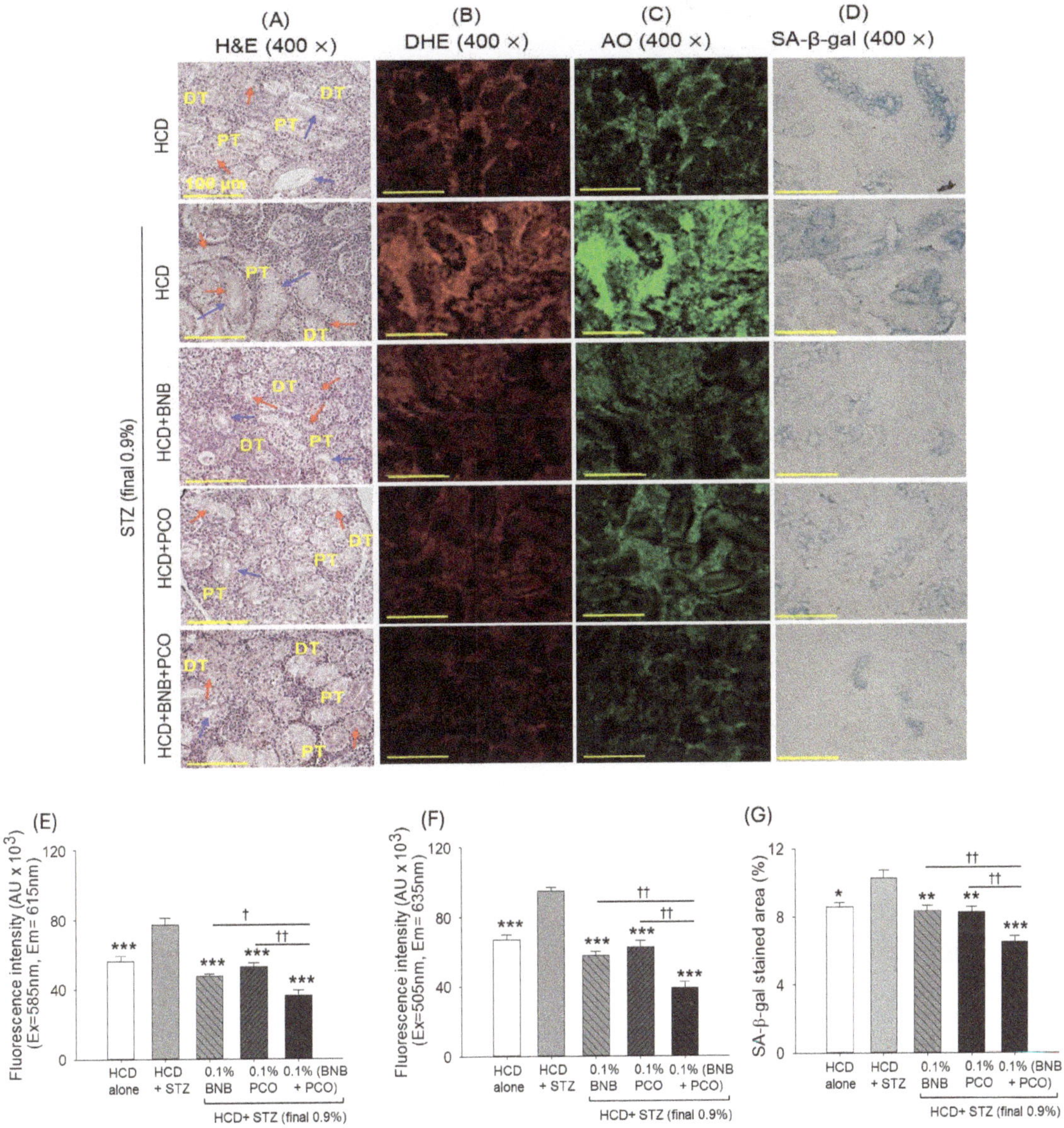

Figure 9. Effect of banaba leaf extract and policosanol (alone or in combination) on the kidney histology of the streptozotocin-treated hyperlipidemia zebrafish (n = 3). (**A**) Hematoxylin and eosin (H&E) staining. PT and DT represent the proximal and distal tubules; the blue and red arrows describe the enlarged tubular lumen and luminal debris. (**B**) Dihydroethidium (DHE) and (**C**) acridine orange (AO) fluorescent staining were used to determine ROS and apoptosis, respectively. (**D**) Senescence-associated β-galactosidase (SA-β-gal) staining. (**E**,**F**) illustrate the quantification of DHE and AO fluorescence intensity, respectively. (**G**) Percentage quantification of the SA-β-gal-positive area. Abbreviations: HCD (high cholesterol diet), STZ (streptozotocin), BNB (banaba), and PCO (policosanol). The symbols *, **, and *** underline the statistical significance at $p < 0.05$, $p < 0.01$, and $p < 0.001$, respectively, vs. the HCD+STZ group. † and †† indicate statistical significance at $p < 0.05$ and $p < 0.01$ vs. the BNB+PCO group.

The DHE (Figure 9B,E) and AO (Figure 9C,F) staining revealed the highest red and green color fluorescence intensity corresponding to the ROS production and apoptosis in the kidney section of the STZ+BNB group. The supplementation with both policosanol and banaba protected the kidney from excessive ROS generation and apoptosis, evidenced by a 39% and a 31.7% reduction in DHE and a 40.1% and a 33.9% reduction in AO fluorescence intensity in the banaba- and policosanol-consuming groups, respectively, compared to the STZ+BNB group. However, the combined supplementation with banaba+policosanol emerged as having a stronger impact, reflected by a 23.3% and a 31.1% reduction in DHE and a 33.3% and a 37.7% reduction in AO fluorescence intensity compared to the fluorescence intensities quantified in the policosanol- and banaba-consuming groups, respectively.

Similarly, the HCD+STZ-induced cellular senescence was prevented by the consumption of banaba and policosanol (Figure 9D,G). Contrary to the individual supplementation, the combined supplementation with banaba and policosanol displayed a ~22.9% ($p < 0.01$) reduction in senescence-positive cells compared to the banaba- and policosanol-supplemented groups and a 36.8% ($p < 0.01$) reduction in SA-β-gal-positive cells compared to the HCD+STZ group. The study outcome confirms the superior effect of the combination of banaba and policosanol over their individual effect to protect the HCD+STZ-induced nephrotoxicity.

3. Discussion

CML is a typical advanced glycation end-product (AGE) and is well recognized to induce several detrimental effects [27,28] through the induction of oxidative stress and inflammation. Similarly, we observed high ROS generation levels in the CML-injected embryos that led to the teratogenic effect and apoptotic cell death of the embryos. The CML-induced ROS generation and apoptosis were substantially inhibited by the exposure to banaba, consequently preventing developmental deformities and rescuing the embryos from CML-mediated death. Results endorsed by earlier studies document the strong antioxidant properties of banaba and its phytoconstituents that directly scavenge the free radicals [29] and modulate cellular antioxidants through the activation of Nrf-2 [30], an important signaling molecule that regulates the expression of antioxidants like superoxide dismutase (SOD), catalase, reduced glutathione (GSH), and glutathione S-transferase (GST) [31]. Not restricted to embryos, the severe CML-induced toxicity to adult zebrafish was substantially undermined by the exposure to banaba, highlighting the strong curative effect of banaba which can rescue the zebrafish from the CML-arrested swimming activity and CML-induced mortality. Probably, the strong antioxidant and anti-inflammatory action of banaba is behind the protection of adult zebrafish from CML-triggered paralysis. This postulation is supported by earlier findings describing an association between acute inflammation and paralytic disorders [32]. As the banaba plays a substantial role in curtailing the generation of proinflammatory IL-6 [24] and other inflammatory markers [24,33], it consequently rescues the zebrafish from the acute CML-imposed paralysis. This finding aligns with previous studies that have deciphered the effect of tocilizumab (an IL-6 inhibitor) on restoring zebrafish swimming ability impaired by the administration of CML [32].

MDA is an important lipid peroxidation marker that documents the status of oxidative stress [34]. Similarly, the plasma sulfhydryl content is an important stress marker [35,36], and its diminished level has been associated with a variety of disease conditions [37]. CML-impaired MDA levels and plasma sulfhydryl content are effectively restored by the exposure to banaba, attesting the protective effect of banaba on CML-induced oxidative stress. Consistently, the elevated plasma FRA and PON activity in response to banaba attests the significant role of banaba in boosting the antioxidant status and is consistent with the accumulating literature describing the impact of banaba on the antioxidant variables [24]. However, to the best of our knowledge, this is the first report describing the effect of banaba on PON functionality, an important antioxidant associated with HDL, a versatile molecule with a multifaceted role including antioxidant and anti-inflammatory properties [38]. The results of this study, performed on embryos and adult zebrafish, highlight the protective effect of banaba in alleviating CML-induced oxidative stress.

Encouraged by these promising findings, the study was expanded to evaluate the effects of banaba on hyperlipidemic and hyperglycemic (diabetic) conditions induced by HCD+STZ in zebrafish. Additionally, the efficacy of banaba was compared with that of policosanol and their combination to identify the most effective formulation for mitigating chronic pathological conditions in the hyperlipidemic diabetic zebrafish. Supplementation with HCD is an efficient way to cause dyslipidemia [39]; likewise, STZ-induced type 2 diabetes, achieved through the reduction of insulin secretion from the pancreatic β-cells and its impact on insulin resistance [40], leads to hyperglycemia and associated disorders in a variety of model organisms [41,42], including the zebrafish [43]. An elevated glucose level was detected in the HCD+STZ group, such an increase being substantially prevented through the consumption of banaba, policosanol, and the combination of banaba+policosanol, attesting the impact of these supplements in protecting the organisms from STZ-induced hyperglycemia. AMP-activated protein kinase (AMPK) and phosphatidylinositol 3-kinase/protein kinase B (PI3K/Akt) are important signaling pathways that influence insulin secretion and enhance insulin sensitization, thus playing a critical role in diminishing hyperglycemic conditions. Fortunately, policosanol has a positive impact on these pathways [44] and, thus, effectively controls STZ-induced hyperglycemia. Similarly, banaba has a notable effect on glucose metabolism and insulin sensitization [23], leading to hypoglycemic effects. The effect of corosolic acid (an important component of banaba) on the activation of the AMPK signaling pathway [26], protein kinase B (Akt), and insulin receptor substance (IRS)-I phosphorylation [26,45] has been recognized as an important event modulating the insulin signal transduction, thus having a hypoglycemic effect. In addition, corosolic acid plays a role in inhibiting α-glucosidase [26,46] and α-amylase [26] enzymatic activity, consequently affecting the post-prandial glucose level. Compared to the individual supplementation, the combination of banaba+policosanol exhibited a markedly enhanced hypoglycemic effect, potentially due to their synergistic interaction that modulates the protective molecular events effectively, leading to an improved glycemic control in the zebrafish subjected to HCD+STZ-induced hyperglycemia. Despite the numerous essential developmental processes, such as glucose metabolism, which are comparable to those observed in humans [47], zebrafish differ in many aspects, for example in their insulin regulation and pancreatic function not being identical to that of humans. Nonetheless, it is evident from the present preclinical findings that the BNB+PCO combination has a substantial protective effect against STZ-triggered diabetic conditions in hyperlipidemic zebrafish and may elicit a similar response to that of human subjects. However, a clinical study needs to be conducted to establish the efficacy of BNB+PCO in dealing with diabetic conditions in human subjects.

The effects of banaba and policosanol, both of which were substantially and synergistically improved by their combination, were noticed in relation to the amputated tail fin regeneration and glucose lowering effect under the chronic hyperlipidemic and diabetic conditions imposed by HCD+STZ in the zebrafish. There has been no study, so far, describing the effect of banaba on wound healing and tissue regeneration; however, some preliminary studies have documented the tissue regenerative effect of policosanol against CML-induced chronic wounds [15,16]. The substantially lower glucose level associated with the combination of banaba+policosanol compared to that associated with their individual supplementation is the key contributor to the better tail fin regeneration effect. The notion is in accordance with reports documenting high-glucose environments leading to intense inflammation and having an impact on the vascular endothelial growth factor tissue regeneration and delayed wound healing [48,49]. In addition, hyperglycemia led to the protein glycation resulting in the formation of the AGE product, which leads to ROS generation and elevated inflammation via the nuclear factor kappa-light-chain-enhancer of activated B cells (NFκB) and increases apoptosis in fibroblasts and keratinocytes, leading to the inhibition of tissue repair processes [50]. Beyond its hypoglycemic properties, banaba exhibits significant antioxidant and anti-inflammatory properties [24], while policosanol demonstrates a potent antiglycation effect and tissue regeneration effect [15,16]; together, these events work synergistically to ameliorate HCD+STZ-induced adversities, thereby prompting an enhanced tissue regeneration. The positive effect of corosolic acid (an important component of banaba) [51] and policosanol [17,18] has been noticed against dyslipidemia; similarly, we noticed a significant reduction in TC, TGs, and LDL-C in response to banaba and policosanol. Earlier, it has been described that hexacosanol (a major LCAA of policosanol) modulates the activity of 3-hydroxy-3-methyl-glutaryl-coenzyme A reductase (HMG-CoA), a main rate-limiting enzyme of cholesterol biosynthesis [52]. In contrast to banaba and policosanol alone, the combination of BNB+PCO elicited a significantly larger reduction of the HCD+STZ-elevated TC, TG, and LDL-C levels, suggesting that the synergisms between policosanol and banaba exert a counter effect against HCD+STZ-triggered dyslipidemia.

Also, banaba or policosanol significantly elevated the HDL-C level; however, the most pronounced effect was observed following the combined supplementation with banaba+policosanol, emphasizing the role of their association in elevating HCD+STZ-reduced HDL-C levels. Policosanol has been well-documented as positively influencing HDL-C levels through various mechanisms, including cholesteryl ester transfer protein (CETP) inhibition [16,20] and upregulation of apolipoprotein A (apoA-I) [20], a key structural protein component of HDL. Additionally, previous studies suggest that corosolic acid has a modulatory effect on HDL-C [51], though the underlining mechanism remains unclear. Taken together, we hypothesize that the combination of banaba and policosanol (BNB+PCO) may synergistically enhance apoA-I expression and inhibit CETP activity more efficiently than either banaba or policosanol alone, leading to a greater improvement in HDL-C levels. Nevertheless, future comprehensive studies are necessary to confirm the notion. The present results of the blood lipid profile align with previous studies documenting the effect of policosanol [17,18] and banaba [51] in countering dyslipidemia, though no study has, so far, been conducted describing the efficacy of the banaba+policosanol combination in mitigating aggravated dyslipidemia caused by HCD+STZ. The elevated HDL-C levels in the banaba+policosanol group may be an additional reason for better tissue regeneration, as HDL-C has been closely linked to chronic wound healing [53]. Supporting this, a clinical study highlights the positive role of HDL-C in diabetic wound healing [54]. Furthermore, studies have demonstrated that the direct application of HDL-C to the wound sites significantly accelerates healing in both diabetic and non-diabetic conditions [55,56], highlighting the importance of HDL-C in tissue regeneration and wound healing.

The effect of hyperglycemia on the augmented free radicals and decreased antioxidants are the typical hallmark of diabetic conditions [57]. Perpetually, we noticed the disturbed plasma oxidative and antioxidant variables in response to the HCD+STZ treatment, such attributes being substantially restored by the consumption of banaba or policosanol. However, the most promising effect, entailing the lowest MDA levels and significantly elevated sulfhydryl content, FRA activity, and PON activity, was noticed in the banaba+policosanol-supplemented group, underscoring the synergetic positive effect of the combination against HCD+STZ-induced stress.

High cholesterol and hyperglycemia are the key contributors to liver injury and fatty liver disease [58]. The high lipid accumulation in the liver impairs its antioxidant capacity, leading to intensified oxidative stress and inflammation in the fatty liver disease [59]. During hyperglycemic and hyperlipidemic conditions, endoplasmic reticulum (ER) stress occurs in hepatocytes that modulate NFκB and c-Jun N-terminal kinase (JNK) signaling, leading to severe inflammation [59]. In the present work, we also witnessed substantial fatty liver changes, higher neutrophil counts, and a higher IL-6 production in the HCD+STZ groups, with the abovementioned phenomena prevented by the supplementation with banaba and policosanol; however, a significantly higher protection was observed when banaba and policosanol were consumed concurrently. The better effect of banaba+policosanol can be justified by their joint effect that leads to different cellular pathways converging in an effective way to prevent hepatic damage. Policosanol (Raydel®) also has an impact on ROS generation [16], similarly to banaba, due to its antioxidant properties [24,26] preventing oxidative stress stimulated by a variety of factors. Oxidative stress has been recognized as a major culprit in inducing apoptotic cell death [60]. In the present study, both policosanol and banaba were found to be effective in preventing oxidative stress; however, the prevention of oxidative stress was significantly higher when banaba and policosanol were used in combination (BNB+PCO), due to their distinct modes of action working synergistically. Due to the lower oxidative stress status, significantly lower apoptosis (as measured by the AO fluorescence staining) was observed in the BNB+PCO group compared to the groups supplemented with banaba or policosanol alone. The statement is supported by an earlier report which describes oxidative stress as a major provocatory event of apoptosis [60]. Also, oxidative stress has a substantial effect on the induction of senescence [61]. Herein, the BNB+PCO group exhibited reduced senescence, likely due to BNB+PCO's enhanced ability to inhibit oxidative stress.

High liver cholesterol and hyperglycemia have adverse effects on the kidney, leading to diabetic nephropathy [62]. Policosanol is known for its kidney-protective role [63]. Similarly, few studies have documented corosolic acid's (a main component of banaba) impact in protecting against diabetic nephropathy [64]. Herein, the significantly higher protective effect of banaba in combination with policosanol compared to their individual effect was observed against HCD+STZ-induced kidney damage. The distinct properties of policosanol (an antiglycation and hypoglycemic agent) [16,44] and banaba (a hypoglycemic, antioxidant, and anti-inflammatory agent) [23,24] work together in a synergistic manner, leading to better protective roles against kidney damage. The study outcomes are in accordance with earlier reports documenting antiglycation, antioxidant, and hypoglycemic effects as being important events to prevent diabetic nephropathy [65]. Also, kidneys from the banaba+policosanol-consuming group displayed higher efficacy in reducing HCD+STZ-induced ROS generation than the banaba or policosanol groups. The banaba+policosanol group consistently displayed the highest protective effect in mitigating the HCD+STZ-induced apoptosis and senescence. The better antiapoptotic and senescence effect can be attributed to the higher inhibitory effect of banaba+policosanol on the kidney ROS generation, which has been recognized as the inducer of apoptosis [60] and senescence [61].

4. Materials and Methods

4.1. Materials

The banaba leaf extract (batch no. UO/LSD-1825/02/23-24) was purchased from Umalaxmi Organics Pvt. Ltd. (Jodhpur, Rajasthan, India). The banaba leaves were dried, finely ground into a powder, and subjected to extraction using absolute ethanol. The ethanol extract was collected, and the solvent was removed through low-temperature heat streaming to obtain the dried powdered extract. No external additives or antioxidants were introduced during the extraction process or during the storage of the extract. The final extract was analyzed for microbial and heavy metal contamination, as well as for the quantification of its critical phytoconstituent (corosolic acid). A detailed specification and certificate of analysis of the used banaba extract is provided in the Supplementary Table S1. Policosanol (Raydel®, Sydney, Australia) was purified to at least >90% purity from sugarcane wax and procured from the National Center for Scientific Research (CNIC, Havana, Cuba). The used policosanol was a typical mixture of eight long-chain aliphatic alcohols (LCAA, C24-C34); a detailed specification of the policosanol product is presented in our previous report [18]. Dihydroethidium (Cat#37291), acridine orange (Cat#A9231), *N*-ε-carboxymethyllysine (Cat#14580-5g), 5-bromo-4-chloro-3-indolyl-β-D-galactopyranoside (Cat# B42525), oil red O (Cat#O0625), and 2-phenoxyethanol (Sigma P1126; St. Louis, MO, USA) were procured from Sigma Aldrich (St. Louis, MO, USA). All the other chemicals and reagents were of analytical grade and used as supplied unless otherwise stated.

4.2. *Zebrafish Husbandry and Production of Embryos*

A young zebrafish (*Danio rerio*, 16 weeks old) was cultured in a water tank equipped with a circulating water supply following the standard guidelines for Animal Use and Care adopted by the Raydel Research Institute (approval code RRI-23-2007, approval date 27 July 2023). The zebrafish were fed normal terabit (ND) and maintained under alternating light (14 h) and dark (10 h) photo periods.

To produce embryos, male and female zebrafish were placed in the breeding tank and separated from each other using the perforated physical divider. After 16 h, the divider was removed, allowing the male and female zebrafish to breed uninterruptedly. Following 30 min of mating, the embryos were collected, washed with water, and used for further study.

4.3. *Microinjection of Zebrafish Embryos*

Zebrafish embryos [1.5 h post fertilization (hpf)] were segregated into four different groups (n = 100/group). Group I embryos were microinjected (10 nL) with phosphate-buffered saline (PBS), while the embryos in group II were injected with 500 ng of CML/10 nL of PBS. Group IV and V embryos received 5 ng and 10 ng of banaba suspended in 10 nL of PBS containing 500 ng of CML. Microinjection was performed under a stereomicroscope (Motic SMZ 168; Hong Kong, China) using microcapillary needles and a pneumatic picopump (PV8830; World Precision Instruments, Sarasota, FL, USA) equipped with a magnetic manipulator (MM33; Kanetc, Bensenville, IL, USA). Embryos in the different groups were monitored under a stereomicroscope (Motic SMZ 168; Hong Kong, China) up to 72 h post injection to examine their survivability, hatching, and developmental deformities. The selection of the 5 ng and 10 ng doses of banaba was based on preliminary experiments where banaba doses ranging from 0 to 25 ng were injected into zebrafish embryos in the presence of CML (500 ng) following a survivability analysis 48 h post injection. The results revealed a protective effect of banaba that significantly improved with the increasing concentration of banaba up to 10 ng. At higher doses (15, 20, and 25 ng), the effect was similar and was comparable to that observed under the 10 ng dose. Consequently, the 10 ng dose of banaba was selected as the optimal high dose for the microinjection studies, while the 5 ng dose was selected to assess the dose-dependent effect.

4.4. *Acute Toxicity in Adult Zebrafish*

Acute toxicity in adult zebrafish (16 weeks old) was induced through an intraperitoneal injection of 250 μg of CML (equivalent to 3 mM)/10 μL of 50% ethanol in PBS. Zebrafish (n = 30) were randomly allocated to three different groups. Zebrafish (n = 10) were injected with 10 μL of PBS (PBS alone group). Similarly, zebrafish (n = 10/group) were injected with 250 μg of CML suspended in 10 μL of 50% ethanol in PBS (3 mM CML + 50% EtOH group) and 250 μg of CML suspended in 10 μL of 50% ethanol in PBS containing 8 μg of the banaba extract (3 mM CML+50% EtOH+banaba group). Among all the groups, the intraperitoneal injection was given by using a 28-gauge needle after anaesthetizing the zebrafish by drenching them in 2-phenoxyethanol (0.1% *v*/*v*). The zebrafish were constantly monitored until 90 min post injection to assess survivability and swimming activity following the OECD 2019 guidelines [66].

4.5. Blood Analysis for Malondialdehyde (MDA) Levels and Antioxidant Variables

The zebrafish from all the groups were sacrificed 90 min post injection using the hypothermic shock method [67], and blood was immediately collected. The oxidative status of the plasm was assessed by quantifying the malondialdehyde (MDA) level using a thiobarbituric acid reactive substance (TBARS) assay [68]. In brief, 1 mg/mL equivalent plasma was suspended in 20 μL of PBS and subsequently blended with 50 μL of trichloroacetic acid (20%) and 100 μL of thiobarbituric acid (0.67%) and incubated at 95 °C for 10 min. Finally, an absorbance of 560 nm was recorded, and the results were quantified by using the MDA standard (0.5–50 μM).

The plasma antioxidant variables were determined by assessing the ferric ion reduction ability (FRA), the sulfhydryl content, and the paraoxonase (PON) activity. The plasma FRA was determined by the method described earlier, with slight amendments [68]. Briefly, 1 mg/mL protein equivalent plasma was dissolved in 20 μL of PBS and mixed with 180 μL of FRA reagents [68]. Following 1 h of incubation at room temperature, an absorbance of 593 nm was recorded.

The sulfhydryl content was assessed using the 5,5-dithiol-bis-(2-nitrobenzoic acid) (DTNB) method [68]. Briefly, 50 μL of plasma (1.0 mg/mL protein) was mixed with 50 μL of DTNB (4 mg/mL). Following 2 h of incubation at room temperature, an absorbance of 412 nm was recorded to measure the chromogenic product 5-thiol-2-nitrobenzoic acid (TNB), with the results expressed as nmol/mg of protein employing the $13.6 \times 10^3\ M^{-1}\ cm^{-1}$ molar absorbance coefficient (ε) of TNB.

Paraoxonase (PON) activity was assessed by mixing 40 μL of plasma (1.0 mg/mL equivalent protein) with 160 μL of paraoxon ethyl (0.15 g/mL) [68]. Following a 2 h incubation at 25 °C, an absorbance of 415 nm was recorded to quantify the formed product *p*-nitrophenol, and the PON activity was expressed as μU/L/min using the $1.7 \times 10^4\ M^{-1}\ cm^{-1}$ molar absorbance coefficient (ε) of *p*-nitrophenol.

The liver function biomarkers in the plasma, i.e., aspartate aminotransferase (AST) and alanine aminotransferase (ALT), were assessed using the commercial detection kit, following the manufacturers' guidelines; a detailed methodology is provided in the Supplementary Method S1.

4.6. Formulation of Different Diets

The normal diet (ND), tetrabit, a regular diet of zebrafish, was mixed with cholesterol (final 4%, *w*/*w*) to make a high-cholesterol (HCD) diet. The HCD was infused with banaba leaf extract (final 0.1% *w*/*w*), policosanol (final 0.1% *w*/*w*), and 0.1% each of banaba and policosanol to make three different dietary formulations named HCD+BNB, HCD+PCO, and HCD+BNB+PCO, respectively. The 0.1% dose was selected based on our previous study [69], where 0.1% policosanol displayed the optimal effect against high-cholesterol diet-induced dyslipidemia and associated adverse events. Furthermore, for the comparative evaluation, a similar amount of banaba (i.e., 0.1%) was used.

4.7. Induction of Hyperglycemia in Zebrafish and Tail Fin Regeneration

Adult zebrafish (18 weeks old, n = 60) were fed exclusively with HCD for 8 weeks (56 days) to induce hyperlipidemia following tail fin amputation using the earlier described method [70]. In brief, the zebrafish were anaesthetized by submerging them in a 0.1% 2 phenoxyethanol solution, followed by tail amputation using a sterilized surgical blade near the dermal rays of the tail fin. The tail-fin-amputated hyperlipidemic zebrafish (n = 60) were randomly divided into five groups (n = 12/group) (Figure 10). The zebrafish in group I were exclusively fed with HCD. At the same time, the zebrafish in groups II to V received the four injections of streptozotocin (STZ, 10 µL, final 0.9%) at one-day intervals and were fed with HCD alone (HCD+STZ group), HCD+banaba (HCD+STZ+BNB group), HCD+policosanol (HCD+STZ+PCO group), and HCD+banaba+policosanol (HCD+STZ+BNB+PCO group). Tail fin regeneration across all groups was measured on days 0, 4, 6, 10, and 14 under a stereomicroscope connected with a digital camera, and the tail fin regeneration area was quantified using the Image J software (https://imagej.net/ij, 1.53 version, accessed on 6 June 2023).

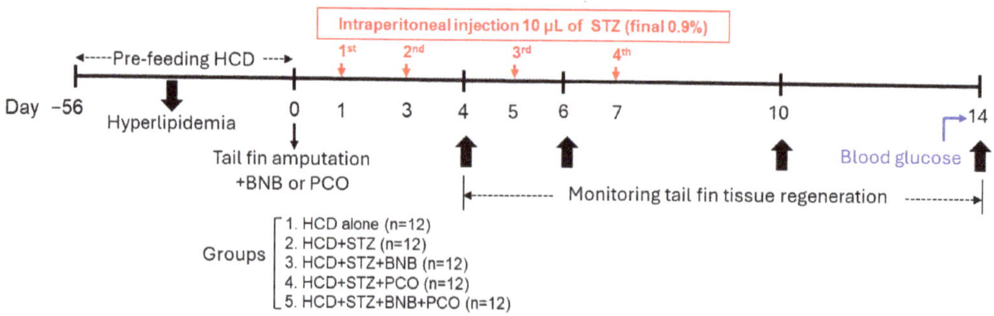

Figure 10. Study layout of the development of hyperlipidemia in adult zebrafish with and without hyperglycemia induction by streptozotocin and tail fin regeneration. Abbreviations: HCD (high cholesterol diet), STZ (streptozotocin), BNB (banaba leaf extract), and PCO (policosanol). HCD was prepared by mixing cholesterol and tetrabits, a brand name of the zebrafish diet which was purchased from Tetrabit Gmbh, Melle, Germany, and contains 47.5% crude protein, 6.5% crude fat, 2.0% crude fiber, and 10.5% crude ash, as well as vitamin A (29,770 IU/kg), vitamin D3 (1860 IU/kg), vitamin E (200 mg/kg), and vitamin C (137 mg/kg).

4.8. Blood Analysis and Collection of Organs

After 14 days of intervention with different diets, the zebrafish (group I–V) were sacrificed by hypothermic shock and blood was immediately collected. The liver and kidney from the different groups were surgically exiced and preserved in 10% formalin for the histological analysis.

Blood from the different groups was analyzed for the glucose level using a blood detection kit (ASAN Pharma. Co., Ltd., Hwaseong, Republic of Korea) following the manufacturer's guidelines. The total blood cholesterol (TC), triglycerides (TGs), and high-density lipoproteins (HDL-C) were quantified by employing the commercial lipoprotein quantification kits following the method suggested by the manufacturers. The liver function biomarkers aspartate aminotransferase (AST) and alanine aminotransferase (ALT) were assessed using the commercial detection kit following the guidelines provided by the manufacturers. A detailed methodology is provided in the Supplementary Method S1.

Blood MDA, sulfhydryl content, and FRA and PON activity were assessed using the methodology described in Section 4.5.

4.9. Histological Analysis and Cellular Senescence

The tissues (liver and kidney) were fixed in the FSC 22 clear frozen solution (Leica) and processed for cryo-sectioning using the cryo-microtome (Leica CM1510 S, Leica biosystem, Nussloch, Germany) to obtain a tissue section (7 μm thick). The tissue section was processed for hematoxylin and eosin (H&E) staining to assess the histological changes in the liver and kidney.

Fatty liver changes in the hepatic section were examined by oil red O (ORO) staining [67]. In brief, the hepatic tissue section was stained with an ORO solution (0.25 mL, 0.3%). After incubation under mild heating conditions (5 min, 60 °C), the stained section was rinsed thoroughly with water and examined under a microscope.

Cellular senescence was detected using the senescence-associated β galactosidase (SA-β-gal) assay [71]. In brief, the tissue section was stained with a 5-bromo-4-choloro-3-indolyl-β-D-galactopyranoside (X-gal, 0.1%) solution [71]. The tissue section was visualized under a microscope for the detection of blue-stained senescence-positive cells after 16 h of staining.

4.10. Immunohistochemistry (IHC) and Fluorescence Imaging

The interleukin (IL)-6 was detected in the hepatic section using IHC [72]. The tissue section was flooded with the 200× time diluted anti-IL-6 antibody (ab9324, Abcam, London, UK). Following 16 h of incubation under cool conditions, the section was developed using an EnVisin+system HRP polymer kit (Code K4001, Dako, Glostrup, Denmark).

For fluorescence imaging to detect ROS generation and apoptosis, a tissue section (7 μm) was stained with dihydroethidium (DHE, 30 μM) and acridine orange (AO, 5 μg/mL) [67]. Following 30 min of incubation in the dark, the tissue section was visualized using fluorescence microscopy at the excitation/emission wavelength of 585/615 nm for DHE and 505/535 nm for AO.

4.11. Statistical Analysis

One-way and two-way analyses of variance (ANOVA), followed by Tukey's post-hoc analyses, were conducted using the SPSS software (version 29.0; Chicago, IL, USA) to establish the statistical difference between the multivariate groups. The two-tailed Student's *t*-test was utilized to establish pairwise statistical differences between the groups. All the data depicted in the graphs were obtained from the triplicate experiments and are represented as the mean ± SEM.

5. Conclusions

Both banaba and policosanol displayed substantial effects in alleviating hyperglycemia and dyslipidemia in diabetic hyperlipidemic zebrafish. However, these effects accelerated greatly in a synergistic manner through the combination of banaba and policosanol. Similarly, the combination of banaba+policosanol prompted tissue regeneration and had a substantial inhibitory effect on the oxidative variables via the augmentation of the antioxidant parameters. Due to the substantial hypoglycemic effect and antioxidant property combination of banaba+policosanol, the latter effectively protected against fatty liver changes and hepatic IL-6 generation in the diabetic hyperlipidemic zebrafish. Likewise, the banaba+policosanol supplementation safeguarded the kidney from oxidative stress, apoptosis, and cellular senescence actuated by the diabetic hyperlipidemic conditions. The findings confirm the superior efficacy of the banaba+policosanol combination compared to their individual supplementation in alleviating the metabolic stress induced by diabetic hyperlipidemic conditions. As a future prospect, studies will be conducted to compare the effects of the banaba+policosanol combination with standard antidiabetic drugs. Additionally, genomics and proteomics studies will be explored to decode the protective molecular mechanism exerted by banaba+policosanol. Given the promising preclinical findings in zebrafish, a human clinical trial will be planned to further assess the potential efficacy of banaba+policosanol in managing diabetic hyperlipidemic conditions.

Supplementary Materials: The following supporting information can be downloaded at: https://www.mdpi.com/article/10.3390/ph18030362/s1, Supplementary Table S1: A certificate of analysis of the used banaba extract. Method S1: Methodology for the quantification of plasma lipid profile and hepatic function biomarkers.

Author Contributions: Conceptualization, K.-H.C.; methodology, S.H.L., Y.L., A.B. and J.-E.K.; data curation, writing—original draft preparation, K.-H.C.; writing—review and editing, K.-H.C., supervision, K.-H.C. All authors have read and agreed to the published version of the manuscript.

Funding: This research received no external funding.

Institutional Review Board Statement: The animal study protocol was approved by the Committee of Animal Care and Use of Raydel Research Institute (approval code RRI-23-001, approval date 27 July 2023).

Informed Consent Statement: Not applicable.

Data Availability Statement: The data used to support the findings of this study are available from the corresponding author upon reasonable request.

Conflicts of Interest: The authors declare no conflict of interest.

References

1. Saeedi, P.; Petersohn, I.; Salpea, P.; Malanda, B.; Karuranga, S.; Unwin, N.; Colagiuri, S.; Guariguata, L.; Motala, A.A.; Ogurtsova, K.; et al. Global and regional diabetes prevalence estimates for 2019 and projections for 2030 and 2045: Results from the International Diabetes Federation Diabetes Atlas. *Diabetes Res. Clin. Pract.* **2019**, *157*, 107843. [CrossRef] [PubMed]
2. Abduh, M.S.; Alzoghaibi, M.A.; Alzoghaibi, A.M.; Bin-Ammar, A.; Alotaibi, M.F.; Kamel, E.M.; Mahmoud, A.M. Arbutin ameliorates hyperglycemia, dyslipidemia and oxidative stress and modulates adipocytokines and PPARγ in high-fat diet/streptozotocin-induced diabetic rats. *Life Sci.* **2023**, *321*, 121612. [CrossRef] [PubMed]
3. Kawahito, S.; Kitahata, H.; Oshita, S. Problems associated with glucose toxicity: Role of hyperglycemia-induced oxidative stress. *World J. Gastroenterol.* **2009**, *15*, 4137–4142. [CrossRef]
4. Maddatu, J.; Anderson-Baucum, E.; Evans-Molina, C. Smoking and the risk of type 2 diabetes. *Transl. Res.* **2017**, *184*, 101–107. [CrossRef]
5. Kahn, S.E.; Cooper, M.E.; Del Prato, S. Pathophysiology and treatment of type 2 diabetes: Perspectives on the past, present, and future. *Lancet* **2014**, *383*, 1068–1083. [CrossRef] [PubMed]
6. Mohamed, J.; Nazratun Nafizah, A.H.; Zariyantey, A.H.; Budin, S.B. Mechanisms of diabetes-induced liver damage: The role of oxidative stress and inflammation. *Sultan Qaboos Univ. Med. J.* **2016**, *16*, e132–e141. [CrossRef]
7. Giri, B.; Dey, S.; Das, T.; Sarkar, M.; Banerjee, J.; Dash, S.K. Chronic hyperglycemia mediated physiological alteration, and metabolic distortion leads to organ dysfunction, infection, cancer progression and other pathophysiological consequences: An update on glucose toxicity. *Biomed. Pharmacother.* **2018**, *107*, 306–328. [CrossRef]
8. Bertoni, A.G.; Hundley, W.G.; Massing, M.W.; Bonds, D.E.; Burke, G.L.; Goff, D.C., Jr. Heart failure prevalence, incidence, and mortality in the elderly with diabetes. *Diabetes Care* **2004**, *27*, 699–703. [CrossRef]
9. Levinthal, G.N.; Tavill, A.S. Liver disease and diabetes mellitus. *Clin. Diabetes* **1999**, *17*, 73–81.
10. Sharma, S.; Schaper, N.; Rayman, G. Microangiopathy: Is it relevant to wound healing in diabetic foot disease? *Diabetes Metab. Res. Rev.* **2020**, *36*, e3244. [CrossRef]
11. Khalid, M.; Petroianu, G.; Adem, A. Advanced glycation end products and diabetes mellitus: Mechanisms and perspectives. *Biomolecules* **2022**, *12*, 542. [CrossRef]
12. Blahova, J.; Martiniakova, M.; Babikova, M.; Kovacova, V.; Mondockova, V.; Omelka, R. Pharmaceutical drugs and natural therapeutic products for the treatment of Type 2 diabetes mellitus. *Pharmaceuticals* **2021**, *14*, 806. [CrossRef] [PubMed]
13. Alam, F.; Islam, M.A.; Kamal, M.A.; Gan, S.H. Updates on managing type 2 diabetes mellitus with natural products: Towards antidiabetic drug development. *Curr. Med. Chem.* **2018**, *25*, 5395–5431. [CrossRef] [PubMed]
14. Chen, Z.Y.; Jiao, R.; Ma, K.Y. Cholesterol-lowering nutraceuticals and functional foods. *J. Agric. Food Chem.* **2008**, *56*, 8761–8773. [CrossRef]

15. Lee, E.Y.; Yoo, J.A.; Lim, S.M.; Cho, K.H. Anti-aging and tissue regeneration ability of policosanol along with lipid-lowering effect in hyperlipidemic zebrafish via enhancement of high-density lipoprotein functionality. *Rejuvenation Res.* **2016**, *19*, 149–158. [CrossRef]
16. Lim, S.M.; Yoo, J.A.; Lee, E.Y.; Cho, K.H. Enhancement of high-density lipoprotein cholesterol functions by encapsulation of policosanol exerts anti-senescence and tissue regeneration effects via improvement of anti-glycation, anti-apoptosis, and cholesteryl ester transfer inhibition. *Rejuvenation Res.* **2016**, *19*, 59–70. [CrossRef] [PubMed]
17. Throne Research. Monograph. Policosanol. *Altern. Med. Rev.* **2004**, *9*, 312–317.
18. Cho, K.-H.; Nam, H.-S.; Baek, S.-H.; Kang, D.-J.; Na, H.; Komatsu, T.; Uehara, Y. Beneficial effect of Cuban policosanol on blood pressure and serum lipoproteins accompanied with lowered glycated hemoglobin and enhanced high-density lipoprotein functionalities in a randomized, placebo-controlled, and double-blinded trial with healthy Japanese. *Int. J. Mol. Sci.* **2023**, *24*, 5185. [CrossRef]
19. Olatunji, L.K.; Jimoh, A.O.; Tukur, U.M.; Imam, M.U. A review of the effects of policosanol on metabolic syndrome. *Clin. Complement. Med. Pharmacol.* **2022**, *2*, 100058. [CrossRef]
20. Kim, J.-Y.; Kim, S.-M.; Kim, S.-J.; Lee, E.-Y.; Kim, J.-R.; Cho, K.-H. Consumption of policosanol enhances HDL functionality via CETP inhibition and reduces blood pressure and visceral fat in young and middle-aged subjects. *Int. J. Mol. Med.* **2017**, *39*, 889–899. [CrossRef]
21. Uehara, Y.; Komatsu, T.; Sasaki, K.; Abe, S.; Nakashima, S.; Yamamoto, T.; Kim, J.-E.; Cho, K.-H. Cuban policosanol improves high-density lipoprotein cholesterol efflux capacity in healthy Japanese subjects. *Front. Nutr.* **2024**, *10*, 1297008. [CrossRef] [PubMed]
22. Crespo, N.; Illnait, J.; Mas, R.; Fernandez, L.; Fernandez, J.; Castano, G. Comparative study of the efficacy and tolerability of policosanol and lovastatin in patients with hypercholesterolemia and noninsulin dependent diabetes mellitus. *Int. J. Clin. Pharmacol. Res.* **1999**, *29*, 117–127.
23. Stohs, S.J.; Miller, H.; Kaats, G.R. A review of the efficacy and safety of banaba (*Lagerstroemia speciosa* L.) and corosolic acid. *Phytother. Res.* **2012**, *26*, 317–324. [CrossRef] [PubMed]
24. Mousa, A.M.; El-Sammad, N.M.; Abdel-Halim, A.H.; Anwar, N.; Khalil, W.K.B.; Nawwar, M.; Hashim, A.N.; Elsayed, E.A.; Hassan, S.K. *Lagerstroemia speciosa* (L.) pers leaf extract attenuates lung tumorigenesis via alleviating oxidative stress, inflammation and apoptosis. *Biomolecules* **2019**, *9*, 871. [CrossRef]
25. Teng, H.; Yuan, B.; Gothai, S.; Arulselvan, P.; Song, X.; Chen, L. Dietary triterpenes in the treatment of type 2 diabetes: To date. *Trends Food Sci. Technol.* **2018**, *72*, 34–44. [CrossRef]
26. Singh, L.S.; Singh, W.S. Multifaceted therapeutic potential of corosolic acid: A novel bioactive compound. *Obes. Med.* **2024**, *49*, 100548. [CrossRef]
27. Lee, B.H.; Hsu, W.H.; Hsu, Y.W.; Pan, T.M. Suppression of dimerumic acid on hepatic fibrosis caused from carboxymethyl-lysine (CML) by attenuating oxidative stress depends on Nrf2 activation in hepatic stellate cells (HSCs). *Food Chem. Toxicol.* **2013**, *62*, 413–419. [CrossRef]
28. Liu, X.; Zheng, L.; Zhang, R.; Liu, G.; Xiao, S.; Qiao, X.; Wu, Y.; Gong, Z. Toxicological evaluation of advanced glycation end product Nε-(carboxymethyl)lysine: Acute and subacute oral toxicity studies. *Regul. Toxicol. Pharmacol. RTP* **2016**, *77*, 65–74. [CrossRef]
29. Pareek, A.; Suthar, M.; Rathore, G.S.; Bansal, V.; Kumawat, T. In vitro antioxidant studies of *Lagerstroemia speciosa* leaves. *Pharmacogn. J.* **2010**, *2*, 357–360. [CrossRef]
30. Tidke, P.S.; Patil, C.R. Nrf2 activator corosolic acid meliorates alloxan induced diabetic nephropathy in mice. *Asian Pac. J. Trop. Biomed.* **2017**, *7*, 797–804. [CrossRef]
31. Wang, L.; Zhang, X.; Xiong, X.; Zhu, H.; Chen, R.; Zhang, S.; Chen, G.; Jian, Z. Nrf2 regulates oxidative stress and Its role in cerebral ischemic stroke. *Antioxidants* **2022**, *11*, 2377. [CrossRef] [PubMed]
32. Cho, K.-H.; Nam, H.-S.; Kim, J.-E.; Na, H.-J.; del Carmen Dominguez-Horta, M.; Martinez-Donato, G. CIGB-258 exerts potent anti-inflammatory activity against carboxymethyllysine-induced acute inflammation in hyperlipidemic zebrafish via the protection of apolipoprotein AI. *Int. J. Mol. Sci.* **2023**, *24*, 7044. [CrossRef]
33. Priya, T.T.; Sabu, M.C.; Jolly, C.I. Free radical scavenging and anti-inflammatory properties of *Lagerstroemia speciosa* (L). *Inflammopharmacology* **2008**, *16*, 182–187. [CrossRef] [PubMed]
34. Gaweł, S.; Wardas, M.; Niedworok, E.; Wardas, P. Malondialdehyde (MDA) as a lipid peroxidation marker. *Wiad. Lek.* **2004**, *57*, 453–455.
35. Bourgonje, A.R.; Abdulle, A.E.; Bourgonje, M.F.; Binnenmars, S.H.; Gordijn, S.J.; Bulthuis, M.L.C.; la Bastide-van Gemert, S.; Kieneker, L.M.; Gansevoort, R.T.; Bakker, S.J.L.; et al. Serum free sulfhydryl status associates with new-onset chronic kidney disease in the general population. *Redox Biol.* **2021**, *48*, 102211. [CrossRef] [PubMed]

36. Bourgonje, A.R.; Bourgonje, M.F.; Post, A.; Gemert, S.L.B.-V.; Kieneker, L.M.; Bulthuis, M.L.; Gordijn, S.J.; Gansevoort, R.T.; Bakker, S.J.; Mulder, D.J.; et al. Systemic oxidative stress associates with new-onset hypertension in the general population. *Free Radic. Biol. Med.* **2022**, *187*, 123–131. [CrossRef]
37. Hu, M.-L. Measurement of protein thiol groups and glutathione in plasma. *Methods Enzymol.* **1994**, *233*, 380–385. [CrossRef]
38. Mcgrowder, D.; Riley, C.; Morrison, E.Y.S.A.; Gordon, L. The role of high-density lipoproteins in reducing the risk of vascular diseases, neurogenerative disorders, and cancer. *Cholesterol* **2011**, *2011*, 496925. [CrossRef]
39. Tréguier, M.; Briand, F.; Boubacar, A.; André, A.; Magot, T.; Nguyen, P.; Krempf, M.; Sulpice, T.; Ouguerram, K. Diet-induced dyslipidemia impairs reverse cholesterol transport in hamsters. *Eur. J. Clin. Investig.* **2011**, *41*, 921–928. [CrossRef]
40. Bagaméry, F.; Varga, K.; Kecsmár, K.; Vincze, I.; Szökő, É.; Tábi, T. Lack of insulin resistance in response to streptozotocin treatment in neuronal SH-SY5Y cell line. *J. Neural Transm.* **2020**, *127*, 71–80. [CrossRef]
41. Gheibi, S.; Kashfi, K.; Ghasemi, A. A practical guide for induction of type-2 diabetes in rat: Incorporating a high-fat diet and streptozotocin. *Biomed. Pharmacother.* **2017**, *95*, 605–613. [CrossRef]
42. Furman, B.L. Streptozotocin-induced diabetic models in mice and rats. *Curr. Protoc.* **2021**, *1*, e78. [CrossRef]
43. Lin, B.; Ma, J.; Fang, Y.; Lei, P.; Wang, L.; Qu, L.; Wu, W.; Jin, L.; Sun, D. Advances in zebrafish for diabetes mellitus with wound model. *Bioengineering* **2023**, *10*, 330. [CrossRef] [PubMed]
44. Amini, M.R.; Kazeminejad, S.; Jalalzadeh, M.; Majd, S.S.; Kavyani, Z.; Askari, G.; Hekmatdoost, A. The effects of policosanol supplementation on blood glucose: A systematic review and dose-response meta-analysis of randomized controlled trials. *Diabetes Res. Clin. Pract.* **2024**, *212*, 111709. [CrossRef]
45. Yang, J.; Leng, J.; Li, J.J.; Tang, J.F.; Li, Y.; Liu, B.L.; Wen, X.D. Corosolic acid inhibits adipose tissue inflammation and ameliorates insulin resistance via AMPK activation in high-fat fed mice. *Phytomedicine Int. J. Phytother. Phytopharm.* **2016**, *23*, 181–190. [CrossRef] [PubMed]
46. Hou, W.; Li, Y.; Zhang, Q.; Wei, X.; Peng, A.; Chen, L.; Wei, Y. Triterpene acids isolated from *Lagerstroemia speciosa* leaves as α-glucosidase inhibitors. *Phytother. Res.* **2009**, *23*, 614–618. [CrossRef] [PubMed]
47. Sharchil, C.; Vijay, A.; Ramachandran, V.; Bhagavatheeswaran, S.; Devarajan, R.; Koul, B.; Yadav, D.; Balakrishnan, A. Zebrafish: A model to study and understand the diabetic nephropathy and other microvascular complications of Type 2 diabetes mellitus. *Vet. Sci.* **2022**, *9*, 312. [CrossRef]
48. Dasari, N.; Jiang, A.; Skochdopole, A.; Chung, J.; Reece, E.M.; Vorstenbosch, J.; Winocour, S. Updates in diabetic wound healing, inflammation, and scarring. *Semin. Plast. Surg.* **2021**, *35*, 153–158. [CrossRef]
49. Wang, K.; Ge, Y.; Yang, Y.; Li, Z.; Liu, J.; Xue, Y.; Zhang, Y.; Pang, X.; Ngan, A.H.W.; Tang, B. Vascular endothelial cellular mechanics under hyperglycemia and its role in tissue regeneration. *Regen. Biomater.* **2024**, *11*, rbae004. [CrossRef]
50. Accipe, L.; Abadie, A.; Neviere, R.; Bercion, S. Antioxidant activities of natural compounds from caribbean plants to enhance diabetic wound healing. *Antioxidants* **2023**, *12*, 1079. [CrossRef]
51. Cannarella, R.; Garofalo, V.; Calogero, A.E. Anti-dyslipidemic and anti-diabetic properties of corosolic acid: A narrative review. *Endocrines* **2023**, *4*, 616–629. [CrossRef]
52. Lee, J.H.; Jia, Y.; Thach, T.T.; Han, Y.; Kim, B.; Wu, C.; Kim, Y.; Seo, W.D.; Lee, S.J. Hexacosanol reduces plasma and hepatic cholesterol by activation of AMP-activated protein kinase and suppression of sterol regulatory element-binding protein-2 in HepG2 and C57BL/6J mice. *Nutr. Res.* **2017**, *43*, 89–99. [CrossRef] [PubMed]
53. Chen, L.; Ma, W.; Chen, D.; Wang, C.; Gao, Y.; Ran, X. Association of high-density lipoprotein cholesterol and wound healing in patients with diabetic foot ulcers. *Chin. Med. J.* **2022**, *135*, 110–112. [CrossRef]
54. Ikura, K.; Hanai, K.; Shinjyo, T.; Uchigata, Y. HDL cholesterol as a predictor for the incidence of lower extremity amputation and wound-related death in patients with diabetic foot ulcers. *Atherosclerosis* **2015**, *239*, 465–469. [CrossRef] [PubMed]
55. Tan, J.T.M.; Prosser, H.C.; Dunn, L.L.; Vanags, L.Z.; Ridiandries, A.; Tsatralis, T.; Leece, L.; Clayton, Z.E.; Yuen, S.C.G.; Robertson, S.; et al. High-density lipoproteins rescue diabetes-impaired angiogenesis via scavenger receptor class B type I. *Diabetes* **2016**, *65*, 3091–3103. [CrossRef] [PubMed]
56. Tsatralis, T.; Ridiandries, A.; Robertson, S.; Vanags, L.Z.; Lam, Y.T.; Tan, J.T.M.; Ng, M.K.; Bursill, C.A. Reconstituted high-density lipoproteins promote wound repair and blood flow recovery in response to ischemia in aged mice. *Lipids Health Dis.* **2016**, *15*, 150. [CrossRef]
57. Cheng, K.-Y.; Lin, Z.-H.; Cheng, Y.-P.; Chiu, H.-Y.; Yeh, N.-L.; Wu, T.-K.; Wu, J.-S. Wound healing in streptozotocin-induced diabetic rats using atmospheric-pressure argon plasma Jet. *Sci. Rep.* **2018**, *8*, 12214. [CrossRef]
58. Wang, Q.; Wei, S.; Zhou, S.; Qiu, J.; Shi, C.; Liu, R.; Zhou, H.; Lu, L. Hyperglycemia aggravates acute liver injury by promoting liver-resident macrophage NLRP3 inflammasome activation via the inhibition of AMPK/mTOR-mediated autophagy induction. *Immunol. Cell Biol.* **2020**, *98*, 54–66. [CrossRef]
59. Mu, W.; Cheng, X.-F.; Liu, Y.; Lv, Q.-Z.; Liu, G.-L.; Zhang, J.-G.; Li, X.-Y. Potential nexus of non-alcoholic fatty liver disease and type 2 diabetes mellitus: Insulin resistance between hepatic and peripheral tissues. *Front. Pharmacol.* **2019**, *9*, 1566. [CrossRef]
60. Kannan, K.; Jain, S.K. Oxidative stress and apoptosis. *Pathophysiology* **2000**, *7*, 153–163. [CrossRef]

61. Faraonio, R. Oxidative stress and cell senescence process. *Antioxidants* **2022**, *11*, 1718. [CrossRef] [PubMed]
62. Kawanami, D.; Matoba, K.; Utsunomiya, K. Dyslipidemia in diabetic nephropathy. *Ren. Replace. Ther.* **2016**, *2*, 16. [CrossRef]
63. Elnagar, G.M.; Elseweidy, M.M.M.; Elkomy, N.M.; Keshawy, M.M.; Fathy, O.M.; Sobh, M.S.; Mahmoud, Y.K. Policosanol ameliorates renal inflammation and pyroptosis in hypercholesterolemic rabbits via modulation of HMGB1/PI3K/mTOR/NLRP3/Caspase-1 pathway. *J. Funct. Foods* **2022**, *97*, 105250. [CrossRef]
64. Li, X.-Q.; Tian, W.; Liu, X.-X.; Zhang, K.; Huo, J.-C.; Liu, W.-J.; Li, P.; Xiao, X.; Zhao, M.-G.; Cao, W. Corosolic acid inhibits the proliferation of glomerular mesangial cells and protects against diabetic renal damage. *Sci. Rep.* **2016**, *6*, 26854. [CrossRef]
65. Mestry, S.N.; Dhodi, J.B.; Kumbhar, S.B.; Juvekar, A.R. Attenuation of diabetic nephropathy in streptozotocin-induced diabetic rats by *Punica granatum* Linn. leaves extract. *J. Tradit. Complement. Med.* **2017**, *7*, 273–280. [CrossRef]
66. OECD. Test No. 203: Fish, Acute Toxicity Testing. In *OECD Guidelines for the Testing of Chemicals, Section 2*; OECD Publishing: Paris, France, 2019.
67. Cho, K.-H.; Kim, J.-E.; Bahuguna, A.; Kang, D.-J. Long-term supplementation of ozonated sunflower oil improves dyslipidemia and hepatic inflammation in hyperlipidemic zebrafish: Suppression of oxidative stress and inflammation against carboxymethyllysine toxicity. *Antioxidants* **2023**, *12*, 1240. [CrossRef]
68. Cho, K.-H.; Kim, J.-E.; Lee, M.-S.; Bahuguna, A. Oral supplementation of ozonated sunflower oil augments plasma antioxidant and anti-Inflammatory abilities with enhancement of high-density lipoproteins functionality in rats. *Antioxidants* **2024**, *13*, 529. [CrossRef]
69. Cho, K.-H.; Kim, J.-E.; Nam, H.-S.; Baek, S.-H.; Bahuguna, A. Consumption of policosanol (Raydel®) improves hepatic, renal, and reproductive functions in zebrafish: In vivo comparison study among Cuban, Chinese, and American policosanol. *Pharmaceuticals* **2023**, *17*, 66. [CrossRef]
70. Cho, K.-H.; Kim, J.-H.; Nam, H.-S.; Kang, D.-J. Efficacy comparison study of human epidermal growth factor (EGF) between Heberprot-P® and Easyef® in adult zebrafish and embryo under presence or absence combination of diabetic condition and hyperlipidemia to mimic elderly patients. *Geriatrics* **2022**, *7*, 45. [CrossRef]
71. Cho, K.-H.; Bahuguna, A.; Kang, D.-J.; Kim, J.-E. Prolonged supplementation of ozonated sunflower oil bestows an antiaging effect, improves blood lipid profile and spinal deformities, and protects vital organs of zebrafish (*Danio rerio*) against age-related degeneration: Two-years consumption study. *Antioxidants* **2024**, *13*, 123. [CrossRef]
72. Shull, L.C.; Sen, R.; Menzel, J.; Goyama, S.; Kurokawa, M.; Artinger, K.B. The conserved and divergent roles of Prdm3 and Prdm16 in zebrafish and mouse craniofacial development. *Dev. Biol.* **2020**, *461*, 132–144. [CrossRef] [PubMed]

pharmaceuticals

MDPI

Article

BuZhong YiQi Formula Alleviates Postprandial Hyperglycemia in T2DM Rats by Inhibiting α-Amylase and α-Glucosidase In Vitro and In Vivo

Xin-Xin Zeng [1], Liang Wang [1], Ming-Yu Wang [1], Zhen-Ran Hu [1], Xiang-Ke Li [1], Guo-Jun Fei [1], Ling Ling [1], Yu-Ting Fan [1] and Ze-Min Yang [1,2,*]

1 Department of Biochemistry and Molecular Biology, School of Basic Medical Sciences, Guangdong Pharmaceutical University, Guangzhou 510006, China; zengxinxin27@163.com (X.-X.Z.); liang7982023@163.com (L.W.); wmy112222@163.com (M.-Y.W.); 2112255029@stu.gdpu.edu.cn (Z.-R.H.); kekeli123123@163.com (X.-K.L.); feiguojun2024@163.com (G.-J.F.); lingl6963@163.com (L.L.); 2112255030@stu.dgpu.edu.cn (Y.-T.F.)

2 Guangdong Provincial Key Laboratory of Pharmaceutical Bioactive Substances, 280 Waihuan Road East in Guangzhou Higher Education Mega Center, Guangzhou 510006, China

* Correspondence: yangzm@gdpu.edu.cn

Abstract: Background/Objectives: BuZhong YiQi Formula (BZYQF) can alleviate type 2 diabetes mellitus (T2DM). However, its efficacy in managing postprandial hyperglycemia in T2DM needs to be further confirmed, and its underlying mechanism and pharmacodynamic material basis have not been sufficiently investigated. **Methods:** A T2DM rat model was induced to measure postprandial glycemic responses following glucose and starch ingestion. In vitro assays of enzymatic inhibition and the kinetic mode were performed to evaluate the inhibitory effect of BZYQF on α-amylase and α-glucosidase activities. The main constituent contents of BZYQF in a simulated digestion assay were measured to screen the active constituents in BZYQF against α-amylase and α-glucosidase activities via Pearson correlation and multiple linear regression analyses. Finally, the total flavonoids were purified from BZYQF to perform in vitro activity validation, and the flavonoid constituent activity was verified through molecular docking. **Results:** In vivo assays showed that BZYQF significantly reduced the blood glucose values of CON rats but not T2DM rats after glucose ingestion, while BZYQF significantly reduced the blood glucose levels by 15 min after starch ingestion in CON and T2DM rats, with more significant decreases in blood glucose levels in T2DM rats. In vitro enzymatic assays showed that BZYQF could inhibit the activities of α-amylase and α-glucosidase in competitive and non-competitive modes and in an uncompetitive mode, respectively. Furthermore, BZYQF showed a stronger inhibitory effect on α-glucosidase activity than on α-amylase activity. Simulated digestion showed that simulated gastric fluid and intestinal fluid changed the main constituent contents of BZYQF and their inhibition rates against α-amylase and α-glucosidase activities, and similar results were rarely found in simulated salivary fluid. Pearson correlation and multiple linear regression analyses revealed that the total flavonoids were the active constituents in BZYQF inhibiting α-amylase and α-glycosidase activities. This result was verified by examining the total flavonoids purified from BZYQF. A total of 1909 compounds were identified in BZYQF using UPLC-MS/MS, among which flavones were the most abundant and consisted of 467 flavonoids. Molecular docking showed that flavonoids in BZYQF were bound to the active site of α-amylase, while they were bound to the inactive site of α-glucosidase. This result supported the results of the enzyme kinetic assay. **Conclusions:** BZYQF significantly alleviated postprandial hyperglycemia in T2DM rats by inhibiting α-amylase and α-glycosidase activities, in which flavonoids in BZYQF were the active constituents.

 https://doi.org/10.3390/ph18020201

Keywords: postprandial glycemic responses; enzyme kinetics; simulated digestion; total flavonoids; molecular docking

1. Introduction

Type 2 diabetes mellitus (T2DM) is caused by insufficient insulin and peripheral insulin resistance, resulting in hyperglycemia [1]. The International Diabetes Federation projections outline that approximately 783 million people will be living with T2DM by the year 2045. In addition, T2DM often leads to several complications, including nephropathy, retinopathy, neuropathy and cardiovascular diseases, which are the major causes of mortality in T2DM patients [2]. Epidemiological studies have suggested that postprandial hyperglycemia may be an independent risk factor of cardiovascular disease and mortality in T2DM patients [3]. Therefore, it is particularly important for T2DM patients to reduce postprandial hyperglycemia and maintain stable blood glucose levels.

The theory of traditional Chinese medicine (TCM) considers that T2DM belongs to the category of "Xiaoke disease", with its main cause being spleen and stomach deficiency. As a TCM term, spleen and stomach deficiency refers to the impairment of the patient's spleen and stomach functions, manifested by weakened digestion, absorption, and metabolism of nutrients. The latest evidence shows that TCMs, including Chinese traditional patent medicines, empirical formulas, and monomers, not only demonstrate clinical efficacy comparable to that of existing Western drugs in managing hypoglycemia but also offer fewer adverse effects and a multitarget therapeutic approach [4]. BuZhong YiQi Formula (BZYQF) is a classic formula for treating spleen and stomach deficiency. BZYQF is composed of eight Chinese herbs: *Astragalus membranaceus*, *Glycyrhiza uralensis*, *Ginseng quinquefolium*, *Atractylodes macrocephala*, *Angelica sinensis*, *Cimicifuga heracleifolia*, *Bupleurum chinense*, and *Citrus reticulata*. Modern pharmacological studies have found that all the herbs *Astragalus membranaceus*, *Ginseng quinquefolium*, *Atractylodes macrocephala*, and *Citrus reticulata*, as well as their constituents in BZYQF, exhibit hypoglycemic effects [5–8]. Clinical observations have found that BZYQF could significantly improve fasting blood glucose, Hb A1c, and 2 h postprandial blood glucose in patients with T2DM [9]. These studies have revealed the hypoglycemic effects of BZYQF in T2DM rats and patients. However, these studies have mainly focused on fasting blood glucose, with limited reports on the role of BZYQF in managing postprandial hyperglycemia in T2DM.

Postprandial blood glucose generally refers to the blood glucose level measured 1 or 2 h after a meal. In this process, α-amylase in the salivary glands and pancreas hydrolyses dietary starch into maltose, maltotriose, isomaltose, and α-limit dextrin, which consists of four to nine glucose residues. Subsequently, α-glucosidase in intestinal mucosa hydrolyses maltose and maltotriose into glucose. The released glucose is absorbed into the bloodstream by the transporters of SGLT-1 and GLUT2, resulting in an increase in blood glucose levels. Therefore, the inhibition of α-amylase and α-glucosidase activities prevents a sudden surge in glucose, leading to lower postprandial hyperglycemia [10]. Acarbose, a drug that inhibits α-amylase and α-glucosidase inhibitors, has been widely used to control postprandial hyperglycemia in T2DM patients. However, acarbose causes gastrointestinal side effects, including diarrhea, abdominal pain, and flatulence [11]. Therefore, it is urgent to discover novel α-amylase and α-glucosidase inhibitors with fewer side effects.

In this study, we characterized the chemical constituents in BZYQF using UPLC-MS/MS analysis and evaluated the effect of BZYQF on postprandial hyperglycemia in T2DM rats. Subsequently, we investigated the inhibitory effect of BZYQF on α-amylase and α-glucosidase activities in vitro. Finally, we measured the main constituent contents of BZYQF during simulated digestion and screened the active constituents in BZYQF that inhibit α-amylase and α-glycosidase activities using Pearson's correlation analysis, multiple linear regression analysis, and molecular docking. The present study provides experimental evidence for the treatment of T2DM with BZYQF through the inhibition of α-amylase and α-glucosidase activities.

2. Results

2.1. Chemical Constituents of BZYQF

A total of 1909 primary compounds were identified in BZYQF through a widely targeted metabolic profiling analysis (Figure 1 and Supplementary Material). The primary compounds accounting for more than 5% were flavones, phenolic acids, amino acids, and their derivatives, alkaloids, lipids, terpenoids, organic acids, lignans, and coumarins. Among them, flavones had the highest proportion at almost 25% and consisted of 467 secondary flavonoids. These flavonoids mainly included flavones, xanthone alcohols, isoflavones, dihydroflavonoids, chalcones, and other flavonoids. The content of calycosin-7-O-β-D-glucoside, an isoflavone from *Astragalus membranaceus*, was 0.83 mg/g pills, which was the highest content among the flavonoids in BZYQF (Supplementary Material).

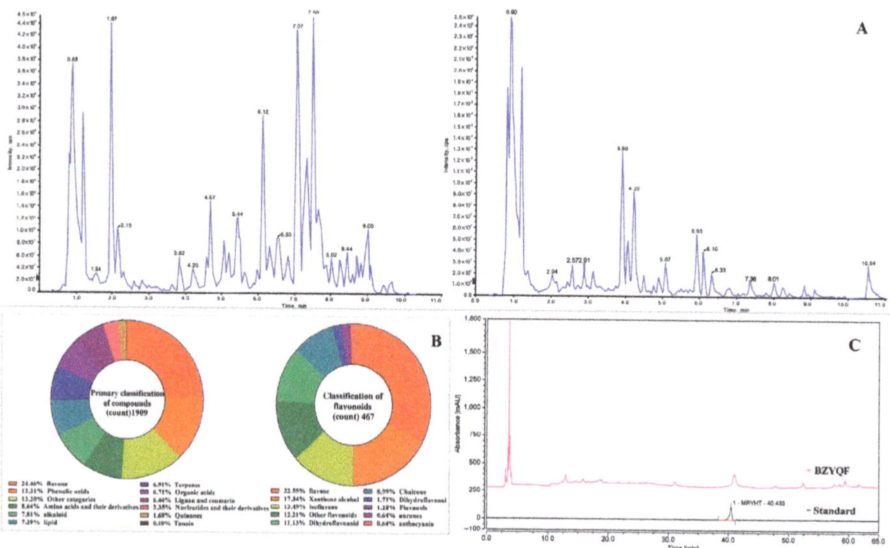

Figure 1. Chemical constituent characterization of BZYQF. (**A**) Total Ion Chromatograms of positive ion mode (left) and negative ion mode (right); (**B**) Primary and secondary classification of compounds identified in BZYQF; (**C**) HPLC chart for determination of calycosin-7-O-β-D-glucoside (MRYHT) content in BZYQF.

The Qquantification of the main constituents in BZYQF revealed that the total carbohydrate content was 146.72 ± 2.59 mg/g; the reducing sugar content was 86.22 ± 1.11 mg/g; the polysaccharide content was 60.50 ± 3.12 mg/g; the total flavonoid content was 23.45 ± 4.39 mg/g; the total polyphenol content was 123.79 ± 2.68 mg/g; and the total saponin content was 8.11 ± 3.05 mg/g.

2.2. BZYQF Ameliorated Postprandial Hyperglycemia in T2DM Rats

To evaluate the effect of BZYQF on postprandial hyperglycemia in T2DM rats, in vivo postprandial glycemic responses following starch and glucose ingestion were observed.

The results of postprandial glycemic responses following the ingestion of starch and glucose solutions without BZYQF intervention are shown in Figure 2A,F. Following the ingestion of glucose and starch solutions, the blood glucose values of CON rats significantly increased and peaked at 15 min, followed by a rapid decline to near baseline level. Furthermore, the blood glucose values at any time point and AUC of CON rats did not differ between the ingestion of the two solutions. This finding reveals that both starch and glucose solutions could rapidly increase the blood glucose levels of CON rats, and there was no difference in glycemic response between the two solutions. Following the ingestion of glucose and starch solutions, the blood glucose values of T2DM rats significantly increased and peaked at 15 min, followed by a decline. Moreover, the blood glucose values of T2DM rats differed over time between the ingestion of the two solutions. Specifically, the blood glucose values of T2DM rats at 45 and 60 min after the ingestion of starch solution were significantly lower than those after the ingestion of glucose solution, and the AUC of the former was significantly lower than that of the latter. This finding reveals that both starch and glucose solutions could rapidly increase the blood glucose levels of T2DM rats, but the glycemic response of starch solution was lower than that of glucose solution. In addition, the blood glucose values and AUC of T2DM rats were significantly higher than those of CON rats after the ingestion of the two solutions. This result suggests that CON rats were able to rapidly digest starch and utilize glucose, thereby controlling blood glucose stability, while T2DM rats showed weakened glucose metabolism due to impaired starch digestion and glucose uptake.

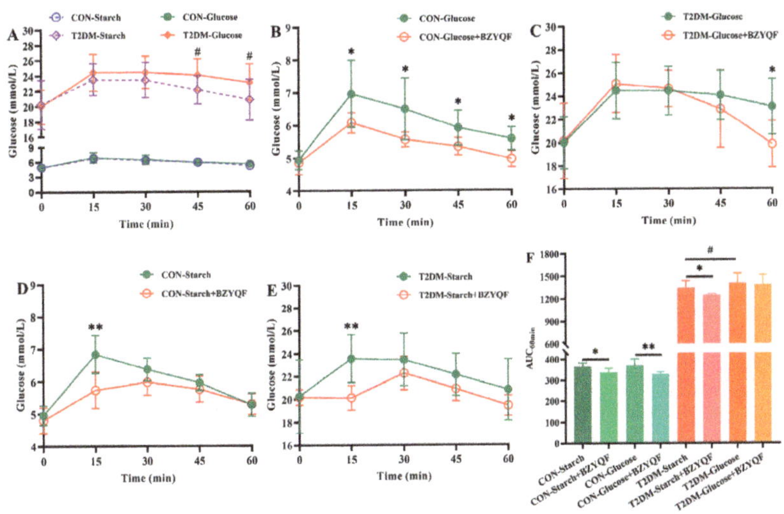

Figure 2. Blood glucose value and AUC of experimental rats after the ingestion of glucose and starch solutions. (**A**) Blood glucose value of experimental rats after the ingestion of glucose and starch solutions without BZYQF; (**B**) Blood glucose value of CON rats after the ingestion of glucose solution; (**C**) Blood glucose value of T2DM rats after the ingestion of glucose solution; (**D**) Blood glucose value of CON rats after the ingestion of starch solution; (**E**) Blood glucose value of T2DM rats after the ingestion of starch solution; (**F**) the AUC of experimental rats after the ingestion of glucose and starch solutions. * $p < 0.05$, ** $p < 0.01$, compared with starch or glucose solution without BZYQF; # $p < 0.05$, compared with glucose solution.

The results of postprandial glycemic responses following the ingestion of glucose solution with BZYQF intervention are shown in Figure 2B,C,F. BZYQF significantly reduced the blood glucose values and AUC of CON rats at all time points after the ingestion of glucose solution, while BZYQF only significantly decreased the blood glucose value of T2DM rats at 60 min after the ingestion of glucose solution. These results suggest that BZYQF was able to better control the blood glucose values of CON rats to the baseline level within 60 min by regulating glucose metabolism (such as by promoting insulin secretion and glucose uptake). At the same time, due to impaired glucose metabolism in T2DM rats, BZYQF had no effect on their blood glucose values after the ingestion of glucose solution in a short period of time (within 45 min), but it might have a certain improvement effect after a prolonged intervention time. The results of postprandial glycemic responses following the ingestion of starch solution with BZYQF intervention are shown in Figure 2D–F. BZYQF significantly reduced the blood glucose values of CON and T2DM rats at 15 min, and delayed the peak of their blood glucose values from the 15 min to 30 min time point. BZYQF had no effect on the blood glucose values at other time points after the ingestion of starch solution. Furthermore, the AUC of CON and T2DM rats significantly decreased after BZYQF intervention. These results suggest that BZYQF reduced postprandial blood glucose levels in CON and T2DM rats at 15 min after the ingestion of starch solution by inhibiting starch hydrolysis. In addition, BZYQF caused a greater drop in blood glucose values at 15 min in T2DM rats than in CON rats (the delta blood glucose value decreased 2.02-fold from 1.88 to 0.93 in CON rats, and the delta blood glucose value reduced 9.65-fold from 3.28 to 0.34 in T2DM, $p < 0.05$). This finding indicates that after the ingestion of starch solution, BZYQF caused a more significant reduction in postprandial blood glucose levels in T2DM rats compared to CON rats.

2.3. *BZYQF Inhibited α-Amylase and α-Glucosidase Activities In Vitro*

To determine the inhibitory effect of BZYQF on the activities of α-amylase and α-glucosidase, in vitro enzyme inhibition assays were performed. The results are shown in Figure 3. The results demonstrate that the inhibitory effect of BZYQF on the activities of α-amylase and α-glucosidase steeply increased with an increase in its concentration, and then increased at a slower rate. The IC50 values of BZYQF against α-amylase and α-glucosidase activities were 53.51 ± 2.32 mg/mL and 10.70 ± 0.06 mg/mL, respectively. The IC50 values of acarbose against α-amylase and α-glucosidase were 2.12 ± 0.07 mg/mL and 0.09 ± 0.00 mg/mL, respectively. These results reveal that BZYQF and acarbose had notable inhibitory effects on the activities of α-amylase and α-glucosidase, and their inhibitory effects on the activity of α-glucosidase were stronger than those of α-amylase.

2.4. *BZYQF Inhibited α-Amylase and α-Glucosidase Activities Through Different Kinetic Modes*

To confirm the inhibition modes of α-amylase and α-glucosidase by BZYQF, the enzyme kinetic parameters, Km and Vmax, were determined using Lineweaver–Burk plots. The results are shown in Figure 4 and Table 1. For α-amylase, all lines fit linearly and intersect in the third quadrant. The values of Km and Vmax decrease simultaneously with an increase in the BZYQF concentration, while the slope of the straight line increases from 30.53 to 40.81, indicating that BZYQF could bind to α-amylase in mixed competition mode. This mode means that some compounds in BZYQF could bind to active sites of α-amylase in a competitive mode, while others bound to the inactive sites of α-amylase in a non-competitive mode. For α-glucosidase, all lines fit linearly and are parallel. The values of Km and Vmax decrease simultaneously with an increase in the BZYQF concentration, while the slope of the straight line remains almost constant, indicating that BZYQF could bind to an α-glucosidase–substrate complex in an uncompetitive mode. These results suggest that BZYQF inhibited α-amylase and α-glucosidase activities in different kinetic modes.

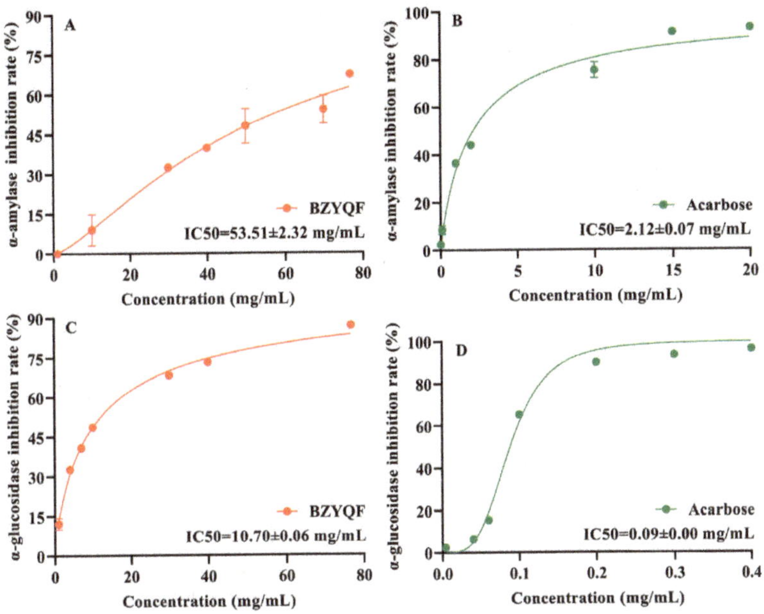

Figure 3. The IC50 values of BZYQF and acarbose for α-amylase and α-glucosidase inhibition. (**A**) the IC50 values of BZYQF for α-amylase inhibition; (**B**) the IC50 values of acarbose for α-amylase inhibition; (**C**) the IC50 values of BZYQF for α-glucosidase inhibition; (**D**) the IC50 values of acarbose for α-glucosidase inhibition.

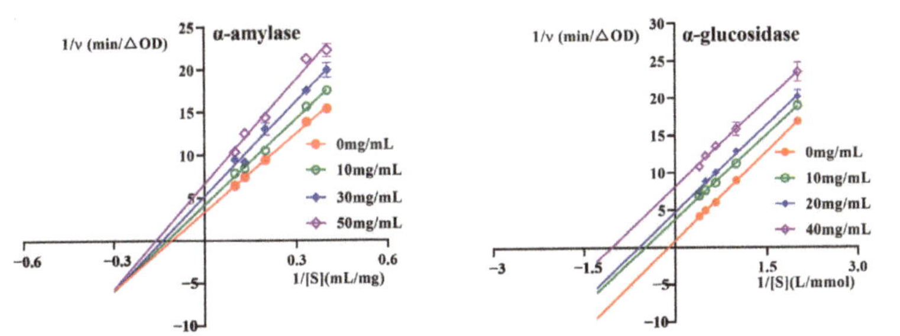

Figure 4. Lineweaver–Burk plots of α-amylase and α-glucosidase inhibitions by BZYQF.

Table 1. Kinetic parameters of α-amylase and α-glucosidase inhibitions by BZYQF.

Enzyme	BZYQF Con. (mg/mL)	Km (mg/mL)	Vmax (ΔOD/min)	Slope
α-amylase	0	9.16 ± 0.94	0.30 ± 0.02	30.53 ± 0.95
	10	8.08 ± 1.07	0.24 ± 0.02	33.52 ± 1.47
	30	7.13 ± 2.03	0.19 ± 0.04	36.94 ± 3.66
	50	6.18 ± 1.51	0.15 ± 0.02	40.81 ± 3.85
α-glucosidase	0	9.36 ± 1.39	1.18 ± 0.22	7.96 ± 0.12
	10	2.03 ± 0.22	0.27 ± 0.02	7.56 ± 0.29
	20	1.67 ± 0.25	0.21 ± 0.03	7.79 ± 0.48
	40	0.95 ± 0.15	0.12 ± 0.01	7.70 ± 0.69

2.5. In Vitro Simulated Digestion Changed the Main Constituent Contents of BZYQF and Their Inhibition Rates for α-Amylase and α-Glucosidase

To explore the influence of digestive fluids on BZYQF, in vitro simulated digestion was performed. The changes in the main constituent contents of BZYQF during in vitro simulated salivary–gastrointestinal digestion are shown in Figure 5A–F. The contents of total carbohydrate and reducing sugar demonstrated no significant change, while the polysaccharide content notably decreased during salivary digestion. Interestingly, the contents of total carbohydrate and reducing sugar significantly increased during gastric digestion, while their contents notably decreased after intestinal digestion. On the contrary, the polysaccharide content clearly reduced during gastric digestion but showed no significant change after intestinal digestion. The total flavonoid and total polyphenol contents demonstrated no significant change during salivary digestion. However, the total flavonoid content gradually decreased after gastrointestinal digestion, while the total polyphenol content markedly increased after intestinal digestion. In addition, the total saponin content demonstrated no significant change during salivary–gastrointestinal digestion. These results suggest that the main constituent contents of BZYQF were less affected by SSF, but their contents were greatly influenced by SGF and SIF.

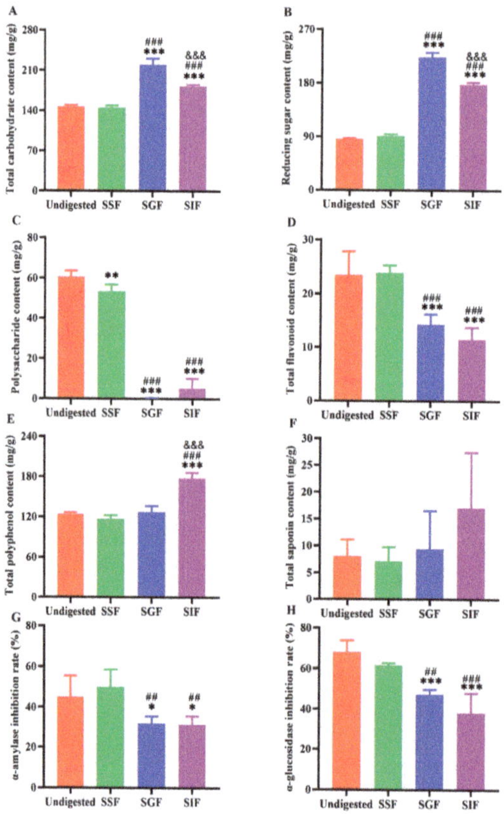

Figure 5. The main constituent contents of BZYQF and their inhibition rates for α-amylase and α-glucosidase during in vitro simulated digestion. (**A**) Total carbohydrate content; (**B**) Reducing sugar content; (**C**) Polysaccharide content; (**D**) Total flavonoid content; (**E**) Total polyphenol content; (**F**) Total saponin content; (**G**) the α-amylase inhibition rate; (**H**) the α-glucosidase inhibition rate. * $p < 0.05$, ** $p < 0.01$, *** $p < 0.001$, compared with undigested group; ## $p < 0.01$, ### $p < 0.001$, compared with SSF group; &&& $p < 0.001$, compared with SGF group.

The changes in the inhibition rates of α-amylase and α-glucosidase by BZYQF during in vitro simulated salivary–gastrointestinal digestion are shown in Figure 5G,H. The inhibition rates of α-amylase and α-glucosidase by BZYQF showed no significant change during salivary digestion. Interestingly, the inhibition rates of α-amylase and α-glucosidase significantly decreased during gastric digestion. These results suggest that the inhibition rates of α-amylase and α-glucosidase by BZYQF are closely related to its main constituent contents.

2.6. The Total Flavonoids Played an Important Role in the Inhibition of α-Amylase and α-Glucosidase Activities by BZYQF

To clarify the active constituents of BZYQF in the inhibition of α-amylase and α-glucosidase activities, we performed Pearson correlation analysis and multiple linear regression analysis between the inhibition rate of α-amylase and α-glucosidase and the main constituent contents of BZYQF. As illustrated in Figure 6, the total flavonoid content was highly correlated with the inhibition rates of α-amylase ($r = 0.90$) and α-glycosidase ($r = 0.87$), with the highest correlation coefficients among all factors. As listed in Table 2, the formula generated by the multiple linear regression analysis was as follows: the inhibition rate of α-amylase = 0.319 + 0.294 × total flavonoid and the inhibition rate of α-glucosidase = 0.532 + 0.236 × total flavonoid. The non-significant coefficients ($p > 0.05$) were removed from the analysis, showing that the response variables were only dependent on the factor of total flavonoids and were positively influenced by this factor. The factors of total carbohydrates, reducing sugar, polysaccharides, total polyphenols, and total saponins were not significant, showing no significant influence on the response variables. The R^2 values indicate that the variability in the inhibition rates of α-amylase and α-glycosidase could be explained by the fitting of the model, as their values are greater than 85% (85.0% and 85.6%, respectively). These results suggest that the total flavonoids might be the active constituents of BZYQF in the inhibition of α-amylase and α-glucosidase activities.

Table 2. Summary output of the multiple linear regression analysis performed between the inputs (the main constituent contents of BZYQF) and the output (the inhibition rates of α-amylase or α-glucosidase).

Enzyme	Variables	Regression Coefficient	p Value	95% CI (Lower ~ Upper)
α-amylase	Intercept	0.319	0.000	0.194 ~ 0.445
	Total carbohydrate	-	-	-
	Reducing sugar	0.014	0.200	−0.008 ~ 0.036
	Polysaccharide	0.023	0.266	−0.019 ~ 0.065
	Total flavonoid	0.294	0.010	0.082 ~ 0.507
	Total polyphenol	−0.057	0.072	−0.120 ~ 0.006
	Total saponin	0.111	0.427	−0.177 ~ 0.400
α-glucosidase	Intercept	0.532	0.000	0.448 ~ 0.616
	Total carbohydrate	-	-	-
	Reducing sugar	−0.010	0.191	−0.024 ~ 0.005
	Polysaccharide	0.017	0.228	−0.011 ~ 0.045
	Total flavonoid	0.236	0.003	0.094 ~ 0.378
	Total polyphenol	−0.018	0.386	−0.060 ~ 0.024
	Total saponin	−0.131	0.168	−0.324 ~ 0.061

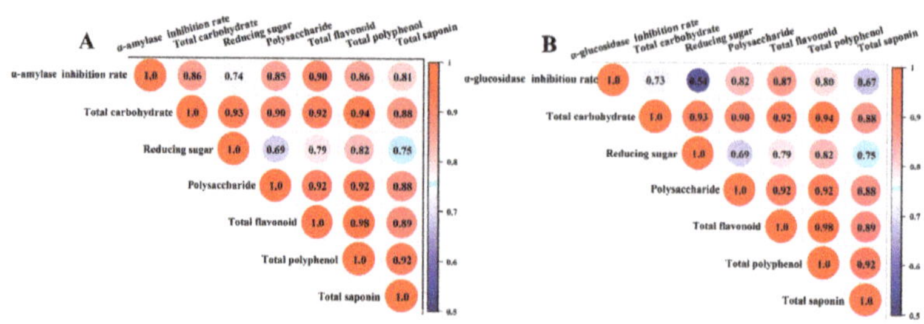

Figure 6. Pearson correlation coefficient (r) between the main constituent contents of BZYQF and their inhibition rates of α-amylase (**A**) or α-glucosidase (**B**).

2.7. Purification of Total Flavonoids and In Vitro Activity Validation

To verify the biological activity of the total flavonoids, they were extracted and isolated from BZYQF to measure the main constituent content and perform in vitro inhibition assays of α-amylase and α-glucosidase. As shown in Figure 7A, after the isolation of D101 macroporous resin, the total carbohydrate, reducing sugar, and polysaccharide contents significantly decreased, while the total flavonoid, total polyphenol, and total saponin contents remarkably increased in the purified total flavonoids compared with BZYQF. Furthermore, the total flavonoid content increased 12.44-fold from 23.45 to 291.94 mg/g crude drug (equivalent to 625.23 mg/g dry powder) with the most significant increase. After purification, flavonoids and polyphenols were the main constituents of the purified total flavonoids. As illustrated in Figure 7B,C, the IC50 values of the purified total flavonoids against α-amylase and α-glucosidase activities were 27.37 ± 3.27 mg/mL and 0.31 ± 0.03 mg/mL, respectively. As indicated in Figure 7D,E, in the purified total flavonoids, the total flavonoid content was highly correlated with the inhibition rates of α-amylase (r = 0.94) and α-glycosidase (r = 0.83), with the highest correlation coefficients among all factors. As listed in Table 3, in the purified total flavonoids, the formula generated from multiple linear regression analysis was as follows: the inhibition rate of α-amylase = 0.046 × total flavonoid and the inhibition rate of α-glucosidase = 0.219 + 0.051 × total flavonoid. Their R^2 values were greater than 80% (93.1% and 80.6%, respectively). These results suggest that the purified total flavonoid had stronger inhibitory effects on the activities of α-amylase and α-glucosidase than BZYQF, which is closely related to the increase in the total flavonoid content.

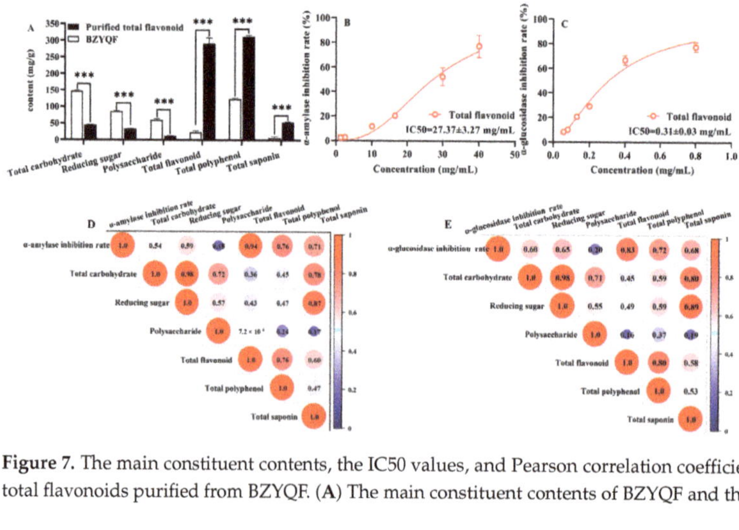

Figure 7. The main constituent contents, the IC50 values, and Pearson correlation coefficients of the total flavonoids purified from BZYQF. (**A**) The main constituent contents of BZYQF and the purified

total flavonoids; (**B**,**C**) the IC50 values of the purified total flavonoids for α-amylase and α-glucosidase inhibition; (**D**,**E**) Pearson correlation coefficients between the main constituent contents of the purified total flavonoids and their inhibition rates of α-amylase (**D**) or α-glucosidase (**E**). *** $p < 0.001$, compared with BZYQF.

Table 3. Summary output of the multiple linear regression analysis performed between the inputs (the main constituent contents of the total flavonoids purified from BZYQF) and the output (the inhibition rates of α-amylase or α-glucosidase).

Enzyme	Variables	Regression Coefficient	*p* Value	95% CI (Lower ~ Upper)
α-amylase	Intercept	0.003	0.957	−0.099 ~ 0.104
	Total carbohydrate	-	-	-
	Reducing sugar	−0.025	0.492	−0.103 ~ 0.053
	Polysaccharide	0.081	0.201	−0.051 ~ 0.213
	Total flavonoid	0.046	0.001	0.024 ~ 0.068
	Total polyphenol	0.003	0.696	−0.012 ~ 0.018
	Total saponin	0.111	0.251	−0.092 ~ 0.313
α-glucosidase	Intercept	0.219	0.018	0.046 ~ 0.392
	Total carbohydrate	-	-	-
	Reducing sugar	0.122	0.135	−0.045 ~ 0.289
	Polysaccharide	−0.155	0.216	−0.415 ~ 0.106
	Total flavonoid	0.051	0.017	0.011 ~ 0.091
	Total polyphenol	−0.005	0.735	−0.037 ~ 0.027
	Total saponin	−0.217	0.285	−0.645 ~ 0.211

2.8. Molecular Docking of Flavonoids in BZYQF with α-Amylase and α-Glycosidase

Molecular docking was performed to further understand the binding mechanism between flavonoids in BZYQF and α-amylase/α-glycosidase, and the associated structures were characterized using Discovery Studio. Out of the 467 flavonoids identified in BZYQF, 197 of them were able to bind to α-amylase or α-glycosidase. Among them, 187 flavonoids could bind to α-amylase and α-glycosidase simultaneously, including 5 dihydroflavonols, 18 chalcones, 32 flavonols, 71 flavones, 44 isoflavones, and 17 dihydroflavones. As presented in Figure 8, the binding of 187 flavonoids to the two enzymes was mainly characterized by low (interaction energy > −40) and medium (−60 < interaction energy < −40) binding intensities. Among them, the number and percentage of flavonoids with moderate binding intensity to α-glycosidase were significantly higher than those of flavonoids bound to α-amylase. In addition, the average interaction energy of all of these flavonoids to α-glucosidase was significantly lower than their average interaction energy to α-amylase. Similar results were found in other secondary flavonoids, with the exception of isoflavones, in which a low binding intensity predominated. These results suggest that flavonoids in BZYQF more strongly bound to α-glycosidase than to α-amylase.

As shown in Figure 9A,C,E, similarly to the themaltotriose substrate, flavonoids of BZYQF (Robinin was shown) docked into the active site of α-amylase, exhibiting competitive binding behavior. When bound to α-amylase (interaction energy < −40), flavonoids of BZYQF were mainly surrounded by 13 amino acid residues of Glu 233, Lys 200, Asp 197, Asp 300, Tyr 151, Gln 63, His 201, Ala 198, Leu 162, Ile 235, Trp 62, Trp 59, and His 305. In these cases, five main interactions—Pi–anion, Pi–Pi (including stacked and T-shape), Pi–alkyl, hydrogen bonds, and carbon hydrogen bonds—were formed between flavonoids of BZYQF and α-amylase. In the proportion of amino acid residues in these five interactions, the proportions of Glu233, Asp197, Asp300, and His201 were higher than those of other amino acid residues, exceeding 50%. Moreover, the first three amino acid residues formed three interactions—Pi–anion, hydrogen bonds, and carbon hydrogen bonds—while the amino acid residue of His201 formed two interactions—Pi–Pi and carbon hydrogen bonds—between flavonoids of BZYQF and α-amylase. On binding to α-amylase, flavonoids of BZYQF hampered the access of the substrate or occupied the binding site of starch, which further suppressed the activity of α-amylase.

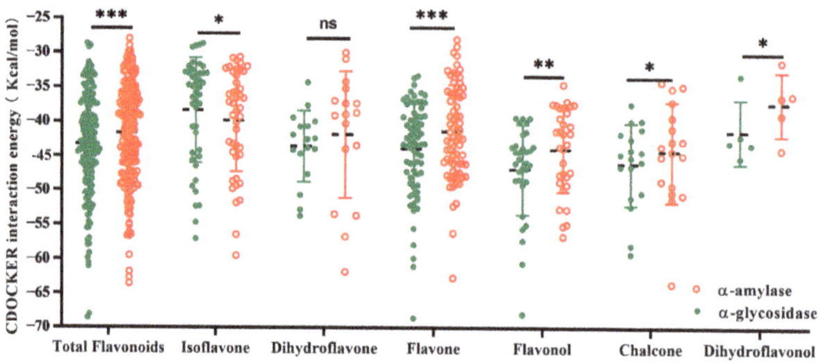

Figure 8. Interaction energy of flavonoids in BZYQF with α-amylase and α-glycosidase. * $p < 0.05$, ** $p < 0.01$, *** $p < 0.001$; ns, not statistically significant.

As shown in Figure 9B,D,F, unlike the substrate of maltose, flavonoids of BZYQF (Sudachiin C was shown) interacted with the essential amino acid residues located in the non-catalytic site of α-glucosidase, exhibiting a non-competitive or uncompetitive binding behavior. When bound to α-glycosidase (interaction energy < −40), flavonoids of BZYQF were mainly surrounded by 15 amino acid residues: Glu 856, Ile 823, Arg 725, Lyd 348, Glu 721, Arg 854, Glu 748, Gly 855, Gly 747, Pro 825, Leu 712, Ala 749, Tyr 822, His 708, and Ala 719. In these cases, five main interactions—Pi–anion, Pi–Pi, Pi–alkyl, hydrogen bonds, and carbon hydrogen bonds—were also formed between flavonoids of BZYQF and α-glycosidase. In the proportion of amino acid residues in these five interactions, the proportions of Glu748, Glu856, Tyr 822, and His 708 were higher than those of other amino acid residues, exceeding 50%. Moreover, the amino acid residues of Glu748 and Glu856 formed three interactions—Pi–anion, hydrogen bonds, and carbon hydrogen bonds—while the amino acid residues of Tyr 822 and His 708 formed two interactions—Pi–Pi and Pi–alkyl—between flavonoids of BZYQF and α-glycosidase. These amino acid residues increased the stability of the inhibitor–enzyme complex, exposing the inhibitory ability of flavonoids of BZYQF. On binding to α-glycosidase, flavonoids of BZYQF probably perturbed the protein structure and inhibited α-glucosidase in a non-competitive or uncompetitive mode, thus altering the enzyme activity.

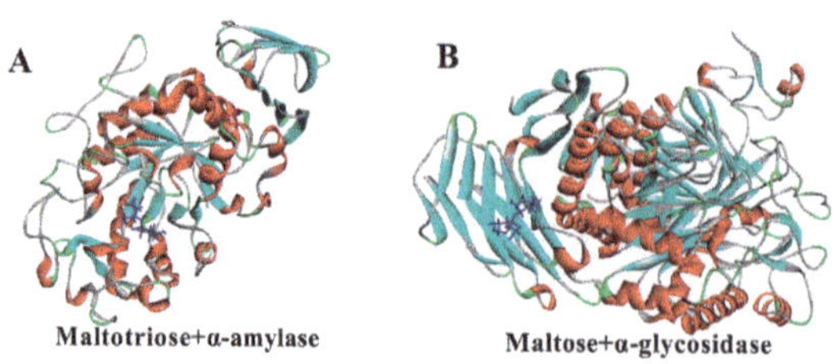

Figure 9. *Cont.*

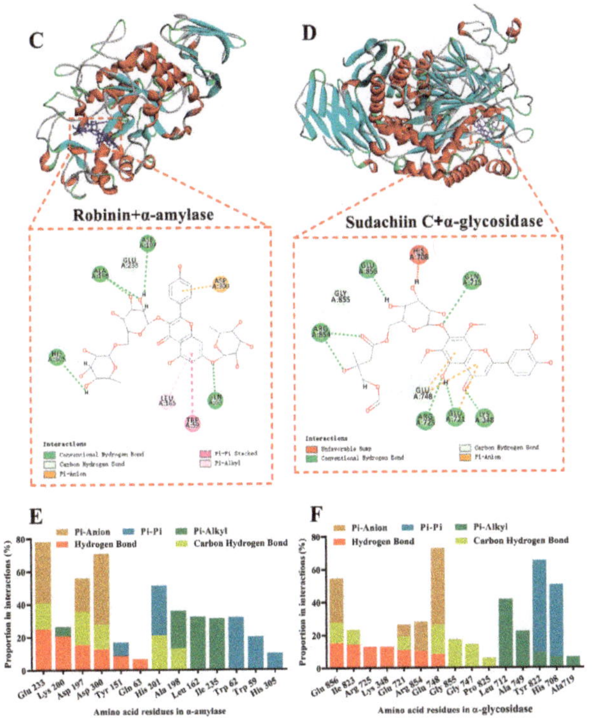

Figure 9. The docked diagrams and the proportion of amino acid residues in interactions based on the predicted optimal binding mode of flavonoids in BZYQF to α-amylase and α-glucosidase. (**A**,**B**) Three-dimensional diagrams of the substrates of maltotriose and maltose binding to α-amylase and α-glucosidase, respectively; (**C**,**D**) Three-dimensional and two-dimensional diagrams of flavonoids in BZYQF binding to α-amylase and α-glucosidase; Robinin and Sudachiin C are shown here; (**E**,**F**) The proportions of amino acid residues (interaction energy < −40, accounting for >5% of amino acid residues) in interactions, which formed between flavonoids of BZYQF and α-amylase or α-glucosidase. Among all flavonoids of BZYQF, Robinin and Sudachiin C had the lowest interaction energy to α-amylase (−73.7461) and α-glycosidase (−68.5875), respectively.

3. Discussion

The present study found that BZYQF could significantly reduce postprandial hyperglycemia after the ingestion of starch solution in T2DM rats. The molecular mechanism may involve BZYQF inhibiting the activities of α-amylase and α-glycosidase, reducing glucose production and thereby preventing a sudden increase in blood glucose levels. Through multiple linear regression analysis and molecular docking, we speculated that the main constituents of BZYQF that inhibited α-amylase and α-glycosidase activities were total flavonoids. Moreover, this speculation was verified by analyzing the total flavonoids isolated from BZYQF. This study provides a theoretical basis for BZYQF to control postprandial hyperglycemia in T2DM.

Postprandial hyperglycemia is one of the central symptoms of T2DM. Controlling postprandial hyperglycemia can not only minimize blood glucose fluctuation but also reduce the risk of cardiovascular disease. However, the changes in postprandial blood glucose levels are closely associated with the composition of food and the efficiency of the body's carbohydrate metabolism. Monosaccharide foods can be absorbed directly by the intestines, causing a rapid increase in blood glucose levels. Polysaccharide-rich foods such as starch must be enzymatically digested in the mouth and intestines to be converted into monosaccharides before absorption, resulting in a more consistent and gradual increase in blood glucose levels compared to monosaccharide foods. In addition, glucose was absorbed into the bloodstream via the SGLT1 and GLUT2 transporters in the small intestine, resulting in an increase in postprandial blood glucose [12]. The increased blood glucose stimulated pancreatic β-cells to secrete insulin, which, in turn, activated peripheral tissues to uptake glucose, thus lowering postprandial blood glucose to maintain glucose homeostasis. Therefore, the changes in postprandial blood glucose levels were influenced by food, digestive enzyme activity, glucose transporters, and the function of insulin. At present, in the clinical treatment of T2DM, most drugs target insulin and glucose transporters, such as metformin, thiazolidinediones, GLP-1 receptor agonists, SGLT-1 inhibitors, etc., while few drugs target digestive enzymes. Acarbose, as an α-glycosidase inhibitor, had a prominent effect on controlling postprandial hyperglycemia. However, its side effects, such as gastrointestinal complaints, allergic reactions, and damage to liver function, were also evident. Therefore, studying the glycemic capacity of carbohydrate-containing foods and screening for digestive enzyme inhibitors with low side effects remain important for the control of postprandial hyperglycemia in T2DM. BZYQF has been used as a classic formula of TCM in China for hundreds of years. It has been widely used to regulate subhealth and impaired spleen and stomach functions [13] and has excellent therapeutic effects in improving digestion and immune deficiency [14–16]. Clinical studies have found that BZYQF could improve fasting blood glucose and pancreatic islet function in patients with T2DM [17]. However, research on the role of BZYQF in regulating postprandial hyperglycemia in T2DM is limited. The present study found that following the ingestion of glucose and starch solutions, the blood glucose values of CON rats increased significantly from 5 mM to 7 mM, and those of T2DM rats increased from 20 mM to 25 mM. This result is supported by the reports of Momtazi-Borojen et al. [18] and Liu et al. [19], in which the blood glucose value of CON or T2DM rats had a similar increase from the low value to the highest value in an oral glucose tolerance test. These results indicate that the concentrations of glucose/starch solutions used in this study were effective. Furthermore, this study found that the blood glucose level and AUC of T2DM rats were significantly higher than those of CON rats. This result is also confirmed by a large number of animal experiments [20–23]. Interestingly, the blood glucose levels of CON rats had no difference between the ingestion of glucose and starch solutions, while T2DM rats had lower blood glucose levels following the ingestion of starch solution than those following the ingestion of glucose solution. These results suggest that CON rats were able to rapidly digest starch and utilize glucose, whereas T2DM rats exhibited abnormal carbohydrate metabolism, manifested by a reduced ability to digest starch and utilize glucose. As is well known, T2DM rats have insufficient insulin secretion and insulin resistance, and there are increased expressions of GLUT2 and SGLT-1 in the intestine of T2DM rats [24–26]. In addition, this study also found that after BZYQF intervention, BZYQF could significantly reduce the blood glucose levels at 15 min after the ingestion of starch solution and within 0–60 min after the ingestion of glucose solution in CON rats. However, BZYQF could only reduce the blood glucose levels at 15 min after the ingestion of starch solution and had no effect on the blood glucose levels within 0–45 min after the ingestion of glucose solution in T2DM rats. These results suggest that BZYQF could better stabilize postprandial blood glucose levels in CON rats and significantly reduce postprandial blood glucose following the ingestion of starch solution in CON and T2DM rats. BZYQF could reduce postprandial blood glucose levels following the ingestion of glucose solution in CON rats but not in T2DM rats. This might be because BZYQF regulated glucose uptake and improved insulin secretion and sensitivity in CON rats, while it did not improve impaired glucose utilization and insulin function in T2DM rats in the short term. Clinical observations have shown that

BZYQF could improve insulin sensitivity and reduce hyperglycemia in T2DM patients [17]. Moreover, our previous research on *Astragalus membranaceus* (the most important Chinese herbs in BZYQF) found that after treatment for 8 weeks, Astragalus polysaccharides could promote insulin secretion, improve insulin resistance, and reduce the expressions of SGLT-1 and GLUT2 in the intestine of T2DM rats [27]. Notably, BZYQF could significantly reduce blood glucose levels at 60 min after the ingestion of glucose solution in T2DM rats. This result indicates that prolonging the intervention time of BZYQF had a certain improvement effect on glucose utilization in T2DM rats. In the present study, BZYQF simultaneously reduced the blood glucose levels at 15 min after the ingestion of starch solution in CON and T2DM rats, with a more significant decrease in blood glucose levels in T2DM rats. This result suggests that BZYQF could inhibit the activity of digestive enzymes and that T2DM rats exhibit defects in starch digestion. In addition, after intervention with BZYQF, the peak of blood glucose levels in CON and T2DM rats was delayed from 15 min to 30 min after the ingestion of starch solution, while similar results were not observed in rats that ingested glucose solution. This further confirms that BZYQF could inhibit the process of starch digestion into glucose. Clinical studies have found that ZBYQF reduces postprandial glucose levels within 2 h [9]. Thus, it can be seen that BZYQF could significantly reduce postprandial hyperglycemia in T2DM rats, and its mechanism might be related to the improvement of glucose metabolism, especially the inhibition of digestive enzyme activity.

Digestive enzymes, particularly α-amylase and α-glucosidase, are key enzymes involved in the hydrolysis of dietary starch to produce glucose, which has been closely linked to elevated postprandial blood glucose [28]. α-amylase catalyzes the hydrolysis of α-1,4-glycosidic bonds of starch, glycogen, and various oligosaccharides. α-glucosidase catalyzes the breaking of glycosidic bonds and the subsequent release of glucose from the non-reducing ends of oligosaccharide chains [28,29]. When dietary starch is ingested, it is first hydrolyzed by salivary α-amylase in the mouth and pancreatic α-amylase in the small intestine, yielding smaller oligomers such as maltose and maltotriose. Subsequently, these oligomers are further degraded into glucose molecules by other hydrolyzing enzymes, such as α-glucosidase, in the small intestine. Finally, glucose is transported into the bloodstream via the transporters of GLUT2 and SGLT1. Therefore, the inhibition of these enzyme activities could reduce postprandial blood glucose levels by delaying the digestion of carbohydrates into glucose. The IC50 value refers to the semi-inhibitory concentration of the measured antagonist. It represents the concentration at which a drug inhibits enzyme activity by 50%. In the drug screening process, IC50 values are used to preliminarily screen potential drug candidate molecules and determine their activity against specific targets. Usually, a smaller IC50 value indicates that the drug has a stronger inhibitory effect. Enzyme kinetics studies have shown that inhibition consists of both reversible and irreversible inhibition. Between the two, reversible inhibition is more important as it only slows down the digestive process but does not permanently block it. By slowing down the digestive process, glucose would be produced at a more consistent rate, thereby preventing blood sugar spikes [30]. Reversible inhibition includes three types: competitive, non-competitive, and uncompetitive. In competitive inhibition, the inhibitor and substrate have similar structures and compete for binding to the active sites of the enzyme. In non-competitive inhibition, both the substrate and the inhibitor bind to the enzyme at completely independent sites. In contrast, uncompetitive inhibitors do not bind to the free enzyme, but only to the enzyme–substrate complex [31,32]. Acarbose, which has been widely used in the clinical treatment of diabetes, is a classic inhibitor, binding competitively to α-amylase and α-glucosidase. The present study found that BZYQF had a good inhibitory effect on the activities of α-amylase and α-glucosidase in vitro, although the IC50 values of BZYQF against the two enzymes were higher than those of acarbose. Similarly to acarbose, BZYQF showed a stronger inhibitory effect on α-glucosidase than on α-amylase. In contrast to acarbose, BZYQF bound to α-amylase in a mixed competition mode, while it bound to α-glucosidase in an uncompetitive mode. Some studies have reported that a single constituent in BZYQF had inhibitory effects on α-amylase and α-glucosidase, although the inhibitory effects of BZYQF for the two enzymes have not been reported yet. Our previous study showed that *Astragalus* polysaccharides exerted an inhibitory effect on α-amylase in a dose-dependent manner [33]. Other research has reported that *Astragalus* polysaccharides and isoflavones have an inhibitory effect on α-glucosidase [34,35]. Licorice extracts have shown important anti-amylase and anti-glucosidase activities [36,37], among which glycyrrhizic acid inhibited α-glucosidase activity in a mixed competition mode [38]. *Codonopsis pilosula* (Franch.) Nannf. has been shown to have a strong inhibitory effect against mammalian α-glucosidase, which could significantly reduce the postprandial blood glucose level in diabetic mice in an oral starch tolerance test [39]. Therefore, BZYQF could lower postprandial blood glucose by inhibiting the activities of α-amylase and α-glucosidase, but the active constituents that inhibited enzyme activity need to be further determined.

Widely targeted metabolomic analysis and molecular docking have been widely used to identify active constituents in herbs and formulas. The results of our metabolomics analysis show that flavonoids accounted for the highest proportion among the 1909 compounds identified in BZYQF, accounting for over 40%, although their contents were not abundant. Using UPLC-QE-MS analysis, Xin Su et al. [40] also found that the chemical constituents of BZYQF included large amounts of flavonoids. In vitro simulated digestion assays simulated the physiological conditions of digestion in vivo and have been widely used in pharmacology to study and understand the changes, interactions, and bioavailability of chemical compounds. The present study found that the main constituent contents of BZYQF, excluding polysaccharides, did not significantly change during digestion with SSF, suggesting that SSF has a weak effect on BZYQF. The polysaccharide content decreased during salivary digestion, indicating that some polysaccharides could be hydrolyzed by amylase. During digestion with SGF, the total carbohydrate and reducing sugar contents in BZYQF increased, while polysaccharide contents decreased, indicating that glycans and polysaccharides were broken down into monosaccharides or oligosaccharides in SGF. Jing Kun Yan et al. [41] found that after digestion with SGF, the reducing sugar contents increased significantly, which might be due to the strong acidic environment in SGF disrupting glycosidic bonds, leading to an increase in reducing sugars. In this study, during digestion with SIF, the total carbohydrate and reducing sugar contents in BZYQF decreased. This could be because the small intestinal fluid affected the conformation and stability of polysaccharides, thereby leading to a reduction in reducing sugar content [42]. This study also found that the total flavonoid content of BZYQF significantly decreased after digestion with SGF, while there was no change after digestion with SIF. This result suggests that flavonoids in BZYQF could be degraded by the strong acids in SGF. A similar result was reported by Zhang et al. [43], where the total flavonoid content in the ethanol extract from camphor seed kernels decreased after gastric digestion. In addition, the present study found that the total polyphenol content in BZYQF increased during digestion with SIF, and the total saponin content in BZYQF had no significant change during salivary–gastrointestinal digestion. This result suggests that the total polyphenols in BZYQF could be influenced by SIF, while the total saponins in BZYQF were not affected by simulated digestive fluid. The increase in total polyphenol content could be due to the degradation of macromolecular polyphenols, releasing simpler polyphenolic acids. These polyphenol derivatives release active functional groups and react with Folin–Ciocalteu reagents to increase the total polyphenol content [44]. In vitro enzyme inhibition assays revealed that the inhibition rates of BZYQF against α-amylase and α-glucosidase varied with the changes in its main constituent contents during simulated digestion. Notably, the trend in changes in the BZYQF inhibition rates of α-amylase and α-glucosidase was consistent with the trend in changes in its total flavonoid content. Furthermore, correlation analysis and multiple linear regression analysis showed that the total flavonoid content in BZYQF was significantly positively correlated with its inhibition rates against α-amylase and α-glycosidase. These results indicate that the total flavonoids were the active constituents of BZYQF in inhibiting α-amylase and α-glycosidase activities. Subsequently, we extracted and isolated the total flavonoids from BZYQF and found that the IC50 values of the purified total flavonoids against α-amylase and α-glucosidase activities were significantly lower than those of BZYQF. This result indicates that the purified total flavonoids had stronger enzyme inhibitory activities than BZYQF, which further verified the inhibitory effects of total flavonoids in BZYQF on the activities of α-amylase and α-glucosidase. Finally, our molecular docking results indicate that 40% of the flavonoids in BZYQF could bind to α-amylase and α-glycosidase simultaneously and that these flavonoids bound more strongly to α-glycosidase than to α-amylase. This result is consistent with the lower IC50 values of BZYQF and the purified total flavonoids against α-glycosidase than their IC50 values against α-amylase. In addition, the molecular docking site of this study showed that flavonoids in BZYQF were bound to the inactive site of α-glucosidase while they were bound to the active site of α-amylase. This result is consistent with the results of the enzyme kinetics assay, in which BZYQF inhibited α-glucosidase activity in an uncompetitive mode, and α-amylase activity, in a mixed competition and non-competition mode. At the same time, this result also suggests that among the main constituents in BZYQF that inhibited α-amylase activity, in addition to flavonoids, other chemical constituents such as polysaccharides and polyphenols could exert their effects in a non-competitive mode. Our previous study found that *Astragalus* polysaccharides had an inhibitory effect on α-amylase activity [33]. A review confirmed that polyphenols from various extracts, such as gallic acid, caffeic acid, and kaempferol, inhibited α-amylase activity in a non-competitive mode [45]. In addition, several studies have shown that flavonoids have a strong inhibitory effect on α-glucosidase and a moderate inhibitory effect on α-amylase, making them promising candidates for antidiabetic drugs [46–48]. However, no consensus has been reached regarding the mode by which flavonoids inhibit α-glucosidase and α-amylase. This could be due to the differences in plant flavonoid sources and detection methods used in different studies [46]. Overall, flavonoids play an important role in the inhibition of α-glucosidase and α-amylase activity in BZYQF.

4. Materials and Methods

4.1. Preparation of BZYQF

BZYQF was purchased from JiuZhiTang Co., Ltd. (National Medical Approval No. Z43020143, Changsha, China). It was composed of 8 Chinese herbs, including 200 g of *Astragalus membranaceus* (Fisch.) Bunge (honey roasted), 100 g of *Glycyrhiza uralensis* Fisch. (honey roasted), 60 g of *Codonopsis pilosula* (Franch.) Nannf., 60 g of *Atractylodes macrocephala* Koidz. (stir fried), 60 g of *Angelica sinensis [Oliv.] Diels.*, 60 g of *Cimicifuga heracleifolia* Kom, 60 g of *Bupleurum chinense* DC., 60 g of *Citrus reticulata* Blanco., 40 g of *Ziziphus jujuba* Mill, and 20 g of *Zingiber offcinale* Roscoe. BZYQF was manufactured in accordance with the drug standards of the Ministry of Health for Traditional Chinese Medicine Formulations (Volume 7). A brief introduction is as follows: the volatile oil was extracted from *Zingiber officinale* and *Citrus reticulata*. The remaining residues were boiled twice in water with *Astragalus membranaceus, Atractylodes macrocephala, Cimicifuga heracleifolia, Bupleurum chinense, Ziziphus jujuba*, and one half of *Glycyrhiza uralensis*, for 3 h and 2 h, respectively. The decoction was collected and filtered. The filtrate was concentrated into a thick paste with a relative density of 1.3–1.35. The *Codonopsis pilosula*, *Angelica sinensis*, and the other half of *Glycyrhiza uralensis* were crushed into fine powder. All the above pastes, powders, and volatile oils were mixed to make BZYQF pills.

4.2. Characterization of Chemical Constituents in BZYQF

A chemical constituent analysis of BZYQF was conducted using the widely targeted metabolomic techniques reported by Chen et al. [49]. A brief introduction is as follows: BZYQF was ground into powder (30 Hz, 1.5 min) using a grinder (MM 400, Retsch, Haan, Germany) after being freeze-dried in a lyophilizer (Scientz-100F, Ningbo, China). A measure of 50 mg of sample powder was added to 1200 μL of pre-cooled 70% methanolic aqueous solution and vortexed for 30 s once every 30 min a total of 6 times. After centrifugation at 12,000× *g* for 3 min, the supernatant was filtered with a microporous membrane (0.22 μm pore size) for UPLC-MS/MS analysis. The UPLC analytical conditions were as follows: the injection volume was 2 μL; the flow velocity was set as 0.35 mL/min; the column oven was set at 40 °C; an Agilent SB-C18 column (1.8 μm, 2.1 mm × 100 mm, Agilent, Santa Clara, CA, USA) was used; and the mobile phase consisted of solvent A, pure water with 0.1% formic acid, and solvent B, acetonitrile with 0.1% formic acid. Sample measurements were carried out using a gradient program as follows: the initial conditions of 95% A and 5% B were used. A linear gradient to 5% A and 95% B was then programmed within 9 min, and a composition of 5% A and 95% B was maintained for 1 min. Subsequently, a composition of 95% A and 5.0% B was adjusted within 1.1 min and maintained for 2.9 min. The effluent was alternatively connected to an ESI-Triple Quadrupole-Linear Ion Trap (QTRAP)-MS (Qtrap 5500, AB Sciex, Framingham, MA, USA). The operating parameters of the ESI source were as follows: the source temperature was 500 °C; the ion spray voltage (IS) was 5500*V* (positive ion mode)/−4500*V* (negative ion mode); ion source gas I (GSI), gas II (GSII), and curtain gas (CUR) were set at 50, 60, and 25 psi, respectively; collision-activated dissociation (CAD) was set to high; QQQ scans were performed using the MRM model; and collision gas (nitrogen) was set to medium. The DP (declustering potential) and CE (collision energy) for individual MRM transitions were acquired through DP and CE optimization. A specific set of MRM ion pairs were monitored at each period according to the eluted metabolites during this period. The primary and secondary metabolites were determined using secondary spectral information and the self-created database MWDB (Metware database, Wuhan, China).

The content of calycosin-7-O-β-D-glucoside, an isoflavone isolated from *Astragalus membranaceus* in BZYQF, was determined using HPLC (UltiMate3000, Thermo, Waltham, MA, USA). After treatment with methanol, BZYQF and the standard samples of calycosin-7-O-β-D-glucoside were filtered using a 0.22 μm microporous filter membrane, and the filtrate was analyzed using HPLC. The HPLC analytical conditions were as follows: the injection volume was 20 μL; the flow velocity was set as 1 mL/min; the column oven was set at 30 °C; an Agilent Durashell C18(L) column (1.5 μm, 4.6 mm × 250 mm) was used; and the mobile phase was acetonitrile with 0.1% phosphoric acid solution (3:97). Sample measurements were performed using gradient elution with a wavelength range of 200–400 nm.

4.3. Quantitative Determination of the Main Constituents in BZYQF

BZYQF pills were crushed and then incubated in water at 90 °C at a solid/liquid ratio of 1:30 for 1 h. After centrifugation at 3000× *g* for 10 min, the supernatant was used for subsequent experiments, including the following assays for quantitation, enzyme inhibition, and simulated digestion.

The total carbohydrate content was determined using the phenol–sulfuric acid method [50]. BZYQF solutions or standard solutions (1 mL) were mixed with 0.5 mL of 6% phenol solution and 2.5 mL of concentrated sulfuric acid. The mixture was placed into boiling water for 15 min and quickly cooled to room temperature with cold water. The absorbance at 490 nm was measured on a microplate reader (ELx800, BIOTEK, Winooski, VT, USA). The total carbohydrate content was calculated from a standard glucose curve and expressed as a glucose equivalent (mg/g crude drug).

The reducing sugar content was determined using the 3,5-dinitrosalicylic acid method [50]. BZYQF solutions or standard solutions (2 mL) were mixed with 2 mL of 3,5-dinitrosalicylic acid. The mixture was placed into boiling water for 5 min and quickly cooled to room temperature. The total volume of the mixture was supplemented to 25 mL by adding 21 mL of distilled water. The absorbance at 520 nm was measured on a microplate reader (ELx800, BIOTEK, Vermont, USA). The reducing sugar content was calculated from a standard glucose curve and expressed as a glucose equivalent (mg/g crude drug).

The polysaccharide content was calculated as the difference between the total carbohydrate content and reducing sugar content.

The total flavonoid content was determined using a colorimetric method with minor modifications [51]. BZYQF solutions or standard solutions (1 mL) were mixed with 0.3 mL of 5% $NaNO_2$ solution (w/v) and incubated for 6 min at room temperature. Then, 0.3 mL of 5% $Al(NO_3)_3$ solution (w/v) was added and incubated for 6 min at room temperature. Finally, 4 mL of 4% NaOH (w/v) was added and incubated for 15 min at room temperature. The absorbance at 510 nm was determined on a microplate reader (ELx800, BIOTEK, Vermont, USA). The total flavonoid content was calculated from a standard rutin curve and expressed as a rutin equivalent (mg/g crude drug).

The total polyphenol content was determined using Singleton's method [52], with minor modifications. BZYQF solutions or standard solutions (1 mL) were mixed with 0.25 mL of 50% Folin–Ciocalteu reagent and 0.75 mL of 20% sodium carbonate solution. The mixture was kept in the dark at room temperature for 30 min. The absorbance at 740 nm was measured on the microplate reader (ELx800, BIOTEK, Vermont, USA). The total polyphenol content was calculated from a standard gallic acid curve and expressed as a gallic acid equivalent (mg/g crude drug).

The total saponin content was determined using Milad Hadidi et al.'s method [53], with minor modifications. BZYQF solutions or standard solutions (1 mL) were mixed with 0.5 mL of 8% vanillin ethanol solution (w/v) and 5 mL of 72% sulfuric acid. The mixture was heated for 10 min at 60 °C, followed by cooling on ice for 5 min. The absorbance at 520 nm was measured on a microplate reader (ELx800, BIOTEK, Vermont, USA). The total saponin content was calculated from a standard ginsenoside curve and expressed as a ginsenoside equivalent (mg/g crude drug).

4.4. Induction of T2DM Rats

Male Sprague Dawley (SD) rats (190–210 g) were provided by the Medical Experimental Animal Center of Guangdong Province, with production license number SCXK (Guangdong) 2022-0002. SD rats were bred in the Experimental Animal Center of Guangdong Pharmaceutical University at a relative humidity of 65% ± 5% and 20 ± 2 °C room temperature with a 12/12 h light/dark cycle. The present study strictly complied with animal welfare ethics about the reasonable use of animal numbers and measures to reduce animal suffering, and it was approved by the Laboratory Animal Ethics Committee of Guangdong Pharmaceutical University (approval number gdpulacspf2022203). T2DM induction was performed according to references for previously validated models [54,55]. After adaptive feeding for 3 days, SD rats were randomly divided into two groups: control

(CON, $n = 8$) and T2DM ($n = 8$). During the experiment, the rats in the CON group were fed a basal diet (25% flour, 25% cornmeal, 25% wheat, 10% bean power, 8% fish flour, 4% bone meal, 2% yeast, and 1% refined salt), while the rats in the T2DM group were fed a high-sugar and high-fat diet (20% casein, 17.8% lard, 16.8% sucrose, 10% maltodextrin, 7.3% corn starch, 5% cellulose, 5% mineral mix S10026B, 2.5% soybean oil, 1% vitamin mix ain-76A, 0.3% L-cystine, and 0.2% choline bitartrate). After feeding for 8 weeks, the rats in the T2DM group received a single intraperitoneal injection of 35 mg/kg streptozotocin (STZ, Sigma, Saint Louis, MO, USA), and the rats in the CON group were injected with an equivalent volume of citrate buffer after fasting for 12 h. After STZ injection for one week, orbital blood was collected to measure fasting blood glucose (FBG). The T2DM rat model was successfully induced when rats had FBG $\geq$ 11.1 mmol/L and lower fasting blood insulin and HOMA-IS than CON rats, accompanied by typical symptoms such as polydipsia, polyphagia, polyuria, and weight loss. After completing the experiment on postprandial glycemic responses following carbohydrate ingestion, experimental rats were anesthetized through the intraperitoneal injection of 10% pelltobarbitalum natricum. After anesthesia was determined through the pain reflex and cornea reflex, experimental rats were sacrificed by draining blood from the abdominal aorta.

4.5. *Postprandial Glycemic Responses Following Carbohydrate Ingestion*

In vivo postprandial glycemic responses following the ingestion of starch and glucose solutions were recorded according to our previous method [33] and Mandel AL and Breslin PA's method [56], with minor modifications. The four independent experiments were conducted in the mornings on separate days. After fasting for 12 h, each rat was administered 0.5 g/kg (7.5% solution) of glucose/starch solution in the control condition, and 0.5 g/kg of glucose/starch solution + 8 g/kg BZYQF in the experimental condition through a single oral dose. The blood glucose value was measured in serum samples from the tail vein at 0, 15, 30, 45, and 60 min. The area under the curve (AUC) was calculated using the trapezoid method. The glucose and starch solutions were equal in terms of energy provided. Before use, soluble starch was dissolved in a small amount of boiling water and then prepared to a concentration of 7.5%. This starch was processed to obtain a solution that was not noticeably different in viscosity from the glucose solution. A BZYQF dosage of 8 g/kg was selected according to the reference confirmed by our preliminary experimental results [57]. One hour after a meal is an important stage for food digestion and absorption, during which blood glucose rapidly increases and reaches its peak, reflecting individual blood glucose fluctuations. Hence, the present study mainly observed the 1 h postprandial blood glucose change.

4.6. *In Vitro Inhibition Assays of α-Amylase and α-Glucosidase*

The inhibition assay of α-amylase and α-glucosidase was carried out according to the method described by Yuxue Zheng et al. [58] with some modification. Briefly, 50 μL measures of α-amylase (meilunbio Co., Ltd., Dalian, China, 10 U/mL, dissolved in phosphate-buffered saline with pH 6.9) were mixed thoroughly with 50 μL measures of BZYQF solutions (0, 1, 10, 30, 40, 50, 70, 77 mg/mL, dissolved in double distilled water) and incubated for 10 min at 37 °C. Then, 0.1 mL of soluble starch (Macklin Biochemical Technology Co., Ltd., Shanghai, China, 1%, dissolved in double-distilled water) was added and incubated for 10 min at 37 °C. Finally, 0.1 mL of DNS reagent (3,5-dinitrosalicylic acid, Phygene Biotechnology Co., Ltd., Fuzhou, China) was added and incubated for 5 min at 100 °C for color development. The absorbance of the colored complex was recorded at 540 nm using an Elx-800 microplate reader (BioTek, Vermont, USA).

The inhibitory assay of α-glucosidase was performed as follows. Briefly, 50 μL of α-glucosidase (Yuanye Bio-Technology Co., Ltd., Shanghai, China, 4.4 U/mL, dissolved in PBS with pH 6.9) was mixed thoroughly with 50 μL of BZYQF (0, 1, 4, 7, 10, 30, 40, 77 mg/mL, dissolved in double-distilled water) and incubated for 10 min at 37 °C. Then, 0.1 mL of pNPG solution (2.5 mmol/L) as the substrate was added and incubated for 10 min at 37 °C. Finally, the reaction was terminated by adding 0.1 mL of 0.2 mol/L Na_2CO_3. The absorbance of the solution was recorded at 450 nm using an Elx-800 microplate reader (BioTek, Vermont, USA).

The inhibition rate of BZYQF for α-amylase and α-glucosidase was calculated according to Equation (1):

$$\text{Inhibition\%} = \frac{(\text{Acontrol} - \text{Acontrol blank}) - (\text{Asample} - \text{Asample blank})}{\text{Acontrol} - \text{Acontrol blank}} \quad (1)$$

where $A_{control}$, $A_{control\ blank}$, A_{sample}, and $A_{sample\ blank}$ represent the absorbance values of the sample with enzymes and PBS, PBS without enzymes, BZYQF with enzymes, and BZYQF without enzymes, respectively. Acarbose was used as a positive control. All samples were measured in triplicate. The IC50 value is the concentration of BZYQF required for 50% inhibition of the α-amylase/α-glucosidase activity.

4.7. Kinetic Inhibition Mode of α-Amylase and α-Glucosidase

The inhibition mode of α-amylase and α-glucosidase by BZYQF was determined using the Lineweaver–Burk plot method at specific enzyme concentrations and reaction times [58]. The concentrations of the starch solution ranged from 2.5 to 10.0 mg/mL, while the concentrations of the pNPG solution ranged from 0.5 to 2.5 mmol/L, and the crude drug concentrations of BZYQF solutions ranged from 0 to 50 mg/mL. The assay was performed as mentioned in Section 4.6. The Michaelis constant (Km) and maximal velocity (Vmax) were obtained from the plots.

4.8. In Vitro Simulated Digestion of BZYQF

The in vitro simulated digestion procedure was carried out according to the INFOGEST protocol with some modifications [59]. Simulated salivary fluid (SSF), simulated gastric fluid (SGF), and simulated intestinal fluid (SIF) were purchased from Yuanye Bio-Technology Co., Ltd. (Shanghai, China). A measure of 8 mL of SSF, including KCl, KSCN, NaH_2PO_4, Na_2SO_4, NaCl, $NaHCO_3$, amylase, uric acid, and mucin, was preheated in water for 5 min at 37 °C and added to 16 mL of BZYQF solution (as mentioned in Section 4.3). The mixture was incubated for 5 min at 37 °C. After the incubation, 8.0 mL of the digested sample was taken out and immediately placed in boiling water for 5 min to inactivate the enzymes. The remaining 16 mL of digestion mixture was retained to simulate gastric digestion.

Hydrochloric acid of 6 mol/L was added to the digestion mixture of saliva to bring the pH to 2.0. A measure of 8 mL of SGF, including NaCl, KCl, $CaCl_2$, NH_4Cl, NaH_2PO_4, glucose, glucuronic acid, HCl, urea, BSA, pepsin, and mucin, was preheated in water for 5 min at 37 °C and added to the digestion mixture of saliva with pH 2.0. Then, the mixture was incubated for 2 h at 37 °C. After the incubation, 8 mL of the digested sample was taken out and immediately placed in boiling water for 5 min to kill the enzymes. The remaining 16 mL of digestion mixture was retained to simulate intestinal digestion.

The pH in the gastric digestion mixture was adjusted to 7.0 with 6 mol/L sodium hydroxide. A measure of 8 mL of SIF, including NaCl, KCl, $CaCl_2$, NaOH, $NaHCO_3$, phosphate, and pancreatin, was preheated in water for 5 min at 37 °C and added to the gastric digestion mixture with pH 7.0. Then, the mixture was incubated for 2 h at 37 °C.

After the incubation, 8 mL of the digested sample was taken out and immediately placed in boiling water for 5 min to inactivate the enzymes.

During the in vitro simulated digestion, ultrapure water was added to the simulated digestive fluids as a no-BZYQF control. BZYQF solution was mixed with ultrapure water as a control without simulated digestive fluids. All experiments were repeated six times.

4.9. Extraction and Isolation of Total Flavonoids and In Vitro Activity Validation

The extraction and isolation of total flavonoids were carried out according to the method reported by Yao et al. [60], with some modifications. The BZYQF pills were crushed to a powder and were extracted exhaustively with 50% aqueous ethanol (with a liquid-to-material ratio of 30:1, v/w) at 50 °C for 1 h through reflux extraction on three occasions. After centrifugation at 3000× g for 10 min, the supernatant was concentrated under reduced pressure in a rotary evaporator at 40 °C, and the crude extracts were obtained. These crude extracts were then chromatographed on a glass column (60 cm × 3 cm, containing 150 g of D101 macroporous resin) with a 0.2 L bed volume (BV) for 7 h of adsorption. After reaching adsorption equilibrium, distilled water was used to wash the D101 macroporous resin until the effluent was almost colorless. Finally, 3.5 BV of 50% aqueous ethanol was used to rinse the adsorbent with an elution rate of 1 mL/min. The elution of 50% aqueous ethanol was collected in separate test tubes with 30 mL/tube, and then concentrated and dried. The purified total flavonoid was used to determine the main constituent content and perform in vitro inhibition assays of α-amylase and α-glucosidase as described in Sections 4.3 and 4.6.

4.10. Molecular Docking

Molecular docking was applied to speculate the possible binding site(s) between flavonoids of BZYQF and α-amylase/α-glucosidase. The crystal structures of α-amylase (PDB code: 5E0F) and α-glucosidase (PDB code: 5NN8) were downloaded from the RCSB Protein Data Bank "https://www.rcsb.org/ (accessed on 2 May 2024)". The 2D structures of flavonoids in BZYQF were downloaded from the PubChem "https://pubchem.ncbi.nlm.nih.gov/ (accessed on 10 May 2024)", TCMSP "https://www.tcmsp-e.com/#/home (accessed on 10 May 2024)" and ZINC "https://zinc20.docking.org/ (accessed on 10 May 2024)" databases. Autodock version 4.2.6 was used to remove the cofactors, water molecules, and heteroatoms from 5E0F and 5NN8 and obtain a stable receptor for flavonoids of BZYQF. The optimized protein structures of 5NN8 and 5E0F were imported into Discovery Studio 2019 "http://www.discoverystudio.net (accessed on 12 May 2024)" for batch docking with pre-processed flavonoids in BZYQF. The CDOCKER module of Discovery Studio 2019 was used to analyze the interaction energy of α-amylase and α-glucosidase with flavonoids in BZYQF. The parameters (e.g., binding sites of amino acid residues and interactions) were obtained based on the docking results with CDOCKER interaction energy of <−40 Kcal/mol.

4.11. Statistical Analysis

The comparison analysis of multiple groups was conducted using one-way ANOVA with Tukey's post hoc test, while the comparison between two groups was conducted using Student's t-test with GraphPad Prism version 8 (GraphPad Software, La Jolla, CA, USA). The active constituents in BZYQF inhibiting the activities of α-amylase and α-glucosidase were identified through Pearson correlation analysis and multiple linear regression analysis using Origin Pro 2021 (OriginLab, Northampton, MA, USA) and SPSS version 22.0 (IBM SPSS, New York, NY, USA), respectively. The 50% inhibitory concentration (IC50) of BZYQF against the activities of α-amylase and α-glucosidase was calculated through nonlinear regression using GraphPad Prism version 8. $p < 0.05$ was considered statistically significant. All data are presented as the mean ± standard deviation ($\overline{x} \pm SD$).

5. Conclusions

In summary, the present study demonstrated that BZYQF could significantly reduce postprandial hyperglycemia following the ingestion of starch solution in T2DM rats by inhibiting α-amylase and α-glycosidase activities. An in vitro enzyme kinetic assay suggested that BZYQF inhibited α-glucosidase activity in the uncompetitive mode and inhibited α-amylase activity in the competitive and non-competitive modes. Furthermore, BZYQF had a stronger inhibitory effect on α-glucosidase activity than on α-amylase activity. These results were also theoretically validated through molecular docking results. The Pearson correlation and multiple linear regression analysis results revealed that the total flavonoids in BZYQF were the active constituents inhibiting α-amylase and α-glycosidase activities. This result was verified by examining the total flavonoids purified from BZYQF. Overall, the present study provided a theoretical basis for the use of BZYQF as an adjuvant therapy in T2DM. In addition, the effect of the total flavonoids in BZYQF on postprandial hyperglycemia in T2DM rats needs further confirmation through in vivo experiments.

Supplementary Materials: The following supporting information can be downloaded at https://www.mdpi.com/article/10.3390/ph18020201/s1: Figure S1: Content of calycosin-7-O-β-D-glucoside in BZYQF; Figure S2: Content of standard (calycosin-7-O-β-D-glucoside); Figure S3: MRM_detection_of_multimodal_maps-N; Figure S4: MRM_detection_of_multimodal_maps-P; Figure S5: MWXS-23-777-01-a_QC_MS_TIC-N; Figure S6: MWXS-23-777-01-a_QC_MS_TIC-P; Table S1: All compounds were identified in BZYQF by UPLC-MSMS.

Author Contributions: Conceptualization, Z.-M.Y.; methodology, L.W., M.-Y.W., Z.-R.H., X.-K.L., G.-J.F., L.L. and Z.-M.Y.; software, L.W.; validation, Z.-R.H.; formal analysis, X.-X.Z.; investigation, L.L. and Y.-T.F.; data curation, X.-X.Z. and Z.-M.Y.; writing—original draft preparation, X.-X.Z.; writing—review and editing, Z.-M.Y.; visualization, L.W., Z.-R.H., X.-K.L., G.-J.F. and Z.-M.Y.; supervision, Z.-M.Y.; project administration, M.-Y.W.; funding acquisition, Z.-M.Y. All authors have read and agreed to the published version of the manuscript.

Funding: This research was funded by the National Natural Science Foundation of China (grant number 82174105, 81102703); the Natural Science Foundation of Guangdong Province (grant number 2017A030313837); the Science and Technology Planning Project of Guangdong Province (grant number 2013A032500005); and the College Student Innovation Training Program in China (grant number 202410573003).

Institutional Review Board Statement: The animal study protocol was approved by the Ethics Committee of Guangdong Pharmaceutical University (protocol code: gdpulacspf2022203 and date of approval: May 2023).

Informed Consent Statement: Not applicable.

Data Availability Statement: The datasets used and/or analyzed during the current study are available from the corresponding author on reasonable request.

Conflicts of Interest: The authors declare no conflicts of interest.

References

1. ElSayed, N.A.; Aleppo, G.; Aroda, V.R.; Bannuru, R.R.; Brown, F.M.; Bruemmer, D.; Collins, B.S.; Hilliard, M.E.; Isaacs, D.; Johnson, E.L.; et al. 2. Classification and Diagnosis of Diabetes: Standards of Care in Diabetes-2023. *Diabetes Care* **2023**, *46*, S19–S40. [CrossRef]
2. Eid, S.; Sas, K.M.; Abcouwer, S.F.; Feldman, E.L.; Gardner, T.W.; Pennathur, S.; Fort, P.E. New insights into the mechanisms of diabetic complications: Role of lipids and lipid metabolism. *Diabetologia* **2019**, *62*, 1539–1549. [CrossRef]

3. Bonora, E.; Muggeo, M. Postprandial blood glucose as a risk factor for cardiovascular disease in Type II diabetes: The epidemiological evidence. *Diabetologia* **2001**, *44*, 2107–2114. [CrossRef]
4. Ni, Y.; Wu, X.; Yao, W.; Zhang, Y.; Chen, J.; Ding, X. Evidence of traditional Chinese medicine for treating type 2 diabetes mellitus: From molecular mechanisms to clinical efficacy. *Pharm. Biol.* **2024**, *62*, 592–606. [CrossRef] [PubMed]
5. Chen, X.; Chen, C.; Fu, X. Hypoglycemic activity in vitro and vivo of a water-soluble polysaccharide from Astragalus membranaceus. *Food Funct.* **2022**, *13*, 11210–11222. [CrossRef] [PubMed]
6. Guo, J.; Tao, H.; Cao, Y.; Ho, C.T.; Jin, S.; Huang, Q. Prevention of Obesity and Type 2 Diabetes with Aged Citrus Peel (Chenpi) Extract. *J. Agric. Food Chem.* **2016**, *64*, 2053–2061. [CrossRef]
7. Xu, J.; Liu, H.; Su, G.; Ding, M.; Wang, W.; Lu, J.; Bi, X.; Zhao, Y. Purification of ginseng rare sapogenins 25-OH-PPT and its hypoglycemic, antiinflammatory and lipid-lowering mechanisms. *J. Ginseng Res.* **2021**, *45*, 86–97. [CrossRef] [PubMed]
8. Yang, L.; Yu, H.; Hou, A.; Man, W.; Wang, S.; Zhang, J.; Wang, X.; Zheng, S.; Jiang, H.; Kuang, H. A Review of the Ethnopharmacology, Phytochemistry, Pharmacology, Application, Quality Control, Processing, Toxicology, and Pharmacokinetics of the Dried Rhizome of Atractylodes macrocephala. *Front. Pharmacol.* **2021**, *12*, 727154. [CrossRef]
9. Lai, L.; Hu, T.; Peng, L. Analysis of the Dialectical Addition and Subtraction of Buzhong Yiqi Decoction on the Level of Blood Glucose Control and the Improvement of TCM Syndrome Scores in Patients with Type 2 Diabetes. *Diabetes New World* **2021**, *24*, 34–37. [CrossRef]
10. Tolmie, M.; Bester, M.J.; Apostolides, Z. Inhibition of α-glucosidase and α-amylase by herbal compounds for the treatment of type 2 diabetes: A validation of in silico reverse docking with in vitro enzyme assays. *J. Diabetes* **2021**, *13*, 779–791. [CrossRef] [PubMed]
11. Dirir, A.M.; Daou, M.; Yousef, A.F.; Yousef, L.F. A review of alpha-glucosidase inhibitors from plants as potential candidates for the treatment of type-2 diabetes. *Phytochem. Rev.* **2022**, *21*, 1049–1079. [CrossRef] [PubMed]
12. Proença, C.; Ribeiro, D.; Freitas, M.; Fernandes, E. Flavonoids as potential agents in the management of type 2 diabetes through the modulation of α-amylase and α-glucosidase activity: A review. *Crit. Rev. Food Sci. Nutr.* **2022**, *62*, 3137–3207. [CrossRef] [PubMed]
13. Zheng, X.F.; Tian, J.S.; Liu, P.; Xing, J.; Qin, X.M. Analysis of the Restorative Effect of Bu-Zhong-Yi-Qi-Tang in the Spleen-Qi Deficiency Rat Model Using 1H-NMR-Based Metabonomics. *J. Ethnopharmacol.* **2014**, *151*, 912–920. [CrossRef] [PubMed]
14. Hu, L.F.; Yamamoto, M.; Chen, J.L.; Duan, H.F.; Du, J.; He, L.L.; Shi, D.F.; Yao, X.S.; Nagai, T.; Kiyohara, H.; et al. Integrating network pharmacology and experimental verification to decipher the immunomodulatory effect of Bu-Zhong-Yi-Qi-Tang against poly (I:C)-induced pulmonary inflammation. *Front. Pharmacol.* **2022**, *13*, 1015486. [CrossRef]
15. Mayu, I.; Yosuke, T.; Haruna, H.; Kayako, S.; Satoshi, I.; Yuki, N.; Michiko, S.; Takayuki, N.; Hiroaki, K. Inulooligosaccharides in Atractylodis lanceae rhizoma and Atractylodis rhizoma of hochuekkito formula are essential for regulation of the pulmonary immune system of immuno-compromised mice. *Tradit. Kampo Med.* **2020**, *7*, 96–107. [CrossRef]
16. Zhang, Y.G.; Niu, J.T.; Zhang, S.J.; Si, X.L.; Bian, T.T.; Wu, H.W.; Li, D.H.; Sun, Y.J.; Jia, J.; Xin, E.D.; et al. Comparative study on the gastrointestinal- and immune- regulation functions of Hedysari Radix Paeparata Cum Melle and Astragali Radix Praeparata cum Melle in rats with spleen-qi deficiency, based on fuzzy matter-element analysis. *Pharm. Biol.* **2022**, *60*, 1237–1254. [CrossRef]
17. Li, N.; Duan, C.; Hu, M. Effect of Buzhong Yiqi decoction on blood glucose and islet function in patients with type 2 diabetes. *Shanxi J. Tradit. Chin. Med.* **2019**, *35*, 21–23.
18. Momtazi-Borojeni, A.A.; Jaafari, M.R.; Abdollahi, E.; Banach, M.; Sahebkar, A. Impact of PCSK9 Immunization on Glycemic Indices in Diabetic Rats. *J. Diabetes Res.* **2021**, *2021*, 4757170. [CrossRef] [PubMed]
19. Liu, K.-F.; Niu, C.-S.; Tsai, J.-C.; Yang, C.-L.; Peng, W.-H.; Niu, H.-S. Comparison of area under the curve in various models of diabetic rats receiving chronic medication. *Arch. Med. Sci.* **2022**, *18*, 1078–1087. [CrossRef]
20. Chewchinda, S.; Leakaya, N.; Sato, H.; Sato, V.H. Antidiabetic effects of (Lour.) corner heartwood extract. *J. Tradit. Compl. Med.* **2021**, *11*, 68–74. [CrossRef] [PubMed]
21. Io, F.; Gunji, E.; Koretsune, H.; Kato, K.; Sugisaki-Kitano, M.; Okumura-Kitajima, L.; Kimura, K.; Uchida, S.; Yamamoto, K. SGL5213, a novel and potent intestinal SGLT1 inhibitor, suppresses intestinal glucose absorption and enhances plasma GLP-1 and GLP-2 secretion in rats. *Eur. J. Pharmacol.* **2019**, *853*, 136–144. [CrossRef] [PubMed]
22. Ramkumar, S.; Thulasiram, H.V.; RaviKumar, A. Improvement in serum amylase and glucose levels in diabetic rats on oral administration of bisdemethoxycurcumin from *Curcuma longa* and limonoids from *Azadirachta indica*. *J. Food Biochem.* **2021**, *45*, e13674. [CrossRef]
23. Zhao, X.; Tao, J.; Zhang, T.; Jiang, S.; Wei, W.; Han, H.; Shao, Y.; Zhou, G.; Yue, H. Resveratroloside Alleviates Postprandial Hyperglycemia in Diabetic Mice by Competitively Inhibiting α-Glucosidase. *J. Agric. Food Chem.* **2019**, *67*, 2886–2893. [CrossRef] [PubMed]
24. Burant, C.F.; Flink, S.; DePaoli, A.M.; Chen, J.; Lee, W.S.; Hediger, M.A.; Buse, J.B.; Chang, E.B. Small intestine hexose transport in experimental diabetes. Increased transporter mRNA and protein expression in enterocytes. *J. Clin. Investig.* **1994**, *93*, 578–585. [CrossRef]

25. Dyer, J.; Wood, I.S.; Palejwala, A.; Ellis, A.; Shirazi-Beechey, S.P. Expression of monosaccharide transporters in intestine of diabetic humans. *Am. J. Physiol. Gastrointest. Liver Physiol.* **2002**, *282*, G241–G248. [CrossRef]
26. Fiorentino, T.V.; Suraci, E.; Arcidiacono, G.P.; Cimellaro, A.; Mignogna, C.; Presta, I.; Andreozzi, F.; Hribal, M.L.; Perticone, F.; Donato, G.; et al. Duodenal Sodium/Glucose Cotransporter 1 Expression Under Fasting Conditions Is Associated With Postload Hyperglycemia. *J. Clin. Endocrinol. Metab.* **2017**, *102*, 3979–3989. [CrossRef] [PubMed]
27. Ze-Min, Y.; Ying, W.; Siyu, C. Astragalus polysaccharide alleviates type 2 diabetic rats by reversing the glucose transporters and sweet taste receptors/GLP-1/GLP-1 receptor signaling pathways in the intestine-pancreatic axis. *J. Funct. Foods* **2021**, *76*, 104310. [CrossRef]
28. Shori, A.B. Screening of antidiabetic and antioxidant activities of medicinal plants. *J. Integr. Med.* **2015**, *13*, 297–305. [CrossRef]
29. Borges de Melo, E.; da Silveira Gomes, A.; Carvalho, I. α- and β-Glucosidase inhibitors: Chemical structure and biological activity. *Tetrahedron* **2006**, *62*, 10277–10302. [CrossRef]
30. Campbell, L.K.; White, J.R.; Campbell, R.K. Acarbose: Its role in the treatment of diabetes mellitus. *Ann. Pharmacother.* **1996**, *30*, 1255–1262. [CrossRef]
31. Masson, P.; Mukhametgalieva, A.R. Partial Reversible Inhibition of Enzymes and Its Metabolic and Pharmaco-Toxicological Implications. *Int. J. Mol. Sci.* **2023**, *24*, 12973. [CrossRef] [PubMed]
32. Whiteley, C.G. Mechanistic and kinetic studies of inhibition of enzymes. *Cell Biochem. Biophys.* **2000**, *33*, 217–225. [CrossRef]
33. Chen, S.; Tang, S.; Wang, Y.; Yang, Z. Effect of Astragalus Polysaccharides on Postprandial 1 Hour Blood Glucose in Type 2 Diabetic Rats. *Tradit. Chin. Drug Res. Clin. Pharmacol.* **2020**, *31*, 396–401. [CrossRef]
34. Liu, Y.; Nyberg, N.T.; Jäger, A.K.; Staerk, D. Facilitated Visual Interpretation of Scores in Principal Component Analysis by Bioactivity-Labeling of 1H-NMR Spectra-Metabolomics Investigation and Identification of a New α-Glucosidase Inhibitor in Radix Astragali. *Molecules* **2017**, *22*, 411. [CrossRef]
35. Zhu, Z.Y.; Zhang, J.Y.; Chen, L.J.; Liu, X.C.; Liu, Y.; Wang, W.X.; Zhang, Y.M. Comparative evaluation of polysaccharides isolated from Astragalus, oyster mushroom, and yacon as inhibitors of α-glucosidase. Chin. *J. Nat. Med.* **2014**, *12*, 290–293. [CrossRef]
36. Al-Hmadi, H.B.; Majdoub, S.; El Mokni, R.; Angeloni, S.; Mustafa, A.M.; Caprioli, G.; Zengin, G.; Maggi, F.; Hammami, S. Metabolite profiling, enzyme inhibitory activity and antioxidant potential of different extracts from Glycyrrhiza foetida Desf. (Fabaceae, Galegeae, Glycyrrhizinae). *Fitoterapia* **2024**, *173*, 105792. [CrossRef]
37. Yang, L.; Jiang, Y.; Zhang, Z.X.; Hou, J.M.; Tian, S.K.; Liu, Y. The anti-diabetic activity of licorice, a widely used Chinese herb. *J. Ethnopharmacol.* **2020**, *263*, 113216. [CrossRef]
38. Zhang, W.; Li, T.; Zhang, X.J.; Zhu, Z.Y. Hypoglycemic effect of glycyrrhizic acid, a natural non-carbohydrate sweetener, on streptozotocin-induced diabetic mice. *Food Funct.* **2020**, *11*, 4160–4170. [CrossRef] [PubMed]
39. Jia, W.J.; Bi, Q.M.; Jiang, S.R.; Tao, J.H.; Liu, L.Y.; Yue, H.L.; Zhao, X.H. Hypoglycemic activity of *Codonopsis pilosula* (Franch.) Nannf. in vitro and in vivo and its chemical composition identification by UPLC-Triple-TOF-MS/MS. *Food Funct.* **2022**, *13*, 2456–2464. [CrossRef]
40. Su, X.; Luo, L. UPLC-QE-MS combined network pharmacological to analyze the mechanism and experimental verification of BuzhongYiqi pill in the treatment of ulcerative colitis. *Chin. J. Clin. Pharmacol. Ther.* **2024**, *29*, 241–251.
41. Yan, J.K.; Chen, T.T.; Wang, L.; Wang, Z.W.; Li, C.; Chen, W.Y.; Liu, C.H.; Li, L. In vitro simulated digestion affecting physicochemical characteristics and bioactivities of polysaccharides from barley (*Hordeum vulgare* L.) grasses at different growth stages. *Int. J. Biol. Macromol.* **2022**, *219*, 876–885. [CrossRef] [PubMed]
42. Fang, C.; Chen, G.; Kan, J. Characterization and in vitro simulated gastrointestinal digestion and fermentation of Mentha haplocalyx polysaccharide. *Int. J. Biol. Macromol.* **2022**, *222*, 360–372. [CrossRef]
43. Zhang, G.; Yan, X.; Wu, S.; Ma, M.; Yu, P.; Gong, D.; Deng, S.; Zeng, Z. Ethanol extracts from *Cinnamomum camphora* seed kernel: Potential bioactivities as affected by alkaline hydrolysis and simulated gastrointestinal digestion. *Food Res. Int.* **2020**, *137*, 109363. [CrossRef]
44. Tarko, T.; Duda-Chodak, A.; Soszka, A. Changes in Phenolic Compounds and Antioxidant Activity of Fruit Musts and Fruit Wines during Simulated Digestion. *Molecules* **2020**, *25*, 5574. [CrossRef]
45. Martinez-Gonzalez, A.I.; Díaz-Sánchez, A.G.; de la Rosa, L.A.; Vargas-Requena, C.L.; Bustos-Jaimes, I.; Alvarez-Parrilla, E. Polyphenolic Compounds and Digestive Enzymes: In Vitro Non-Covalent Interactions. *Molecules* **2017**, *22*, 669. [CrossRef]
46. Lam, T.P.; Tran, N.N.; Pham, L.D.; Lai, N.V.; Dang, B.N.; Truong, N.N.; Nguyen-Vo, S.K.; Hoang, T.L.; Mai, T.T.; Tran, T.D. Flavonoids as dual-target inhibitors against α-glucosidase and α-amylase: A systematic review of in vitro studies. *Nat. Prod. Bioprospect.* **2024**, *14*, 4. [CrossRef]
47. Yang, J.; Li, H.; Wang, X.; Zhang, C.; Feng, G.; Peng, X. Inhibition Mechanism of α-Amylase/α-Glucosidase by Silibinin, Its Synergism with Acarbose, and the Effect of Milk Proteins. *J. Agric. Food Chem.* **2021**, *69*, 10515–10526. [CrossRef] [PubMed]

48. Zhao, Y.; Kongstad, K.T.; Jäger, A.K.; Nielsen, J.; Staerk, D. Quadruple high-resolution α-glucosidase/α-amylase/PTP1B/radical scavenging profiling combined with high-performance liquid chromatography-high-resolution mass spectrometry-solid-phase extraction-nuclear magnetic resonance spectroscopy for identification of antidiabetic constituents in crude root bark of *Morus alba* L. *J. Chromatogr. A* **2018**, *1556*, 55–63. [CrossRef]
49. Chen, W.; Gong, L.; Guo, Z.; Wang, W.; Zhang, H.; Liu, X.; Yu, S.; Xiong, L.; Luo, J. A novel integrated method for large-scale detection, identification, and quantification of widely targeted metabolites: Application in the study of rice metabolomics. *Mol. Plant* **2013**, *6*, 1769–1780. [CrossRef]
50. Zhang, J.; Gong, Z.; Wang, W.; Jia, F.; Cui, W.; Wang, Y. Method for Detecting Polysaccharide in Water Extraction from Flammulina Velutipes. *Farm Prod. Process.* **2017**, 31–34. [CrossRef]
51. Shen, Y.; Jin, L.; Xiao, P.; Lu, Y.; Bao, J.S. Total phenolics, flavonoids, antioxidant capacity in rice grain and their relations to grain color, size and weight. *J. Cereal Sci.* **2009**, *49*, 106–111. [CrossRef]
52. Singleton, V.L. Analysis of total phenols and other oxidation substrates and their antioxidants by means of Folin-Ciocalteu reagent. *Methods Enzymol.* **1999**, *299*, 152–178.
53. Hadidi, M.; Ibarz, A.; Pagan, J. Optimisation and kinetic study of the ultrasonic-assisted extraction of total saponins from alfalfa (*Medicago sativa*) and its bioaccessibility using the response surface methodology. *Food Chem.* **2020**, *309*, 125786. [CrossRef] [PubMed]
54. Luo, M.J.; Wang, Y.; Chen, S.Y.; Yang, Z.M. Astragalus Polysaccharides Alleviate Type 2 Diabetic Rats by Reversing the Expressions of Sweet Taste Receptors and Genes Related to Glycolipid Metabolism in Liver. *Front. Pharmacol.* **2022**, *13*, 916603. [CrossRef]
55. Zhuo, J.; Zeng, Q.; Cai, D.; Zeng, X.; Chen, Y.; Gan, H.; Huang, X.; Yao, N.; Huang, D.; Zhang, C. Evaluation of type 2 diabetic mellitus animal models via interactions between insulin and mitogen-activated protein kinase signaling pathways induced by a high fat and sugar diet and streptozotocin. *Mol. Med. Rep.* **2018**, *17*, 5132–5142. [CrossRef]
56. Mandel, A.L.; Breslin, P.A. High endogenous salivary amylase activity is associated with improved glycemic homeostasis following starch ingestion in adults. *J. Nutr.* **2012**, *142*, 853–858. [CrossRef]
57. Dong, Y.X.; Li, T.H.; Wang, S.S.; Hu, Y.H.; Liu, Y.; Zhang, F.; Sun, T.S.; Zhang, C.J.; Du, Q.H.; Li, W.H. Bu zhong Yiqi Decoction ameliorates mild cognitive impairment by improving mitochondrial oxidative stress damage via the SIRT3/MnSOD/OGG1 pathway. *J. Ethnopharmacol.* **2024**, *331*, 118237. [CrossRef] [PubMed]
58. Zheng, Y.; Tian, J.; Yang, W.; Chen, S.; Liu, D.; Fang, H.; Zhang, H.; Ye, X. Inhibition mechanism of ferulic acid against α-amylase and α-glucosidase. *Food Chem.* **2020**, *317*, 126346. [CrossRef]
59. Brodkorb, A.; Egger, L.; Alminger, M.; Alvito, P.; Assunção, R.; Ballance, S.; Bohn, T.; Bourlieu-Lacanal, C.; Boutrou, R.; Carrière, F.; et al. INFOGEST static in vitro simulation of gastrointestinal food digestion. *Nat. Protoc.* **2019**, *14*, 991–1014. [CrossRef]
60. Yao, X.; Zhu, L.; Chen, Y.; Tian, J.; Wang, Y. In vivo and in vitro antioxidant activity and α-glucosidase, α-amylase inhibitory effects of flavonoids from *Cichorium glandulosum* seeds. *Food Chem.* **2013**, *139*, 59–66. [CrossRef]

pharmaceuticals

Article

Syringaldehyde Alleviates Cardiac Hypertrophy Induced by Hyperglycemia in H9c2 Cells Through GLP-1 Receptor Signals

Yingxiao Li [1], Chao-Tien Hsu [2], Ting-Ting Yang [3] and Kai-Chun Cheng [4,*]

1 Department of Anatomy, College of Medicine, I-Shou University, Kaohsiung 824005, Taiwan; yxli0809@isu.edu.tw
2 Department of Pathology, E-Da Hospital, I-Shou University, Kaohsiung 824005, Taiwan; ed103797@edah.org.tw
3 School of Chinese Medicine for Post Baccalaureate, College of Medicine, I-Shou University, Kaohsiung 824005, Taiwan; tingting@isu.edu.tw
4 Department of Pharmacy, College of Pharmacy and Health Care, Tajen University, Pingtung 90741, Taiwan
* Correspondence: kc-cheng@tajen.edu.tw

Abstract: Background: Cardiac hypertrophy is a significant complication of diabetes, often triggered by hyperglycemia. Glucagon-like peptide-1 (GLP-1) receptor agonists alleviate cardiac hypertrophy, but their efficacy diminishes under GLP-1 resistance. Syringaldehyde (SA), a natural phenolic compound, may activate GLP-1 receptors and mitigate hypertrophy. This study explores SA's therapeutic potential in hyperglycemia-induced cardiac hypertrophy in H9c2 cardiomyocytes. **Methods:** H9c2 cells were exposed to high glucose to induce hypertrophy. Cells were treated with varying SA concentrations, and hypertrophic biomarkers were analyzed using ELISA, qPCR, and Western blot. **Results:** SA reduced cell size and hypertrophic biomarkers in a dose-dependent manner while increasing GLP-1 receptor expression and cAMP levels. These effects were attenuated in GLP-1-resistant cells, highlighting the role of GLP-1 receptor activation. AMPK activation was essential, as its inhibition abolished SA's effects. SA also decreased O-linked N-acetylglucosamine transferase (OGT) expression via AMPK activation, contributing to reduced hypertrophy. **Conclusions:** SA alleviates hyperglycemia-induced cardiac hypertrophy in H9c2 cells by activating the GLP-1 receptor and AMPK signaling pathway.

Keywords: AMPK; cardiac hypertrophy; diabetes complications; GLP-1 resistance; O-linked N-acetylglucosamine transferase (OGT); syringaldehyde

1. Introduction

Diabetic cardiomyopathy (DCM) is a common consequence of diabetes characterized by hypertrophy in cardiomyocytes in response to prolonged exposure to elevated glucose levels [1]. Cardiac hypertrophy is characterized by cellular hypertrophy resulting from age and/or neurohumoral stimulation, and it is regarded as an independent risk factor for heart failure. Consequently, it may be categorized into pathological or physiological processes [2–4]. Furthermore, atrial natriuretic peptide (ANP), brain/B-type natriuretic peptide (BNP), and β-myosin heavy chain (β-MHC) serve as markers of hypertrophy progression [5]. The goal of treatment for hypertrophic cardiomyopathy is to reduce the risk of heart failure. However, there has been no confirmed effective treatment for DCM [6].

Glucagon-like peptide-1 (GLP-1) is a member of the incretin hormone family, which is released from the stomach to induce insulin secretion after consuming nutrients [7]. Moreover, cardiomyocytes express the GLP-1 receptor (GLP-1R) [8]. GLP-1R activation has been extensively studied for its dual role in managing diabetes-related complications and reducing cardiac hypertrophy [9]. In clinical trials, GLP-1R agonists have been shown to stabilize and decrease blood glucose levels while also promoting weight loss [10]. Moreover, these agonists exhibit direct cardioprotective [11] and renal protective effects [12], achieved by reducing oxidative stress, improving myocardial energy efficiency, and modulating inflammatory pathways [13]. Recent studies have highlighted additional benefits of GLP-1R agonists. Semaglutide has been found to ameliorate cardiac remodeling in male mice by optimizing energy substrate utilization through the Creb5/NR4a1 axis [14]. Similarly, exendin-4 (EX-4) has been shown to reduce infarct size and myocardial stiffness in animal models of acute myocardial infarction [15]. Another GLP-1 agonist, liraglutide, has demonstrated the ability to decrease intracellular calcium overload in myocardial injury induced by hydrogen peroxide in vitro [16]. Clinically, liraglutide has been found to improve reperfusion injury in patients with ST-segment elevation myocardial infarction [17]. Both liraglutide [18] and EX-4 [19] protect the heart from cardiac hypertrophy by activating the AMP-activated protein kinase (AMPK) pathway. These findings indicate a potential link between GLP-1 expression and AMPK activation.

Natural products have been identified as potential GLP-1R agonists [20]. Syringaldehyde (SA), a natural phenolic aldehyde with antioxidant properties, has a unique structure consisting of a benzene ring substituted with two methoxy groups and an aldehyde group, making it a promising dual-function GLP-1 receptor modulator [21]. SA has been shown to regulate enzyme activity, protein dynamics, and transcription factors associated with diabetes, inflammation, cancer, and angiogenesis [22,23]. Research indicates that SA improves glucose metabolism and alleviates diabetes through GLP-1 receptor activation [24]. In addition, SA exhibited cardioprotective effects in a myocardial infarction model, indicating its potential in cardiovascular therapy [25]. Similarly, other natural compounds, such as geniposide [26] and catalpol [27], have also demonstrated GLP-1 receptor activation, with geniposide further showing cardioprotective effects by reducing cardiac hypertrophy via the AMPK signaling pathway [19].

This study aims to investigate whether SA can mitigate cardiac hypertrophy under high-glucose conditions, potentially offering new therapeutic strategies for diabetes-related cardiac complications. H9c2 cells, which are immortalized cardiomyocyte-like cells commonly used for in vitro cardiac injury models [28], were employed in this study. Using an established model [24], we examined SA's effects on glucose-induced cardiac hypertrophy, providing insights into its potential as a GLP-1 receptor agonist in cardiomyocytes [29].

2. Results

2.1. *Syringaldehyde (SA) Activated GLP-1 Receptors in Cardiomyocytes and Alleviated Cardiac Hypertrophy Induced by Hyperglycemia in H9c2 Cells*

SA is recognized to be non-invasive in cardiomyocytes and has been demonstrated to promote the mRNA level of the GLP-1 receptor in H9c2 cells [24]. The concentration of SA treatment was derived from preliminary experiments. SA has increased the protein level of the GLP-1 receptor in a dose-dependent manner in hypertrophic cardiomyocytes as shown by Western blot analysis (Figure 1a). SA treatment also resulted in a concentration increase for both calcium influx and cyclic AMP (cAMP) levels (Figure 1b,c). However, the increase in cAMP levels was inhibited by pretreatment with exendin 9–39 (EX9), a GLP-1 receptor antagonist (Figure 1d). The impact of SA as a GLP-1 receptor agonist was assessed in H9c2 cells.

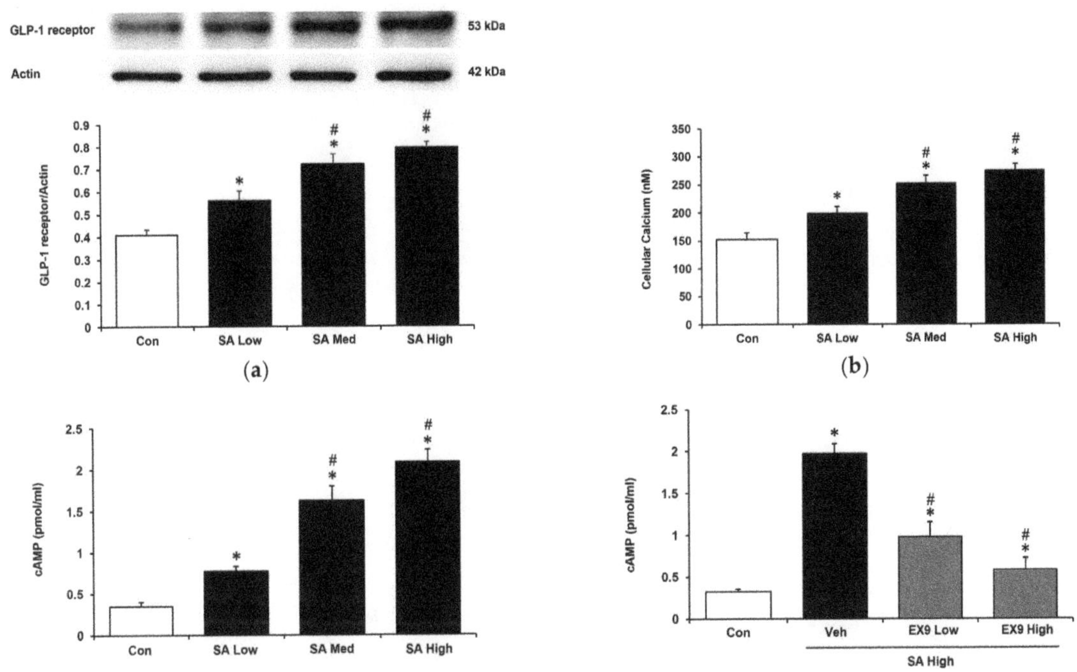

Figure 1. Syringaldehyde (SA) increases the expression of the GLP-1 receptor in H9c2 cells with hypertrophy. (**a**) Changes in GLP-1 receptor protein levels induced via SA administration at concentrations of 0.1 μM (low), 0.5 μM (medium), and 1 μM (high). (**b**) Changes in calcium influx induced via SA administration at different concentrations. (**c**) Levels of cellular cyclic AMP (cAMP) in cells subjected to different concentrations of SA. (**d**) The cellular cAMP level induced by SA at 1 μM was inhibited, following 30 min pretreatment with Ex 9 at concentrations of 0.1 μM or 0.5 μM. The sample size was 6 except for the Western blotting analysis (n = 4). Statistical significance was indicated as follows: * $p < 0.05$ vs. control (Con); # $p < 0.05$ vs. vehicle (Veh).

Hypertrophy was induced in H9c2 cells by incubation in a medium containing 30 mmol/L glucose for 48 h, following the protocol established in our previous study [29]. The morphological changes in cells subjected to various treatments were observed in Figure 2d. High glucose incubation led to a significant increase in cell size and hypertrophic biomarkers, including ANPs, BNPs, and β-MHC. Treatment with SA ameliorated the hypertrophic size in a dose-dependent manner (Figure 2a). Furthermore, the expression levels of hypertrophic biomarkers (ANPs, BNPs, and β-MHC) were significantly reduced, following the administration of SA at medium and high concentrations (Figure 2b,c). These findings suggest that SA exhibits a protective effect against hyperglycemia-induced cardiac hypertrophy in H9c2 cells.

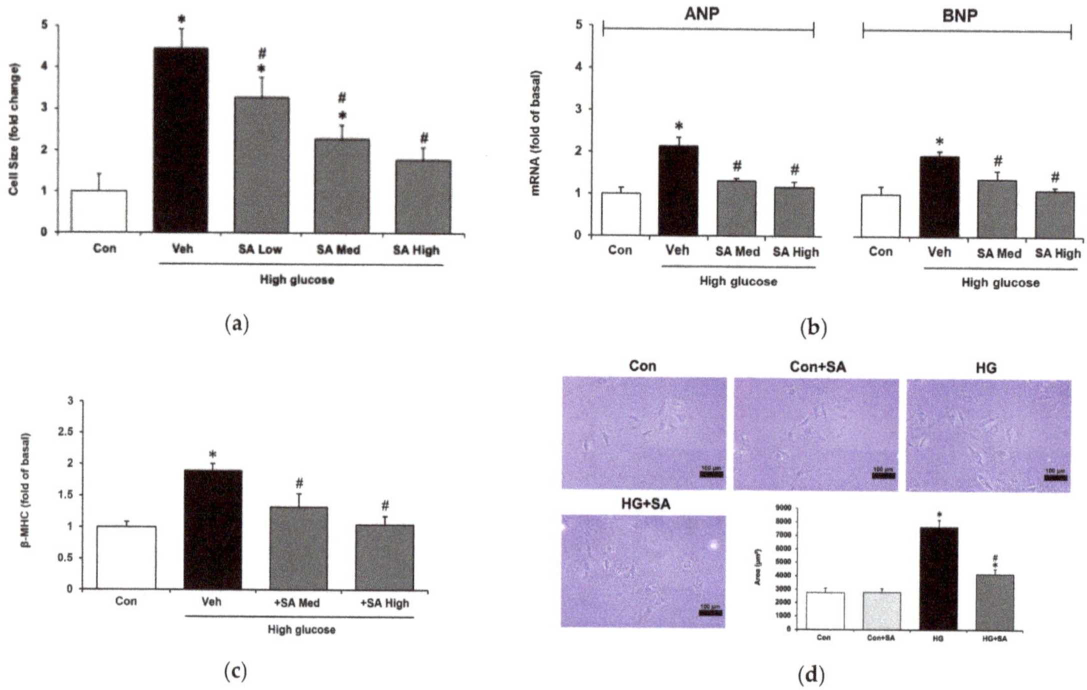

Figure 2. Syringaldehyde (SA) ameliorated the hyperglycemia-induced hypertrophy of H9c2 cells. (**a**) Changes in the size of the hypertrophic cells treated with syringaldehyde at different concentrations of 0.1 μM (low), 0.5 μM (medium), and 1 μM (high). * $p < 0.05$ vs. control (Con). # $p < 0.05$) vs. vehicle (Veh). Gene expression levels of (**b**) the gene expression levels of ANP (Con: 1 ± 0.2; Veh: 2.1 ± 0.2; SA Med: 1.3 ± 0.1; SA High: 1.2 ± 0.1), BNP (Con: 1 ± 0.2; Veh: 1.9 ± 0.1; SA Med: 1.4 ± 0.2; SA High: 1.1 ± 0.1) and (**c**) β-MHC (Con: 1 ± 0.1; Veh: 1.9 ± 0.1; SA Med: 1.3 ± 0.2; SA High: 1 ± 0.1) in hypertrophic cells administered various concentrations of SA or without treatment. * $p < 0.05$ vs. control (Con). # $p < 0.05$) vs. vehicle (Veh). (**d**) The size of the H9c2 cells was observed using light microscopy (scale bar: 100 μm). Control cells in a normal culture (Con) were not modified with SA at 1 μM (Con + SA), as indicated in the upper panel. * $p < 0.05$ vs. normal cells (Con). # $p < 0.05$) vs. high glucose-induced hypertrophic cell (HG). Values for each indicator are expressed as fold changes in gene expressions of ANP, BNP, and β-MHC, relative to the control group. Fold change is calculated as follows: fold change = data of the experimental group/data of the control group.

2.2. *Effects of Syringaldehyde (SA) Were Ablated in H9c2 Cells with GLP-1 Resistance*

Previous studies have suggested that under hyperglycemic conditions, the cardioprotective effects of GLP-1 are significantly impaired, which is referred to as GLP-1 resistance [30]. In the current study, the results demonstrated that the efficacy of EX-4 was markedly diminished in H9c2 cells with GLP-1 resistance (Figure 3a), suggesting a loss of responsiveness to the GLP-1 agonist. Furthermore, SA was unable to ameliorate cardiac hypertrophy in GLP-1-resistant H9c2 cells (Figure 3a). However, as shown in Figure 3a, metformin retained its ability to reduce cell size in hypertrophic cells, even under conditions of GLP-1 resistance.

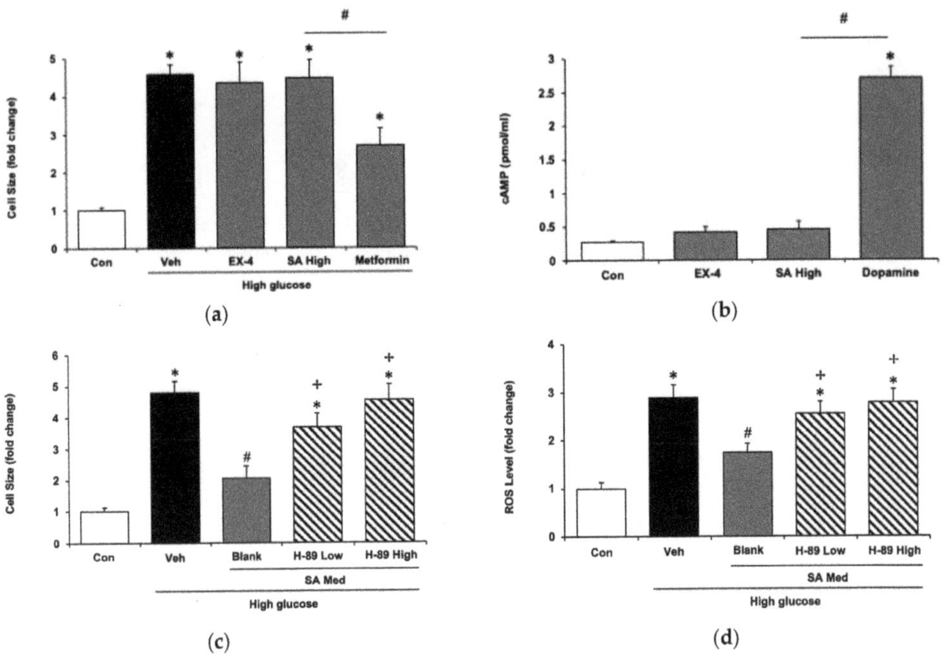

Figure 3. The signaling pathway for syringaldehyde (SA) alleviated cardiac hypertrophy in H9c2 cells. (**a**) Changes in cell size in hypertrophic cardiomyocytes with GLP-1 resistance. Cells were treated with or without SA at 1 μM (high dose), exendin-4 (EX-4) at 0.5 μM, and metformin at 5 μM, respectively. (**b**) SA and EX-4 failed to stimulate cAMP levels in H9c2 cells with GLP-1 resistance, whereas dopamine at 5 μM elevated cAMP levels in these cells. (**c**) A decrease in hypertrophic cell size due to SA at 0.5 μM (a medium dose) was reversed via pretreatment with H-89 at doses of 0.5 μM (low) or 1 μM (high). (**d**) Changes in cellular ROS levels in high glucose-induced hypertrophic cells with or without SA treatment. The inhibition of PKA by H-89 (1 μM) reversed the ROS-lowering effect of SA. Values for each indicator are expressed as fold changes in cell size, gene expressions of ANP, BNP, and β-MHC, relative to the control group. Results are presented as the mean ± SE from independent experiments, n = 6. Statistical significance: * $p < 0.05$ vs. normal control (Con). # $p < 0.05$ vs. vehicle (Veh). † $p < 0.05$ vs. hypertrophic cells treated with SA at 0.5 μM (Blank).

Additionally, the increase in cAMP due to SA was also ablated in H9c2 cells with GLP-1 resistance (Figure 3b). However, the effect of dopamine on H9c2 cells with GLP-1 resistance was unchanged (Figure 3b). This means that, like exendin-4, the regular GLP-1 receptor is essential to the effect of SA in H9c2 cells.

2.3. Protein Kinase A (PKA) Is Involved in the Activation of the GLP-1 Receptor in H9c2 Cells

Protein kinase A (PKA), also known as cAMP-dependent protein kinase, plays a pivotal role in cellular signaling pathways. The cAMP–PKA signaling cascade is critically involved in metabolic regulation [31]. SA may alleviate cardiac hypertrophy in H9c2 cells after GLP-1 receptor activation. To determine whether PKA plays a role in the signaling pathway mediated by SA, we employed H-89, a specific PKA inhibitor, as previously described [32]. As shown in Figure 3c, the effects of SA were dose-dependently reversed by H-89. The dose of H-89 administered was able to inhibit PKA [33]. Interestingly, the same dose of H-89 was able to reverse the reduction in the reactive oxygen species (ROS) by SA in H9c2 cells incubated with high glucose levels (Figure 3d). As in a previous study [34], ROS were increased by high glucose levels in H9c2 cells. SA was found to reduce ROS levels that were increased due to hyperglycemia. ROS were involved in the progression from compensating hypertrophy to heart failure. In the advanced stage of cardiac hypertrophy, ROS induced damage to the myocardium, resulting in myocardial dysfunction or injury [35].

2.4. Role of AMPK in Cardiac Effects of Syringaldehyde (SA)

GLP-1R agonist could activate AMPK signaling to prevent glucotoxicity in cardiomyocyte [36]. We applied AMPK siRNA to investigate the role of AMPK in the SA-induced alleviation of cardiac hypertrophy in H9c2 cells. As shown in Figure 4a, as a positive control, exendin-4 failed to modify the size of H9c2 cells in the absence of AMPK. Similarly, SA-induced action in scramble cells was reduced to zero in the absence of AMPK. The same results were observed in metformin-treated H9c2 cells. Moreover, the expression of the hypertrophic gene was changed in the same manner; reductions in the mRNA levels of each gene by SA were ablated in the absence of AMPK, as shown in Figure 4b,c. Finally, the expression of O-linked b-N-acetylglucosamine transferase (OGT) was promoted by high glucose levels, and it was reduced by a 1 μM (high)dose of SA. Interestingly, the effect of SA was reversed by the administration of compound C (Figure 4d) at the dose able to inhibit AMPK [37].

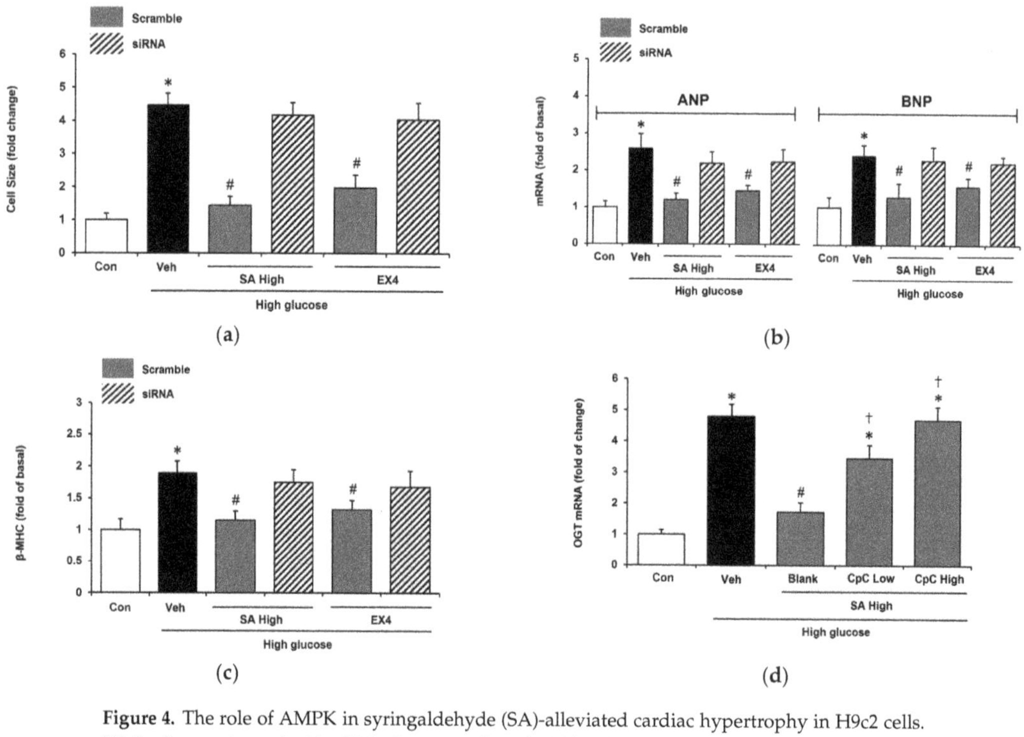

Figure 4. The role of AMPK in syringaldehyde (SA)-alleviated cardiac hypertrophy in H9c2 cells. H9c2 cells were treated with a high glucose medium for 48 h. siRNA was used to ablate the expression of AMPK and H9c2 cells that received with same volume of scramble. (**a**) Changes in cell size due to SA at 1 μM (high) were, like the effect of EX-4, reversed by AMPK ablation. Additionally, the effects of metformin were also removed in AMPK-silenced cells. (**b**) The changes in gene expression levels of ANP (Con: 1 ± 0.2; Veh: 2.6 ± 0.4; SA High + scramble: 1.2 ± 0.2; SA High + siRNA: 2.2 ± 0.3;

EX4+ scramble: 1.4 ± 0.1; EX4 + siRNA: 2.2 ± 0.3), and BNP (Con: 1 ± 0.3; Veh: 2.4 ± 0.3; SA High + scramble: 1.3 ± 0.4; SA High + siRNA: 2.3 ± 0.4; EX4+ scramble: 1.6 ± 0.2; EX4 + siRNA: 2.2 ± 0.4). (**c**) The changes in gene expression levels of β-MHC (Con: 1 ± 0.2; Veh: 1.9 ± 0.2; SA High + scramble: 1.2 ± 0.1; SA High + siRNA: 1.7 ± 0.2; EX4+ scramble: 1.3 ± 0.1; EX4 + siRNA: 1.7 ± 0.3). (**d**) The expression of O-linked b-N-acetylglucosamine transferase (OGT) was promoted by high glucose levels and reduced by SA at a 1 μM (high) dose. The effect of SA was reversed by compound C (CpC) at doses of 5 μM (low) and 10 μM (high). The value of each indicator shown in a column is the mean ± standard error of the mean (SEM) per group; n = 6. Values for each indicator are expressed as fold changes in cell size, cAMP levels, and ROS levels relative to the control group. Fold change is calculated as follows: fold change = data of the experimental group/data of the control group. * $p < 0.05$ vs. normal control (Con). # $p < 0.05$ vs. vehicle (Veh). † $p < 0.05$ vs. hypertrophic cell administered with SA 1 μM (Blank).

3. Discussion

In this study, SA demonstrated the ability to alleviate hyperglycemia-induced cardiac hypertrophy in cardiomyocytes, an effect that appeared to be dependent on the activation of the GLP-1 receptor. Furthermore, SA increased the protein expression level of the GLP-1 receptor in a dose-dependent manner. This was accompanied by a parallel increase in cAMP levels. Notably, the elevation in cAMP levels induced by SA was significantly diminished by the administration of Ex 9-39, a GLP-1 receptor antagonist at a dose sufficient to block receptor activity [38]. These findings indicate that SA activates the GLP-1 receptor in H9c2 cells and exerts protective effects against cardiac hypertrophy.

Myocardial hypertrophy is characterized by an enlargement in cell size and increased expression of embryonic genes, including ANP, BNP, and β-MHC, which can be considered three biomarkers of cardiomyocyte hypertrophy [39,40]. Hypertrophic gene expression in cardiomyocytes is promoted by oxidative stress, insulin resistance, and hyperglycemia [41]. Aortic stenosis, hypertension, and genetic abnormalities, such as hypertrophic cardiomyopathy, may cause maladaptive cardiac hypertrophy, while physiological cardiac hypertrophy is adaptive [42]. Hypertrophic enlargement is characterized by an increase in the cell size of cardiomyocytes [43]. Various sources of ROS have been identified in cardiac cells [42]. LVT hypertrophy (LVH) and heart failure caused by pressure overload have been linked to an increase in oxidative stress and, therefore, an increase in ROS production in the heart. Furthermore, it has been shown that the emergence of cellular remodeling and hypertrophy is linked to increased ROS production. It has been observed that ROS are involved in the progression from compensated hypertrophy to heart failure. It seems that ROS are injurious to the myocardium and cause damage or injury in the latter stages of cardiac hypertrophy [35]. According to the current findings, functional communication between endothelial cells and cardiomyocytes is caused by both direct and indirect processes that result from redox signaling both within and between these cells [44]. However, as including these parameters seemed unnecessary, cultured cardiomyocyte H9c2 cells were used in the present study. A direct reduction in cardiac hypertrophy due to SA was observed in the H9c2 cells. A similar reduction due to SA was also observed in hypertrophic biomarkers, including ANP, BNP, and β-MHC. As a result, SA might have reduced the heart hypertrophy identified in vitro.

The potential mechanism by which SA alleviates cardiac hypertrophy in vitro was examined. A previous study demonstrated that under high-glucose conditions, H9c2 cells exhibit a reduction in GLP-1R expression, resulting in compromised cardioprotective effects of GLP-1 [30]. These cells were subsequently referred to as GLP-1-resistant H9c2 cells [45]. In the present study, the GLP-1-resistant phenotype was confirmed by Western blot analysis, which revealed significantly reduced levels of GLP-1 receptor expression. Although the real mechanism remained unclear, which was likely mediated by Protein Kinase C (PKC) [30] or induced by β-Arrestin [45], this cell model was suitable for examining the role of the

GLP-1 receptor. EX-4, an analog of the GLP-1 receptor [15], was able to alleviate cardiac hypertrophy in H9c2 cells after the activation of the GLP-1 receptor [19]. The loss of EX-4 action in this cell model indicated the successful manipulation of the GLP-1 receptor. Interestingly, SA-induced action was also markedly reduced in H9c2 cells with GLP-1 resistance. However, metformin-induced changes were not modified by manipulating the GLP-1 receptor. Additionally, an increase in cAMP due to EX-4 was also reversed in cells with GLP-1 resistance. The same results were observed in SA-treated cells. However, the cAMP-increasing effect of dopamine through another specific receptor [46] was not modified. Therefore, GLP-1 receptor activation via SA is a critical influencing factor that is fully consistent with previous reports [24].

AMPK is a serine–threonine kinase that mainly acts as a metabolic sensor to regulate anabolic and catabolic processes in the heart [47]. In cardiac hypertrophy, AMPK has been suggested to be the key target of agents such as Geniposide [38]. Several upstream signal transduction molecules, including liver kinase B1 (LKB1) and calcium/calmodulin-activated protein kinase kinase 2 (CaMKK2), may activate AMPK through phosphorylation [48]. AMPK has been proposed as an inhibitor of cardiac hypertrophy because it suppresses protein synthesis and ROS generation [49]. The downstream signal pathways of AMPK have been identified as the MAPK family, which includes ERK1/2, p38, and JNK1/2 [50]. The development of pathological cardiac hypertrophy is significantly influenced by these signals [51]. AMPK is a stress-activated kinase [49]. AMPK localized within the intercalated disk of the heart may regulate directional cell migration by modulating the dynamic instability of the microtubule (MT) [52]. Therefore, AMPK has been demonstrated to regulate the cell shape and aspect ratio of cardiomyocytes by modulating the turnover of MTs [53]. This is consistent with the view that the microtubule cytoskeleton is a sensitive target of AMPK [54].

In cardiomyocytes, AMPK is known to reduce ROS production [49] and improve endoplasmic reticulum (ER) stress [55]. Both effects have been widely used to support the role of AMPK in cardiac hypertrophy [38]. AMPK is also known to be linked with autophagy [56]. AMPK may recruit Unc-51-like kinase 1 (ULK1) to activate autophagy [57]. Numerous physiological stressors, including oxidative damage, ER stress, and food constraints, may trigger autophagy, which usually occurs at low basal levels to preserve cellular homeostasis [56]. By removing damaged cells or undesirable macromolecules and organelles, autophagy helps maintain cellular homeostasis, which may negatively impact the structure of the whole heart [58]. Some natural products, such as berberine [59], dihydromyricetin [60], resveratrol [61] and irisin [62], induce autophagy as a mechanism for reducing cardiac hypertrophy. The original objective of autophagy in cardiac tissue was to preserve cardiac structure and function by providing energy, removing ROS, and controlling protein quality to adjust to internal environmental disturbances. However, excessive autophagy harms the heart by increasing cell death [56]. Autophagy modulation has been investigated [63] because higher dosing and long-term treatment with agents may drive excessive autophagy that damages the heart. Therefore, inhibiting excess autophagy using natural products such as Tanshinone IIA [64] has become a popular approach.

The association of N-Acetylglucosamine (GlcNAc) with cardiac hypertrophy is widely acknowledged [65]. GlcNAc, an amide derivative of the monosaccharide glucose, is formed through the reaction between glucosamine and acetic acid, and its levels are elevated in cardiac hypertrophy [66]. The modification of serine and threonine residues by GlcNAc, known as O-GlcNAcylation (OGN), is a dynamic process involving the addition and removal of the monosaccharide. This process is mediated by O-linked β-N-acetylglucosamine transferase (OGT) and O-linked β-N-acetylglucosaminase (OGA), respectively [67]. Elevated OGN plays a crucial role in mitigating myocardial remodeling,

fibrosis, and hypertrophy induced by short-term exposure to intermittent hypoxia [68]. OGN modulates myocardial hypertrophy through various molecular mechanisms, including the hyperglycemia-induced upregulation of ERK1/2 and cyclin D2 [69]. Additionally, activation of the AMPK pathway has been shown to suppress cardiac hypertrophy in vivo by reducing OGN levels [70]. Therefore, AMPK and OGN are common subjects in research on cardiac hypertrophy. It was recently proposed that SA may improve cardiac hypertrophy in H9c2 cells through AMPK to reduce OGT expression, which is consistent with a recent report that AMPK improved cardiac hypertrophy by reducing OGN [70] (Figure 5).

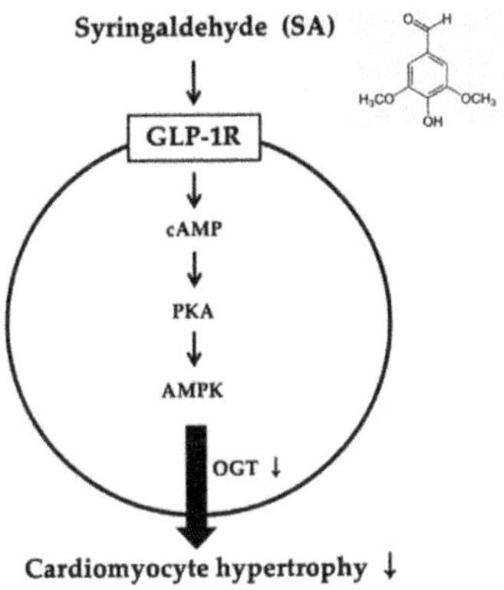

Figure 5. The schematic diagram that presents how syringaldehyde alleviates cardiac hypertrophy.

Compared to other GLP-1R agonists, SA can shorten the α-amylase reaction time and reduce glucose absorption, offering comparable efficacy with potentially fewer side effects [71]. Furthermore, SA has been shown to suppress oxidative stress and inflammatory responses, particularly in myocardial infarction patients, further emphasizing its therapeutic potential and favorable safety profile [72]. Beyond its role in diabetes management, recent studies have also highlighted SA's anticancer properties, including its ability to inhibit the proliferation of triple-negative breast cancer (TNBC) cells [73]. These findings suggest that exploring SA's efficacy and safety in animal models of TNBC, as well as its long-term effects on tumor recurrence and metastasis, could be valuable.

In comparison to existing GLP-1 receptor agonists, such as exenatide and liraglutide, SA offers dual functionality by modulating the GLP-1 receptor while simultaneously reducing oxidative stress and inflammation. This makes SA a promising candidate for addressing both glycemic control and the secondary complications of diabetes, such as cardiovascular disease. Unlike synthetic peptide-based agonists that require injection due to their susceptibility to enzymatic breakdown, SA, as a naturally occurring compound, offers the advantages of potentially fewer side effects and broader accessibility when developed as a dietary supplement.

This study is limited to evaluating the effects of SA in hypertrophic H9c2 cells, without incorporating primary cardiomyocytes or in vivo models, which hinders the extrapolation of the results to clinical settings. Additionally, changes in protein levels related to cellular signaling pathways should be examined. Future experiments will systematically collect protein samples for WB analysis to validate findings at the protein level, while studies involving primary cardiomyocytes and in vivo models will also be undertaken. Furthermore, long-term efficacy studies are necessary to assess the sustained therapeutic potential of SA, which will be investigated in subsequent research.

4. Materials and Methods

4.1. Materials

Syringaldehyde (SA) (purity: 98%), H-89, compound C, exendin-4 (EX-4), exendin 9–39 (EX9), metformin, and other chemicals or reagents were obtained from Sigma-Aldrich (St. Louis, MO, USA).

4.2. Culture of Cardiac Cells

The H9c2 cardio myoblast cell line (BCRC No. 60096) was cultured in Dulbecco's modified Eagle's medium (DMEM, pH 7.2; Gibco-BRL Life Technologies, Gaithersburg, MD, USA) with 10% fetal bovine serum (FBS, Gibco-BRL Life Technologies, Gaithersburg, MD, USA), in accordance with our previous method [74]. Cells were maintained at 37 °C in a humidified atmosphere with 5% CO_2. The cells were seeded at a density of 60,000 cells/cm^2. Cell passage numbers were strictly controlled (passages 3–10) to minimize variability, and a consistent cell source was used throughout the experiments. The medium was replaced on the second day. Experiments were performed in triplicate to ensure reproducibility, and culture conditions were standardized to mitigate variability.

4.3. Induction of Cardiac Hypertrophy in H9c2 Cells

A cellular model of cardiac hypertrophy was generated using a high-glucose medium containing 33 mM glucose and 2% FBS. H9c2 cells were incubated with high glucose concentrations for 48 h after achieving 70% confluence, as described previously [29]. D-glucose (Sigma-Aldrich, St. Louis, MO, USA) was dissolved in a normal medium to produce a solution with a concentration of 30 mmol/L glucose. SA was incubated for 1 h before the addition of glucose at a high concentration. The concentrations and treatment durations of SA were determined based on our preliminary experiments [24], which demonstrated their ability to induce significant biological effects while avoiding cytotoxicity. Moreover, our preliminary results showed that H9c2 cells exhibit hypertrophic responses similar to those of primary rat neonatal cardiomyocytes, consistent with previous studies [75]. Thus, the current study utilized H9c2 cells to investigate the hypertrophic response of cardiomyocytes [29].

4.4. Induction of GLP-1 Resistance in H9c2 Cells

GLP-1 resistance in H9c2 cells was established following the methodology described in a prior study [30]. H9C2 cells were maintained in either high glucose (HG, 33 mM) or normal glucose (NG, 5 mM) conditions for 21 days, with the culture media replaced every 48 h without subculturing the cells. Hypoxia/re-oxygenation injury in H9C2 cells was induced by subjecting them to hypoxic conditions (95% N_2, 5% CO_2) in an anaerobic system (Thermo Forma) at 37 °C for 6 h, followed by 10 h of re-oxygenation under normoxic conditions (95% ambient air, 5% CO_2). H9c2 cells in a control group were maintained under normal conditions for the same duration. Exendin-4 (EX-4 50 nM) was applied one hour before cell collection to verify the effectiveness of the induction [45]. Depending on the experimental design, syringaldehyde (SA, 0.5 μM or 1 μM), metformin (5 μM), dopamine (5 μM), or H-89 (0.5 μM or 1 μM) were added individually or in combination one hour prior to harvesting the cells.

4.5. Detection of Cellular ROS

The intracellular reactive oxygen species (ROS) levels were measured using 2′,7′-dichlorodihydrofluorescein diacetate (DCFH-DA; Sigma-Aldrich), following an established protocol [76]. H9c2 cells were treated with the test compound at a specified concentration for 24 h. After treatment, the cells were washed twice with phosphate-buffered saline

(PBS) to remove residual compounds. Subsequently, the cells were incubated with 10 μM DCFH-DA in PBS for 30 min at 37 °C. After incubation, the cells were harvested using trypsin-ethylenediaminetetraacetic acid (EDTA) solution, centrifuged at 200× *g* for 5 min, and resuspended in 0.5 mL of PBS. The fluorescence intensity of the DCF, a marker for ROS levels, was visualized using a fluorescence microscope (Olympus, Tokyo, Japan). Quantification of fluorescence intensity was performed using ImageJ software (version 1.43, Vector Laboratories, Burlingame, CA, USA). The ROS levels were expressed as the ratio of the fluorescence intensity of treated samples to that of control cells, ensuring accurate comparison [77].

4.6. *Cardiomyocyte Transfections*

To investigate the interaction between SA and AMPK signaling pathways, H9c2 cells were first induced to develop hypertrophy. Subsequently, siRNA transfections were conducted as previously described [78]. The transfection reagent and siRNAs targeting AMPK (GCATATGCTGCAGGTAGAT) were obtained from Dharmacon (Horizon Discovery, Lafayette, CO, USA). Cells were transfected with either AMPKα1-specific siRNA (100 nM) or an equivalent amount of scrambled siRNA using Lipofectamine 2000 (0.15%, *v*/*v*, Thermo Fisher Scientific, Waltham, MA, USA) for 12 h. After that, lipofectamine 2000 was removed by changing into a fresh medium containing 10% FBS. The cells were then administered with drugs and further analysis following transfection.

4.7. *Quantitative Reverse-Transcription Polymerase Chain Reaction (qRT-PCR) of O-Linked N-Acetylglucosamine Transferase (OGT)*

As with the biomarkers of hypertrophy, ANP, BNP, and β-MHC [29], the expression of OGT was determined via qRT-PCR as described in our previous report [24]. Total RNA was extracted by using a TRIzol reagent (Invitrogen, Carlsbad, CA, USA). qRT-PCR primers were acquired from Roche (Roche Diagnostics GmbH, Mannheim, Germany). Approximately, 200 ng of total RNA was reverse-transcribed into cDNA. As in the previous study [78], the primers used in the experiment were as follows:

ANP	F: 5′-CACAGATCTGATGGATTTCAAGA-3′;
	R: 5′-CCTCATCTTCTACCGGCATC-3′;
BNP	F: 5′-GTCAGTCGCTTGGGCTGT-3′;
	R: 5′-CCAGAGCTGGGGAAAGAAG-3′;
β-MHC	F: 5′-CATCCCCAATGAGACGAAGT-3′;
	R: 5′-GGGAAGCCCTTCCTACAGAT-3′
Ogt	F: 5′-G GCTATGTGAGTT CTGACTTCGG-3′
	R: 5′-GATTGGCTTCCGCCATCACCTT-3′,
Gapdh	F: 5′-CATCACTGCCACCCAGAAGACTG-3′
	R: 5′-ATGCCAGTGAGCTTCCCGTTCAG-3′

The concentration of each qRT-PCR product was determined by comparison with a corresponding standard curve to ensure quantitative accuracy [24].

4.8. *Western Blot Analysis*

H9C2 cells subjected to various treatments were harvested and lysed for Western blot analysis [24]. Primary antibodies used were anti-GLP-1R (1:200, Abcam, Cambridge, UK) and anti-β-Actin (1:5000, Abcam, Cambridge, UK) as a loading control. Membranes were incubated with the primary antibodies overnight at 4 °C. After washing with TBST, the membranes were incubated with horseradish peroxidase-conjugated goat anti-rabbit IgG secondary antibodies (1:5000, Santa Cruz, CA, USA) for 1 h at room temperature. Protein bands were visualized using an enhanced chemiluminescence (ECL) detection system (Amersham, UK). Densitometric analysis of the protein bands was conducted using ImageJ software (version 1.43; NIH, Bethesda, MD, USA) to quantify relative protein expression levels.

4.9. Detection of Intracellular Calcium Level

The intracellular calcium concentration $[Ca^{2+}]i$ changes were measured using the fluorescent probe fura-2, as previously detailed [79]. Cells were harvested and suspended in PBS, after which 5 μM Fura-2 was added for staining. Following incubation, the fluorescence intensity was measured using a fluorescence spectrofluorometer (Hitachi F-2000, Tokyo, Japan). Background fluorescence from unloaded cells was subtracted from all measurements to ensure accuracy. The intracellular calcium concentration was then calculated according to the previous study [79].

4.10. Statistical Analysis

For each experimental group, results are presented as the mean ± standard error of the mean (SEM) based on the designated sample size. Data were analyzed using SPSS statistical software version 21 (SPSS Inc., Chicago, IL, USA). An unpaired *t*-test was used to assess the differences between the two groups, while a one-way analysis of variance (ANOVA) followed by Tukey's post hoc test was applied to compare differences among more than two groups. Statistical significance was established at $p < 0.05$.

5. Conclusions

Syringaldehyde demonstrates the potential to attenuate hyperglycemia-induced cardiac hypertrophy in H9c2 cells, primarily by activating the GLP-1 receptor. This mechanism involves the AMPK signaling pathway and the suppression of OGT expression. This study represents a preliminary investigation into the therapeutic potential of SA. Overall, this study highlights the potential of SA to advance herbal medicine and serve as a novel therapeutic strategy for managing cardiac hypertrophy in diabetes.

Author Contributions: Conceptualization, C.-T.H. and K.-C.C.; methodology, T.-T.Y.; investigation, Y.L.; data curation, Y.L. and K.-C.C.; writing—original draft preparation, Y.L.; writing—review and editing, K.-C.C.; supervision, K.-C.C.; project administration, K.-C.C. All authors have read and agreed to the published version of the manuscript.

Funding: This research received no external funding.

Institutional Review Board Statement: Not applicable.

Informed Consent Statement: Not applicable.

Data Availability Statement: The data presented in this study are available from the corresponding author upon reasonable request.

Conflicts of Interest: The authors declare no conflicts of interest.

References

1. Zuo, L.; Youtz, D.J.; Wold, L.E. Particulate matter exposure exacerbates high glucose-induced cardiomyocyte dysfunction through ROS generation. *PLoS ONE* **2011**, *6*, e23116. [CrossRef] [PubMed]
2. Braunwald, E. The war against heart failure: The Lancet lecture. *Lancet* **2015**, *385*, 812–824. [CrossRef] [PubMed]
3. D'Ascenzi, F.; Pelliccia, A.; Corrado, D.; Cameli, M.; Curci, V.; Alvino, F.; Natali, B.M.; Focardi, M.; Bonifazi, M.; Mondillo, S. Right ventricular remodelling induced by exercise training in competitive athletes. *Eur. Heart J. Cardiovasc. Imaging* **2016**, *17*, 301–307. [CrossRef]
4. Driver, J.A.; Djousse, L.; Logroscino, G.; Gaziano, J.M.; Kurth, T. Incidence of cardiovascular disease and cancer in advanced age: Prospective cohort study. *BMJ* **2008**, *337*, a2467. [CrossRef]

5. Bernardo, B.C.; Weeks, K.L.; Pretorius, L.; McMullen, J.R. Molecular distinction between physiological and pathological cardiac hypertrophy: Experimental findings and therapeutic strategies. *Pharmacol. Ther.* **2010**, *128*, 191–227. [CrossRef]
6. Voulgari, C.; Papadogiannis, D.; Tentolouris, N. Diabetic cardiomyopathy: From the pathophysiology of the cardiac myocytes to current diagnosis and management strategies. *Vasc. Health Risk Manag.* **2010**, *6*, 883–903. [CrossRef] [PubMed]
7. Drucker, D.J. The biology of incretin hormones. *Cell Metab.* **2006**, *3*, 153–165. [CrossRef] [PubMed]
8. Ban, K.; Noyan-Ashraf, M.H.; Hoefer, J.; Bolz, S.S.; Drucker, D.J.; Husain, M. Cardioprotective and vasodilatory actions of glucagon-like peptide 1 receptor are mediated through both glucagon-like peptide 1 receptor-dependent and -independent pathways. *Circulation* **2008**, *117*, 2340–2350. [CrossRef]
9. Ma, X.; Liu, Z.; Ilyas, I.; Little, P.J.; Kamato, D.; Sahebka, A.; Chen, Z.; Luo, S.; Zheng, X.; Weng, J.; et al. GLP-1 receptor agonists (GLP-1RAs): Cardiovascular actions and therapeutic potential. *Int. J. Biol. Sci.* **2021**, *17*, 2050–2068. [CrossRef] [PubMed]
10. Popoviciu, M.S.; Paduraru, L.; Yahya, G.; Metwally, K.; Cavalu, S. Emerging Role of GLP-1 Agonists in Obesity: A Comprehensive Review of Randomised Controlled Trials. *Int. J. Mol. Sci.* **2023**, *24*, 10449. [CrossRef] [PubMed]
11. Tsapas, A.; Avgerinos, I.; Karagiannis, T.; Malandris, K.; Manolopoulos, A.; Andreadis, P.; Liakos, A.; Matthews, D.R.; Bekiari, E. Comparative Effectiveness of Glucose-Lowering Drugs for Type 2 Diabetes: A Systematic Review and Network Meta-analysis. *Ann. Intern. Med.* **2020**, *173*, 278–286. [CrossRef]
12. Thomas, M.C. The potential and pitfalls of GLP-1 receptor agonists for renal protection in type 2 diabetes. *Diabetes Metab.* **2017**, *43* (Suppl. S1), 2S20–2S27. [CrossRef] [PubMed]
13. Zhong, J.; Chen, H.; Liu, Q.; Zhou, S.; Liu, Z.; Xiao, Y. GLP-1 receptor agonists and myocardial metabolism in atrial fibrillation. *J. Pharm. Anal.* **2024**, *14*, 100917. [CrossRef]
14. Ma, Y.L.; Kong, C.Y.; Guo, Z.; Wang, M.Y.; Wang, P.; Liu, F.Y.; Yang, D.; Yang, Z.; Tang, Q.Z. Semaglutide ameliorates cardiac remodeling in male mice by optimizing energy substrate utilization through the Creb5/NR4a1 axis. *Nat. Commun.* **2024**, *15*, 4757. [CrossRef] [PubMed]
15. Timmers, L.; Henriques, J.P.; de Kleijn, D.P.; Devries, J.H.; Kemperman, H.; Steendijk, P.; Verlaan, C.W.; Kerver, M.; Piek, J.J.; Doevendans, P.A.; et al. Exenatide reduces infarct size and improves cardiac function in a porcine model of ischemia and reperfusion injury. *J. Am. Coll. Cardiol.* **2009**, *53*, 501–510. [CrossRef] [PubMed]
16. Palee, S.; Chattipakorn, S.C.; Chattipakorn, N. Liraglutide preserves intracellular calcium handling in isolated murine myocytes exposed to oxidative stress. *Physiol. Res.* **2017**, *66*, 889–895. [CrossRef]
17. Chen, W.R.; Chen, Y.D.; Tian, F.; Yang, N.; Cheng, L.Q.; Hu, S.Y.; Wang, J.; Yang, J.J.; Wang, S.F.; Gu, X.F. Effects of Liraglutide on Reperfusion Injury in Patients With ST-Segment-Elevation Myocardial Infarction. *Circ. Cardiovasc. Imaging* **2016**, *9*, e005146. [CrossRef] [PubMed]
18. Wang, J.; Fan, S.; Xiong, Q.; Niu, Y.; Zhang, X.; Qin, J.; Shi, Y.; Zhang, L. Glucagon-like peptide-1 attenuates cardiac hypertrophy via the AngII/AT1R/ACE2 and AMPK/mTOR/p70S6K pathways. *Acta Biochim. Biophys. Sin.* **2021**, *53*, 1189–1197. [CrossRef]
19. Zhou, Y.; He, X.; Chen, Y.; Huang, Y.; Wu, L.; He, J. Exendin-4 attenuates cardiac hypertrophy via AMPK/mTOR signaling pathway activation. *Biochem. Biophys. Res. Commun.* **2015**, *468*, 394–399. [CrossRef]
20. Yaribeygi, H.; Jamialahmadi, T.; Moallem, S.A.; Sahebkar, A. Boosting GLP-1 by Natural Products. *Adv. Exp. Med. Biol.* **2021**, *1328*, 513–522. [CrossRef] [PubMed]
21. Upadhyay, D.; Banerjee, R.; Kallijarvi, J.; Purhonen, J. Protocol for quantification of UDP-GlcNAc using an enzymatic microplate assay. *STAR Protoc.* **2024**, *5*, 102817. [CrossRef]
22. Cheemanapalli, S.; Anuradha, C.M.; Madhusudhana, P.; Mahesh, M.; Raghavendra, P.B.; Kumar, C.S. Exploring the Binding Affinity of Novel Syringic Acid Analogues and Critical Determinants of Selectivity as Potent Proteasome Inhibitors. *Anticancer Agents Med. Chem.* **2016**, *16*, 1496–1510. [CrossRef] [PubMed]
23. Velu, P.; Vinothkumar, V.; Babukumar, S.; Ramachandhiran, D. Chemopreventive effect of syringic acid on 7,12-dimethylbenz(a)anthracene induced hamster buccal pouch carcinogenesis. *Toxicol. Mech. Methods* **2017**, *27*, 631–640. [CrossRef] [PubMed]
24. Lee, J.; Li, Y.; Cheng, J.T.; Liu, I.M.; Cheng, K.C. Development of Syringaldehyde as an Agonist of the GLP-1 Receptor to Alleviate Diabetic Disorders in Animal Models. *Pharmaceuticals* **2024**, *17*, 538. [CrossRef] [PubMed]
25. Shahzad, S.; Mateen, S.; Mubeena Mariyath, P.M.; Naeem, S.S.; Akhtar, K.; Rizvi, W.; Moin, S. Protective effect of syringaldehyde on biomolecular oxidation, inflammation and histopathological alterations in isoproterenol induced cardiotoxicity in rats. *Biomed. Pharmacother.* **2018**, *108*, 625–633. [CrossRef]
26. Guo, L.X.; Xia, Z.N.; Gao, X.; Yin, F.; Liu, J.H. Glucagon-like peptide 1 receptor plays a critical role in geniposide-regulated insulin secretion in INS-1 cells. *Acta Pharmacol. Sin.* **2012**, *33*, 237–241. [CrossRef] [PubMed]
27. Jia, Y.; Gong, N.; Li, T.F.; Zhu, B.; Wang, Y.X. Peptidic exenatide and herbal catalpol mediate neuroprotection via the hippocampal GLP-1 receptor/beta-endorphin pathway. *Pharmacol. Res.* **2015**, *102*, 276–285. [CrossRef] [PubMed]
28. Asadi, F.; Razmi, A.; Dehpour, A.R.; Shafiei, M. Tropisetron inhibits high glucose-induced calcineurin/NFAT hypertrophic pathway in H9c2 myocardial cells. *J. Pharm. Pharmacol.* **2016**, *68*, 485–493. [CrossRef] [PubMed]

29. Cheng, K.C.; Chang, W.T.; Kuo, F.Y.; Chen, Z.C.; Li, Y.; Cheng, J.T. TGR5 activation ameliorates hyperglycemia-induced cardiac hypertrophy in H9c2 cells. *Sci. Rep.* **2019**, *9*, 3633. [CrossRef] [PubMed]
30. Pan, X.; Chen, J.; Wang, T.; Zhang, M.; Wang, H.; Gao, H. Essential Role Of High Glucose-Induced Overexpression Of PKCbeta And PKCdelta In GLP-1 Resistance In Rodent Cardiomyocytes. *Diabetes Metab. Syndr. Obes.* **2019**, *12*, 2289–2302. [CrossRef]
31. Depre, C.; Ponchaut, S.; Deprez, J.; Maisin, L.; Hue, L. Cyclic AMP suppresses the inhibition of glycolysis by alternative oxidizable substrates in the heart. *J. Clin. Investig.* **1998**, *101*, 390–397. [CrossRef]
32. Liu, C.; Ke, P.; Zhang, J.; Zhang, X.; Chen, X. Protein Kinase Inhibitor Peptide as a Tool to Specifically Inhibit Protein Kinase A. *Front. Physiol.* **2020**, *11*, 574030. [CrossRef]
33. Fan, S.; Xiong, Q.; Zhang, X.; Zhang, L.; Shi, Y. Glucagon-like peptide 1 reverses myocardial hypertrophy through cAMP/PKA/RhoA/ROCK2 signaling. *Acta Biochim. Biophys. Sin.* **2020**, *52*, 612–619. [CrossRef]
34. Bugyei-Twum, A.; Advani, A.; Advani, S.L.; Zhang, Y.; Thai, K.; Kelly, D.J.; Connelly, K.A. High glucose induces Smad activation via the transcriptional coregulator p300 and contributes to cardiac fibrosis and hypertrophy. *Cardiovasc. Diabetol.* **2014**, *13*, 89. [CrossRef] [PubMed]
35. Sawyer, D.B.; Siwik, D.A.; Xiao, L.; Pimentel, D.R.; Singh, K.; Colucci, W.S. Role of oxidative stress in myocardial hypertrophy and failure. *J. Mol. Cell Cardiol.* **2002**, *34*, 379–388. [CrossRef] [PubMed]
36. Balteau, M.; Van Steenbergen, A.; Timmermans, A.D.; Dessy, C.; Behets-Wydemans, G.; Tajeddine, N.; Castanares-Zapatero, D.; Gilon, P.; Vanoverschelde, J.L.; Horman, S.; et al. AMPK activation by glucagon-like peptide-1 prevents NADPH oxidase activation induced by hyperglycemia in adult cardiomyocytes. *Am. J. Physiol. Heart Circ. Physiol.* **2014**, *307*, H1120–H1133. [CrossRef]
37. Xie, Z.; Yang, C.; Xu, T. Hesperetin attenuates LPS-induced the inflammatory response and apoptosis of H9c2 by activating the AMPK/P53 signaling pathway. *Immun. Inflamm. Dis.* **2023**, *11*, e973. [CrossRef]
38. Ma, Z.G.; Dai, J.; Zhang, W.B.; Yuan, Y.; Liao, H.H.; Zhang, N.; Bian, Z.Y.; Tang, Q.Z. Protection against cardiac hypertrophy by geniposide involves the GLP-1 receptor / AMPKalpha signalling pathway. *Br. J. Pharmacol.* **2016**, *173*, 1502–1516. [CrossRef] [PubMed]
39. Kehat, I.; Molkentin, J.D. Molecular pathways underlying cardiac remodeling during pathophysiological stimulation. *Circulation* **2010**, *122*, 2727–2735. [CrossRef] [PubMed]
40. Boudina, S.; Abel, E.D. Diabetic cardiomyopathy revisited. *Circulation* **2007**, *115*, 3213–3223. [CrossRef]
41. Grubic Rotkvic, P.; Planinic, Z.; Liberati Prso, A.M.; Sikic, J.; Galic, E.; Rotkvic, L. The Mystery of Diabetic Cardiomyopathy: From Early Concepts and Underlying Mechanisms to Novel Therapeutic Possibilities. *Int. J. Mol. Sci.* **2021**, *22*, 5973. [CrossRef]
42. Bazgir, F.; Nau, J.; Nakhaei-Rad, S.; Amin, E.; Wolf, M.J.; Saucerman, J.J.; Lorenz, K.; Ahmadian, M.R. The Microenvironment of the Pathogenesis of Cardiac Hypertrophy. *Cells* **2023**, *12*, 1780. [CrossRef] [PubMed]
43. Wan, S.; Wang, S.; Yang, X.; Cui, Y.; Guan, H.; Xiao, W.; Liu, F. Regulation of H9C2 cell hypertrophy by 14-3-3eta via inhibiting glycolysis. *PLoS ONE* **2024**, *19*, e0307696. [CrossRef]
44. Zhang, M.; Shah, A.M. ROS signalling between endothelial cells and cardiac cells. *Cardiovasc. Res.* **2014**, *102*, 249–257. [CrossRef]
45. Pan, X.; Li, C.; Gao, H. High Glucose Attenuates Cardioprotective Effects of Glucagon-Like Peptide-1 Through Induction of Mitochondria Dysfunction via Inhibition of beta-Arrestin-Signaling. *Front. Physiol.* **2021**, *12*, 648399. [CrossRef]
46. Yang, Y. Functional Selectivity of Dopamine D(1) Receptor Signaling: Retrospect and Prospect. *Int. J. Mol. Sci.* **2021**, *22*, 11914. [CrossRef] [PubMed]
47. Arad, M.; Seidman, C.E.; Seidman, J.G. AMP-activated protein kinase in the heart: Role during health and disease. *Circ. Res.* **2007**, *100*, 474–488. [CrossRef]
48. Yan, Y.; Zhou, X.E.; Xu, H.E.; Melcher, K. Structure and Physiological Regulation of AMPK. *Int. J. Mol. Sci.* **2018**, *19*, 3534. [CrossRef] [PubMed]
49. Zaha, V.G.; Young, L.H. AMP-activated protein kinase regulation and biological actions in the heart. *Circ. Res.* **2012**, *111*, 800–814. [CrossRef] [PubMed]
50. Chen, Y.; Ge, Z.; Huang, S.; Zhou, L.; Zhai, C.; Chen, Y.; Hu, Q.; Cao, W.; Weng, Y.; Li, Y. Delphinidin attenuates pathological cardiac hypertrophy via the AMPK/NOX/MAPK signaling pathway. *Aging* **2020**, *12*, 5362–5383. [CrossRef] [PubMed]
51. Esposito, G.; Prasad, S.V.; Rapacciuolo, A.; Mao, L.; Koch, W.J.; Rockman, H.A. Cardiac overexpression of a G(q) inhibitor blocks induction of extracellular signal-regulated kinase and c-Jun NH(2)-terminal kinase activity in in vivo pressure overload. *Circulation* **2001**, *103*, 1453–1458. [CrossRef]
52. Chen, C.Y.; Caporizzo, M.A.; Bedi, K.; Vite, A.; Bogush, A.I.; Robison, P.; Heffler, J.G.; Salomon, A.K.; Kelly, N.A.; Babu, A.; et al. Suppression of detyrosinated microtubules improves cardiomyocyte function in human heart failure. *Nat. Med.* **2018**, *24*, 1225–1233. [CrossRef] [PubMed]
53. Yashirogi, S.; Nagao, T.; Nishida, Y.; Takahashi, Y.; Qaqorh, T.; Yazawa, I.; Katayama, T.; Kioka, H.; Matsui, T.S.; Saito, S.; et al. AMPK regulates cell shape of cardiomyocytes by modulating turnover of microtubules through CLIP-170. *EMBO Rep.* **2021**, *22*, e50949. [CrossRef]

54. Fassett, J.T.; Hu, X.; Xu, X.; Lu, Z.; Zhang, P.; Chen, Y.; Bache, R.J. AMPK attenuates microtubule proliferation in cardiac hypertrophy. *Am. J. Physiol. Heart Circ. Physiol.* **2013**, *304*, H749–H758. [CrossRef]
55. Terai, K.; Hiramoto, Y.; Masaki, M.; Sugiyama, S.; Kuroda, T.; Hori, M.; Kawase, I.; Hirota, H. AMP-activated protein kinase protects cardiomyocytes against hypoxic injury through attenuation of endoplasmic reticulum stress. *Mol. Cell Biol.* **2005**, *25*, 9554–9575. [CrossRef]
56. Li, Z.; Wang, J.; Yang, X. Functions of autophagy in pathological cardiac hypertrophy. *Int. J. Biol. Sci.* **2015**, *11*, 672–678. [CrossRef]
57. Xie, Z.; Dong, Y.; Scholz, R.; Neumann, D.; Zou, M.H. Phosphorylation of LKB1 at serine 428 by protein kinase C-zeta is required for metformin-enhanced activation of the AMP-activated protein kinase in endothelial cells. *Circulation* **2008**, *117*, 952–962. [CrossRef] [PubMed]
58. Li, L.; Xu, J.; He, L.; Peng, L.; Zhong, Q.; Chen, L.; Jiang, Z. The role of autophagy in cardiac hypertrophy. *Acta Biochim. Biophys. Sin.* **2016**, *48*, 491–500. [CrossRef]
59. Hang, W.; He, B.; Chen, J.; Xia, L.; Wen, B.; Liang, T.; Wang, X.; Zhang, Q.; Wu, Y.; Chen, Q.; et al. Berberine Ameliorates High Glucose-Induced Cardiomyocyte Injury via AMPK Signaling Activation to Stimulate Mitochondrial Biogenesis and Restore Autophagic Flux. *Front. Pharmacol.* **2018**, *9*, 1121. [CrossRef]
60. Meng, G.; Yang, S.; Chen, Y.; Yao, W.; Zhu, H.; Zhang, W. Attenuating effects of dihydromyricetin on angiotensin II-induced rat cardiomyocyte hypertrophy related to antioxidative activity in a NO-dependent manner. *Pharm. Biol.* **2015**, *53*, 904–912. [CrossRef]
61. Gurusamy, N.; Lekli, I.; Mukherjee, S.; Ray, D.; Ahsan, M.K.; Gherghiceanu, M.; Popescu, L.M.; Das, D.K. Cardioprotection by resveratrol: A novel mechanism via autophagy involving the mTORC2 pathway. *Cardiovasc. Res.* **2010**, *86*, 103–112. [CrossRef] [PubMed]
62. Li, R.L.; Wu, S.S.; Wu, Y.; Wang, X.X.; Chen, H.Y.; Xin, J.J.; Li, H.; Lan, J.; Xue, K.Y.; Li, X.; et al. Irisin alleviates pressure overload-induced cardiac hypertrophy by inducing protective autophagy via mTOR-independent activation of the AMPK-ULK1 pathway. *J. Mol. Cell Cardiol.* **2018**, *121*, 242–255. [CrossRef]
63. Wang, X.; Cui, T. Autophagy modulation: A potential therapeutic approach in cardiac hypertrophy. *Am. J. Physiol. Heart Circ. Physiol.* **2017**, *313*, H304–H319. [CrossRef]
64. Wen, L.; Cheng, X.; Fan, Q.; Chen, Z.; Luo, Z.; Xu, T.; He, M.; He, H. TanshinoneIIA inhibits excessive autophagy and protects myocardium against ischemia/reperfusion injury via 14-3-3eta/Akt/Beclin1 pathway. *Eur. J. Pharmacol.* **2023**, *954*, 175865. [CrossRef]
65. Jones, S.P.; Zachara, N.E.; Ngoh, G.A.; Hill, B.G.; Teshima, Y.; Bhatnagar, A.; Hart, G.W.; Marban, E. Cardioprotection by N-acetylglucosamine linkage to cellular proteins. *Circulation* **2008**, *117*, 1172–1182. [CrossRef]
66. Lunde, I.G.; Aronsen, J.M.; Kvaloy, H.; Qvigstad, E.; Sjaastad, I.; Tonnessen, T.; Christensen, G.; Gronning-Wang, L.M.; Carlson, C.R. Cardiac O-GlcNAc signaling is increased in hypertrophy and heart failure. *Physiol. Genom.* **2012**, *44*, 162–172. [CrossRef]
67. Mannino, M.P.; Hart, G.W. The Beginner's Guide to O-GlcNAc: From Nutrient Sensitive Pathway Regulation to Its Impact on the Immune System. *Front. Immunol.* **2022**, *13*, 828648. [CrossRef] [PubMed]
68. Nakagawa, T.; Furukawa, Y.; Hayashi, T.; Nomura, A.; Yokoe, S.; Moriwaki, K.; Kato, R.; Ijiri, Y.; Yamaguchi, T.; Izumi, Y.; et al. Augmented O-GlcNAcylation attenuates intermittent hypoxia-induced cardiac remodeling through the suppression of NFAT and NF-kappaB activities in mice. *Hypertens. Res.* **2019**, *42*, 1858–1871. [CrossRef]
69. Ding, F.; Yu, L.; Wang, M.; Xu, S.; Xia, Q.; Fu, G. O-GlcNAcylation involvement in high glucose-induced cardiac hypertrophy via ERK1/2 and cyclin D2. *Amino Acids* **2013**, *45*, 339–349. [CrossRef]
70. Gelinas, R.; Mailleux, F.; Dontaine, J.; Bultot, L.; Demeulder, B.; Ginion, A.; Daskalopoulos, E.P.; Esfahani, H.; Dubois-Deruy, E.; Lauzier, B.; et al. AMPK activation counteracts cardiac hypertrophy by reducing O-GlcNAcylation. *Nat. Commun.* **2018**, *9*, 374. [CrossRef] [PubMed]
71. Weng, L.; Chen, T.H.; Zheng, Q.; Weng, W.H.; Huang, L.; Lai, D.; Fu, Y.S.; Weng, C.F. Syringaldehyde promoting intestinal motility with suppressing alpha-amylase hinders starch digestion in diabetic mice. *Biomed. Pharmacother.* **2021**, *141*, 111865. [CrossRef] [PubMed]
72. Shahzad, S.; Mateen, S.; Kausar, T.; Naeem, S.S.; Hasan, A.; Abidi, M.; Nayeem, S.M.; Faizy, A.F.; Moin, S. Effect of syringic acid and syringaldehyde on oxidative stress and inflammatory status in peripheral blood mononuclear cells from patients of myocardial infarction. *Naunyn Schmiedebergs Arch. Pharmacol.* **2020**, *393*, 691–704. [CrossRef] [PubMed]
73. Jin, X.X.; Mei, Y.N.; Shen, Z.; Zhu, J.F.; Xing, S.H.; Yang, H.M.; Liang, G.; Zheng, X.H. A chalcone-syringaldehyde hybrid inhibits triple-negative breast cancer cell proliferation and migration by inhibiting CKAP2-mediated FAK and STAT3 phosphorylation. *Phytomedicine* **2022**, *101*, 154087. [CrossRef] [PubMed]
74. Li, Y.X.; Cheng, K.C.; Liu, I.M.; Niu, H.S. Myricetin Increases Circulating Adropin Level after Activation of Glucagon-like Peptide 1 (GLP-1) Receptor in Type-1 Diabetic Rats. *Pharmaceuticals* **2022**, *15*, 173. [CrossRef]
75. Watkins, S.J.; Borthwick, G.M.; Arthur, H.M. The H9C2 cell line and primary neonatal cardiomyocyte cells show similar hypertrophic responses in vitro. *In Vitro Cell Dev. Biol. Anim.* **2011**, *47*, 125–131. [CrossRef]

76. Ullah, I.; Park, H.Y.; Kim, M.O. Anthocyanins protect against kainic acid-induced excitotoxicity and apoptosis via ROS-activated AMPK pathway in hippocampal neurons. *CNS Neurosci. Ther.* **2014**, *20*, 327–338. [CrossRef]
77. Lo, S.H.; Hsu, C.T.; Niu, H.S.; Niu, C.S.; Cheng, J.T.; Chen, Z.C. Ginsenoside Rh2 Improves Cardiac Fibrosis via PPARdelta-STAT3 Signaling in Type 1-Like Diabetic Rats. *Int. J. Mol. Sci.* **2017**, *18*, 1364. [CrossRef] [PubMed]
78. Wang, Z.P.; Shen, D.; Che, Y.; Jin, Y.G.; Wang, S.S.; Wu, Q.Q.; Zhou, H.; Meng, Y.Y.; Yuan, Y. Corosolic acid ameliorates cardiac hypertrophy via regulating autophagy. *Biosci. Rep.* **2019**, *39*, BSR20191860. [CrossRef] [PubMed]
79. Cheng, K.C.; Chang, W.T.; Li, Y.; Cheng, Y.Z.; Cheng, J.T.; Chen, Z.C. GW0742 activates peroxisome proliferator-activated receptor delta to reduce free radicals and alleviate cardiac hypertrophy induced by hyperglycemia in cultured H9c2 cells. *J. Cell Biochem.* **2018**, *119*, 9532–9542. [CrossRef] [PubMed]

pharmaceuticals

MDPI

Article

Application of Integrated Optical Density in Evaluating Insulin Expression in the Endocrine Pancreas During Chronic Ethanol Exposure and β-Carotene Supplementation: A Novel Approach Utilizing Artificial Intelligence

Cristian Sandoval [1,2,3,*], Luciano Canobbi [4], Álvaro Orrego [4], Camila Reyes [4], Felipe Venegas [4], Ángeles Vera [4], Francisco Torrens [5], Bélgica Vásquez [6,7], Karina Godoy [8], Mauricio Zamorano [2], José Caamaño [3] and Jorge Farías [2,*]

1 Escuela de Tecnología Médica, Facultad de Salud, Universidad Santo Tomás, Los Carreras 753, Osorno 5310431, Chile

2 Departamento de Ingeniería Química, Facultad de Ingeniería y Ciencias, Universidad de La Frontera, Temuco 4811230, Chile; mauricio.zamorano@ufrontera.cl

3 Departamento de Medicina Interna, Facultad de Medicina, Universidad de La Frontera, Temuco 4811230, Chile; jose.caamano@ufrontera.cl

4 Carrera de Tecnología Médica, Facultad de Medicina, Universidad de La Frontera, Temuco 4811230, Chile; l.canobbi01@ufromail.cl (L.C.); a.orrego03@ufromail.cl (Á.O.); c.reyes24@ufromail.cl (C.R.); f.venegas04@ufromail.cl (F.V.); a.vera08@ufromail.cl (Á.V.)

5 Institut Universitari de Ciència Molecular, Universitat de València, 46071 València, Spain; torrens@uv.es

6 Departamento de Ciencias Básicas, Facultad de Medicina, Universidad de La Frontera, Temuco 4811230, Chile; belgica.vasquez@ufrontera.cl

7 Centro de Excelencia en Estudios Morfológicos y Quirúrgicos (CEMyQ), Facultad de Medicina, Universidad de La Frontera, Temuco 4811230, Chile

8 Núcleo Científico y Tecnológico en Biorecursos (BIOREN), Universidad de La Frontera, Temuco 4811230, Chile; karina.godoy@ufrontera.cl

* Correspondence: cristian.sandoval@ufrontera.cl (C.S.); jorge.farias@ufrontera.cl (J.F.)

Abstract: Background: β-carotene is an essential antioxidant, providing protection against type 2 diabetes mellitus, cardiovascular illnesses, obesity, and metabolic syndrome. This study investigates the impact of β-carotene on biochemical parameters and pancreatic insulin expression in mice exposed to ethanol. Methods: Thirty-six C57BL/6 mice (*Mus musculus*) were divided into six groups: 1. C (control), 2. LA (3% alcohol dose), 3. MA (7% alcohol dose), 4. B (0.52 mg/kg body weight/day β-carotene), 5. LA+B (3% alcohol dose + 0.52 mg/kg body weight/day β-carotene), and 6. MA+B (7% alcohol dose plus 0.52 mg/kg body weight/day β-carotene). After 28 days, the animals were euthanized for serum and pancreatic tissue collection. Biochemical analysis and pancreatic insulin expression were performed. One-way ANOVA was used. Results: The B, LA+B, and MA+B groups improved insulin levels and decreased HOMA-β versus the C group, with the LA+B and MA+B groups also showing lower ADH and ALDH levels than their nonsupplemented counterparts ($p < 0.05$). The B, LA+B, and MA+B groups showed a greater β-cell mass area compared to the unsupplemented groups. Additionally, the LA+B and MA+B groups demonstrated significantly increased β-cell area and integrated optical density compared to the LA and MA groups, respectively ($p < 0.001$). Conclusions: In mice, β-cell loss led to increased glucose release due to decreased insulin levels. β-carotene appeared to mitigate ethanol's impact on these cells, resulting in reduced insulin degradation when integrated optical density was used. These findings suggest that antioxidant supplementation may be beneficial in treating ethanol-induced type 2 diabetes in animal models.

Keywords: alcohol intake; insulin; antioxidant treatment; chronic alcohol consumption

1. Introduction

Alcohol consumption poses a significant public health concern, with an estimated annual cost of EUR 155 billion attributed to related issues [1]. It is widely recognized as a major risk factor for both acute and chronic pancreatitis, contributing to approximately 50% to 80% of all documented cases [2]. Recent research highlights alcohol as the predominant factor responsible for pancreatitis in the United States [3].

However, studies indicate that less than 5% of individuals who chronically consume large amounts of alcohol are at risk of developing pancreatitis [4]. This discrepancy suggests that the development of alcohol-induced pancreatitis may require additional risk factors, influenced by genetic or environmental variables [5,6].

The complex and multifaceted effects of alcohol on the pancreas contribute to an incomplete understanding of the etiology of alcohol-induced pancreatitis. Alcohol is believed to damage pancreatic acinar cells, ductal epithelium, and stellate cells, potentially promoting pancreatic fibrosis [7,8]. Alcohol-induced pancreatitis is likely to develop only when compensatory mechanisms are exhausted or when other genetic or environmental stresses increase pancreatic vulnerability. Findings from animal models support this hypothesis, suggesting that the pancreas can mitigate alcohol-induced damage by initiating an adaptive stress response [9,10].

Pancreatic acinar cells metabolize alcohol through both oxidative and nonoxidative pathways [11–15]. The metabolic breakdown of alcohol in these cells generates toxic byproducts, including fatty acid ethyl esters (FAEEs), acetaldehyde, and reactive oxygen species (ROS), which contribute to cellular damage [11,16,17]. This oxidative stress destabilizes zymogen granules and lysosomes, as well as disrupts other organelle functions within the cell [4,11,18].

Chronic pancreatitis is marked by recurring abdominal pain and is frequently accompanied by symptoms such as nausea and weight loss [19]. Persistent pancreatic damage reduces the secretion of enzymes essential for digestion and fat absorption, leading to a progressive decline in digestive function. Additionally, the destruction of pancreatic β-cells, which produce, store, and release insulin, increases the risk of diabetes development [20].

Diabetes mellitus (DM) is a common chronic metabolic disorder characterized by elevated blood glucose levels, arising from either insufficient insulin production or impairments in insulin signaling [21,22]. As a growing global public health challenge, diabetes incidence is anticipated to rise significantly in the coming decades, driven in part by aging populations worldwide [23].

Both type 1 and type 2 diabetes (T2DM) involve pancreatic dysfunction, impairing the β-cells' capacity to meet increased insulin demands [24]. A family history of diabetes is widely recognized as a significant risk factor for developing T2DM and pre-diabetes [25–27].

Evidence suggests that β-carotene supplementation enhances GSH concentration by stimulating the activity of GSH synthetase. Previous research has shown that adding β-carotene can stop the loss of GSH caused by ethanol by raising the amount of GSH inside cells [28,29]. These studies indicate that it may be due to the stimulation of GSH synthetase activity caused by β-carotene. Therefore, β-carotene supplementation may serve as an effective approach to mitigate liver damage resulting from excessive alcohol consumption and to prevent the progression of alcoholic disease to more severe conditions [14].

Previous studies have shown that ethanol exposure induces oxidative stress and apoptosis, leading to tissue damage, while β-carotene supplementation (0.52 mg/kg BW/day) can alleviate ethanol-induced injury by reducing oxidative stress and inhibiting apoptosis in tissues [30]. Additional findings also report an increase in serum total amylase levels and a decrease in lipase levels in groups receiving 7% alcohol plus β-carotene supplementation compared to those without it [15]. Histological analysis further revealed that perilobular parenchyma, intralobular parenchyma, and fibrosis scores were lower in the 7% alcohol plus β-carotene group compared to the groups given 3% alcohol, 7% alcohol, or 3% alcohol plus β-carotene [15]. These findings suggest that antioxidant therapy could be beneficial in addressing the effects of ethanol exposure in animal models.

β-carotene, a member of the carotene family, is among the most prevalent carotenoids in food sources and is also present in the human body. About 17–45% of the consumed β-carotene remains intact in organisms, indicating its significant bioavailability, which refers to its effective absorption and utilization capacity [31]. Research indicates that β-carotene serves as a safeguard against several conditions, including type 2 diabetes mellitus (T2DM), cardiovascular disease, obesity, and metabolic syndrome (MetS) [32–34]. β-carotene is noted for its ability to enhance expression and secretion, which in turn improves insulin sensitivity [35].

The consumption of β-carotene is linked to several outcomes, including a decrease in the size of adipocytes and overall body adipose tissue; a decline in proinflammatory markers, low-density lipoprotein cholesterol (LDL-c), and very-low-density lipoprotein cholesterol (VLDL-c); and an increase in high-density lipoprotein cholesterol (HDL-c) [36–39]. Furthermore, they have the potential to enhance insulin resistance and maintain insulin receptors [37,39]. These actions take place to manage oxidative stress, which plays a role in all of the diseases mentioned [40].

β-carotene has the ability to modulate lipid and carbohydrate metabolism, thereby enhancing the function of pancreatic cells and improving hyperglycemic conditions. The regulation of β-pancreatic cell functions stimulates insulin secretion, regulates lipid metabolism, and alleviates oxidative and inflammatory stress [39,41,42].

The American Diabetes Association defines diabetes as a condition marked by the degeneration of insulin- and glucagon-producing cells. Histological examination reveals fibrosis, the shrinkage of pancreatic acini, chronic inflammation, the deformation of pancreatic ducts with narrowed regions, and damage to ß- and α-cells [14,15,43].

Thus, a comprehensive histological evaluation is essential. In particular, assessing insulin activity requires a multifaceted approach involving the analysis of serum biochemical markers alongside the measurement of insulin production in pancreatic islets [15]. This assessment may include evaluating the dimensions of the pancreatic islets or calculating their integrated optical density (IOD), with average values typically presented per cell [44,45]. The final evaluation involves staining the pancreatic islets with specific markers, such as immunohistochemistry staining, followed by image capture with a light microscope equipped with specialized optical filters. The IOD quantifies the light absorption across the entire pancreatic islet as captured in the images.

The cellular IOD serves as a quantitative metric. Previous research utilizing immunohistochemistry and Sirius Red staining on liver tissue observed significant increases in IOD levels following moderate alcohol consumption and carotene supplementation [14]. Additionally, IOD can be instrumental in identifying morphologically and functionally distinct cell subpopulations by maintaining consistent light contrast in imaging [14,45]. Consequently, the IOD analysis of cell dynamics may correlate with various pathophysiological states, offering valuable insights into disease processes.

Previous research has documented the effects of alcohol on the pancreas; however, the potential benefits of antioxidant supplementation during chronic ethanol exposure remain insufficiently understood. This study aimed to evaluate glucose and insulin serum levels, as well as insulin expression within the endocrine pancreas, in C57BL/6 mice subjected to ethanol exposure and/or β-carotene supplementation.

2. Results

2.1. Biochemistry

Table 1 presents the biochemical analyses of insulin, glucose, ADH, ALDH, HOMA-β, and HOMA-IR indices. The LA+B group showed significantly lower HOMA-β levels than the C, LA, MA, and B groups, while the MA+B group displayed reduced insulin and HOMA-β levels but higher glucose levels relative to the C group ($p < 0.05$). β-carotene supplementation improved the insulin levels and decreased HOMA-β versus the C group, with the LA+B and MA+B groups also showing lower ADH and ALDH levels than their nonsupplemented counterparts ($p < 0.05$).

Table 1. Biochemical evaluation of male C57BL/6 mice following ethanol consumption and β-carotene supplementation.

	Media ± SD						
	C (n = 6)	LA (n = 6)	MA (n = 6)	B (n = 6)	LA+B (n = 6)	MA+B (n = 6)	p
Insulin (µU/mL)	28.60 ± 5.45	16.44 ± 7.27 [a]	14.96 ± 5.01 [a]	24.27 ± 9.58 [abc]	11.34 ± 3.91 [ad]	9.46 ± 1.55 [acd]	<0.001
Glucose (mmol/L)	9.03 ± 0.53	13.45 ± 1.27 [a]	15.11 ± 0.45 [ab]	14.63 ± 0.84 [ab]	13.46 ± 0.43 [acd]	14.31 ± 0.86 [a]	<0.001
ADH (nmol/min/mL)	20.42 ± 2.52	33.03 ± 3.42 [a]	36.15 ± 2.74 [a]	23.22 ± 5.58 [bc]	26.09 ± 3.16 [abc]	29.83 ± 3.51 [acd]	<0.001
ALDH (pmol/min/mL)	11.81 ± 1.82	15.81 ± 1.62 [a]	17.04 ± 1.78 [a]	11.21 ± 1.30 [bc]	14.25 ± 1.67 [acd]	15.81 ± 1.77 [ad]	<0.001
HOMA-β	104.41 ± 21.30	33.34 ± 15.51 [a]	25.77 ± 6.77 [a]	43.53 ± 15.51 [a]	22.77 ± 7.38 [a]	17.61 ± 3.19 [ad]	<0.001
HOMA-IR	11.44 ± 1.49	9.83 ± 4.59	10.06 ± 2.76	15.84 ± 6.04	6.79 ± 2.21 [d]	6.01 ± 0.85 [d]	<0.001

[a] significant differences ($p < 0.05$) with the C group. [b] significant differences ($p < 0.05$) with the LA group. [c] significant differences ($p < 0.05$) with the MA group. [d] significant differences ($p < 0.05$) with the B group. Differences were analyzed by one-way ANOVA.

2.2. Immunohistochemistry

The immunohistochemical localization of insulin was observed in the endocrine pancreas across all the experimental groups (Figure 1). The histological analysis revealed variations in immunolabeling patterns and intensity among the groups. The C group exhibited a normal morphology of the beta-pancreatic islets, with the cells showing strong positive immunostaining (Figure 1A).

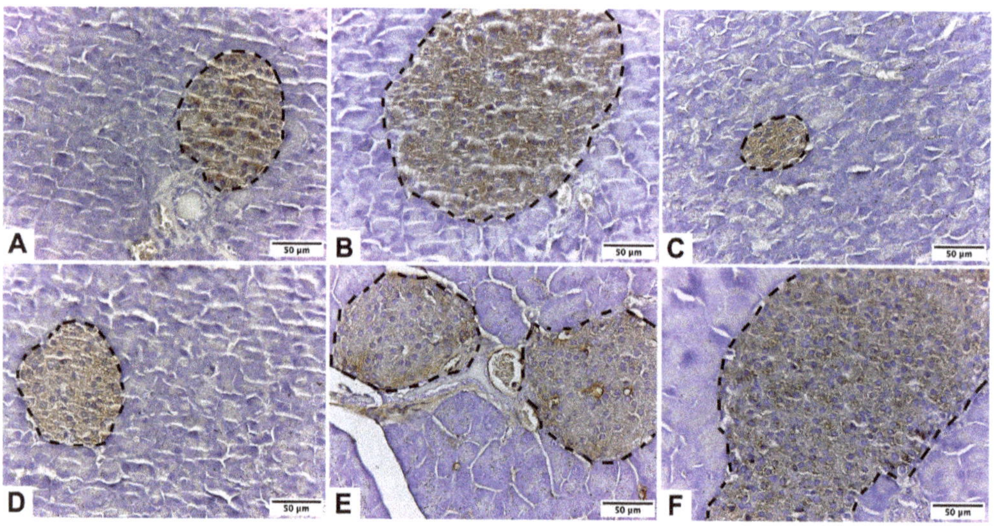

Figure 1. Pancreas of male C57BL/6 mice stained with anti-insulin IgG Guinea pig primary antibody. Insulin expression in the endocrine pancreas was observed in groups: control (**A**); low-dose alcohol (**B**); moderate-dose alcohol (**C**); β-carotene (**D**); low-dose alcohol + β-carotene (**E**); and moderate-dose alcohol + β-carotene (**F**). Pancreatic islets are in the segmented lines.

Figure 1D–F illustrate an association between β-carotene supplementation and an increase in both the number and size of the pancreatic islets. Notably, no insulin marker immunoreactivity was detected outside the beta-pancreatic islets or the endocrine pancreas. Among the groups, the MA+B group displayed the highest immunostaining intensity (Figure 1D).

2.3. *Area*

The groups supplemented with β-carotene (B, LA+B, and MA+B) exhibited at least a 30% increase in the β-cell mass area compared to those without β-carotene supplementation (C, LA, and MA) (Table 2). In ethanol-consuming mice (LA and MA vs. LA+B and MA+B, respectively), β-carotene supplementation led to a 30–50% restoration of the median β-cell mass relative to the C and MA+B groups ($p < 0.05$).

Table 2. Analysis of area and integrated optical density properties of β-cell in pancreatic islets of C57BL/6 mice.

	Media ± SD						
	C (n = 6)	LA (n = 6)	MA (n = 6)	B (n = 6)	LA+B (n = 6)	MA+B (n = 6)	*p*
Area (μm^2)	194.78 ± 38.30	270.44 ± 107.99 [a]	69.24 ± 22.61 [ab]	429.50 ± 246.77 [ac]	330.79 ± 117.64 [ac]	1028.27 ± 356.19 [ac]	<0.001
Integrated optical density (lum/μm^2)	26,006.67 ± 5063.97	35,661.82 ± 13,921.15 [a]	9722.07 ± 3049.34 [ab]	51,611.28 ± 29,343.24 [ac]	43,537.44 ± 15,480.09 [ac]	54,324.13 ± 29,600.55 [ac]	<0.001

[a] significant differences ($p < 0.05$) with the C group. [b] significant differences ($p < 0.05$) with the LA group. [c] significant differences ($p < 0.05$) with the MA group. A total of 144 pancreatic islets were evaluated, 24 pancreatic islets by group. Differences were analyzed by one-way ANOVA.

2.4. *Integrated Optical Density Analysis*

The immunohistochemistry analysis demonstrated the immunolabeling of β-cells throughout different regions of the beta-pancreatic islets in all the experimental groups. The concentration and intensity of insulin within the islets were higher in the groups supplemented with β-carotene (Table 2).

3. Discussion

3.1. *Summary of Key Findings and Interpretation*

Studies have shown a positive correlation between higher alcohol consumption and an increased incidence of T2DM [46]. In contrast, research also suggests that moderate alcohol intake may be linked to a reduced risk of T2DM [47]. Animal model studies investigating insulin production after ethanol exposure indicate that antioxidants can be effective in managing elevated blood glucose levels [14,48].

Although the specific mechanisms through which alcohol influences insulin remain unclear, numerous studies have identified a U-shaped or J-shaped relationship between alcohol consumption and insulin sensitivity or plasma insulin concentrations [49–52]. In individuals with T2DM, insulin production continues during the early stages of the disease; however, the body becomes resistant to insulin's effects, as reflected in our results. Initially, the pancreas compensates for this resistance by increasing insulin synthesis, but eventually, it reaches a threshold where it can no longer produce adequate insulin.

3.2. *Biochemistry*

The HOMA-IR is considered a straightforward, cost-effective, and trustworthy indicator of insulin resistance, whereas the HOMA-β index has been identified as an effective measure of β-cell function [53]. Our results show that the groups that regularly consumed low and moderate amounts of ethanol had a lower HOMA-IR index and better insulin sensitivity (Table 1), which is in line with what other researchers have found. Nonetheless, the HOMA-β index in the mice subjected to prolonged ethanol consumption varies from what has been previously stated.

Chronic alcoholics experience an increase in alcohol metabolism [54]. This is often regarded as a significant factor contributing to alcohol-induced injury [55]. The primary enzymes involved in alcohol metabolism include alcohol dehydrogenase (ADH), mitochondrial aldehyde dehydrogenase (ALDH), and cytochrome P450 2E1 (CYP2E1). The alcohol is broken down into acetaldehyde by ADH and then further converted into acetate by ALDH. Therefore, significant toxicity caused by ethanol may be linked to the functions of ADH and ALDH [56].

3.3. Immunohistochemistry

Immunocytochemistry is a highly effective and sensitive method for detecting insulin and assessing its expression levels in pancreatic islets [57]. In this study, immunohistochemical labeling proved to be a valuable tool for identifying and distinguishing insulin-expressing cells in the pancreatic islets of C57BL/6 mice. The results showed that the islets predominantly contain insulin-producing cells with a lobular shape, consistent with the findings from previous studies [58,59].

This study employed ethanol exposure to induce diabetes in C57BL/6 mice. In the male mice of this strain, ethanol administration leads to elevated blood glucose levels, indicating that ethanol exerts a cytotoxic effect on pancreatic β-cells, likely through the generation of free radicals. The resulting destruction of β-cells reduces or entirely depletes insulin, thereby causing hyperglycemia [60]. However, in the mice that received β-carotene supplementation alongside ethanol, there was a notable increase in both the number and size of pancreatic islets (Figure 1D–F). The MA+B group exhibited the highest immunostaining intensity among the groups, as shown in Figure 1D. These findings suggest that β-carotene, as an antioxidant, may reduce free radical presence and mitigate ethanol's cytotoxic effects on pancreatic cells.

3.4. Integrated Optical Density Analysis

Analyzing the mean gray value of each object within a digital image allows for the calculation of optical density (OD), a measurable parameter. Integrated optical density (IOD) represents the relationship between OD and a specific area of an image [61]. Pixel density quantifies the number of pixels per unit area, enabling an assessment of the object of interest relative to the image background. IOD facilitates the evaluation of immunohistochemical labeling by measuring color variations at the pixel level, which are then converted into numerical values to establish a quantifiable parameter.

In C57BL/6 mice, Table 2 presents the measured area and IOD characteristics of pancreatic islets. IOD properties varied across the experimental groups, with each group demonstrating statistically significant differences from the C group ($p < 0.05$). Notably, the β-cell mass area was larger in the β-carotene-supplemented groups (B, LA+B, and MA+B) compared to the unsupplemented groups (C, LA, and MA) (Table 2). Additionally, the β-carotene-supplemented groups showed elevated insulin concentration and potency in the islets, as displayed in Table 1.

Insulin resistance is defined as an inadequate response of tissues to insulin's action in the bloodstream and is widely recognized as a key indicator for the development of metabolic disorders such as T2DM and metabolic syndrome [62]. Previous studies have explored the relationship between carotenoid consumption and impaired glucose tolerance, finding an inverse linear correlation between the concentrations of β-carotene and lycopene and the level of glucose tolerance, as shown by glucose tolerance test results [59]. These findings suggest that carotenoids may improve insulin sensitivity. Studies by Facchini et al. and Sugiura et al. have shown that lower plasma carotenoid levels are associated with higher insulin resistance in healthy individuals [63,64].

In this study, insulin expression in the pancreatic islets varied among the groups. The LA group demonstrated increased β-cell area and IOD (270.44 ± 107.99 μm^2 and 35661.82 ± 13921.15 lum/μm^2, respectively) compared to the C group (194.78 ± 38.30 μm^2 and 26006.67 ± 5063.97 lum/μm^2, respectively), potentially indicating heightened insulin sensitivity ($p < 0.001$). Although no significant differences in the serum glucose levels were found between the LA and C groups using the same experimental models, the LA group exhibited lower serum insulin content relative to the C group [60].

When β-carotene was administered concurrently with ethanol (in the LA+B and MA+B groups), there was a significant increase in the β-cell area and IOD compared to the groups without the β-carotene supplementation (LA and MA), although no differences were observed in the serum insulin or glucose levels. This effect could be attributed to several potential mechanisms: (1) β-carotene may reduce ethanol-induced β-cell damage while increasing insulin sensitivity [11,12,16]; (2) β-carotene alone may enhance insulin sensitivity [52,65,66]; or (3) β-carotene could mitigate ethanol damage in β-cells while jointly enhancing insulin sensitivity with ethanol [11,12,16,52,65,66].

3.5. Limitations

Our data offer new insights into the relationship between alcohol-induced diabetes and antioxidant therapies, specifically β-carotene. However, this study has a limitation in that it does not examine the interactions between alcohol metabolism byproducts and other pancreatic hormones, such as glucagon, somatostatin, amylin, or pancreatic polypeptide, in the context of antioxidant treatments. Future research should, therefore, focus on investigating the effects of β-carotene in cultured pancreatic cells and identifying the specific molecules and signaling pathways involved. Nevertheless, our findings suggest that β-carotene exposure may mitigate ethanol-induced damage to β-cells and enhance insulin sensitivity, even during ethanol consumption.

4. Materials and Methods

4.1. Sample Size

The study was a comparative analysis of independent groups, with parameters set at an alpha of 0.10, beta of 0.05, standard deviation of 0.05, a minimum detectable difference between groups of 0.1, and an anticipated follow-up loss proportion of 0.2 [67–69]. The sample size calculation was conducted using the G*Power 3.1.9.7 Software (Heinrich-Heine-Universität Düsseldorf, Düsseldorf, Germany).

4.2. Animals

Thirty-six male C57BL/6 mice (*Mus musculus*), aged fifty days, were obtained from the Public Health Institute of Chile. They were housed in the Animal Facility at the Center of Excellence in Morphological and Surgical Studies (CEMyQ), Universidad de La Frontera, for 30 days to acclimate to their environment. During this period, the mice were provided with a standard laboratory diet (AIN-93M) and water ad libitum. Lighting conditions were maintained on a 12 h light/dark cycle from 08:00 to 20:00 and 20:00 to 08:00. Animal care followed the guidelines from the Institute for Laboratory Animal Research's Committee for the Update of the Guide for the Care and Use of Laboratory Animals [70].

On the first day of the experiment, the mice were divided into six groups (n = 6 per group):

Control group (Group C): No alcohol or β-carotene administration.

Low-dose alcohol group (Group LA): Administered 3% *v*/*v* alcohol ad libitum for 28 days based on studies suggesting low alcohol intake enhances insulin sensitivity [49,71–73].

Moderate-dose alcohol group (Group MA): Administered 7% *v*/*v* alcohol ad libitum for 28 days, as moderate intake is also linked to increased insulin sensitivity [49,71–73].

β-carotene group (Group B): Administered 0.52 mg/kg body weight/day β-carotene for 28 days, as this dose has been shown to mitigate alcohol-induced liver damage by reducing oxidative stress and inhibiting apoptosis [30].

Low-dose alcohol + β-carotene group (Group LA+B): Administered low-dose alcohol plus 0.52 mg/kg body weight/day β-carotene for 28 days.

Moderate-dose alcohol + β-carotene group (Group MA+B): Administered moderate-dose alcohol plus 0.52 mg/kg body weight/day β-carotene for 28 days. Figure 2 illustrates the experimental design.

Chronic ethanol was administered using a modified Lieber–DeCarli liquid diet [71,73], while β-carotene was provided orally at a dosage of 0.52 mg/kg body weight per day [15]. This experimental model has been previously applied in animal studies [14,15,18,60].

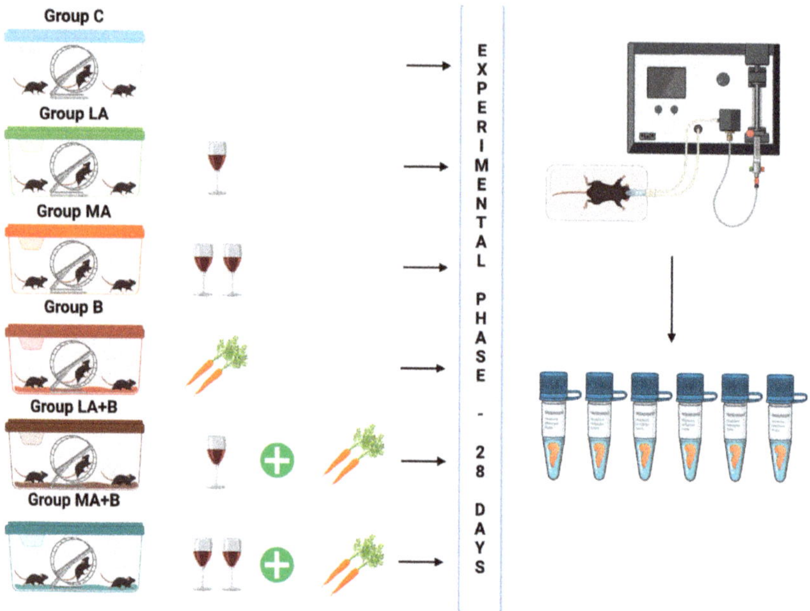

Figure 2. Summary of the experimental design of the study. In this schematic representation, one glass of wine corresponds to an administration of a 28-day 3% alcohol dose, and two glasses of wine correspond to an administration of a 28-day 7% alcohol dose. Also, the carrots correspond to an administration of 28-day 0.52 mg/kg body weight/day of β-carotene. After the experimental phase, the animals were euthanized and samples (the blood and tissues) were obtained.

4.3. Alcoholism and Treatments

A chronic plus single binge ethanol consumption (referred to as Lieber–DeCarli alcoholic diet) was used [71,74,75].

The ethanol groups were provided a liquid diet containing either 3% (LA or LA+B) or 7% (MA or MA+B) alcohol over a period of 28 days, while the control groups (C or B) were pair-fed an equivalent control diet for the same duration. On day 29, the mice in the ethanol groups were administered a single oral dose of ethanol (5 g/kg body weight, 20% ethanol), while the control groups received isocaloric dextrin maltose. Ethanol was sourced from Merck KGaA (107017, Darmstadt, Germany). The liquid diets were freshly prepared and administered daily [76].

β-carotene was administered in a dose of 0.52 mg/kg body weight/day (C9750, Sigma-Aldrich Co., St. Louis, MO, USA). β-carotene was diluted in water for the groups C, LA, MA, and B, whereas alcohol was used for the dissolution in the groups LA+B and MA+B. β-carotene was administered once a day by oral gavage (C9750, Sigma-Aldrich Co., St. Louis, MO, USA).

4.4. Euthanasia

On day 28, the animals were deprived of food for 6 h and then euthanized with sodium pentobarbital.

4.5. Biochemical Analyses

Centrifugation at 3500 rpm for 15 min separated the serum, which we then stored at −80 °C until analysis. In the biochemical analysis, we used a colorimetric kit (Sigma-Aldrich Co., St. Louis, MO, USA) to quantify the physiological concentration of glucose and a mouse-specific ELISA kit (Sigma-Aldrich Co., St. Louis, MO, USA) to measure insulin levels. The enzymatic activity of ADH and ALDH was assessed using the respective kit provided by Sigma-Aldrich Co. (St. Louis, MO, USA).

4.6. Homeostasis Model Assessment of β-Cell Function (HOMA-SS)

The HOMA-ß index was determined using Equation (1) [77]:

$$\frac{\left[20 \times \text{fasting insulin}\left(\frac{\text{uU}}{\text{mL}}\right)\right]}{\left[\text{fasting glucose}\left(\frac{\text{mmoL}}{\text{L}}\right) - 3.5\right]} \tag{1}$$

4.7. Homeostasis Model Assessment of Insulin Resistance (HOMA-IR)

The HOMA-IR index was determined using Equation (2) [78]:

$$\frac{\left[\text{fasting insulin}\left(\frac{\text{uU}}{\text{mL}}\right) \times \text{fasting glucose}\left(\frac{\text{mmoL}}{\text{L}}\right)\right]}{22.5} \tag{2}$$

4.8. Processing and Staining of Pancreas

To ensure random sampling, multiple sections were obtained from each pancreas, capitalizing on the tissue's isotropic characteristics. After a 48 h fixation in 4% buffered formalin (1.27 mol/L formaldehyde in 0.1 M phosphate buffer, pH 7.2; Sigma-Aldrich, St. Louis, MO, USA), the samples were dehydrated and embedded in Paraplast Plus (Sigma-Aldrich, St. Louis, MO, USA). Each block was sectioned into four groups, with 5 µm cuts spaced 120 µm apart using a microtome (Leica® RM2255, Leica Biosystems, Nussloch, Germany).

4.9. Immunohistochemistry

In summary, the paraffin sections were hydrated using a series of alcohols in decreasing concentrations following the standard procedure for traditional histological staining. Subsequently, they were immersed in distilled water for a duration of five minutes to restore their moisture content. Each histological section was washed in 1× PBS (Sigma-Aldrich Co., St. Louis, MO, USA) twice. They were treated with H_2O_2 (*v*/*v*) (ab64264, Abcam, Cambridge, UK) for 15 min to block the activity of endogenous peroxidase. Then, antigenic recovery was performed with HistoReveal (ab103720, Abcam, Cambridge, UK) for 10 min at room temperature. Next, each histological section was washed in 1× PBS three times. Then, the unspecific background was blocked using Protein Block (ab64207, Abcam, Cambridge, UK) for 15 min at room temperature. Each washing was performed with 1× PBS three times. First, the sections were incubated with anti-insulin IgG Guinea pig primary antibody (ab7842, Abcam, Cambridge, UK), dilution 1:50, in PBS overnight at 4 °C under a wet chamber. Second, each washing was performed with 1× PBS, four times. After washing with PBS, the sections were incubated with a biotinylated goat anti-polyvalent antibody (ab64207, Abcam, Cambridge, UK) for 10 min at room temperature in a wet chamber. Next, each wash was performed with 1× PBS four times. Then, the sections were incubated with streptavidin peroxidase (ab64207, Abcam, Cambridge, UK) for 10 min at room temperature. Afterward, each washing was performed with 1× PBS, four times. Finally, they were incubated with diaminobenzidine-peroxidase (ab64207, Abcam, Cambridge, UK) for visualization for ten minutes and washed with 1× PBS four times. The nuclear counterstain was performed with Harris hematoxylin (Sigma-Aldrich Co., St. Louis, MO, USA) for 50 s. The slides were dehydrated using a series of alcohols (Sigma-Aldrich Co., St. Louis, MO, USA) in increasing concentrations, following the standard procedure for traditional histological staining. A total of four pancreatic islets by slide were observed under a light microscope (Leica® LED750, Leica Biosystems, Nussloch, Germany) and photographed (Leica® ICC50W, Leica Biosystems, Nussloch, Germany). A total of 144 pancreatic islets were evaluated. For each immunohistochemical reaction, negative controls were used, which were incubated in PBS, omitting the primary antibody (ab7842, Abcam, Cambridge, UK). Table 3 shows the labeled process used for positive and negative control. The immunolabeling was quantified by the area (mm^2) occupied in each field, and the IOD analysis was expressed as lum/μm^2 [79]. Both measurements were made using the Image-ProPremier 9.1 software (Media Cybernetics, Warrendale, PA, USA). Figure 3 shows the positive and negative controls.

Table 3. Labeled process used for positive and negative controls to determine insulin in pancreatic islets of C57BL/6 mice.

	Block Peroxidase	Antigenic Recovery	Unspecific Background	Primary Antibody	Secondary Antibody	Labeled	Detection
Positive control (protein of interest)	H_2O_2	HistoReveal	Protein Block	Anti-insulin IgG guinea pig primary antibody	Biotinylated goat anti-polyvalent antibody	Streptavidin peroxidase	Diaminobenzidine-peroxidase
Negative control (without protein of interest)	H_2O_2	HistoReveal	Protein Block	Saline solution	Biotinylated goat anti-polyvalent antibody	Streptavidin peroxidase	Diaminobenzidine-peroxidase
Samples (pancreas cuts)	H_2O_2	HistoReveal	Protein Block	Anti-insulin IgG guinea pig primary antibody	Biotinylated goat anti-polyvalent antibody	Streptavidin peroxidase	Diaminobenzidine-peroxidase

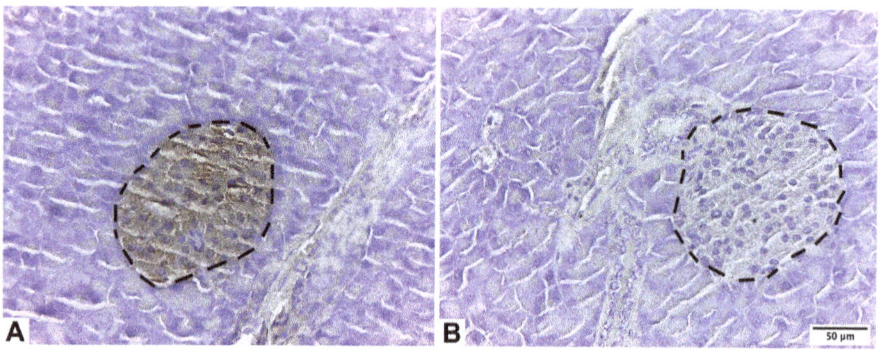

Figure 3. Exocrine pancreas of male C57BL/6 mice. Positive control for pancreatic islets stained with anti-insulin IgG Guinea pig primary antibody (**A**); negative control for pancreatic islets stained with primary antibody (anti-insulin IgG Guinea pig primary antibody was omitted) (**B**). Pancreatic islets are in segmented lines.

4.10. Statistical Analysis

Levene's test was applied to assess the homoscedasticity of variances, while the Kolmogorov–Smirnov test was used to evaluate data normality. These tests were conducted to assess disparities in the quantitative data. Group differences were analyzed using one-way ANOVA, followed by either Dunnett's T3 test or Tukey's post hoc HSD test, as appropriate. Statistical significance was determined at a *p*-value of less than 0.05 using IBM SPSS Statistics, Version 21 (IBM Corp., Armonk, NY, USA).

5. Conclusions

Insulin expression in pancreatic islets varied among the groups. In mice, β-cell loss led to increased glucose release due to decreased insulin levels. β-carotene appeared to mitigate ethanol's impact on these cells, resulting in reduced insulin degradation. In the pancreatic islets of the C57BL/6 mice, β-carotene exposure improved insulin sensitivity and lessened ethanol-induced β-cell damage. These findings suggest that antioxidant supplementation may be beneficial in treating ethanol-induced T2DM in animal models. Further research is necessary to better understand the interaction between alcohol consumption and antioxidant therapy, including studies using specific cell lines and clinical trials.

Author Contributions: C.S., B.V., K.G., J.C. and J.F. carried out the conception and design of the research. C.S., B.V., K.G. and J.F. have participated in the experimental phase. L.C., Á.O., C.R., F.V. and Á.V. carried out the immunohistochemistry and integrated optical density analysis. C.S., F.T. and K.G. performed the statistical analysis. C.S., L.C., Á.O., C.R., F.V., Á.V., F.T., B.V., K.G., M.Z., J.C. and J.F. wrote the original draft preparation. C.S., L.C., Á.O., C.R., F.V., Á.V., F.T., B.V., K.G., M.Z., J.C. and J.F. wrote the review and editing. C.S. and J.F. carried out the supervision and project administration. C.S., K.G., M.Z. and J.F. participated in obtaining funding. All authors have read and agreed to the published version of the manuscript.

Funding: This research was partially financed by Universidad de La Frontera, GI23-0021 Project; Universidad de La Frontera, DI22–0007 Project; and Universidad de La Frontera, PDT22-0001 Project and ANID, FONDECYT INI 11240623 Project.

Institutional Review Board Statement: The animal study protocol was approved by the Scientific Ethics Committee of the Universidad de La Frontera (N°034/22).

Informed Consent Statement: Not applicable.

Data Availability Statement: The original data presented in the study are openly available in FigShare at https://doi.org/10.6084/m9.figshare.27130587.v1 (accessed on 2 November 2024).

Acknowledgments: The authors thank SmartC-BIOREN (Service Management Analytical Research and Training Center), CCSS210005 Project, and Agencia Nacional de Investigación y Desarrollo de Chile (ANID). In addition, we would like to thank Isabela Pérez Núñez for her technical support to the Universidad de La Frontera, GI23-0021 Project.

Conflicts of Interest: The authors declare no conflicts of interest.

References

1. Anderson, P.; Dalziel, K.; Davies, E.; Fitzsimmons, D.; Hale, J.; Hughes, A.; Isaac, J.; Onishchenko, K.; Phillips, C.; Pockett, R. Survey of digestive health across Europe: Final report. Part 2: The economic impact and burden of digestive disorders. *United Eur. Gastroenterol. J.* **2014**, *2*, 544–546. [CrossRef] [PubMed]
2. Żorniak, M.; Beyer, G.; Mayerle, J. Risk Stratification and Early Conservative Treatment of Acute Pancreatitis. *Visc. Med.* **2019**, *35*, 82–89. [CrossRef] [PubMed]
3. Conwell, D.L.; Banks, P.A.; Sandhu, B.S.; Sherman, S.; Al-Kaade, S.; Gardner, T.B.; Anderson, M.A.; Wilcox, C.M.; Lewis, M.D.; Muniraj, T.; et al. Validation of Demographics, Etiology, and Risk Factors for Chronic Pancreatitis in the USA: A Report of the North American Pancreas Study (NAPS) Group. *Dig. Dis. Sci.* **2017**, *62*, 2133–2140. [CrossRef] [PubMed]
4. Lankisch, P.G.; Apte, M.; Banks, P.A. Acute pancreatitis. *Lancet* **2015**, *386*, 85–96. [CrossRef]
5. Whitcomb, D.C.; LaRusch, J.; Krasinskas, A.M.; Klei, L.; Smith, J.P.; Brand, R.E.; Neoptolemos, J.P.; Lerch, M.M.; Tector, M.; Sandhu, B.S.; et al. Alzheimer's Disease Genetics Consortium; Alkaade, S.; Amann, S.T.; Anderson, M.A.; Baillie, J.; et al. Alzheimer's Disease Genetics Consortium. Common genetic variants in the CLDN2 and PRSS1-PRSS2 loci alter risk for alcohol-related and sporadic pancreatitis. *Nat. Genet.* **2012**, *44*, 1349–1354. [CrossRef]
6. Pandol, S.J.; Lugea, A.; Mareninova, O.A.; Smoot, D.; Gorelick, F.S.; Gukovskaya, A.S.; Gukovsky, I. Investigating the pathobiology of alcoholic pancreatitis. *Alcohol Clin. Exp. Res.* **2011**, *35*, 830–837. [CrossRef]
7. Maléth, J.; Balázs, A.; Pallagi, P.; Balla, Z.; Kui, B.; Katona, M.; Judák, L.; Németh, I.; Kemény, L.V.; Rakonczay, Z., Jr.; et al. Alcohol disrupts levels and function of the cystic fibrosis transmembrane conductance regulator to promote development of pancreatitis. *Gastroenterology* **2015**, *148*, 427–439.e16. [CrossRef]
8. Apte, M.V.; Wilson, J.S.; Lugea, A.; Pandol, S.J. A starring role for stellate cells in the pancreatic cancer microenvironment. *Gastroenterology* **2013**, *144*, 1210–1219. [CrossRef]
9. Lugea, A.; Tischler, D.; Nguyen, J.; Gong, J.; Gukovsky, I.; French, S.W.; Gorelick, F.S.; Pandol, S.J. Adaptive unfolded protein response attenuates alcohol-induced pancreatic damage. *Gastroenterology* **2011**, *140*, 987–997. [CrossRef]
10. Lugea, A.; Waldron, R.T.; Pandol, S.J. Pancreatic adaptive responses in alcohol abuse: Role of the unfolded protein response. *Pancreatology* **2015**, *15* (Suppl 4), S1–S5. [CrossRef]
11. Sandoval, C.; Vásquez, B.; Mandarim-de-Lacerda, C.; del Sol, M. Ethanol intake and toxicity: In search of new treatments. *Int. J. Morphol.* **2017**, *35*, 942–949. [CrossRef]
12. Sandoval, C.; Vásquez, B.; Souza-Mello, V.; Mandarim-de-Lacerda, C.; del Sol, M. Role of Alcohol Consumption and Antioxidants on Global Methylation of DNA and Cancer. *Int. J. Morphol.* **2018**, *36*, 367–372. [CrossRef]

13. Wu, H.; Cai, P.; Clemens, D.L.; Jerrells, T.R.; Shakeel Ansari, G.A.; Kaphalia, B.S. Metabolic basis of ethanol-induced cytotoxicity in recombinant HepG2 Cells: Role of nonoxidative metabolism. *Toxicol. Appl. Pharmacol.* **2006**, *216*, 238–247. [CrossRef] [PubMed]
14. Sandoval, C.; Vásquez, B.; Souza-Mello, V.; Adeli, K.; Mandarim-de-Lacerda, C.; del Sol, M. Morphoquantitative effects of oral β-carotene supplementation on liver of C57BL/6 mice exposed to ethanol consumption. *Int. J. Clin. Exp. Pathol.* **2019**, *12*, 1713–1722. [PubMed]
15. Sandoval, C.; Vera, A.; Birditt, K.; Godoy, K.; Carmine, F.; Caamaño, J.; Farías, J. β-Carotene Supplementation Improves Pancreas Function during Moderate Ethanol Consumption: Initial Characterization from a Morphological Overview. *Int. J. Mol. Sci.* **2024**, *25*, 1219. [CrossRef]
16. Apte, M.V.; Wilson, J.S.; Korsten, M.A.; McCaughan, G.W.; Haber, P.S.; Pirola, R.C. Effects of ethanol and protein deficiency on pancreatic digestive and lysosomal enzymes. *Gut* **1995**, *36*, 287–293. [CrossRef]
17. Sandoval, C.; Farías, J.; Zamorano, M.; Herrera, C. Vitamin Supplements as a Nutritional Strategy against Chronic Alcohol Consumption? An Updated Review. *Antioxidants* **2022**, *11*, 564. [CrossRef]
18. Sandoval, C.; Mella, L.; Godoy, K.; Adeli, K.; Farías, J. β-Carotene Increases Activity of Cytochrome P450 2E1 during Ethanol Consumption. *Antioxidants* **2022**, *11*, 1033. [CrossRef]
19. National Institute of Diabetes and Digestive and Kidney Diseases. Symptoms and Causes of Pancreatitis. Available online: https://www.niddk.nih.gov/health-information/digestive-diseases/pancreatitis/symptoms-causes (accessed on 30 June 2024).
20. Kim, J.Y.; Lee, D.Y.; Lee, Y.J.; Park, K.J.; Kim, K.H.; Kim, J.W.; Kim, W.H. Chronic alcohol consumption potentiates the development of diabetes through pancreatic β-cell dysfunction. *World J. Biol. Chem.* **2015**, *6*, 1–15. [CrossRef]
21. Wagner, K.H.; Schwingshackl, L.; Draxler, A.; Franzke, B. Impact of Dietary and Lifestyle Interventions in Elderly or People Diagnosed with Diabetes, Metabolic Disorders, Cardiovascular Disease, Cancer and Micronutrient Deficiency on Micronuclei Frequency—A Systematic Review and Meta-analysis. *Mutat. Res.* **2021**, *787*, 108367. [CrossRef]
22. Roshanravan, N.; Askari, S.F.; Fazelian, S.; Ayati, M.H.; Namazi, N. The Roles of Quercetin in Diabetes Mellitus and Related Metabolic Disorders; Special Focus on the Modulation of Gut Microbiota: A Comprehensive Review. *Crit. Rev. Food Sci. Nutr.* **2021**, *63*, 2990–3003. [CrossRef] [PubMed]
23. Wang, X.; Yang, J.; Qiu, X.; Wen, Q.; Liu, M.; Zhou, D.; Chen, Q. Probiotics, Pre-biotics and Synbiotics in the Treatment of Pre-diabetes: A Systematic Review of Randomized Controlled Trials. *Front. Public Health.* **2021**, *9*, 645035. [CrossRef] [PubMed]
24. Marshall, D.C.; Holloway, M.; Korer, M.; Woodman, J.; Brackenridge, A.; Hussain, S. Do-It-Yourself Artificial Pancreas Systems in Type 1 Diabetes: Perspectives of Two Adult Users, A Caregiver and Three Physicians. *Diabetes Ther.* **2019**, *10*, 1553–1564. [CrossRef] [PubMed]
25. Hu, X.; Wen, J.; Yu, W.; Yang, L.; Pan, W.; Xu, K.; Chen, X.; Li, Q.; Chen, G.; Gu, X. Associations of Early-life Exposure to Famine with Abdominal Fat Accumulation are Independent of Family History of Diabetes and Physical Activity. *Br. J. Nutr.* **2021**, *125*, 943–950. [CrossRef]
26. Li, A.L.; Peng, Q.; Shao, Y.Q.; Fang, X.; Zhang, Y.Y. The Interaction on Hypertension Between Family History and Diabetes and Other Risk Factors. *Sci. Rep.* **2021**, *11*, 4716. [CrossRef]
27. Wu, J.; Zhou, Y.; Hu, H.; Yang, D.; Yang, F. Effects of β-carotene on glucose metabolism dysfunction in humans and type 2 diabetic rats. *Acta Mater. Medica* **2022**, *1*, 138–153. [CrossRef]
28. Lin, W.T.; Huang, C.C.; Lin, T.J.; Chen, J.R.; Shieh, M.J.; Peng, H.C.; Yang, S.C.; Huang, C.Y. Effects of beta- carotene on antioxidant status in rats with chronic alcohol consumption. *Cell Biochem. Funct.* **2009**, *27*, 344–350. [CrossRef]
29. Takeda, S.; Bando, N.; Yamanishi, R. Ingested β-carotene enhances glutathione level and up-regulates the activity of cysteine cathepsin in murine splenocytes. *Biosci. Biotechnol. Biochem.* **2008**, *72*, 1595–1600. [CrossRef]
30. Peng, H.C.; Chen, Y.L.; Yang, S.Y.; Ho, P.Y.; Yang, S.S.; Hu, J.T.; Yang, S.C. The antiapoptotic effects of different doses of β-carotene in chronic ethanol-fed rats. *Hepatobiliary Surg. Nutr.* **2013**, *2*, 132–141. [CrossRef]
31. Shete, V.; Quadro, L. Mammalian metabolism of β-carotene: Gaps in knowledge. *Nutrients* **2013**, *5*, 4849–4868. [CrossRef]
32. Mounien, L.; Tourniaire, F.; Landrier, J.F. Anti-obesity effect of carotenoid: Direct impact on adipose tissue and adipose tissue-driven indirect effects. *Nutrients* **2019**, *11*, 1562. [CrossRef] [PubMed]
33. Rodriguez-Concepcion, M.; Avalos, J.; Bonet, M.L.; Boronat, A.; Lourdes, G.G.; Hornero-Mendez, D.; Limon, M.C.; Meléndez-Martínez, A.J.; Olmedilla-Alonso, B.; Palou, A.; et al. A global perspective on carotenoids: Metabolism, biotechnology, and benefits for nutrition and health. *Prog. Lipid Res.* **2018**, *70*, 62–93. [CrossRef] [PubMed]
34. Perera, C.R.; Yen, G.M. Functional properties of carotenoids in human health. *Int. J. Food Prop.* **2007**, *10*, 201–230. [CrossRef]
35. Rühl, R.; Landrier, J.F. Dietary regulation of adiponectin by direct and indirect lipid activators of nuclear hormone receptors. *Mol. Nutr. Food Res.* **2016**, *60*, 175–184. [CrossRef] [PubMed]
36. Amengual, J.; Gouranton, E.; Helden, Y.G.J.; Hessel, S.; Ribot, J.; Kramer, E.; Kiec-Wilk, B.; Razny, U.; Lietz, A.; Wyss, A.; et al. Beta-carotene reduces body adiposity of mice via BCMO1. *PLoS ONE* **2011**, *6*, e20644. [CrossRef]
37. Beydoun, M.A.; Chen, X.; Jha, K.; Beydoun, H.A.; Zonderman, A.B.; Canas, J.A. Carotenoids, vitamin A, and their association with the metabolic syndrome: A systematic review and meta-analysis. *Nutr. Rev.* **2019**, *77*, 32–45. [CrossRef]
38. Canas, J.A.; Lochrie, A.; McGowan, A.G.; Hossain, J.; Schettino, C.; Balagopal, P.B. Effects of mixed carotenoids on adipokines and abdominal adiposity in children: A pilot study. *J. Clin. Endocrinol. Metab.* **2017**, *102*, 1983–1990. [CrossRef]

39. Asemi, Z.; Alizadeh, S.A.; Ahmad, K.; Goli, M.; Esmailzadeh, A. Effects of beta-carotene fortified symbiotic food on metabolic control of patients with type 2 diabetes mellitus: A double-blind randomized cross-over controlled clinical trial. *Clin. Nutr.* **2016**, *35*, 819–825. [CrossRef]
40. Kim, Y.; Kim, Y.K.; Lim, Y.; Oh, B.; Kim, J.Y.; Bouwman, J.; Kwon, O. Combination of diet quality score, plasma carotenoids, and lipid peroxidation to monitor oxidative stress. *Oxid. Med. Cell Longev.* **2018**, *2018*, 8601028. [CrossRef]
41. Sugiura, M.; Nakamura, M.; Ogawa, K.; Ikoma, Y.; Yano, M. High serum carotenoids associated with lower risk for the metabolic syndrome and its components among Japanese subjects: Mikkabi cohort study. *Br. J. Nutr.* **2015**, *114*, 1674–1682. [CrossRef]
42. Liu, J.; Shi, W.Q.; Cao, Y.; He, L.P.; Guan, K.; Ling, W.H.; Chen, Y.M. Higher serum carotenoid concentrations associated with a lower prevalence of the metabolic syndrome in middle-aged and elderly Chinese adults. *Br. J. Nutr.* **2014**, *112*, 2041–2048. [CrossRef] [PubMed]
43. Witt, H.; Apte, M.V.; Keim, V.; Wilson, J.S. Chronic pancreatitis: Challenges and advances in pathogenesis, genetics, diagnosis, and therapy. *Gastroenterology* **2007**, *132*, 1557–1573. [CrossRef] [PubMed]
44. He, Y.; Shi, B.; Zhao, X.; Sui, J. Sphingosine-1-phosphate induces islet β-cell proliferation and decreases cell apoptosis in high-fat diet/streptozotocin diabetic mice. *Exp Ther Med.* **2019**, *18*, 3415–3424. [CrossRef] [PubMed]
45. Zhang, S.; Wang, Y.; Cui, L.; Deng, Y.; Xu, S.; Yu, J.; Cichello, S.; Serrero, G.; Ying, Y.; Liu, P. Morphologically and Functionally Distinct Lipid Droplet Subpopulations. *Sci. Rep.* **2016**, *6*, 29539. [CrossRef]
46. Cullmann, M.; Hilding, A.; Ostenson, C.G. Alcohol consumption and risk of pre-diabetes and type 2 diabetes development in a swedish population. *Diabet. Med.* **2012**, *29*, 441–452. [CrossRef]
47. Carlsson, S.; Hammar, N.; Grill, V. Alcohol consumption and type 2 diabetes Meta-analysis of epidemiological studies indicates a U-shaped relationship. *Diabetologia* **2005**, *48*, 1051–1054. [CrossRef]
48. Sen, D.B.; Balaraman, R.; Sen, A.K.; Zanwar, A.S.; Greeshma, K.P.; Maheshwari, R.A. Anti-diabetic activity of herbal remedies. *J. Nat. Remedies* **2023**, *23*, 373–381. [CrossRef]
49. Kiechl, S.; Willeit, J.; Poewe, W.; Egger, G.; Oberhollenzer, F.; Muggeo, M.; Bonora, E. Insulin sensitivity and regular alcohol consumption: Large, prospective, cross sectional population study (Bruneck study). *BMJ* **1996**, *313*, 1040–1044. [CrossRef]
50. Lazarus, R.; Sparrow, D.; Weiss, S.T. Alcohol intake and insulin levels: The normative aging study. *Am. J. Epidemiol.* **1997**, *145*, 909–916. [CrossRef]
51. Villegas, R.; Salim, A.; O'Halloran, D.; Perry, I.J. Alcohol intake and insulin resistance. A cross-sectional study. *Nutr. Metab. Cardiovas. Dis.* **2004**, *14*, 233–240. [CrossRef]
52. Sandoval, C.; Herrera, C.; Schulz, M.; Vásquez, B. Relationship Between Ethanol Intake and Insulin Sensitivity Metabolism in Men with no Comorbidities: A Systematic Review. *Int. J. Morphol.* **2021**, *39*, 829–838. [CrossRef]
53. Wallace, T.M.; Levy, J.C.; Matthews, D.R. Use and abuse of HOMA modeling. *Diabetes Care* **2004**, *27*, 1487–1495. [CrossRef] [PubMed]
54. Lieber, C.; DeCarli, L. Hepatic microsomal ethanol-oxidizing system. *J. Biol. Chem.* **1970**, *245*, 2505–2512. [CrossRef] [PubMed]
55. Zakhari, S.; Li, T.K. Determinants of alcohol use and abuse: Impact of quantity and frequency patterns on liver disease. *Hepatology* **2007**, *46*, 2032–2039. [CrossRef] [PubMed]
56. Yoo, Y.; Jung, E.; Kang, H.; Choi, I.; Choi, K.; Jeung, E. The sap of *Acer okamotoanum* decreases serum alcohol levels after acute ethanol ingestion in rats. *Int. J. Mol. Med.* **2011**, *28*, 489–495. [CrossRef] [PubMed]
57. Edlund, H. Developmental biology of the pancreas. *Diabetes* **2001**, *50* (Suppl. 1), S5–S9. [CrossRef]
58. Steiner, D.J.; Kim, A.; Miller, K.; Hara, M. Pancreatic islet plasticity: Interspecies comparison of islet architecture and composition. *Islets* **2010**, *2*, 135–145. [CrossRef]
59. Hawkins, K.L.; Summers, B.A.; Kuhajda, F.P.; Smith, C.A. Immunocytochemistry of normal pancreatic islets and spontaneous islet cell tumors in dogs. *Vet. Pathol.* **1987**, *24*, 170–179. [CrossRef]
60. Sandoval, C.; Vásquez, B.; Vasconcellos, A.; Souza-Mello, V.; Adeli, K.; Mandarim-de-Lacerda, C.; del Sol, M. Oral supplementation of b-carotene benefits the hepatic structure and metabolism in mice exposed to chronic ethanol consumption. *Sains Malays.* **2022**, *51*, 285–296. [CrossRef]
61. Jafari, S.M.S.; Hunger, R.E. IHC Optical Density Score: A New Practical Method for Quantitative Immunohistochemistry Image Analysis. *Appl. Immunohistochem. Mol. Morphol.* **2017**, *25*, e12–e13. [CrossRef]
62. Sluijs, I.; Cadier, E.; Beulens, J.W.; van der A, D.L.; Spijkerman, A.M.; van der Schouw, Y.T. Dietary intake of carotenoids and risk of type 2 diabetes. *Nutr Metab Cardiovasc. Dis.* **2015**, *25*, 376–381. [CrossRef] [PubMed]
63. Facchini, F.S.; Humphreys, M.H.; DoNascimento, C.A.; Abbasi, F.; Reaven, G.M. Relation between insulin resistance and plasma concentrations of lipid hydroperoxides, carotenoids, and tocopherols. *Am. J. Clin. Nutr.* **2000**, *72*, 776–779. [CrossRef] [PubMed]
64. Sugiura, M.; Nakamura, M.; Ogawa, K.; Ikoma, Y.; Yano, M. High-serum carotenoids associated with lower risk for developing type 2 diabetes among Japanese subjects: Mikkabi cohort study. *BMJ Open Diabetes Res. Care.* **2015**, *3*, e000147. [CrossRef] [PubMed]
65. Roohbakhsh, A.; Karimi, G.; Iranshahi, M. Carotenoids in the treatment of diabetes mellitus and its complications: A mechanistic review. *Biomed. Pharmacother.* **2017**, *91*, 31–42. [CrossRef]
66. Marcelino, G.; Machate, D.J.; Freitas, K.C.; Hiane, P.A.; Maldonade, I.R.; Pott, A.; Asato, M.A.; Candido, C.J.; Guimarães, R.C.A. β-Carotene: Preventive Role for Type 2 Diabetes Mellitus and Obesity: A Review. *Molecules* **2020**, *25*, 5803. [CrossRef]
67. Duffau, G. Tamaño muestral en estudios biomédicos. *Rev. Chil. Ped.* **1999**, *70*, 314–324. [CrossRef]

68. Rojo Amigo, A. Cálculo del tamaño muestral en procedimientos de experimentación con animales. Valoración de las incidencias. *Anim. Lab.* **2014**, *62*, 31–33.
69. Bottaro, F. Cómo lidiar con la pérdida en el seguimiento. *Hematologia* **2016**, *20*, 133–137.
70. Committee for the Update of the Guide for the Care and Use of Laboratory Animals, Institute for Laboratory Animal Research, Division on Earth and Life Studies & National Research Council. *Guide for the Care and Use of Laboratory Animals*, 8th ed.; The National Academies Press: Washington, DC, USA, 2011.
71. Furuya, D.T.; Binsack, R.; Machado, U.F. Low ethanol consumption increases insulin sensitivity in Wistar rats. *Braz. J. Med. Biol. Res.* **2003**, *36*, 125–130. [CrossRef]
72. Klatsky, A.L.; Armstrong, M.A.; Friedman, G.D. Alcohol and mortality. *Ann. Intern. Med.* **1992**, *117*, 646–654. [CrossRef]
73. Doll, R.; Peto, R.; Hall, E.; Wheatley, K.; Gray, R. Mortality in relation to consumption of alcohol: 13 years' observations on male British doctors. *BMJ* **1994**, *309*, 911–918. [CrossRef] [PubMed]
74. Diao, Y.; Nie, J.; Tan, P.; Zhao, Y.; Zhao, T.; Tu, J.; Ji, H.; Cao, Y.; Wu, Z.; Liang, H.; et al. Long-term low-dose ethanol intake improves healthspan and resists high-fat diet-induced obesity in mice. *Aging* **2020**, *12*, 13128–13146. [CrossRef] [PubMed]
75. Ki, S.H.; Park, O.; Zheng, M.; Morales-Ibanez, O.; Kolls, J.K.; Bataller, R.; Gao, B. Interleukin-22 treatment ameliorates alcoholic liver injury in a murine model of chronic- binge ethanol feeding: Role of signal transducer and activator of transcription 3. *Hepatology* **2010**, *52*, 1291–1300. [CrossRef]
76. Choi, Y.; Abdelmegeed, M.A.; Song, B.J. Preventive effects of indole-3-carbinol against alcohol-induced liver injury in mice via antioxidant, anti-inflammatory, and anti-apoptotic mechanisms: Role of gut-liver-adipose tissue axis. *J. Nutr. Biochem.* **2018**, *55*, 12–25. [CrossRef] [PubMed]
77. Matthews, D.R.; Hosker, J.P.; Rudenski, A.S.; Naylor, B.A.; Treacher, D.F.; Turner, R.C. Homeostasis model assessment: Insulin resistance and β-cell function from fasting plasma glucose and insulin concentrations in man. *Diabetologia* **1985**, *28*, 412–419. [CrossRef]
78. Vogeser, M.; König, D.; Frey, I.; Predel, H.G.; Parhofer, K.G.; Berg, A. Fasting serum insulin and the homeostasis model of insulin resistance (HOMA-IR) in the monitoring of lifestyle interventions in obese persons. *Clin. Biochem.* **2007**, *40*, 964–968. [CrossRef]
79. Boschi, F.; Rizzatti, V.; Zoico, E.; Montanari, T.; Zamboni, M.; Sbarbati, A.; Colitti, M. Relationship between lipid droplets size and integrated optical density. *Eur. J. Histochem.* **2019**, *63*, 3017. [CrossRef]

pharmaceuticals

MDPI

Article

Adjunctive Therapy with Chinese Herbal Medicine Lowers Risk of Hearing Loss in Type 2 Diabetes Patients: Results from a Cohort-Based Case-Control Study

Hui-Ju Huang [1,†], Hanoch Livneh [2], Chieh-Tsung Yen [3,†], Ming-Chi Lu [4,5], Wei-Jen Chen [6,7,8,9,*] and Tzung-Yi Tsai [10,11,*]

1 Department of Nursing, Dalin Tzu Chi Hospital, Buddhist Tzu Chi Medical Foundation, Chiayi 62247, Taiwan
2 Rehabilitation Counseling Program, Portland State University, Portland, OR 97207-0751, USA
3 Department of Neurology, Dalin Tzu Chi Hospital, Buddhist Tzu Chi Medical Foundation, Chiayi 62247, Taiwan
4 School of Medicine, Tzu Chi University, Hualien 97004, Taiwan
5 Division of Allergy, Immunology and Rheumatology, Dalin Tzu Chi Hospital, Buddhist Tzu Chi Medical Foundation, Dalin Township, Chiayi 62247, Taiwan
6 Department of Chinese Medicine, Dalin Tzuchi Hospital, Buddhist Tzu Chi Medical Foundation, Chiayi 62247, Taiwan
7 Graduate Institute of Sports Science, National Taiwan Sport University, Taoyuan 333325, Taiwan
8 School of Post-Baccalaureate Chinese Medicine, Tzu Chi University, Hualien 97004, Taiwan
9 Center of Sports Medicine, Dalin Tzu Chi Hospital, Buddhist Tzu Chi Medical Foundation, Chiayi 62247, Taiwan
10 Department of Medical Research, Dalin Tzu Chi Hospital, Buddhist Tzu Chi Medical Foundation, Chiayi 62247, Taiwan
11 Department of Environmental and Occupational Health, College of Medicine, National Cheng Kung University, Tainan 70428, Taiwan
* Correspondence: tough2915@hotmail.com (W.-J.C.); dm732024@tzuchi.com.tw (T.-Y.T.); Tel.: +886-5-2648000-5003 (W.-J.C.); +886-5-2648000-3209 (T.-Y.T.); Fax: +886-5-2648006 (W.-J.C. & T.-Y.T.)
† These authors contributed equally to this work.

Abstract: Hearing loss is a frequently observed complication of type 2 diabetes (T2D). Emerging evidence has found that Chinese herbal medicine (CHM) can effectively treat chronic disease; nevertheless, it is unclear if adding CHM to the routine management of T2D would modify sequent risk of hearing loss. This cohort-based case-control study was conducted to address this issue. First, a total of 64,418 subjects aged 20–70 years, diagnosed with T2D between 2002 and 2011, were extracted from a nationwide health claims database. Among them, we identified 4516 cases of hearing loss after T2D by the end of 2013. They were then randomly matched to 9032 controls without hearing loss at a 1:2 ratio. Following conditional logistic regression, we found the addition of CHM to conventional care reduced the risk of developing hearing loss, with an adjusted odds ratio of 0.75 (95% confidence interval: 0.70–0.83). Specifically, taking CHM products for at least two years benefits T2D patients in lowering sequent risk of hearing loss. The findings herein implicated that integrating CHM into conventional care substantially correlated to lower risk of hearing loss for T2D patients, but further basic research is needed to secure the application of finished herbal products.

Keywords: type 2 diabetes; hearing loss; Chinese herbal medicine; cohort-based case-control study; risk

1. Introduction

Today, chronic illness has been regarded as a leading health-related challenge and is a major cause of both death and disability worldwide. For example, there are nearly 530 million people living with diabetes in 2021 worldwide, and approximately 96% of those cases are type 2 diabetes (T2D) [1]. These growing cases of diabetes place a substantial burden on health-care systems. One recent estimate by the International Diabetes

Federation (IDF) shows that present-day health expenditures for the care of diabetes was US$966 billion globally and is forecasted to reach more than US $1054 billion by 2045 [2]. On average, the per-capita healthcare costs for people with diagnosed with T2D is $19,736 US, nearly triple that of those without this condition [3].

Apart from the enormous economic burdens mentioned above, the intrinsic metabolic changes accompanying T2D might be responsible for a wide array of comorbid conditions commonly seen in T2D, including hearing loss. One recent study by Shafiepour and colleagues found that about two-thirds of adults with T2D experienced auditory dysfunction in ancient treatments [4]. Other research has found that people diagnosed with diabetes were more than twice as likely to suffer from hearing impairment as those without diabetes [5]. Hyperglycemia, which is the central cause of diabetes, may insidiously create chemical changes throughout the body that leads to neuronal damage. Reactive oxygen species (ROS) induced by hyperglycemia would lead to the activation of nuclear factor kappa beta (NF-κB) signaling by amplifying the function of caspase family [6,7]. At present, converging scientific consensus is that NF-κB activity is central to the inflammatory response. These include tumor necrosis factor-α (TNF-α), interleukin-1β (IL-1β), and IL-6 [8], all of which play a critical role in the pathogenesis of central auditory dysfunctions [9,10]. For diabetic patients, the concurrent hearing loss can impair speech communication and socialization and thus affect their mental health and quality of life. Notably, prior evidence revealed a positive correlation between hearing loss and suicidal thoughts [11]. With this in mind, adding complementary treatments or interventions to conventional treatment to prevent hearing loss driven by innate inflammatory milieu from hyperglycemia should be explored.

Currently, Chinese herbal medicine (CHM), a special therapy within traditional Chinese medicine, is widely employed in treating or preventing human disease. Several experimental studies have explored the underlying biological activities regulating inflammatory and oxidative stress. For example, one earlier model showed that usage of Bei-Mu correlated with the downregulation of nitric oxide (NO) and pro-inflammatory cytokines [12]. Some multi-herb formulae, like Ping-Wei-San and Ban-Xia-Xie-Xin-Tang, have been indicated to possess beneficial pharmacological activities that included immunostimulant and anti-inflammatory effects, and hence may have the potential as an adjuvant in the treatments for metabolic disorders [13,14]. Despite the reported progress, we still have failed to come up with an alternative therapeutic strategy for preventing or delaying the emergence of auditory dysfunction for those living with T2D. To bridge the gap in existing therapy, we embarked on this cohort-based, case-control study to determine if adding CHM to conventional treatment could reduce the risk of hearing loss in patients with T2D.

2. Results

A total of 13,548 subjects (4516 new cases of hearing cases and 9032 randomly matched controls) were included in the final data analysis (Figure 1). The mean age for both groups was 57.6 years and the mean follow-up period was 7.9 years. Throughout the study period, 29.5% of the cases and 35.2% of the controls ever received CHM treatments. On the whole, over half of enrollees were at the middle-income level and lived in cities. No significant baseline differences existed with regards to demographic data or comorbidities between the two groups. Details of the relevant variables at baseline are shown in Table 1.

Using conditional logistic regression, we observed that those who had a history of CHM use in addition to conventional treatment indeed exhibited a reduced risk of hearing loss in comparison to those who had never used CHM (adjusted OR = 0.75; 95% CI: 0.70–0.83). We also noted that the longer the duration of CHM treatment, the lower the hearing loss risk (Table 2). For example, patients using CHM for at least two years experienced a 42% risk reduction after adjusting for demographics and other clinical characteristics at baseline, implying an exposure–response inverse relationship between CHM use and hearing loss. Collectively, such therapeutic benefits of CHM were present regardless of age or sex (Table 3).

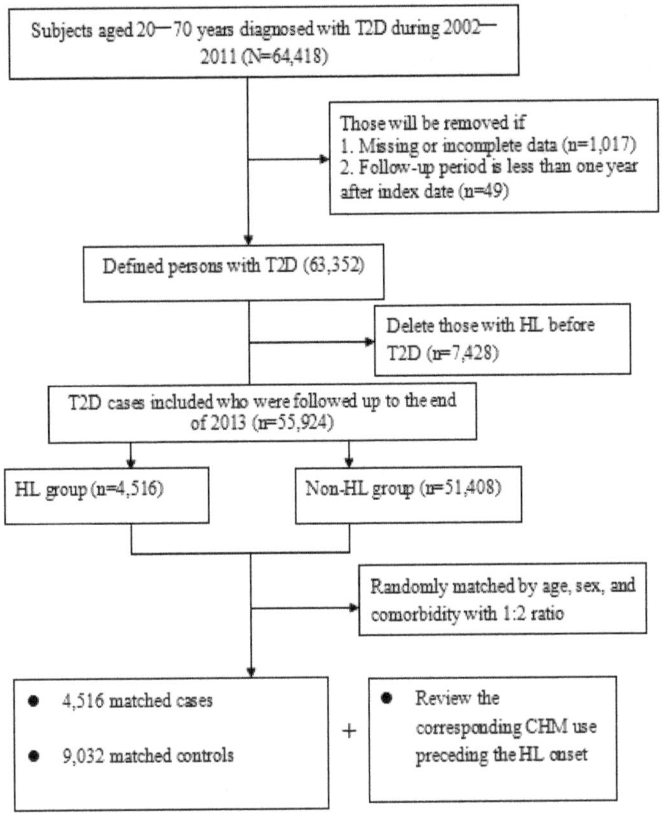

Figure 1. Flowchart of subject selection.

Table 1. Demographic data and selected comorbidities of the two study groups.

Variables	Number (%)	Cases n = 4516 (%)	Controls n = 9032 (%)	*p*
Age (years)				0.79
≤50	3052	1011 (22.4)	2041 (22.6)	
>50	10,496	3505 (77.6)	6991 (77.4)	
Mean (SD)	57.5	57.6 (9.0)	57.4 (7.3)	0.61
Sex				0.99
Female	6651 (49.1)	2217 (49.1)	4434 (49.1)	
Male	6897 (50.9)	2299 (50.9)	4598 (50.9)	
Monthly income				0.89
Low	5001 (36.9)	1655 (36.6)	3346 (37.0)	
Median	7710 (56.9)	2579 (57.1)	5131 (56.8)	
High	837 (6.2)	282 (6.2)	555 (6.1)	
Residential area				0.21
Urban	7834 (57.8)	2622 (58.1)	5212 (57.7)	
Suburban	2028 (15.0)	643 (14.2)	1385 (15.3)	
Rural	3686 (27.2)	1251 (27.7)	2435 (27.0)	
CCI	6.4 (8.1)	6.5 (8.1)	6.3 (8.2)	0.33

SD: standard deviation, CCI: Charlson–Deyo comorbidity index.

Table 2. The association between hearing loss and use of CHM treatment among T2D patients.

CHM Exposure	Patients				Crude OR (95% CI)	Adjusted OR * (95% CI)
	Cases n = 4516		Controls n = 9032			
Non-CHM Users	3184	70.5	5851	64.8	1	1
CHM users	1332	29.5	3181	35.2	0.76 (0.71–0.83)	0.75 (0.70–0.83)
Group 1 (31 days–1 year)	1138	25.2	2622	29.0	0.80 (0.74–0.87)	0.79 (0.73–0.86)
Group 2 (1–2 years)	123	2.7	348	3.9	0.65 (0.53–0.80)	0.64 (0.52–0.80)
Group 3 (more than 2 years)	71	1.6	211	2.3	0.60 (0.47–0.81)	0.58 (0.47–0.79)

* Adjusted for potential confounders including age, residential area, monthly income, and CCI. CHM: Chinese herbal medicine; OR: odds ratio.

Table 3. Risk of hearing loss among T2D patients with and without exposure to CHM use, stratified by age and sex.

Variables	Patients, n (%)	Crude OR (95% CI)	Adjusted OR (95% CI)
Female			
Non-CHM users	1515 (68.3)	1	1
CHM users	702 (31.7)	0.68 (0.62–0.76)	0.66 (0.60–0.74) *
Male			
Non-CHM users	1669 (72.6)	1	1
CHM users	630 (27.4)	0.86 (0.77–0.96)	0.86 (0.76–0.95) *
Aged $\leq$ 50 years			
Non-CHM users	685 (67.8)	1	1
CHM users	326 (32.2)	0.70 (0.60–0.83)	0.69 (0.58–0.81) †
Aged > 50 years			
Non-CHM users	2499 (71.3)	1	1
CHM users	1006 (28.7)	0.78 (0.71–0.85)	0.78 (0.72–0.84) †

* Adjusted for age, residential area, monthly income, and CCI. † Adjusted for sex, residential area, monthly income, and CCI. CHM: Chinese herbal medicine; OR: odds ratio; CI: confidence interval.

By utilizing the forest plot, we summarized the top ten most commonly prescribed single-herb and multi-herb formulae for the treatment of T2D, along with their associated OR against the risk of hearing loss. Out of these, a total of eleven CHM remedies were correlated to a lower likelihood of hearing loss: Bei-Mu, Ge-Gen, Yan-Hu-Suo, Dan-Shen, Hai-Piao-Xiao, Shao-Yao-Gan-Cao-Tang (SYGCT), Ban-Xia-Xie-Xin-Tang (BXXXT), Ping-Wei-San (PWS), Ji-Shen-Shen-Qi-Wan (JSSQW), Ge-Gen-Tang (GGT), and Xue-Fu-Zhu-Yu-Tang (XFZYT) (Figure 2). The relevant ingredients of herbs reported herein is elucidated on Table 4.

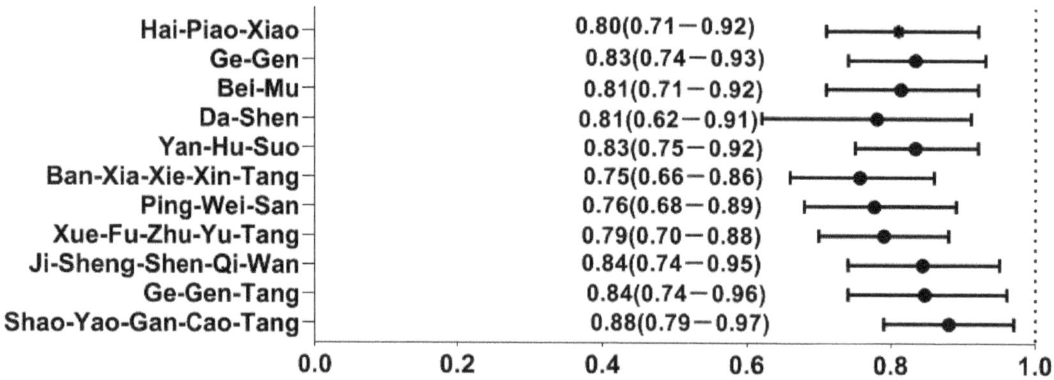

Figure 2. Hearing loss risk determined by multivariate conditional logistic regression across different herbal products. *Y*-axis: Chinese herbal medicines; *X*-axis: odds ratio.

Table 4. The ingredient herbs contained in the most-used single-herb and multi-herb products among T2D persons.

Chinese Herbal Product	Ingredients or Generic Name	Functional Classification
Single-herb products		
Yan-Hu-Suo	*Corydalis yanhusuo*	Used to treat Qi stagnation, blood stasis, chest pain, abdominal pain, amenorrhea, dysmenorrhea, and postpartum stasis
Da-Shen	*Salvia bowleyana*	Invigorates the blood and dispels stasis: for a wide variety of blood stasis disorders in any part of the body. Most commonly used for problems affecting the lower abdomen, chest, or hypochondria.
Tian-Hua-Fen	*Radix Trichosanthis*	Its functions are to clear lung heat, dissolve phlegm, relieve toxicity, and expel pus.
Bei-Mu	*Fritillariae Thunbergii Bulbus*	Eliminate phlegm by cooling, moisten lung to arrest cough, and remove stasis to reduce swelling
Ge-Gen	*Kudzu Root*	Acts to expel pathogenic factors in the muscles to clear heat, vent rashes and nourish the fluids to stop thirst. It also works to raise Yang-Qi and alleviate diarrhoea.
Huang-Qin	*Scutellaria baicalensis*	As an adjuvant therapy of inflammation, diabetes, hypertension, different kinds of cancer and virus related diseases.
Mai-Dong	*Ophiopogon Root*	Nourish yin deficiency, promote body fluid production, nourish the lungs, relieve the mind, and eliminate heart fire.
Shyuan-Shen	*Scrophularia ningpoensis*	Clearing away heat and cooling blood, nourishing Yin and reducing fire, detoxicating and resolving a mass.
Jie-Geng	*Radix Platycodi*	It supports respiratory health and benefits the throat. Jie Geng contains anti-inflammatory, anti-bacterial, expectorant and immune boosting properties.
Hai-Piao-Xiao	*Endoconcha Sepiae Os Sepiae seu Sepiellae*	Controlling acidity, harmonizing the stomach, and alleviating pain
Chuanniuxi	*Cyathula Root*	Activates blood, eliminates stasis. Strengthens tendons and bones. Promotes urination, treats dysuria.
Multi-herb products		
Shu-Jing-Huo-Xie-Tang	*Tang-kuei root, White peony root, Corydalis root, Chin-chiu, Cnidium root, Raw rehmannia root, Peach kernel, Hoelen fungus, Atractylodes root, Citrus peel, Notopterygium root, Fragrant angelica, Scabrous gentiana root, Fang feng root, Achyranthes root, Ginger root, Chinese licorice root*	Clears Heat, cools the blood, nourishes Yin and generates fluids. Breaks up blood stasis and invigorates blood circulation. Strongly dries dampness, tonifies the spleen, induces sweating and expels wind-aampness. Promotes urination and leaches out dampness.
Jia-Wei-Xiao-Yao-San	*Bupleurum Root, Chinese Angelica Root, White Peony Root, White Atractylodes Rhizome, Poria, Licorice Root, Moutan Bark, Gardenia Fruit, Mint Herb, Ginger*	To treat functional dyspepsia.
Shao-Yao-Gan-Cao-Tang	*Rx. Paeoniae Alba, Rx. Glycyrrhizae Preparata Paeonia lactiflora, Glycyrrhiza uralensis*	Antioxidative and antiaggregation effect
Liu-Wei-Di-Huang-Wan	*Rehmannia Root, Fructus Corni, Dioscorea Rhizome, Alisma Rhizome, Moutan cortex, Poria cocos.*	Liver and kidney yin dificiencies, soreness and weakness of the lower back and knees, dizziness, parched mouth and sore throat, heel pain. Enriches the yin and nourishes the kidneys.
Ge-Gen-Tang	*Puerariae radix (Pueraria lobata Ohwi), Ephedrae Herba (Ephedra sinica Stapf), Cinnamomi Ramulus (Cinnamomum cassia Blume), Paeoniae Radix (Paeonia lactiflora Pallas), Glycyrrhizae Radix preparata (Glycyrrhiza uralensis Fischer), Zingiberis Rhizoma (Zingiber officinale Roscoe), and Zizyphi Fructus (Ziziphus jujuba Mill. var. inermis Rehder)*	Induces sweating to release the exterior symptoms and dispel Wind-Cold. It is indicated for stiff neck, headache, muscle aches, alternating chills and fever, sneezing, cough, nasal congestion, runny nose.

Table 4. *Cont.*

Chinese Herbal Product	Ingredients or Generic Name	Functional Classification
Ji-Sheng-Shen-Qi-Wan	*Rehmannia Root, Fructus Corni, Dioscorea Rhizome, Alisma Rhizome, Moutan cortex, Poria cocos, Roasted Aconite, Cinnamon Bark, Achyranthes bidentata, Semen Plantaginis.*	Kidney yang deficiency, lower backache, urinary difficulties./Warms and tonifies kidney yang, regulates water and relieves edema.
Xiao-Qing-Long-Tang	*Herba Ephedrae, Rhizoma Zingiberis, Ramulus Cinnamomi, Radix et Rhizoma Asari, Rhizoma Pinellia, Fructus Schisandrae Chinensis, Radix et Rhizoma Glycyrrhizae, and Radix paeoniae alba.*	Used to treat bronchial asthma and allergic rhinitis.
Xue-Fu-Zhu-Yu-Tang	*Achyranthes bidentata Blume, Angelica sinensis Diels, radix, Citrus aurantium L., fructus, Bupleurum chinense DC., radix, Carthamus tinctorius L., flos, Glycyrrhiza uralensis Fisch., radix and rhizome, Ligusticum chuanxiong Hort., rhizome, Paeonia lactiflora Pall., radix, Prunus persica Stokes, semen, Platycodon grandifloras, A. DC., radix, Rehmannia glutinosa, Libosch., radix*	Invigorate Blood; Expel Blood Stasis; Move Qi; Stop Pain
Chuan-Xiong-Cha-Tiao-San	*Radix Chuanxiong, Herba Schizonepetae, Radix Saposhnikoviae, Rhizoma et Radix Notopterygii, Radix et Rhizoma Glycyrrhizae, Radix Angelicae Dahuricae, Herba Menthae, Radix et Rhizoma Asari*	Dispels wind and clears away heat. It is used for headache, migraine, or headache on the top, aversion to cold and fever, dizziness, nasal obstruction
Ping-Wei-San	*Atractylodes lancea rhizome, Magnolia officinalis bark, Citrus reticulata peel, Glycyrrhiza uralensis root, Zingiber officinale rhizome, Ziziphus jujuba fruit*	For gastroenteritis, intestinal obstruction, coronary artery disease and peptic ulcer
Ban-Xia-Xie-Xin-Tang	*Pinellia ternate, Makino, Panax ginseng, Zingiber officinale Roscoe, Coptis chinensis Franch., Scutellaria baicalensis Georgi, Ziziphus jujuba Mill.*	Treating metabolic diseases, such as nonalcohol fatty liver disease, diabetes mellitus, and obesity.

3. Discussion

Chronic hyperglycemia can cause auditory neuropathy associated with damaged blood vessels and nerves in the inner ear. Today, accumulating evidence shows that people with T2D have a higher risk of hearing loss compared to healthy controls [4,5]. Considering that there are currently no effective therapies for this condition, it is of great importance to understand the impact of CHM on the prevention of incident hearing loss in people with T2D. This cohort-based, case-control study found that T2D patients who receive CHM, combined with conventional care, had a 25% lower chance of developing hearing loss. Notably, a longer duration of CHM treatment was correlated with a remarkable decease in the risk of hearing loss. Despite a lack of comparable studies, the current results should enrich and expand prior literature that supports the benefit of CHM in treating chronic disease [15,16].

After stratification according to age and sex, we observed that females benefited more from CHM treatment than males. There may be several reasons why CHM treatment appeared to be more beneficial in females than in males for the prevention of hearing loss. First, an expanding body of evidence on gender differences concludes that females are more interested in health-related information and more likely to engage in healthy behaviors than males [17,18]. In this case, females may be more willing to follow the prescribed medication regimen as directed by their healthcare provider which, in turn, lowers the subsequent risk of adverse events. Additionally, the release of sex hormones, particularly estrogen, may partially explain this beneficial phenomenon. The female hormone estrogen has been shown to protect the inner ear by amplifying the expression of insulin-like growth factor 1 in the cochlea via the phosphatidylinositol 3′-kinase(*PI3K*)-*Akt* signaling pathway [19], which plays a crucial role in the survival and proliferation of neuronal cells [20].

Another focal contribution of this study was to identify the specific CHM constituents likely to be related to a lower risk of hearing risk in T2D patients. Of the commonly used single-herb products to treat T2D, the most beneficial effects were seen with Bei-Mu, Ge-Gen and Yan-Hu-Suo. The mechanisms with which these herbal products protected against the onset of hearing loss may primarily pertain to the modulation of inflammatory mediators. Based on former reports from the lipopolysaccharide (LPS)- stimulated RAW 264.7 cell model, these herbs were found to inhibit nitric oxide (NO) and regulate the production of proinflammatory cytokines, such as IL-1β, IL-6, and TNF-α, via the suppression of NF-κB activation [21,22], all of which are involved in the pathogenesis of central auditory dysfunction [9,10].

Additionally, both uses of Dan-Shen and Hai-Piao-Xiao were efficient in getting rid of the chance of hearing loss. Dan-Sen is a widely-used single-herb formulation for cardiovascular disease. Tanshinone, a major compound extracted from Dan-Shen, was discovered to possess antioxidant, anti-tumor, and immune-boosting properties by regulating NF-κB and the MAPK pathway in Neuro-2a cells [23]. Hai-Piao-Xiao, on the other hand, has been found to possess neuroprotective properties [24]. In a randomized control trial, a major ingredient of this herb, chitosan, contributed to peripheral sensory nerve regeneration through its profound antioxidant properties [25]. A late meta-analysis focusing on chitosan-injected mice models showed that chitosan exerted a substantial anti-inflammatory effect on active molecules, like TNF-α and IL-1β, via the NF-κB pathway [26]. The pharmacological effects derived from these single-herb formulae collectively might partially explain their beneficial effects on hearing loss in T2D patients.

Among the multi-herb products commonly used to treat T2D, we identified some herb formulae associated with a decreased risk of hearing. SYGCT, for example, has been shown to improve the decreased phosphorylation of glycogen synthase kinase (GSK)-3β among patients with chronic diseases [27]. Today, GSK-3β has been shown to play a role in the regulation of multiple cellular functions, like metabolism, cell motility, apoptosis, and proliferation of inner ear cells [28]. Recent evident found that the GSK-3β inhibitors CHIR99021 and bFGF had the greatest effect on the release of Lgr5-GFP progenitor, which plays a crucial role in the improvement of cochlear hair cell regeneration [29]. In addition, the reason that BXXXT and PWS were commonly prescribed among subjects included in this study is because diabetic patients often suffer from mild to severe gastrointestinal symptoms [30]. Notably, the pharmacological effects of BXXXT, including anti-emetic, anti-diarrheal, anti-oxidative, anti-inflammatory, and anti-lipidemic effects, have been illustrated in modern pharmacological studies [31], thereby lessening the risk of hearing loss at the same time. Furthermore, one former study using an animal experimental model found that the extract of Magnolia officinalis, a major ingredient purified from PWS, could regulate the production of inflammatory mediators through immunoregulatory phagocytosis via the MAPK signaling pathway [32,33]. All of these may point to the possible mechanisms for these herbs.

We also identified several herb products that may have potential for preventing hearing loss, like JSSQW, XFZYT, and GGT. All of these remedies have been shown to regulate cellular responses to inflammation, which in turn decrease the risk of auditory dysfunction after diabetes onset. Regarding JSSQW, it has been demonstrated to be beneficial in ameliorating insulin resistance via the NO pathway [34]. It is well known that an increase in the formation of free radicals, specifically NO, may be linked to necrotic cell death throughout the body [20]. Regarding the positive impact of XFZYT, as compared to untreated controls, rats fed with this herb were found to have notably reduced levels of inflammatory milieu through the inhibition of the PI3K-AKT-mTOR pathway [35]. Beyond that, this inflammasome signaling has been recognized as an important pathway in regulating autophagy and apoptosis in the inner ear cochlea [20]. Lastly, we found positive effects for GGT in preventing hearing loss among T2D patients. A recent review article outlined that puerarin, a major bioactive ingredient isolated from GGT, can significantly inhibit the expression of pro-inflammatory cytokines through the down-regulation of NF-κB/p65 activation and the inhibition of NF-κB activity [36]. The anti-inflammatory effects of these polyherbal formulations may explain the reduction in the development of hearing loss among subjects with T2D.

Despite being a pioneering work, some noteworthy limitations remain. First and foremost, this study was a retrospective analysis based on ICD-9-CM diagnosis codes. Misclassification *error may result in* biased estimates of model parameters. Nevertheless, NHI periodically reviews random charts to verify the accuracy of claims and medical charge data. We believe that misclassification of cases is always present in administrative database research, but this is expected to occur randomly, which in turn gives a conservative estimate of the overall proportion of null p-values. Second, as all data in this study were extracted from a claims-based database, several key factors, such as lifestyle behaviors, family history, and biochemical data, were not available for this study. Thus, residual confounding factors may partly bias the results. Third, information on T2D severity was not available from the database, as we cannot retrieve the relevant laboratory tests from the database. With this aim, we embarked on a sensitivity analysis in which we excluded T2D patients with some comorbidities at baseline, particularly the procedural codes for blindness, amputation, severe kidney failure, hyperglycemia, and hypoglycemia. Upon reanalysis, we still found a beneficial effect of CHM added to existing treatment against the onset of hearing loss, with an adjusted OR of 0.79 (95% CI: 0.72–0.89). Therefore, a bias introduced through diabetic severity is not likely to affect our conclusions. Notwithstanding these limitations, this work is reflective of a population-based investigation that evaluates the association of CHM use with hearing risk in T2D persons via a nationwide health claims database, thus leaving little room for non-response or loss to follow-up. Another strength of this work is the long observation period. With auditory disorder being a major contributor to disability and reduced quality of life, the claims database has the advantages of a 10-year observation period and a large sample size, both of which contributed to a better understanding of the links between diabetes, hearing loss and the effects of CHM. Lastly, the cohort study with a nested case-control approach is an excellent alternative to cohort analysis for determining the causal effects of treatment involved, especially when both treatment and confounding variables may vary over time and when time-varying confounding variables can be influenced by prior treatment or exposure. Hence, the merits of this study may be comparable to the pharmacoepidemiology approach that was carried out under controlled conditions with random allocation of interventions to the groups.

4. Materials and Methods

4.1. Data Source

All population-level data used in this cohort-based, case-control study was from the Longitudinal Health Insurance Database, which covers one million members randomly selected from National Health Insurance (NHI) in Taiwan [37]. With random extraction from all beneficiaries under the NHI program stratified by age and sex, this database was capable of providing a representative sample of the Taiwanese population. The database included encrypted patient data that documented sex, date of birth, medical diagnoses shown with the International Classification of Diseases, Ninth Revision, Clinical Modification (ICD-9-CM) codes, dates of hospital admission and discharge, medical procedures performed, and prescribed medications, including the use of Chinese herbal products. As the data used have been anonymized prior to being released to each researcher, the individual identifying information at any level cannot be obtained from the database. This work was approved by the facility's institutional review board (No. B10004021-3).

4.2. Underlying Cohort Establishment

For this study, we identified 64,418 subjects aged 20 to 70 years from the database and primarily focused on those who had ever sought relevant healthcare services due to T2D between 2002 and 2011 (ICD-9-CM code of 714.0). Patients were classified as T2D and included in the analysis if they had at least one admission code for diabetes or three or more outpatient codes within a 365-day period. The date of the first diagnosis of T2D was viewed as the cohort entry date. To adhere to established research procedures, patients with hearing loss before cohort entry, having been followed for less than one year, or having incomplete data were excluded (n = 8494). The remaining cases were followed up until the earliest occurrence of either hearing loss, death, or by 31 December 2013.

4.3. Ascertainment of Case and Control Groups

The primary outcome was the diagnosis of hearing loss that occurred after T2D onset between 2003 and 2013. Participants were defined as having hearing loss if they had ever received at least two outpatient clinic visits in one year or one hospitalization due to this condition during the study timeframe, as reflected in the use of ICD-9-CM codes 388.2, 388.4, 389.2, 389.9, 389.00, 389.10, or 389.12. The first medical visit of hearing loss was viewed as the index date. Afterwards, each case was randomly matched to two controls without hearing loss on the basis of age, sex, and comorbidities (Figure 1). An index date was assigned to each of these controls corresponding to the date of hearing loss diagnosis in the study group, thus ensuring the identical observational probability in all recruited subjects during the study period.

4.4. Identification of CHM Exposure

Recognition of CHM treatment exposure was based on personal medical records for Chinese medicine practitioners that occurred from the cohort entry to the preceding index date. In this study, CHM users were identified if they had ever received relevant CHM treatments for T2D or its relevant symptoms for more than 30 days. To meticulously assess the exposure–response impact of CHM in the prevention of hearing loss, CHM users were further split into three subgroups based on their prescription days within the study period.

4.5. Measurement of Covariates

Covariates in the statistical model included sex, age, prior medical comorbidities, individual monthly salary, and urbanization of residential area. We first estimated the premium payment category as a proxy of monthly salary, then transformed that to the 25th, 50th, and 75th percentile. In addition, one widely adopted urban–rural classification was used to classify the urbanization of enrollees' residence [38]. This indicator was based on several dimensions of urbanity, such as population density per square kilometer, proportion of persons with college or above educational levels, percentage of the population over 65 years old, proportion of employment in agriculture, and number of medical doctors per 100,000 inhabitants. Then, three groups were designated as urban, suburban, and rural. Medical comorbidities were defined as a condition leading to at least one inpatient visit or two outpatient visits within one year preceding the cohort entry date. The Charlson–Deyo comorbidity index, an approach that took into account both the number and severity of 17 pre-defined comorbid conditions, was used to quantify participants' disease burden from comorbidities [39].

4.6. Evaluation of Data

This study utilized SAS software for Windows Version 9.3 to perform the statistical analysis. Descriptive statistics, such as mean, standard deviation [1], frequency, and percentages, were applied as appropriate. Comparisons of demographic and clinical data between groups with or without CHM use were carried out using the student's *t*-test test for continuous variables or chi-square test for categorical variables, as appropriate. Afterwards, conditional logistic regression was used to calculate odds ratios [OR] with 95% confidence intervals (CI) for the association between CHM usage and subsequent hearing loss incidence. In this process, both crude OR based on a simple model with only use of CHM and adjusted OR for a full model with all the variables shown in Table 1 were presented to better understand how the adjustments affect the impact of CHM treatment. In the meantime, we attempted to outline the 10 most commonly prescribed formulae among the enrolled T2D patients. In all statistical tests, a p-value of 0.05 or lower was considered significant.

5. Conclusions

This is the first work to exploit the cohort-based case-control study to assess the impact of CHM use on the prevention of hearing loss amongst T2D patients. We found that integrating CHM into conventional treatment for diabetes would get rid of the subsequent risk of developing hearing loss by 25%. Furthermore, this therapeutic effect appears to be dose-dependent, with more intensive CHM treatment further reducing the risk for hearing loss. Based on the belief "prevention in itself is preferable to cure", our study suggests that the integration of CHM into routine care of underactive diabetes mellitus may allow for early prevention of hearing loss. At the same time, these encouraging findings provide an impetus for further research that focuses on the adoption of CHM products, as well as in vivo studies, to explore the beneficial mechanisms of CHM in the treatment of chronic, life-changing diseases. Given the high and rising prevalence of hearing loss among T2D groups, for healthcare providers the urgent need to routinely screen for hearing dysfunction and institute complementary therapy for diabetic disease management should be highlighted.

Author Contributions: H.-J.H., H.L. and C.-T.Y. contributed equally to this work. H.-J.H., H.L., C.-T.Y. and T.-Y.T. were involved in the study design and drafted the manuscript; H.L. and T.-Y.T. contributed to data analysis and revised the manuscript; C.-T.Y., H.L., H.-J.H., W.-J.C. and T.-Y.T. contributed to the interpretation of data and provided comments on the final draft of the manuscript; M.-C.L. provided administrative support and draft revisions. All authors have read and agreed to the published version of the manuscript.

Funding: This work did not receive any funding.

Institutional Review Board Statement: This work was approved by the facility's institutional review board (No. B10004021-3).

Informed Consent Statement: Not applicable.

Data Availability Statement: All of the analytical data were retrieved from the National Health Insurance Research Database provided by the Bureau of National Health Insurance, managed by the Department of Health and Welfare, Taiwan. Because of restrictions imposed by the law of "Personal Information Protection Act", the relevant data cannot be publicly obtained. Requisition for usage of datasets should be directed to the Bureau of National Health Insurance and the corresponding author.

Conflicts of Interest: The authors declare that they have no conflicting interests.

References

1. Ong, K.L.; Stafford, L.K.; McLaughlin, S.A.; Boyko, E.J.; Vollset, S.E.; Smith, A.E.; Dalton, B.E.; Duprey, J.; Cruz, J.A.; Hagins, H.; et al. Global, regional, and national burden of diabetes from 1990 to 2021, with projections of prevalence to 2050: A systematic analysis for the Global Burden of Disease Study 2021. *Lancet* **2023**, *402*, 203–234. [CrossRef] [PubMed]
2. Sun, H.; Saeedi, P.; Karuranga, S.; Pinkepank, M.; Ogurtsova, K.; Duncan, B.B.; Stein, C.; Basit, A.; Chan, J.C.N.; Mbanya, J.C.; et al. IDF Diabetes Atlas: Global, regional and country-level diabetes prevalence estimates for 2021 and projections for 2045. *Diabetes Res. Clin. Pract.* **2022**, *183*, 109119. [CrossRef] [PubMed]
3. Parker, E.D.; Lin, J.; Mahoney, T.; Ume, N.; Yang, G.; Gabbay, R.A.; ElSayed, N.A.; Bannuru, R.R. Economic Costs of Diabetes in the U.S. in 2022. *Diabetes Care* **2023**, *47*, 26–43. [CrossRef] [PubMed]
4. Shafiepour, M.; Bamdad, Z.; Radman, M. Prevalence of hearing loss among patients with type 2 diabetes. *J. Med. Life* **2022**, *15*, 772–777. [CrossRef] [PubMed]
5. Horikawa, C.; Kodama, S.; Tanaka, S.; Fujihara, K.; Hirasawa, R.; Yachi, Y.; Shimano, H.; Yamada, N.; Saito, K.; Sone, H. Diabetes and risk of hearing impairment in adults: A meta-analysis. *J. Clin. Endocrinol. Metab.* **2013**, *98*, 51–58. [CrossRef]
6. Sun, J.; Singh, P.; Österlund, J.; Orho-Melander, M.; Melander, O.; Engström, G.; Edsfeldt, A. Hyperglycaemia-associated Caspase-3 predicts diabetes and coronary artery disease events. *J. Intern. Med.* **2021**, *290*, 855–865. [CrossRef]
7. Bhatti, J.S.; Sehrawat, A.; Mishra, J.; Sidhu, I.S.; Navik, U.; Khullar, N.; Kumar, S.; Bhatti, G.K.; Reddy, P.H. Oxidative stress in the pathophysiology of type 2 diabetes and related complications: Current therapeutics strategies and future perspectives. *Free Radic. Biol. Med.* **2022**, *184*, 114–134. [CrossRef]
8. Liu, T.; Zhang, L.; Joo, D.; Sun, S.-C. NF-κB signaling in inflammation. *Signal Transduct. Target Ther.* **2017**, *2*, 17023. [CrossRef]

9. Samaha, N.L.; Almasri, M.M.; Johns, J.D.; Hoa, M. Hearing restoration and the stria vascularis: Evidence for the role of the immune system in hearing restoration. *Curr. Opin. Otolaryngol. Head Neck Surg.* **2021**, *29*, 373–384. [CrossRef]
10. Watson, N.; Ding, B.; Zhu, X.; Frisina, R.D. Chronic inflammation–inflammaging–in the ageing cochlea: A novel target for future presbycusis therapy. *Ageing Res. Rev.* **2017**, *40*, 142–148. [CrossRef]
11. Ahn, J.H.; Yang, J.S.; Jung, J.; Kang, S.; Jung, S.J. Association between hearing loss and suicidal ideation: Discrepancy between pure tone audiometry and subjective hearing level. *J. Affect. Disord.* **2024**, *344*, 495–502. [CrossRef] [PubMed]
12. Li, H.; Hung, A.; Li, M.; Yang, A.W.H. Fritillariae thunbergii bulbus: Traditional uses, phytochemistry, pharmacodynamics, pharmacokinetics and toxicity. *Int. J. Mol. Sci.* **2019**, *20*, 1667. [CrossRef] [PubMed]
13. Li, D.; You, H.J.; Hu, G.J.; Yao, R.Y.; Xie, A.M.; Li, X.Y. Mechanisms of the Ping-wei-san plus herbal decoction against Parkinson's disease: Multiomics analyses. *Front. Nutr.* **2022**, *9*, 945356. [CrossRef] [PubMed]
14. Xia, Q.S.; Gao, Y.; Wen-Bin, W.; Wu, F.; Dong, H.; Xu, L.J.; Fang, K.; Hu, M.L.; Yuan, F.; Lu, F.E.; et al. Ban-xia-xie-xin-tang ameliorates hepatic steatosis by regulating Cidea and Cidec expression in HFD-fed mice. *Phytomedicine* **2022**, *105*, 154351. [CrossRef] [PubMed]
15. Tran, N.; Pham, B.; Le, L. Bioactive compounds in anti-Diabetic plants: From herbal medicine to modern drug discovery. *Biology* **2020**, *9*, 252. [CrossRef]
16. Yen, C.-T.; Livneh, H.; Huang, H.-L.; Lu, M.-C.; Chen, W.-J.; Tsai, T.-Y. Decreased risk of osteoporosis incident in subjects receiving Chinese herbal medicine for Sjögren syndrome treatment: A retrospective cohort study with a nested case-control analysis. *Pharmaceuticals* **2024**, *17*, 745. [CrossRef]
17. Shih, C.C.; Liao, C.C.; Su, Y.C.; Tsai, C.C.; Lin, J.G. Gender differences in traditional Chinese medicine use among adults in Taiwan. *PLoS ONE* **2012**, *7*, e32540. [CrossRef]
18. Aljefree, N.M.; Almoraie, N.M.; Althaiban, M.A.; Hanbazaza, M.A.; Wazzan, H.A.; Shatwan, I.M. Gender differences in knowledge, attitudes, and practices with respect to type 1 diabetes among Saudi public-school teachers. *BMC Public Health* **2023**, *23*, 118. [CrossRef]
19. Williamson, T.T.; Ding, B.; Zhu, X.; Frisina, R.D. Hormone replacement therapy attenuates hearing loss: Mechanisms involving estrogen and the IGF-1 pathway. *Aging Cell* **2019**, *18*, e12939. [CrossRef]
20. Khalin, I.; Alyautdin, R.; Kocherga, G.; Bakar, M.A. Targeted delivery of brain-derived neurotrophic factor for the treatment of blindness and deafness. *Int. J. Nanomed.* **2015**, *10*, 3245–3267. [CrossRef]
21. Eldufani, J.; Blaise, G. The role of acetylcholinesterase inhibitors such as neostigmine and rivastigmine on chronic pain and cognitive function in aging: A review of recent clinical applications. *Alzheimers Dement* **2019**, *5*, 175–183. [CrossRef] [PubMed]
22. Kim, J.H.; Kim, M.; Hong, S.; Kwon, B.; Song, M.W.; Song, K.; Kim, E.Y.; Jung, H.S.; Sohn, Y. Anti-inflammatory effects of Fritillaria thunbergii Miquel extracts in LPS-stimulated murine macrophage RAW 264.7 cells. *Exp. Ther. Med.* **2021**, *21*, 429. [CrossRef] [PubMed]
23. Hung, Y.C.; Pan, T.L.; Hu, W.L. Roles of reactive oxygen Species in anticancer therapy with salvia miltiorrhiza bunge. *Oxid. Med. Cell. Longev.* **2016**, *2016*, 5293284. [CrossRef] [PubMed]
24. Lin, S.K.; Tsai, Y.T.; Lai, J.N.; Wu, C.T. Demographic and medication characteristics of traditional Chinese medicine users among dementia patients in Taiwan: A nationwide database study. *J. Ethnopharmacol.* **2015**, *161*, 108–115. [CrossRef] [PubMed]
25. Neubrech, F.; Sauerbier, M.; Moll, W.; Seegmüller, J.; Heider, S.; Harhaus, L.; Bickert, B.; Kneser, U.; Kremer, T. Enhancing the outcome of traumatic sensory nerve lesions of the hand by additional use of a chitosan nerve tube in primary nerve repair: A randomized controlled bicentric trial. *Plast. Reconstr. Surg.* **2018**, *142*, 415–424. [CrossRef]
26. Ahn, S.-I.; Cho, S.; Choi, N.-J. Effectiveness of chitosan as a dietary supplement in lowering cholesterol in murine models: A meta-analysis. *Mar. Drugs* **2021**, *19*, 26. [CrossRef]
27. Tsai, F.J.; Ho, T.J.; Cheng, C.F.; Shiao, Y.T.; Chien, W.K.; Chen, J.H.; Liu, X.; Tsang, H.; Lin, T.H.; Liao, C.C.; et al. Characteristics of Chinese herbal medicine usage in ischemic heart disease patients among type 2 diabetes and their protection against hydrogen peroxide-mediated apoptosis in H9C2 cardiomyoblasts. *Oncotarget* **2017**, *8*, 15470–15489. [CrossRef]
28. Driver, E.C.; Kelley, M.W. Development of the cochlea. *Development* **2020**, *147*, dev162263. [CrossRef]
29. Shi, F.; Hu, L.; Jacques, B.E.; Mulvaney, J.F.; Dabdoub, A.; Edge, A.S.B. β-Catenin is required for hair-cell differentiation in the cochlea. *J. Neurosci.* **2014**, *34*, 6470–6479. [CrossRef]
30. Bonetto, S.; Gruden, G.; Beccuti, G.; Ferro, A.; Saracco, G.M.; Pellicano, R. Management of dyspepsia and gastroparesis in patients with diabetes. a clinical point of view in the year 2021. *J. Clin. Med.* **2021**, *10*, 1313. [CrossRef]
31. Kim, K.; Ko, S.J.; Cho, S.H.; Kim, J.; Park, J.W. Herbal medicine, Banxia-xiexin tang, for functional dyspepsia: A systematic review and meta-analysis. *Front. Pharmacol.* **2023**, *14*, 1130257. [CrossRef] [PubMed]
32. Chen, H.; Fu, W.; Chen, H.; You, S.; Liu, X.; Yang, Y.; Wei, Y.; Huang, J.; Rui, W. Magnolol attenuates the inflammation and enhances phagocytosis through the activation of MAPK, NF-κB signal pathways in vitro and in vivo. *Mol. Immunol.* **2019**, *105*, 96–106. [CrossRef] [PubMed]
33. Zhang, Z.; Shen, P.; Xie, W.; Cao, H.; Liu, J.; Cao, Y.; Zhang, N. Pingwei san ameliorates dextran sulfate sodium-induced chronic colitis in mice. *J. Ethnopharmacol.* **2019**, *236*, 91–99. [CrossRef] [PubMed]
34. Hu, X.; Sato, J.; Bajotto, G.; Khookhor, O.; Ohsawa, I.; Oshida, Y.; Sato, Y. Goshajinkigan (Chinese herbal medicine niu-che-sen-qi-wan) improves insulin resistance in diabetic rats via the nitric oxide pathway. *Nagoya J. Med. Sci.* **2010**, *72*, 35–42. [PubMed]

35. Xing, Z.; Xia, Z.; Peng, W.; Li, J.; Zhang, C.; Fu, C.; Tang, T.; Luo, J.; Zou, Y.; Fan, R.; et al. Xuefu Zhuyu decoction, a traditional Chinese medicine, provides neuroprotection in a rat model of traumatic brain injury via an anti-inflammatory pathway. *Sci. Rep.* **2016**, *6*, 20040. [CrossRef]
36. Che, C.T.; Wong, M.S.; Lam, C.W. Natural products from Chinese medicines with potential benefits to bone health. *Molecules* **2016**, *21*, 239. [CrossRef] [PubMed]
37. National Health Insurance Database, Taiwan. LHID 2000. Available online: https://dep.mohw.gov.tw/DOS/cp-5119-59201-113.html (accessed on 30 July 2024).
38. Liu, C.Y.; Hung, Y.T.; Chuang, Y.L.; Chen, Y.J.; Weng, W.S.; Liu, J.S.; Liang, K.Y. Incorporating development stratification of Taiwan townships into sampling design of large scale health interview survey (in Chinese). *J. Health Manag.* **2006**, *4*, 1–22. [CrossRef]
39. Deyo, R.A.; Cherkin, D.C.; Ciol, M.A. Adapting a clinical comorbidity index for use with ICD-9-CM administrative databases. *J. Clin. Epidemiol.* **1992**, *45*, 613–619. [CrossRef]

pharmaceuticals

MDPI

Review

Insights into the Therapeutic Use of *Kalanchoe pinnata* Supplement in Diabetes Mellitus

Felix Omoruyi [1,*], Lauren Tatina [2], Lizette Rios [3], Dewayne Stennett [4] and Jean Sparks [1]

1 Department of Health Sciences, Texas A&M University, Corpus Christi, TX 78412, USA; jean.sparks@tamucc.edu
2 School of Osteopathic Medicine, University of the Incarnate Word, San Antonio, TX 78235, USA; lolo.12171998@gmail.com
3 Department of Life Sciences, Texas A&M University, Corpus Christi, TX 78412, USA; lerios@UTMB.EDU
4 The Transitional Year Programme, University of Toronto, Toronto, ON M5S 2E8, Canada; dewayne.stennett@utoronto.ca
* Correspondence: felix.omoruyi@tamucc.edu

Abstract: *Kalanchoe pinnata*, commonly known as the "miracle plant" or "life plant", is a succulent species traditionally used for various health conditions. Recent research investigations have intensified interest in this species due to its diverse repertoire of bioactive constituents, including flavonoids, alkaloids, triterpenes, and glycosides. These compounds have been associated with multiple therapeutic effects, notably antioxidant, anti-inflammatory, and antidiabetic activities. Although several studies have highlighted the positive effects of the extracts of *K. pinnata* on key factors contributing to the pathophysiology and complications of diabetes mellitus, a systematic overview focusing on the use of these extracts and their bioactive constituents in the management of the disease is lacking. This literature review summarizes the phytochemical composition, traditional uses, and recent scientific data supporting the antidiabetic potential of *K. pinnata*, with a particular focus on its effects on glycemic control, as well as inflammatory and oxidative homeostasis, toxicity, safety, and potential clinical implications. The phytochemical constituents discussed include quercetin, kaempferol, apigenin, epigallocatechin gallate (EGCG), avicularin, and bufadienolides, along with a presentation of representative structures. The review also covers the potential mechanisms of action in diabetes mellitus. The survey of available literature highlights the effects of *K. pinnata* on indices of diabetes mellitus, including enhancing insulin sensitivity, mitigating oxidative stress and inflammation, lowering blood glucose levels, and the potential adverse effects. These results point to the promising prospect for *K. pinnata* use in the management of diabetes mellitus and its associated complications, while underscoring the need for more rigorous investigations, including well-controlled clinical trials.

Keywords: diabetes mellitus; *Kalanchoe pinnata*; antioxidants; inflammation; oxidative stress

1. Introduction

According to the World Health Organization (WHO), diabetes mellitus is a chronic condition resulting from either insufficient insulin production or the body's inability to utilize insulin effectively [1]. Insulin, produced by pancreatic beta cells, regulates blood glucose levels. Uncontrolled diabetes mellitus is marked by elevated blood sugar that can subsequently lead to complications such as neuropathy, nephropathy, retinopathy, and atherosclerosis. The International Diabetes Federation (IDF) estimated that 537 million

https://doi.org/10.3390/ph18101518

adults had diabetes in 2021, with projections rising to 643 million by 2030 and 783 million by 2045 [2]. Diabetes mellitus encompasses three main types: Type 1 is caused by the autoimmune or environmental destruction of pancreatic beta cells, leading to absolute insulin deficiency. Type 2 diabetes is characterized by insulin resistance and impaired insulin secretion, resulting from beta-cell dysfunction. Gestational diabetes develops during pregnancy due to hormonal changes that impair insulin production, although blood sugar levels typically normalize after childbirth. The IDF also reported that diabetes caused 6.7 million deaths globally in 2021, with a total estimated health expenditure of 966 billion dollars [2]. As healthcare costs continue to rise, many are turning to alternative medicines for treatment and are combining it with modern medicine. Hence, medicinal plants now play a vital role in global healthcare, especially in the management of diabetes mellitus. Plants have long served as an essential source of therapeutic agents, with over 80% of current drugs derived directly or indirectly from them. Medicinal plants are often favored for their minimal side effects and have been used for centuries in traditional medical systems across many countries worldwide [3].

K. pinnata (Lam.) Pers., a member of the Crassulaceae family, is widely recognized for its medicinal uses across Africa, Asia, and South America. This perennial plant typically grows to a height of 1–1.5 m and features a moist, sturdy, tuberous, hairless stem. Its leaves are thick, simple, and lobed (3 to 5 lobes), while its drooping orange-red flowers are a distinctive feature. Notably, the plant produces vegetative buds—small reddish leaflets—along the leaf margins and stems, which can develop into new plants (Figure 1) [4]. *K. pinnata* is the most widely used species in its genus and has long been integral to traditional and holistic medicine worldwide [5]. It has been employed to treat a wide range of ailments, including wounds, cancer, urolithiasis, hypertension, diabetes, diarrhea, vomiting, respiratory and urinary tract infections, coughs, dysentery, migraines, and rheumatoid disorders [6–9]. Aqueous extracts from the leaves and roots are commonly used in traditional medicine for disease therapy in many regions, including the treatment of diabetes. The plant is known by various names—such as "miracle plant", "air plant", "life plant", "master herb", "cure-all", and "best of luck leaves" reflecting its esteemed status in folk medicine [9,10].

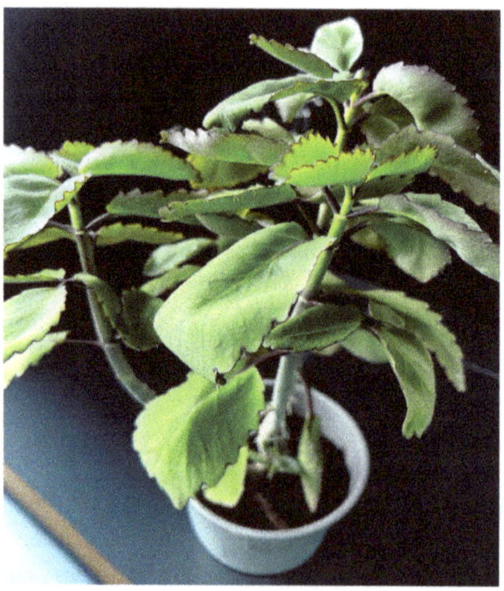

Figure 1. Image of *Kalanchoe pinnata*.

Numerous studies have validated many of its traditional uses, revealing a broad range of therapeutic properties: analgesic, carminative, antiulcer, anti-inflammatory, antimicrobial, antioxidant, hepatoprotective, nephroprotective, cardioprotective, neuroprotective, tocolytic, antimutagenic, antitumor, antinociceptive, anti-edematogenic, immunosuppressive, diuretic, sedative, CNS depressant, muscle relaxant, and bone marrow modulatory effects [6,8,9,11,12]. Due to its potent antioxidant and anti-inflammatory properties, *K. pinnata* has drawn increasing interest in the context of chronic disease management. This review summarizes recent findings and prospects on the therapeutic potential of *K. pinnata* in managing diabetes mellitus.

2. *K. pinnata* Phytochemical Constituents' Role in Diabetes Mellitus

Recent research has unveiled the remarkable phytochemical profile of *K. pinnata*, a plant renowned for its traditional medicinal uses. The phytochemical constituents include flavonoids, polyphenols, triterpenoids of ß-amyrin structure, phytosterols, alkaloids, glycosides, steroids, bufadienolides, lipids, and organic acids [13–15]. These bioactive molecules in the plant contribute to its antimicrobial and overall potential therapeutic properties [6,8]. The bioactive phytomolecules have been identified using Ultraperformance liquid chromatography fusion orbitrap mass spectrometry (UPLC-OT-FTMS) in an aqueous extract of *K. pinnata* leaves, locally grown in the Gulf Coast region of Corpus Christi, South Texas, USA [16]. The five main phytochemicals identified were quercetin, kaempferol, apigenin, epigallocatechin gallate (EGCG), and avicularin (Figure 2), each contributing to the plant's antioxidant and therapeutic potential [16]. The compounds identified shared similarities in their chemical structures, though variations observed among the chemicals were primarily attributed to the presence and positioning of hydroxyl functional groups. These groups were either shifted from the phenol active group or were absent altogether. However, all compounds belonged to the same chemical class known as polyphenols, specifically flavonoids. Among the five main phytochemicals identified, three are flavonols, one is a flavone, and the remaining one is a catechin. Importantly, all compounds are recognized as bioactive molecules with documented antioxidant and anti-inflammatory properties, which may be due to the combined action of the bioflavonoids [16] (Figure 2, Table 1). The presence of various phytochemicals with various biological properties rationalizes the use of *K. pinnata* leaf extracts in folklore medicine [17]. Quercetin, a potent flavonoid found in *K. pinnata*, exhibits antidiabetic properties comparable to those of metformin, a widely used antidiabetic medication, in preclinical models [18]. It improves glycemic control, reduces lipid peroxidation, and protects β-cells by attenuating oxidative and inflammatory pathways [19]. By modulating key signaling pathways, quercetin shields cells from the damaging effects of reactive oxygen species (ROS) and promotes insulin production and release. Its ability to improve hyperglycemia makes it a compelling candidate for diabetes management. Similarly, EGCG, another key phytochemical in *K. pinnata*, has been shown to regulate blood sugar levels. Human trials further support its potential, revealing improvements in insulin sensitivity and metabolic health [20] and thus suggest that EGCG could be a valuable tool in the fight against type 2 diabetes. On the other hand, avicularin, a lesser known yet potent bioactive compound in *K. pinnata*, offers powerful antioxidant benefits. By modulating crucial cellular pathways such as phosphoinositide 3-kinase (PI3K), Akt/PKB, and MAPK [21], avicularin reduces oxidative stress and enhances cell survival. Studies highlight its ability to scavenge hydroxyl radicals, reducing inflammation-induced damage and potentially supporting cell growth [22,23]. Moreover, its positive impact on fasting blood glucose, lipid levels, and β-cell function further underscores its therapeutic promise for diabetic patients. Kaempferol, another flavonoid abundant in *K. pinnata*, has been recognized for its glucose-regulating abilities [24]. Kaempferol regulates lipid metabolism and improves insulin resistance. It also enhances insulin signaling and restores the balance between glucose utilization and production, thereby mitigating glucose toxicity [25]. Research indicates that kaempferol also enhances antioxidant activity by lowering malondialdehyde levels, a marker of oxidative damage [26]. These findings align with previous studies that confirm kaempferol's role in combating oxidative stress and supporting metabolic health. Apigenin and kaempferol have been shown to influence inflammatory pathways. Notably, while both apigenin and kaempferol reduce TNF-α expression and secretion, apigenin uniquely decreases IL-10 levels, whereas kaempferol enhances IL-10 secretion [27]. This intricate interplay suggests that apigenin plays a nuanced role in immune modulation and inflammatory response, which could have implications for managing chronic diseases, including diabetes. Bufadienolides, on the other hand, influence apoptosis and autophagy [28].

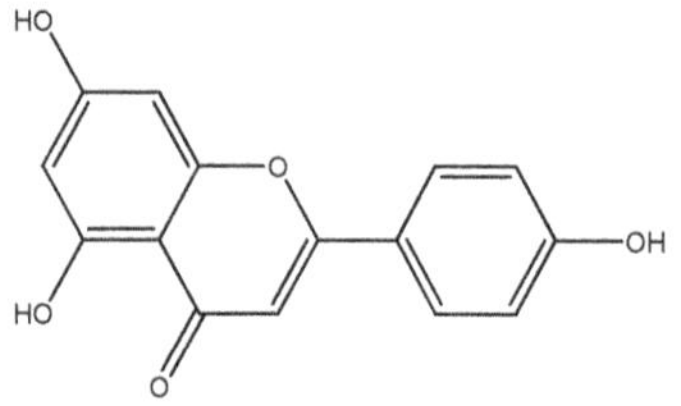

Apigenin

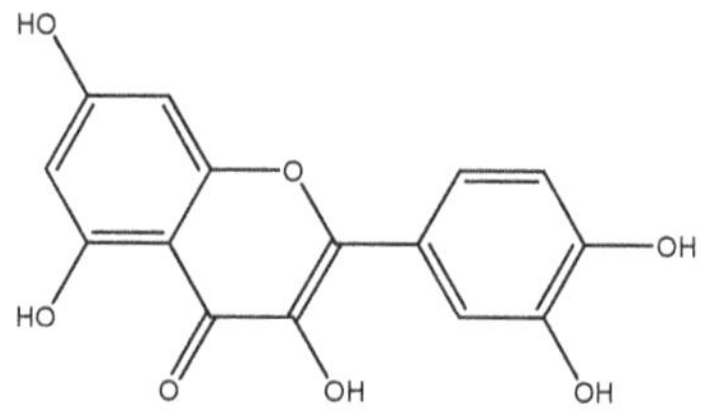

Quercetin

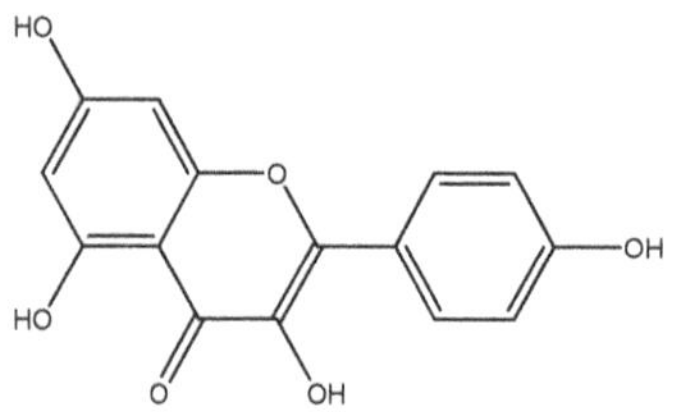

Kaempferol

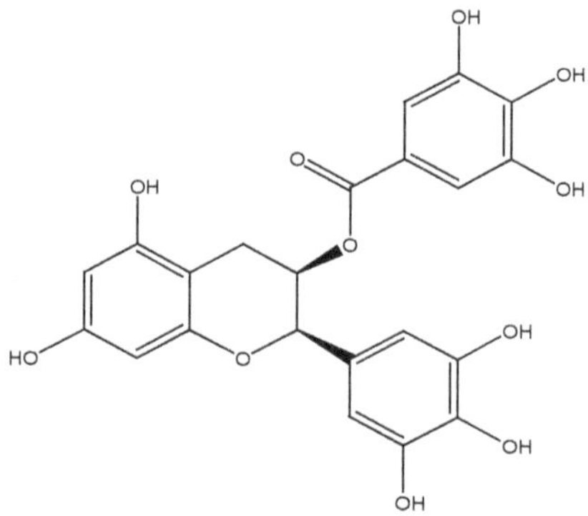

Epigallocatechin gallate (EGCG)

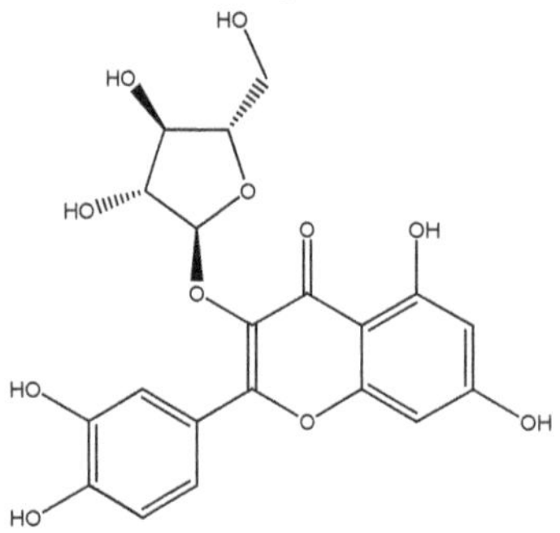

Avicularin

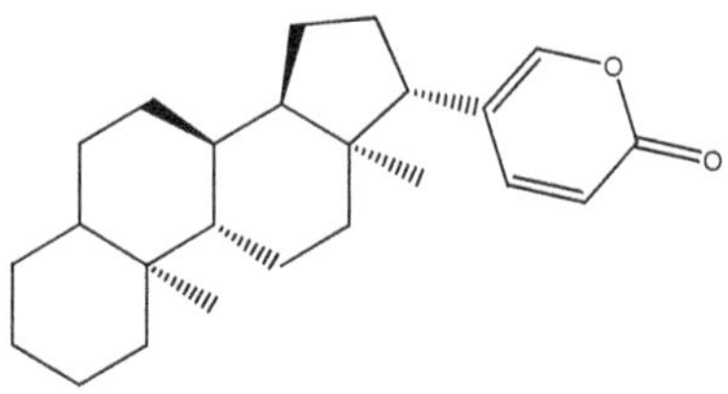

Bufadienolide

Figure 2. Structures of bioactive metabolites present in *K. pinnata* with potential antidiabetic activity.

Table 1. Shows the biological activities of several phytochemicals from *K. pinnata* that suggest antidiabetic potential.

Reference(s)	Bioactive Compound	Mechanism of Antidiabetic Activity
Ozsoy et al., 2020 [19]	Quercetin	1. Improves glycemic control 2. Reduces lipid peroxidation 3. Protects β-cells (by attenuating oxidative and inflammatory pathways)
Liu et al., 2014 [20]	EGCG	1. Regulates blood sugar 2. Improves insulin sensitivity
Williams et al., 2004 [21]	Avicularin	1. Reduces oxidative stress by modulating crucial cellular pathways (PI3K; Akt/PKB; MAPK)
Agüero-Hernández et al., 2020 [24] Yang et al., 2022 [25] de-Araújo et al., 2018 [26] Palacz-Wrobel et al., 2017 [27]	Kaempferol	1. Regulates lipid metabolism 2. Improves insulin resistance 3. Enhances insulin signaling 4. Restores the balance between glucose utilization and production 5. Enhances antioxidant activity 6. Influence inflammatory pathways (reduce TNF-α expression and secretion)
Palacz-Wrobel et al., 2017 [27]	Apigenin	1. Immune modulation and inflammatory response (reduce TNF-α expression and secretion; decreases IL-10 levels)
Huang et al., 2021 [28]	Bufadienolides	1. Influence apoptosis and autophagy

3. Antidiabetic Potentials of *K. pinnata*

Diabetes mellitus is a group of metabolic disorders characterized by chronic hyperglycemia resulting from impaired insulin secretion, insulin action, or both. This condition leads to disturbances in the metabolism of carbohydrates, fats, and proteins, contributing to various metabolic dysfunctions. Millions of people around the world rely on medicinal plants to manage diabetes and other diseases, mainly due to the high cost of conventional treatments and their potential side effects. These plants are commonly used in developing countries, particularly among underprivileged populations, to treat many diseases, including diabetes. According to studies, 80% of people in underdeveloped nations rely on traditional therapies made from plants, which are the most frequently used type of treatment for various health conditions globally [29] (Table 2). Given the global prevalence of diabetes, over 800 medicinal plants have been identified as potential treatment options. However, the use of many of these plants for the therapy of diabetes and other diseases often lacks scientific validation. Critical information, such as proper dosages and potential side effects, remains unknown for many herbal preparations, making herbal medicine a potentially riskier alternative to modern treatments.

Table 2. The diverse range of effects of *K. pinnata* preparations in both in vivo and in vitro models of diabetes.

	Reference	Concentration/Doses	Observed Effects	Potential Benefits/Adverse Effects
1.	Halayal et al., 2024 [29]	In vitro: 0.0–40 μg/mL methanolic extract on 1% starch digestion with time.	Inhibition of alpha-amylase and alpha-glucosidase enzymes.	Potential therapeutic properties of *K. pinnata* in diabetes management.
2.	Singh et al., 2024 [30]	0.5% of *K. pinnata* extract administered to mice for 1 week.	Reduction in lipid levels.	Mitigation of hyperlipidemia and related metabolic disorders associated with diabetes.
3.	Menon et al., 2015 [31]	Aqueous *K. pinnata* leaves 0.14 g/Kg body weight administered to diabetic rats for 4 weeks.	Reduced body weight, blood glucose, cholesterol, IL-6, and increased BUN, IL-1β and TNF-α.	Management of glucose and cholesterol levels in diabetes.
4.	Matthew et al., 2013 [32]	Ethanolic and aqueous extracts of *K. pinnata* stem 300 & 600 mg/Kg body weight) were administered to diabetic rats for 12 days. In vitro: 0.063% & 0.125% ethanolic and aqueous extract on 1% starch digestion with time.	Decreased blood glucose levels occurred in a dose-dependent manner. α-amylase inhibition, but the ethanolic extract was more effective.	Anti-hyperglycemic activity.
5.	Ojewole, 2005 [33]	Aqueous leaf extract of K. *pinnata* was administered to diabetic rats at 25–800 mg/Kg body weight and monitored for 8 h.	Reduced blood glucose levels.	Hypoglycemic properties.
6.	Patil et al., 2013 [34]	Dichloromethane extract of *K. pinnata* leaves was administered to diabetic rats for 45 days. In vitro: rat pancreatic cells treated with 10 μg/mL of *K. pinnata* for 1 h.	Decreased glucose, glycated hemoglobin, lipid profiles & insulin levels. Increased insulin secretion com Parable to glibenclamide 10 μg/mL.	Effective in the therapy of diabetes.
7.	Ramon et al., 2023 [16] & Ramon et al., 2021 [35]	In vitro: Diabetic and non-diabetic skeletal muscle cells treated with combined *K. pinnata* and metformin preparations with combinatorial ratios varying from 5.0 mM metformin-only and 400 μg/mL of K. pinnata-only for 72 h.	Improved oxidative stress, downregulation of IL-6, and may promote inflammation.	May improve diabetes management and potential adverse effects in diabetes care. Immune-modulating activity that may promote beneficial or adverse effects.

K. pinnata has gained attention in diabetes care due to its diverse medicinal properties, particularly its antioxidant, anti-inflammatory, and antihyperglycemic activities. The marked chronic hyperglycemia in diabetes induces oxidative stress and inflammation, contributing to complications such as neuropathy, nephropathy, and retinopathy. Hyperlipidemia has also attracted global attention due to its high prevalence and strong link to several life-threatening conditions, particularly cardiovascular diseases [36–38]. Studies suggest that *K. pinnata* exerts antihyperglycemic effects by modulating glucose metabolism, enhancing insulin sensitivity, and reducing oxidative stress in diabetic models. This makes it a potential candidate for managing diabetes-related complications. Singh & Pattnaik [30] (Table 2) also reported the antihyperlipidemic activity of the extract of *K. pinnata* leaves. Menon et al. [31] (Table 2) reported that the aqueous extract of *K. pinnata* may benefit diabetes management due to its ability to reduce body weight, lower blood glucose (hypoglycemic activity), and lower cholesterol levels. They noted that the decrease in blood glucose may be due to enhanced glycolysis in the liver, as evidenced by elevated pyruvate kinase activity in streptozotocin-induced diabetic rats. They reported an increase in blood urea nitrogen (BUN), which could raise concerns about potential renal damage due to *K. pinnata* supplementation. However, BUN is not the most sensitive marker of renal damage and may be elevated due to various unrelated factors. Additionally, the aqueous extract suppressed interleukin-6 (IL-6), a pro-inflammatory cytokine commonly elevated in diabetes. Goyal et al. [39] reported that administering the ethanolic extract of *K. pinnata* decreased blood glucose levels in diabetic rats. The plant extract also increased pancreatic insulin secretion. Matthew et al. [32] (Table 2) investigated the antidiabetic activity of ethanolic and aqueous extracts of the dried stem of *K. pinnata* in alloxan-induced diabetic rats. Both extracts demonstrated hypoglycemic activity. However, the ethanolic extract showed more inhibitory activity of the α-amylase enzyme than the aqueous extract, while the aqueous extract showed more hypoglycemic activity than the ethanolic extract. Another study revealed that the methanolic extract of the plant leaves exerted inhibitory action on α-amylase and α-glucosidase [29] (Table 2). The extract exhibited higher effectiveness in inhibiting these enzymes than standard acarbose [29,40]. Ojewole [33] (Table 2) also noted a remarkable decrease in the blood glucose levels in diabetic rats administered the aqueous extract of *K. pinnata*. The antidiabetic potential of *K. pinnata* leaves was investigated by Patil et al. [34] (Table 2) using streptozotocin-induced diabetic rats, focusing on the mechanisms underlying its antihyperglycemic effects and insulin secretion enhancement. The study examined four extract fractions: petroleum ether, chloroform, dichloromethane (DCM), and aqueous fractions. Among these, the DCM fraction demonstrated the most potent antihyperglycemic activity. Diabetic rats treated orally with 10 mg/kg body weight of the DCM fraction showed a notable reduction in fasting blood glucose levels, dropping from 228 mg/dL to 116 mg/dL. Glycated hemoglobin levels in this treatment group improved by 8.4% compared to the diabetic control group, which exhibited levels of 12.9%. Additionally, lipid profiles and insulin levels in the DCM-treated group closely resembled those of the non-diabetic control group. The DCM fraction of the plant demonstrated glucose-independent insulin secretagogue action, similar to that of the currently used drug glibenclamide, and therefore needs to be administered just before meals, as is the case with glibenclamide. Phytochemical analysis identified the active component of the DCM fraction as a phenyl alkyl ether derivative. These findings highlight the potential of the *K. pinnata* DCM fraction as a promising therapeutic option for diabetes mellitus, demonstrating its efficacy in promoting insulin secretion and improving glycemic control. Menon et al. [41] hypothesized that *K. pinnata* preparation consumption may act to increase peripheral insulin levels through extra-pancreatic insulin elevation and modulate the insulin–insulin receptor complex that may prolong the half-life of ligand-receptor complex that could sustain signaling similar to the report for AspB10 insulin analog [42]. The phytoconstituents are believed to act synergistically in regulating blood glucose, improving insulin dynamics, and combating oxidative stress, suggesting their potential use in managing diabetes mellitus. Overall, *K. pinnata* demonstrates multifactorial antidiabetic properties, making it a promising natural therapeutic candidate for diabetes management. While these findings are encouraging, more rigorous clinical trials are needed to validate *K. pinnata*'s efficacy and safety in human populations, establish optimal dosages, and develop standardized formulations for therapeutic use.

4. Effect of *K. pinnata* on Antioxidant Activities in Diabetes Mellitus

Oxidative stress is a central contributor to the pathogenesis and progression of diabetes mellitus, particularly through its role in β-cell dysfunction, insulin resistance, and the development of diabetic complications. In this context, *K. pinnata* has garnered increasing scientific interest for its antioxidant properties, which may have therapeutic relevance in diabetes management (Figure 3). Studies have demonstrated that *K. pinnata* extracts possess robust free radical scavenging capacity, primarily attributed to their high content of flavonoids and phenolic acids. These phytochemicals act by neutralizing reactive oxygen species (ROS), thereby preventing oxidative damage to cellular components, including lipids, proteins, and nucleic acids. At the cellular level, antioxidant defense involves both enzymatic and non-enzymatic systems. Enzymes such as manganese superoxide dismutase (Mn-SOD/SOD2), copper-zinc superoxide dismutase (Cu, Zn-SOD/SOD1), catalase (CAT), and glutathione peroxidase (GPX) play pivotal roles in detoxifying ROS, alongside non-enzymatic antioxidants such as glutathione (GSH) (Figure 3), which help maintain redox homeostasis [43]. Ramon et al. [16] reported a remarkable increase in catalase activity following treatment with 400 μg/mL of *K. pinnata* extract in type 2 diabetic human skeletal muscle cells, suggesting its potential to mitigate oxidative damage in type 2 diabetes mellitus. This increase may reflect the synergistic action of multiple bioactive constituents, as also suggested by Uchegbu et al. [17]. Although catalase has a relatively low affinity for hydrogen peroxide (H_2O_2) compared to other peroxidases [44], its upregulation remains critical. Catalase-mediated detoxification of H_2O_2 becomes increasingly essential when peroxidase systems are saturated, thus protecting cells from cumulative oxidative damage. The anti-inflammatory and antioxidant activities of *K. pinnata* have mainly been linked to its natural flavonoid content. Pinheiro et al. [12] assessed the phytochemical profile of *K. pinnata* across different growth stages and geographic regions in Brazil. They observed that younger leaves exhibited higher levels of total phenolics and flavonoids, correlating with increased antioxidant potential. This developmental gradient suggests that phytochemical content, and thus therapeutic efficacy, can vary based on harvest time and environmental conditions, which is particularly relevant for standardizing formulations intended for use in diabetes management. Extraction methods and solvent choice further influence the yield and bioactivity of *K. pinnata* extracts. Saeed et al. [45] demonstrated that supercritical fluid extraction at 5500 psi and 40 °C for 2 h yielded extracts with high concentrations of phenolics and flavonoids, thereby enhancing their antioxidant capacity. Selecting appropriate solvents based on polarity and volatility is essential for preserving these compounds during processing [46]. Collectively, these findings support the potential application of *K. pinnata* as a natural antioxidant agent in the management of diabetes. By modulating oxidative stress pathways and supporting endogenous antioxidant defense mechanisms, *K. pinnata* may provide a complementary strategy to enhance glycemic control and mitigate the risk of oxidative damage associated with chronic hyperglycemia.

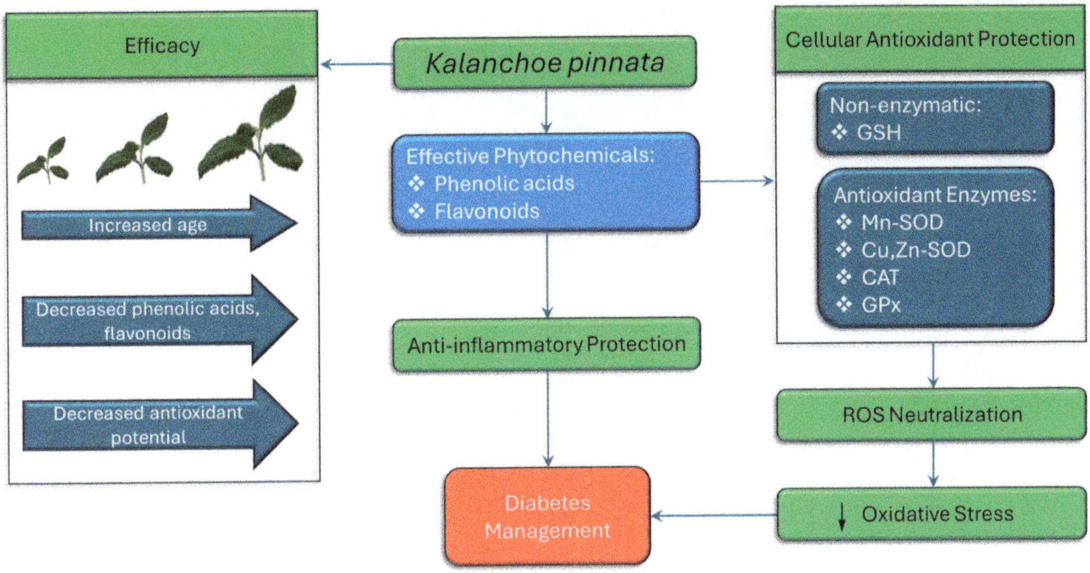

Figure 3. The therapeutic potential of *K. pinnata* in diabetes management, attributed to its antioxidant and anti-inflammatory properties. As the plant ages, levels of phenolic acids and flavonoids decline, resulting in a reduced antioxidant and anti-inflammatory potential and overall efficacy. Antioxidant protection involves both non-enzymatic (GSH) and enzymatic systems (Mn-SOD, Cu, Zn-SOD, CAT, GPx), which collectively neutralize reactive oxygen species (ROS) and reduce oxidative stress. These mechanisms ultimately support better diabetes management by mitigating oxidative damage and inflammation. (↓ denotes decrease).

5. Anti-Inflammatory Potentials of *K. pinnata* in Diabetes Mellitus Management

Inflammation is a complex biological response to harmful stimuli, including pathogens, damaged cells, and irritants. Chronic inflammation is associated with various diseases, including arthritis, diabetes, and cardiovascular disorders. Natural compounds from medicinal plants have gained attention for their potential role in modulating inflammatory pathways. *Kalanchoe pinnata* has been traditionally used to treat inflammation-related conditions. The bioactive compounds responsible for the anti-inflammatory activity of *K. pinnata* include flavonoids, terpenoids, alkaloids, phenolic compounds, and bufadienolides. These secondary metabolites exhibit potent anti-inflammatory effects by inhibiting pro-inflammatory mediators and oxidative stress [47]. The anti-inflammatory effects of *K. pinnata* are attributed to multiple mechanisms, including the inhibition of pro-inflammatory cytokines (Figure 4). Studies indicate that *K. pinnata* extracts reduce levels of key cytokines such as TNF-α, IL-1β [26,48], and IL-6 [34,35] (Table 2), which are involved in inflammatory signaling. The plant extract has also been found to modulate the cyclooxygenase (COX) and lipoxygenase (LOX) pathways and inhibit cyclooxygenase-1 (COX-1) and cyclooxygenase-2 (COX-2) [11,49] and LOX enzymes, reducing the synthesis of inflammatory prostaglandins and leukotrienes. The flavonoids and phenolic compounds also contribute to reducing oxidative stress, a notable factor in chronic inflammation. *K. pinnata* has been reported to suppress the activation of NF-κB, a transcription factor that regulates the expression of pro-inflammatory genes. The extracts also downregulate inducible nitric oxide synthase (iNOS), limiting excessive NO production and contributing to inflammatory damage. Aging and diabetes are associated with elevated systemic levels of IL-1β, TNF-α, and IL-6 [50]. Pro-inflammatory cytokines, such as TNF-α and IL-1β, contribute to atherosclerosis by inducing the expression of E-selectin, intercellular adhesion molecule 1 (ICAM-1), and vascular cell adhesion molecule 1 (VCAM-1) in endothelial cells [51]. Kong et al. [52] identified IL-1β and TNF-α as key mediators in the initiation and progression of atherosclerosis. Conversely, Menon et al. [34] (Table 2) reported elevated IL-1β and TNF-α levels in diabetic rats administered an aqueous *K. pinnata* preparation, indicating that it may not effectively mitigate the risk of atherosclerosis.

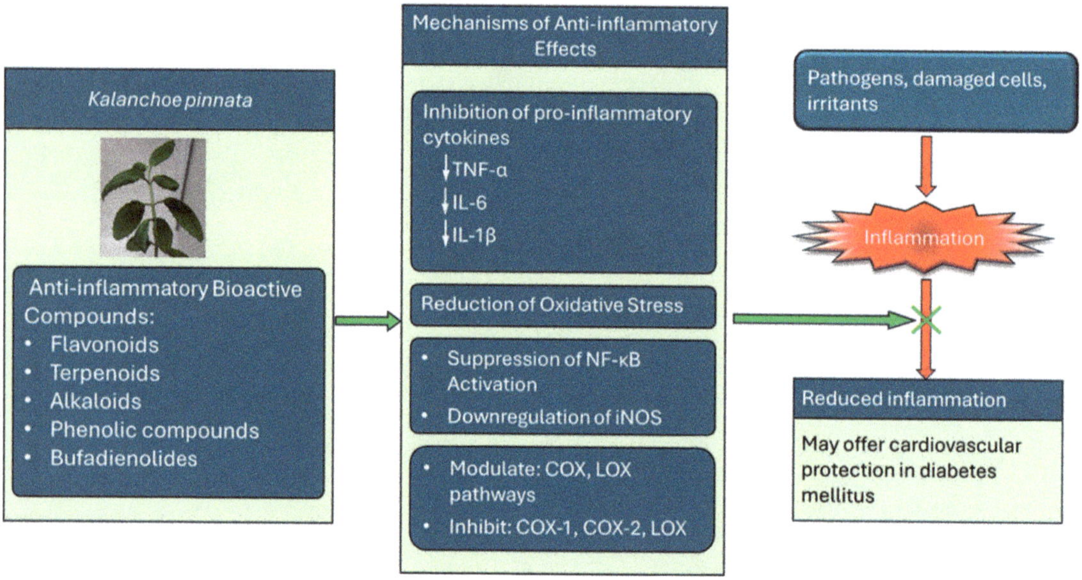

Figure 4. The anti-inflammatory mechanisms of bioactive compounds in *K. pinnata* and its potential cardiovascular benefits in diabetes mellitus. The plant exerts its effects by inhibiting pro-inflammatory cytokines (TNF-α, IL-6, IL-1β), reducing oxidative stress, suppressing NF-κB activation, and downregulating iNOS expression. The compounds also modulate cyclooxygenase (COX) and lipoxygenase (LOX) pathways, inhibiting COX-1, COX-2, and LOX enzymes. Collectively, these actions help block inflammation and improve cardiovascular outcomes in individuals with diabetes (↓ denotes decrease).

However, the aqueous preparation notably reduced the levels of IL-6, a cytokine upregulated in diabetes and known to trigger endothelial dysfunction, which can lead to atherosclerosis [53]. The hypothesis is that IL-6 downregulation may counteract the adverse effects of IL-1β and TNF-α, suggesting that *K. pinnata* may offer cardiovascular protection. Overall, *K. pinnata*'s remarkable anti-inflammatory properties are attributable to its diverse range of bioactive compounds, such as flavonoids, steroids, triterpenoids, and phenolic compounds. Its notable anti-inflammatory activity involves multiple biochemical pathways, including the suppression of cytokines, inhibition of enzymes, and antioxidant effects (Figure 4). The phytochemical profile supports its potential development as a plant-based therapeutic agent.

6. Potential Mechanism of *K. pinnata* Therapy in Diabetes Mellitus

Kalanchoe pinnata extracts have been widely reported to exhibit potent antioxidant and anti-inflammatory properties [26,47], which are particularly relevant in the context of diabetes mellitus, where oxidative stress and chronic low-grade inflammation play central roles in the pathogenesis and progression of the disease. In diabetes, elevated blood glucose levels lead to the overproduction of reactive oxygen species (ROS), which impairs insulin signaling, damages pancreatic β-cells, and contributes to the development of vascular complications. The plant's flavonoid-rich extracts have been shown to regulate redox-sensitive signaling pathways implicated in both cancer and metabolic disorders (Figure 5). One of the central mechanisms by which *K. pinnata* may exert therapeutic effects in diabetes is by modulating intracellular reactive oxygen species (ROS) levels, restoring mitochondrial function, and enhancing the activity of antioxidant defense systems.

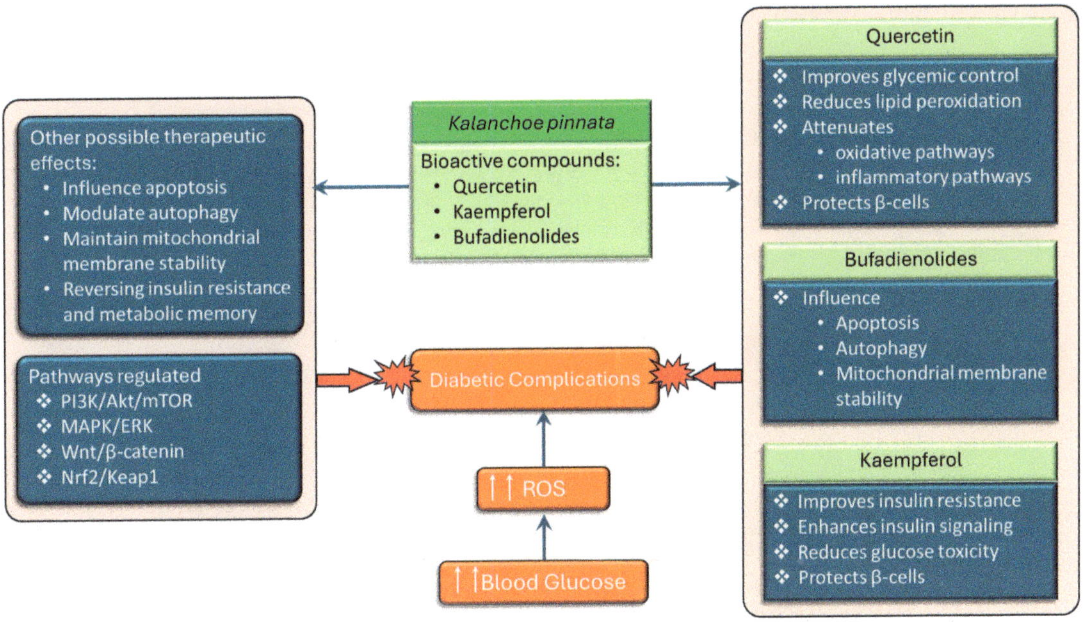

Figure 5. The schematic representation of the potential therapeutic effects of *Kalanchoe pinnata* bioactive compounds, quercetin, kaempferol, and bufadienolides, which exert protective effects by targeting multiple mechanisms. Quercetin improves glycemic control, suppresses oxidative and inflammatory pathways, and protects pancreatic β-cells. Kaempferol enhances insulin signaling, reduces glucose toxicity, and protects β-cells. Bufadienolides influence apoptosis, autophagy, and mitochondrial membrane stability. Collectively, these compounds modulate key signaling pathways (PI3K/Akt/mTOR, MAPK/ERK, Wnt/β-catenin, and Nrf2/Keap1) and may offer additional therapeutic benefits, including the reversal of insulin resistance, modulation of metabolic memory, and stabilization of mitochondrial function (↑↑ denotes increase).

In diabetes, these mechanisms are critical for maintaining β-cell integrity and regulating programmed cell death in insulin-resistant tissues. The modulation of autophagy also holds therapeutic potential, as impaired autophagic flux contributes to β-cell failure and insulin resistance. Importantly, *K. pinnata* and its bioactive compounds regulate multiple cellular signaling pathways that are also dysregulated in diabetes (Figure 5), including the phosphoinositide 3-kinase/protein kinase B/mammalian target of rapamycin (PI3K/Akt/mTOR), mitogen-activated protein kinase/extracellular signal-regulated kinase (MAPK/ERK), wingless/integrated signaling/β-catenin (Wnt/β-catenin), and nuclear factor erythroid 2–related factor 2/kelch-like ECH-associated protein 1 (Nrf2/Keap1) pathways [54]. The PI3K/Akt/mTOR axis plays a pivotal role in insulin signaling, glucose uptake, and lipid metabolism. The activation of this pathway is impaired by insulin resistance resulting in a worsening of insulin resistance and decreased glucose uptake, ultimately leading to hyperglycemia. The MAPK/ERK pathway is involved in cell growth, differentiation and stress response and contributes to disease progression when overactivated in type 2 diabetes by promoting inflammation, insulin resistance and other diabetic complications. Wnt/β-catenin signaling is involved in insulin secretion, β-cell proliferation, and glucose metabolism, and dysregulation of this pathway contributes to the development of type 2 diabetes and its complications. The Nrf2 pathway is a master regulator of antioxidant gene expression. Activation of Nrf2 can restore redox balance and protect against diabetic complications, particularly nephropathy, retinopathy, and cardiomyopathy. Additionally, flavonoids like quercetin and kaempferol may act as epigenetic modulators, potentially reversing insulin resistance and metabolic memory by regulating DNA methylation, histone modification, and non-coding RNAs [54]. This offers a promising avenue for addressing the long-term effects of hyperglycemia even after glucose levels are normalized. These pathways are all potential targets for *K. pinnata* phytochemicals. Taken together, the antioxidant, anti-inflammatory, and signaling-regulatory activities of *K. pinnata* and its key constituents support its potential as an adjunctive therapeutic agent in diabetes management. By mitigating oxidative stress, modulating metabolic signaling pathways, and protecting insulin-producing cells, *K. pinnata* may help reduce the progression of diabetes and its associated complications.

Oufir et al. [55] identified four major bufadienolide components in *K. pinnata* grown in Brazil and Germany: bersaldegenin-1-acetate (1), bersaldegenin-3-acetate (2), bryophyllin A (3), and bersaldegenin-1,3,5-orthoacetate (4). In contrast, Stefanowicz-Hajduk et al. [56] found that bersaldegenin-2-acetate and bersaldegenin-5-acetate were the predominant bufadienolides, along with six additional bufadienolide compounds, in ethanolic extracts of *K. pinnata* cultivated in Poland. These findings suggest that the occurrence and composition of bufadienolides in *K. pinnata* vary with geographical origin. The bufadienolides present in *K. pinnata*, which have been previously studied for their anticancer effects, have been shown to influence apoptosis, autophagy, and mitochondrial membrane stability [28].

7. Organ Protection Properties of *K. pinnata* in Diabetes Mellitus

Organ function is critically important in diabetes management, as chronic hyperglycemia and subsequent oxidative stress can impair multiple organs, including the liver, kidneys, and lungs. Complications such as diabetic nephropathy, non-alcoholic fatty liver disease, and increased susceptibility to infections are well-documented in diabetic individuals. In this context, *K. pinnata* has demonstrated promising protective effects on organ systems implicated in diabetes-related pathology. Several in vivo and in vitro studies have highlighted the hepatoprotective and nephroprotective properties of *K. pinnata* leaf concentrate and ethanolic extract. Yadav and Dixit [57] reported that the administration of *K. pinnata* leaf concentrate remarkably lowered serum bilirubin levels in experimental models, indicating potential in supporting liver detoxification and jaundice management. Moreover, both the leaf concentrates and ethanolic extract reduced thiopental-induced sleep duration in rats exposed to carbon tetrachloride (CCl_4), with histological findings showing that the ethanolic extract more effectively preserved hepatocyte integrity. These hepatoprotective effects are particularly relevant in diabetes, where oxidative stress can accelerate liver injury and metabolic dysregulation. In terms of kidney function, which is commonly compromised in diabetes due to diabetic nephropathy, *K. pinnata* has shown nephroprotective effects. Harlalka et al. [7] demonstrated that an aqueous extract of *K. pinnata* notably reduced blood urea levels and preserved serum and urine creatinine levels in gentamicin-induced nephrotoxicity in rats. The extract also enhanced urine output and maintained body weight, while its antioxidant properties outperformed ascorbic acid in free radical scavenging and inhibition of lipid peroxidation, mechanisms known to be beneficial in slowing the progression of renal damage in diabetes. Further supporting its nephroprotective role, Bigoniya et al. [58] found that *K. pinnata* improved kidney function and reduced renal crystal deposition in a model of sodium glyoxylate-induced nephrolithiasis. These improvements included increased urine volume and decreased excretion of oxalate, citrate, phosphate, and calcium, parameters often dysregulated in individuals with diabetic kidney stones. Histological analysis confirmed reduced tubular damage and inflammation. Emerging nanotechnology-based research also suggests novel applications of *K. pinnata* in diabetes-related urolithiasis. Priya et al. [59] synthesized silver nanoparticles using *K. pinnata* leaf extract and demonstrated dose-dependent inhibition of calcium hydrogen phosphate dihydrate crystal formation in vitro, with up to 84.8% inhibition at a 5% concentration. Similarly, Ranaweera et al. [60] found that *K. pinnata* extract slowed calcium oxalate stone precipitation, enhanced dissolution, and reduced crystal size and density. These findings are significant, as diabetic patients are at higher risk of nephrolithiasis due to altered urinary composition and oxidative stress. Moreover, while the respiratory system is not a classical target of diabetic complications, recent studies suggest an increased risk of pulmonary infections and inflammation in diabetic patients. In this context, *K. pinnata* may offer some protective benefits. Ehi-Omosun & Etunim [61] used bifenthrin to induce interstitial pneumonitis in rats and observed that a 200 mg/kg dose of *K. pinnata* leaf extract effectively mitigated pulmonary tissue damage. Although the higher dose (40,000 mg/kg) offered partial protection, its efficacy was comparatively reduced. These findings suggest a dose-dependent pulmonary protective effect, which may be relevant for preserving respiratory health in diabetic individuals. The organ-protective effects of *K. pinnata*, particularly on the liver and kidneys, are likely mediated by its high content of flavonoids, polyphenols, and organic acids, which exert strong antioxidant and anti-inflammatory actions. Given that diabetes-related complications are largely driven by oxidative stress and metabolic dysregulation, the use of *K. pinnata* as a natural adjunct therapy in diabetes care warrants further exploration. However, extreme caution and supervision must be employed when administering *K. pinnata* as a therapeutic agent, as chronic exposure to its leaf extract can lead to the downregulation of genes essential for proper organ function and defense against infections [62].

8. Toxicity and Safety of *K. pinnata*

Kalanchoe pinnata and other *Kalanchoe* species are important herbs in the traditional medicine of Asia and Africa, commonly used for their reported anti-inflammatory, antimicrobial, antidiabetic, and wound-healing properties. Despite this therapeutic potential, safety and toxicity concerns have been raised, mainly due to the presence of bufadienolides. Oufir et al. [55] quantified bufadienolides in *K. pinnata* leaves grown in Brazil and reported total concentrations ranging from 16.28 to 40.50 mg/100 g dry weight, compared with lower levels of 3.78 to 12.49 mg/100 g dry weight in those grown in Germany. Kolodziejczyk-Czepas and Stochmal [63] highlighted significant gaps in the literature regarding the distribution of bufadienolides across *Kalanchoe* species and their specific plant organs. Toxicological studies have shown mixed findings. Saravanan et al. [64] reported that the median lethal dose (LD_{50}) of ethanolic leaf extract of *K. pinnata* was greater than 2000 mg/kg body weight, indicating low toxicity in rats. Repeated-dose studies revealed no adverse clinical signs, with normal hematological, biochemical, and histopathological results. However, Bhavsar and Chandel [65] reported that fresh leaf juice caused dose-dependent changes in cultured human blood lymphocytes. While 50 mL of juice produced only slight, non-significant increases in sister chromatid exchanges (SCEs)/cell and SCEs/chromosome, the 70 mL led to significant changes in the mitotic index (MI),

SCEs/cell, and SCEs/chromosome. The cell cycle proliferative index, average generation time, and population doubling time values were non-significant for both doses when compared to the controls. They concluded that although the juice can be used pharmaceutically and traditionally, higher doses or prolonged use may induce genotoxic and cytotoxic effects. Chronic exposure of zebrafish embryos to *K. pinnata* per leaf (KPL) extract impaired development and altered behavior in a dose-dependent manner, significantly downregulating genes associated with multiple pathways [62]. The formulation was proposed to cause proteasome degradation, DNA damage, cell cycle arrest, apoptosis, and endocrine dysfunction—potentially leading to developmental delay. Interestingly, it also reduced anxiety-like behaviors, possibly through anti-inflammatory and anti-apoptotic mechanisms that may counteract proteasome inhibition. However, Martins Fernandes Pereira et al. [62] cautioned against the indiscriminate use of KPL extracts during pregnancy, emphasizing the need for further studies on their mechanisms of action and safe dosage. Evidence suggests that the extract may disrupt the endocrine system by inhibiting progesterone-mediated oocyte maturation and interfering with the insulin signaling pathway, potentially leading to mild inflammation, insulin resistance, and obesity [66]. Additionally, KPL may induce DNA damage by impairing replication and repair processes, leading to genetic alterations. If these mutations affect genes that regulate cell growth, they could contribute to cancer development [67]. Bufadienolides themselves are associated with cardiotoxicity. They have been shown to induce atrioventricular block, ventricular arrhythmia, and other cardiac dysfunctions [68,69]. Lin et al. [70] reported that resibufogenin, a bufadienolide, caused arrhythmias and myocardial injury, likely due to its reactive epoxy ring structure, which inhibits the sodium–potassium pump (Na^+/K^+-ATPase) and disrupts ionic homeostasis [71–73]. However, the coexistence of multiple components in traditional Chinese medicine may modify these effects. Synergistic interactions among bufadienolides have been proposed to enhance pharmacological activity, such as anticancer effects against prostate cancer cells, while maintaining a more favorable safety profile [74]. Although *K. pinnata* extract demonstrates a generally favorable safety profile at traditional and experimental therapeutic doses, it may carry potential toxicity risks due to bufadienolides, particularly concerning cardiotoxicity. Hence, the lack of clinical evidence considerably limits the therapeutic use of *K. pinnata*.

9. Potential Clinical Implications of *K. pinnata* Therapy

The collective findings from existing studies highlight the therapeutic potential of *K. pinnata*, particularly its role in preclinical studies in diabetes management. Traditionally used in various medical systems for treating a wide array of conditions, *K. pinnata* has demonstrated protective effects on organs commonly affected by diabetes, including the liver, kidneys, cardiovascular system, and pancreas. The potential clinical applications of *K. pinnata* stem from its rich content of bioactive compounds, including flavonoids, triterpenoids, steroids, bufadienolides, and phenolic acids, which contribute to its diverse therapeutic effects. Preclinical studies have demonstrated that *K. pinnata* can lower fasting blood glucose levels, provide antioxidant protection to pancreatic cells, and exhibit metabolic-regulatory activities and remarkable anti-inflammatory activity, which is believed to be mediated by flavonoids like quercetin. Quercetin inhibits pro-inflammatory enzymes and cytokines. In diabetes care, *K. pinnata* offers a compelling complementary approach. Its ability to modulate oxidative stress, support insulin signaling pathways, and protect against diabetic complications such as nephropathy, hepatopathy, and endothelial dysfunction suggests it may enhance conventional treatment regimens. In some studies, extracts of *K. pinnata* have shown comparable efficacy to standard therapies, often with fewer side effects and potentially lower costs. However, despite promising preclinical data, notable gaps remain in our understanding of *K. pinnata*'s mechanisms of action, safety profile, dose–response relationships, and long-term effects—particularly in the context of diabetes. For example, a recent report by Martins Fernandes Pereira et al. [62] documented gene downregulation in zebrafish following chronic exposure to *K. pinnata*. This finding may have potential health implications in humans. Further research is urgently needed to validate these findings in rigorous clinical trials, explore the effects across different age groups and comorbid conditions, and determine optimal formulations and dosing for therapeutic use. Many patients use *K. pinnata* and other supplements without informing their healthcare providers, thereby increasing the risk of potential drug–supplement interactions. From a clinical perspective, healthcare providers should initiate open conversations with patients about the use of herbal supplements, including *K. pinnata* [75]. To prevent potential adverse outcomes, clinicians should proactively inquire about supplement use and thoroughly assess the patient's overall clinical status, including current medications, metabolic function, and organ health. Additionally, the quality, sourcing, and preparation of *K. pinnata* products are of paramount importance. Adverse side effects associated with herbal supplements often arise not from the herb itself, but from contamination, adulteration, or incorrect labeling. Patients should be encouraged to select products certified by reputable third-party organizations that adhere to Good Manufacturing Practices (GMPs), such as the United States Pharmacopeia (USP), the National Sanitation Foundation (NSF) International, or ConsumerLab. Notably, however, the differences between the doses used in clinical trials and those used in traditional remedies must be considered, along with their varying effects on different age groups. Regulatory resources, such as the NIH's Dietary Supplement Label Database and the FDA's MedWatch program, can also help clinicians and patients identify reliable products and report adverse events. The U.S. National Institutes of Health (NIH) offers several resources describing various *K. pinnata* products currently on the market for researchers and consumers alike. Its Dietary Supplement Label Database includes listings of available *K. pinnata* supplements. For example, Hawaii Pharm provides numerous supplements containing four fl. oz. of plant extract. The NIH National Library of Medicine also offers reliable information about herbal supplements. One such example is RelieveIt@ Regenerating Gel, which contains *K. pinnata* and other medicinal herbs as active ingredients. These sites are valuable resources for healthcare providers when recommending herbal supplements for their patients. Importantly, different species within the *Kalanchoe* genus exhibit remarkable variations in their chemical compositions and should not be used interchangeably. The standardization and identification of bioactive components are critical for ensuring safety and efficacy in diabetes care.

Overall, *K. pinnata* supplementation shows promising therapeutic potential in the management of diabetes. While its traditional use is widespread and some preclinical studies provide supportive evidence, more rigorous studies, including well-controlled human clinical trials, standardization of extracts, and toxicological profiling, are needed to establish its safety, optimal dosage, effects across different age groups and comorbid conditions, and long-term benefits. This literature review is intended for research purposes only and does not recommend therapeutic use without clinical validation. The promising therapeutic potential of *K. pinnata* is primarily based on in vitro and animal studies, which provide only indirect evidence for its safety and effectiveness in humans.

10. Conclusions

Kalanchoe pinnata may hold considerable promise as a natural adjunctive therapy in the management of diabetes mellitus. With continued research, it may contribute meaningfully to integrative therapeutic strategies aimed at improving metabolic control, reducing oxidative and inflammatory damage, and protecting against the development of diabetic complications. As interest in plant-based treatments grows, a thoughtful, evidence-based approach to their use, paired with stringent regulation and patient education, will be crucial to ensure the safe and effective incorporation of these treatments into diabetes care. However, despite the traditional use of *K. pinnata* for diabetes management, clinical trials are lacking, resulting in its current use being mostly complementary.

Author Contributions: Conceptualization, F.O. and J.S.; formal analysis, F.O. and J.S.; writing—original draft preparation, L.R. and L.T.; writing—review and editing, F.O.; preparation of figures, editing and reviewing, D.S.; supervision, F.O. and J.S. All authors have read and agreed to the published version of the manuscript.

Funding: This research received no external funding.

Institutional Review Board Statement: Not applicable.

Informed Consent Statement: Not applicable.

Data Availability Statement: Data sharing is not applicable to this article.

Acknowledgments: Texas A&M University-Corpus Christi supported the publication of this manuscript.

Conflicts of Interest: The authors declare that they have no conflicts of interest.

References

1. World Health Organization. Diabetes. 2023. Available online: https://www.who.int/news-room/fact-sheets/detail/diabetes (accessed on 29 January 2024).
2. International Diabetes Federation (IDF). Diabetes Atlas, Diabetes Around the World. 2021. Available online: https://www.diabetesatlas.org (accessed on 29 January 2024).
3. Balwan, W.K.; Saba, N.; Zargar, J.I. Burden of diabetes and role of medicinal plants in its treatment. *Saudi J. Med. Pharm. Sci.* **2022**, *8*, 355–361. [CrossRef]
4. Okwu, D.E.; Nnamdi, F.U. Two novel flavonoids from *Bryophyllum pinnatum* and their antimicrobial activity. *J. Chem. Pharm. Res.* **2011**, *3*, 1–10.
5. Taylor, L. *Kalanchoe pinnata*. The Tropical Plant Database. Available online: http://www.rain-tree.com/coirama.htm (accessed on 27 September 2024).
6. Mehata, M.S. Green synthesis of silver nanoparticles using *Kalanchoe pinnata* leaves (life plant) and their antibacterial and photocatalytic activities. *Chem. Phys. Lett.* **2021**, *778*, 138760. [CrossRef]
7. Harlalka, G.V.; Patil, C.R.; Patil, M.R. Protective effect of *Kalanchoe pinnata* pers. (*Crassulaceae*) on gentamicin-induced nephrotoxicity in rats. *Indian. J. Pharmacol.* **2007**, *39*, 201–205. [CrossRef]
8. Biswas, S.K.; Chowdhury, A.; Das, J.; Hosen, S.Z.; Uddin, R.; Rahaman, M.S. A review of the traditional medicinal uses of *Kalanchoe pinnata* (*Crassulaceae*). *Int. J. Pharm. Pharmacol.* **2021**, *10*, 1–5.
9. Dogra, P.; Sharma, K.; Bharti, J.; Kumar, N.; Kumar, D. *Kalanchoe pinnata* is a Miraculous Plant: A Review. *J. Biomed. Allied Res.* **2022**, *4*, 1–10. [CrossRef]
10. Phatak, R.S.; Hendre, A.S. Total antioxidant capacity (TAC) of fresh leaves of *Kalanchoe pinnata*. *J. Pharmacogn. Phytochem.* **2014**, *2*, 32–35.
11. Ferreira, R.T.; Coutinho, M.A.; Malvar, D.D.; Costa, E.A.; Florentino, I.F.; Costa, S.S.; Vanderlinde, F.A. Mechanisms underlying the antinociceptive, anti-edematogenic, and anti-inflammatory activity of the main flavonoid from *Kalanchoe pinnata*. *Evid.-Based Complement. Altern. Med.* **2014**, *2014*, 429256. [CrossRef] [PubMed]
12. Pinheiro, G.P.; Clemente, R.C.; Rosini Silva, Á.A.; Pastore, G.M.; de Melo Porcari, A.; Sawaya, A.C. Chemical Profiling and Antioxidant Activity of Extracts from *Kalanchoe* Medicinal Species: Intraspecific Sources of Variation in *Kalanchoe crenata* and *K. pinnata*. *Rev. Bras. Farmacogn.* **2024**, *34*, 818–830. [CrossRef]
13. Siddiqui, S.; Faizi, S.; Siddiqui, B.S.; Sultana, N. Triterpenoids and phenanthrenes from leaves of *Bryophyllum pinnatum*. *Phytochemistry* **1989**, *28*, 2433–2438. [CrossRef]
14. Yamagishi, T.; Haruna, M.; Yan, X.Z.; Chang, J.J.; Lee, K.H. Antitumor agents, 110. *Bryophyllin B*, a novel potent cytotoxic bufadienolide from *Bryophyllum pinnatum*. *J. Nat. Prod.* **1989**, *52*, 1071–1079. [CrossRef] [PubMed]
15. Pattewar, S.V. *Kalanchoe pinnata*: Phytochemical and Pharmacological Profile. *Int. J. Phytopharm.* **2012**, *2*, 993–1000. [CrossRef]

16. Ramon, P.; Bergmann, D.; Abdulla, H.; Sparks, J.; Omoruyi, F. Bioactive Ingredients in *K. pinnata* Extract and Synergistic Effects of Combined *K. pinnata* and Metformin Preparations on Antioxidant Activities in Diabetic and Non-Diabetic Skeletal Muscle Cells. *Int. J. Mol. Sci.* **2023**, *24*, 6211. [CrossRef]
17. Uchegbu, R.I.; Ahuchaogu, A.A.; Amanze, K.O.; Ibe, C.O. Chemical Constituents Analysis of the Leaves of *Bryophyllum pinnatum* by GC-MS. *AASCIT J. Chem.* **2017**, *3*, 19–22.
18. Dhanya, R. Quercetin for managing type 2 diabetes and its complications, an insight into multitarget therapy. *Biomed. Pharmacother.* **2021**, *146*, 112560. [CrossRef]
19. Ozsoy, S.; Becer, E.; Kabadayi, H.; Vatansever, H.S.; Yucecan, S. Quercetin-mediated apoptosis and Cellular Senescence in human Colon cancer. *Anticancer. Agents Med. Chem.* **2020**, *20*, 1387–1396. [CrossRef] [PubMed]
20. Liu, C.Y.; Huang, C.J.; Huang, L.H.; Chen, I.J.; Chiu, J.P.; Hsu, C.H. Effects of Green Tea Extract on Insulin Resistance and Glucagon-Like Peptide 1 in Patients with Type 2 Diabetes and Lipid Abnormalities: A Randomized, Double-Blinded, and Placebo-Controlled Trial. *PLoS ONE* **2014**, *9*, 91163. [CrossRef]
21. Williams, R.J.; Spencer, J.P.E.; Rice-Evans, C. Flavonoids: Antioxidants or signaling molecules? *Free Radic. Biol. Med.* **2004**, *36*, 838–849. [CrossRef]
22. Wang, Y.; Liu, M.; Chen, S.; Wu, Q. *Avicularin* inhibits cell proliferation and induces cell apoptosis in cutaneous squamous cell carcinoma. *Exp. Ther. Med.* **2019**, *19*, 1065–1071. [CrossRef]
23. Lee, J.S.; Lee, A.Y.; Quilantang, N.G.; Geraldino, P.J.L.; Cho, E.J.; Lee, S. Anti-oxidant activity of avicularin and isovitexin from *Lespedeza cuneate*. *J. Appl. Biol. Chem.* **2019**, *62*, 143–147. [CrossRef]
24. Agüero-Hernández, A.L.; Rosales-López, C.; Herrera, C.; Vargas-Picado, A.; Muñoz, R.; Abdelnour-Esquivel, A. Hypoglycemic effect of *Kalanchoe pinnata* (Lam.) Pers. *Leaf Extract. Pharmacogn. J.* **2020**, *12*, 557–561. [CrossRef]
25. Yang, Y.; Chen, Z.; Zhao, X.; Xie, H.; Du, L.; Gao, H.; Xie, C. Mechanisms of Kaempferol in the treatment of diabetes: A comprehensive and latest review. *Front. Endocrinol.* **2022**, *13*, 990299. [CrossRef]
26. de-Araújo, E.; Guerra, G.; Araújo, D.; de Araújo, A.; Fernandes, J.; Júnior, R.D.A.; da Silva, V.; de Carvalho, T.; Ferreira, L.; Zucolotto, S. Gastroprotective and Antioxidant Activity of Kalanchoe brasiliensis and Kalanchoe pinnata Leaf Juices against Indomethacin and Ethanol-Induced Gastric Lesions in Rats. *Int. J. Mol. Sci.* **2018**, *19*, 1265. [CrossRef]
27. Palacz-Wrobel, M.; Borkowska, P.; Paul-Samojedny, M.; Kowalczyk, M.; Fila-Danilow, A.; Suchanek-Raif, R.; Kowalski, J. Effect of apigenin, kaempferol and resveratrol on the gene expression and protein secretion of tumor necrosis factor alpha (TNF-α) and interleukin-10 (IL-10) in RAW-264.7 macrophages. *Biomed. Pharmacother.* **2017**, *93*, 1205–1212. [CrossRef] [PubMed]
28. Huang, H.C.; Chang, W.T.; Lee, M.S.; Chen, H.Y.; Chen, Y.H.; Lin, C.C.; Lin, M.K. Three bufadienolides induce cell death in the human lung cancer cell line CL1-5 mainly through autophagy. *Bioorg Med. Chem. Lett.* **2021**, *31*, 127715. [CrossRef]
29. Halayal, R.Y.; Bagewadi, Z.K.; Aldabaan, N.A.; Shaikh, I.A.; Khan, A.A. Exploring the therapeutic mechanism of potential phytocompounds from *Kalanchoe pinnata* in the treatment of diabetes mellitus by integrating network pharmacology, molecular docking and simulation approach. *Saudi Pharm. J.* **2024**, *32*, 102026. [CrossRef]
30. Singh, R.P.; Pattnaik, A.K. Scientific insights into hyperlipidemia mitigation: A profound examination of isolated bioactive fractions of *Kalanchoe pinnata* (Lam.) leaves and their therapeutic implications using in vitro, in vivo, and in silico study from the characterized compounds using HPTLC MS/MS analysis. *Pharmacogn. Mag.* **2024**, *20*, 863–876.
31. Menon, N.; Sparks, J.; Omoruyi, F. Hypoglycemic and Hypocholesterolemic Activities of the Aqueous Preparation of *Kalanchoe pinnata* Leaves in Streptozotocin-induced Diabetic Rats. *Asian Pac. J. Trop. Biomed.* **2015**, *5*, 3–9. [CrossRef]
32. Matthew, S.; Singh, D.; Jaiswal, S.; Jayakar, M.K.B.; Bhowmik, D. Antidiabetic activity of *Kalanchoe pinnata* (Lam.) Pers. in alloxan-induced diabetic rats. *J. Chem. Pharm. Sci.* **2013**, *6*, 1–7.
33. Ojewole, J.A.O. Antinociceptive, anti-inflammatory and antidiabetic effects of *Bryophyllum pinnatum* (Crassulaceae) leaf aqueous extract. *J. Ethnopharmacol.* **2005**, *99*, 13–19. [CrossRef] [PubMed]
34. Patil, S.B.; Dongare, V.R.; Kulkarni, C.R.; Joglekar, M.M.; Arvindekar, A.U. Antidiabetic activity of *Kalanchoe pinnata* in streptozotocin-induced diabetic rats by glucose-independent insulin secretagogue action. *Pharm. Biol.* **2013**, *51*, 1411–1418. [CrossRef]
35. Ramon, P.; Sparks, J.; Omoruyi, F. Effect of Combined *K. pinnata* and Metformin Preparation on Inflammatory Cytokines in Normal and Diabetic Skeletal Muscle Cells. *J. Med. Food.* **2021**, *24*, 732–740. [CrossRef] [PubMed]
36. Benjamin, B. Screening methods for the evaluation of anti-hyperlipidemic drugs. In *Introduction to Basics of Pharmacology and Toxicology*; Lakshmanan, M., Shewade, D.G., Raj, G.M., Eds.; Springer: Singapore, 2022; pp. 363–369.
37. Kader, M.A.; Rahman, M.M.; Mahmud, S.; Khan, M.S.; Mukta, S.; Zohora, F.T. A comparative study on the anti-hyperlipidemic and antibacterial potency of the shoot and flower extracts of *Melastoma malabathricum* Linn's. *Clin. Phytosci.* **2023**, *9*, 5. [CrossRef]
38. Singh, R.; Nain, S. Anti-hyperlipidemic activity of ethanolic and aqueous extracts of Asparagus racemosus and Chlorophytum borivilianum leaves in albino rats. *Proc. Natl. Acad. Sci. India Sect. B Biol. Sci.* **2023**, *93*, 431–441. [CrossRef]
39. Goyal, P.; Jain, N.; Panwar, N.S.; Singh, G.K.; Nagori, B.P. Investigation of hypoglycemic and antidiabetic activities of ethanol extracts of *Kalanchoe pinnata* leaves in streptozocin-induced diabetic rats. *Int. J. Pharm. Toxicol. Sci.* **2013**, *3*, 9–18.

40. Abchir, O.; Yamari, I.; Nour, H.; Daoui, O.; Elkhattabi, S.; Errougui, A.; Chtita, S. Structure-based Virtual Screening, ADMET analysis, and molecular dynamics simulation of Moroccan natural compounds as candidates α-amylase inhibitors. *ChemistrySelect* **2023**, *8*, e202301092. [CrossRef]
41. Menon, N.; Sparks, J.; Omoruyi, F.O. Oxidative Stress Parameters and Erythrocyte Membrane Adenosine Triphosphatase Activities in Streptozotocin-induced Diabetic Rats Administered Aqueous Preparation of *Kalanchoe pinnata* Leaves. *Pharmacogn. Res.* **2016**, *8*, 85–88.
42. Hansen, B.F.; Danielsen, G.M.; Drejer, K.; Sørensen, A.R.; Wiberg, F.C.; Klein, H.H.; Lundemose, A.G. Sustained signaling from the insulin receptor after stimulation with insulin analogues exhibiting increased mitogenic potency. *Biochem. J.* **1996**, *315*, 271–279. [CrossRef] [PubMed]
43. Kalyanaraman, B. Teaching the basics of redox biology to medical and graduate students: Oxidants, antioxidants and disease mechanisms. *Redox Biol.* **2013**, *1*, 244–257. [CrossRef]
44. Phung, C.D.; Ezieme, J.A.; Turrens, J.F. Hydrogen peroxide metabolism in skeletal muscle mitochondria. *Arch. Biochem. Biophys.* **1994**, *315*, 479–482. [CrossRef]
45. Saeed, K.; Chughtai, M.F.J.; Khaliq, A.; Liaqat, A.; Mehmood, T.; Khalid, M.Z.; Kasongo, E.L.M. Impact of extraction techniques and process optimization on antioxidant and antibacterial potential of *Kalanchoe pinnata* leaf extract. *Int. J. Food Prop.* **2024**, *27*, 909–926. [CrossRef]
46. Tajudin, N.J.; Ismail, I.N. Antimicrobial Activity of *Kalanchoe pinnata*: A review. *MJoSHT* **2022**, *8*, 31–37. [CrossRef]
47. Al-Jumaili, M.H.; Siddique, F.; Abul Qais, F.; Hashem, H.E.; Chtita, S.; Rani, A.; Uzair, M.; Almzaien, K.A. Analysis and prediction pathways of natural products and their cytotoxicity against HeLa cell line protein using docking, molecular dynamics and ADMET. *JBSD* **2023**, *41*, 765–777. [CrossRef]
48. de-Araujo, E.R.D.; Felix-Silva, J.; Xavier-Santos, J.B.; Fernandes, J.M.; Guerra, G.C.B.; de Araujo, A.A.; de Souza Araújo, D.F.; de Santis Ferreira, L.; da Silva Júnior, A.A.; de Freitas Fernandes-Pedrosa, M.; et al. Local anti-inflammatory activity: Topical formulation containing *Kalanchoe brasiliensis* and *Kalanchoe pinnata* leaf aqueous extract. *Biomed. Pharmacother.* **2019**, *113*, 108721. [CrossRef]
49. Hamim, S.I.; Roney, M.; Uddin, M.N.; Issahaku, A.R.; Chhando, K.S.; Aluwi, M.F.; Omar, N.A. Investigating the potential compounds of *Kalanchoe pinnata* plant for the treatment of Inflammation utilizing molecular docking and molecular dynamic simulation approach. *Silico Res. Biomed.* **2025**, *1*, 100007. [CrossRef]
50. Steinbacher, P.; Eckl, P. Impact of oxidative stress on exercising skeletal muscle. *Biomolecules* **2015**, *5*, 356–377. [CrossRef]
51. Haraldsen, G.; Kvale, D.; Lien, B.; Farstad, I.N.; Brandtzaeg, P. Cytokine-regulated expression of E-selectin, intercellular adhesion molecule-1 (ICAM-1), and vascular cell adhesion molecule-1 (VCAM-1) in human microvascular endothelial cells. *J. Immunol.* **1996**, *156*, 2558–2563. [CrossRef] [PubMed]
52. Kong, L.; Luo, C.; Li, X.; Zhou, Y.; He, H. The anti-inflammatory effect of kaempferol on early atherosclerosis in high cholesterol fed rabbits. *Lipids Health Dis.* **2013**, *12*, 115. [CrossRef]
53. Lowenstein, C.; Matsushita, K. The acute phase response and atherosclerosis. *Drug Discov. Today Dis. Mech.* **2004**, *1*, 17–22. [CrossRef]
54. Hernández-Caballero, M.E.; Sierra-Ramírez, J.A.; Villalobos-Valencia, R.; Seseña-Méndez, E. Potential of *Kalanchoe pinnata* as a Cancer Treatment Adjuvant and an Epigenetic Regulator. *Molecules* **2022**, *27*, 6425. [CrossRef] [PubMed]
55. Oufir, M.; Seiler, C.; Gerodetti, M.; Gerber, J.; Fürer, K.; Mennet-von Eiff, M.; Elsas, S.M.; Brenneisen, R.; von Mandach, U.; Hamburger, M.; et al. Quantification of bufadienolides in *Bryophyllum pinnatum* leaves and manufactured products by UHPLC-ESIMS/MS. *Planta Medica* **2015**, *81*, 1190–1197. [CrossRef]
56. Stefanowicz-Hajduk, J.; Hering, A.; Gucwa, M.; Hałasa, R.; Soluch, A.; Kowalczyk, M.; Stochmal, A.; Ochocka, R. Biological activities of leaf extracts from selected Kalanchoe species and their relationship with bufadienolides content. *Pharm. Biol.* **2020**, *58*, 732–740. [CrossRef] [PubMed]
57. Yadav, N.P.; Dixit, V.K. Hepatoprotective activity of leaves of *Kalanchoe pinnata* Pers. *J. Ethnopharmacol.* **2003**, *86*, 197–202. [CrossRef]
58. Bigoniya, P.; Sohgaura, A.K.; Shrivastava, B. Antilithiatic effect of *C. dactylon*, *E. officinalis*, *K. pinnata*, and *B. nutans* ethyl acetate fraction on glyoxylate-induced nephrolithiasis. *FJPS* **2021**, *7*, 79. [CrossRef]
59. Priya, F.J.; Leemarose, A.; Vidhya, S.; Arputharaj, A.; Akshana, S.; Fathima, U.R. A New Frontier Drug Development in Nanomedicine and Its Anti-urolithiatic Activity of *Kalanchoe pinnata*. *Orient. J. Chem.* **2021**, *37*, 444–449. [CrossRef]
60. Ranaweera, S.; Weerasinghe, S.; Tarannum, F.; Walters, K.B. Inhibition and dissolution of calcium oxalate crystals and kidney stones by the extract of *Kalanchoe pinnata*. *J. Med. Plants Res.* **2023**, *17*, 201–217. [CrossRef]
61. Ehi-Omosun, M.B.; Etunim, S.C. Effects of Aqueous Leaf Extract of *Kalanchoe pinnata* on Bifenthrin-Induced Injury in the Lungs of the Adult Wistar Rat. *JASEM* **2023**, *27*, 1159–1164.

62. Martins Fernandes Pereira, K.; de Carvalho, A.C.; Fernandes, B.H.V.; Grecco, S.D.S.; Rodrigues, E.; Fernandes, M.J.D.S.; de Carvalho, L.R.S.; Nakamura, M.U.; Guo, S.; Hernández, R.B. Systems toxicology studies reveal important insights about chronic exposure of zebrafish to *Kalanchoe pinnata* (Lam.) Pers leaf—KPL: Implications for medicinal use. *J. Ethnopharmacol.* **2025**, *338*, 119044. [CrossRef]
63. Kolodziejczyk-Czepas, J.; Stochmal, A. Bufadienolides of *Kalanchoe* species: An overview of chemical structure, biological activity and prospects for pharmacological use. *Phytochem. Rev.* **2017**, *16*, 1155–1171. [CrossRef] [PubMed]
64. Saravanan, V.; Murugan, S.S.; Navaneetha Krishnan, K.R.; Mohana, N.; Sakthive, K.; Sathya, T.N. Toxicological assessment of ethanolic leaves extract of *Kalanchoe pinnata* in rats. *Indian. J. Forensic. Med. Toxicol.* **2021**, *15*, 615–622. [CrossRef]
65. Bhavsar, S.; Chandel, D. Cytotoxic and genotoxic effects of *Kalanchoe pinnata* (Lam.) Pers. fresh leaf juice in the cultured human blood lymphocytes. *Drug. Chem. Toxicol.* **2022**, *45*, 360–366. [CrossRef]
66. Ghosh, S.; Manchala, S.; Raghunath, M.; Sharma, G.; Singh, A.K.; Sinha, J.K. Role of Phytomolecules in the Treatment of Obesity: Targets, Mechanisms and Limitations. *Curr. Top. Med. Chem.* **2021**, *21*, 863–877. [CrossRef]
67. Wiesmüller, L.; Ford, J.M.; Schiestl, R.H. DNA Damage, Repair, and Diseases. *J. Biomed. Biotechnol.* **2002**, *2*, 45. [CrossRef]
68. Bi, Q.R.; Hou, J.J.; Qi, P.; Ma, C.H.; Shen, Y.; Feng, R.H.; Yan, B.P.; Wang, J.W.; Shi, X.J.; Zheng, Y.Y.; et al. Venenum Bufonis induces rat neuroinflammation by activiating NF-κB pathway and attenuation of BDNF. *J. Ethnopharmacol.* **2016**, *186*, 103–110. [CrossRef] [PubMed]
69. Fan, Y.; Zhang, W.; Iqbal, Z.; Li, X.; Lin, Z.; Wu, Z.; Li, Q.; Dong, H.; Zhang, X.; Gong, P.; et al. Rod-shaped mesoporous silica nanoparticles reduce bufalin cardiotoxicity and inhibit colon cancer by blocking lipophagy. *Lipids Health Dis.* **2024**, *23*, 318. [CrossRef]
70. Lin, R.; Ye, Q.; He, Q.; Kim, D.S.; Chen, D.; Jin, L.; Wang, W.; Li, J. Mechanistic analysis of anti-prostate cancer and toxicity-reducing effects of bufadienolides extracts: Comparative efficacy and safety with isolated bioactive compounds. *J. Ethnopharmacol.* **2025**, *352*, 120182. [CrossRef]
71. Moreno, Y.; Banuls, L.; Urban, E.; Gelbcke, M.; Dufrasne, F.; Kopp, B.; Kiss, R.; Zehl, M. Structure-activity relationship analysis of bufadienolide-induced in vitro growth inhibitory effects on mouse and human cancer cells. *J. Nat. Prod.* **2013**, *76*, 1078–1084. [CrossRef] [PubMed]
72. Wang, Y.; Lonard, D.M.; Yu, Y.; Chow, D.C.; Palzkill, T.G.; Wang, J.; Qi, R.; Matzuk, A.J.; Song, X.; Madoux, F.; et al. Bufalin is a potent small-molecule inhibitor of the steroid receptor coactivators SRC-3 and SRC-1. *Cancer Res.* **2014**, *74*, 1506–1517. [CrossRef]
73. Wang, Z.J.; Sun, L.; Heinbockel, T. Resibufogenin and cinobufagin activate central neurons through an ouabain-like action. *PLoS ONE* **2014**, *9*, e113272. [CrossRef] [PubMed]
74. Shao, H.; Li, B.; Li, H.; Gao, L.; Zhang, C.; Sheng, H.; Zhu, L. Novel Strategies for Solubility and Bioavailability Enhancement of Bufadienolides. *Molecules* **2021**, *27*, 51. [CrossRef]
75. Gardiner, P.; Filippelli, A.C.; Low Dog, T. Prescribing botanicals. In *Integrative Medicine*, 4th ed.; Rakel, D., Ed.; Elsevier: Philadelphia, PA, USA, 2018; pp. 979–985.

pharmaceuticals

MDPI

Review

Chaya Leaf: A Promising Approach for Diabetes Management

Fabiola Curiel Ayala [1], Francisco Ignacio García Rodríguez [1], Sandra N. Jimenez-Garcia [2] and Lina Garcia-Mier [1,*]

[1] División de Ciencias de la Salud, Universidad del Valle de México, Campus Querétaro, Blvd. Juriquilla No. 1000, Santa Rosa Jáuregui, Santiago de Querétaro C.P. 76230, QRO, Mexico; fabiola.curiel@uvmnet.edu (F.C.A.); a110167380@my.uvm.edu.mx (F.I.G.R.)

[2] Departamento de Enfermería y Obstetricia, División de Ciencias de la Salud e Ingeniería, Campus Celaya-Salvatierra, Universidad de Guanajuato, Av. Mutualismo Esq. Prolongación Río Lerma S/N, Celaya C.P. 38060, GTO, Mexico; sandra_neli_j@hotmail.com

* Correspondence: linamier@hotmail.com

Abstract: Chaya leaf has long been used in folk medicine and is gaining scientific interest for its potential role in diabetes management. Recent research indicates that chaya leaf may help to regulate glucose, enhance insulin secretion, and reduce related complications, primarily due to the presence of bioactive compounds such as polyphenols and flavonoids. These compounds are believed to enhance insulin sensitivity and offer protection against oxidative stress, a key contributor to diabetes-related complications. Chaya extracts, particularly methanolic and aqueous forms, have shown anti-diabetic effects in animal models, lowering blood glucose, cholesterol, and triglycerides and reducing inflammation; their bioactive compounds, like quercetin, rutin, and ferulic acid, may enhance the insulin response, reduce inflammation, and improve antioxidant activity. Some studies warn of potential interactions with metformin. This review compiles findings from the past five years, drawing from databases such as PubMed, SciELO, ScienceDirect, Dialnet, Web of Science, and Google Scholar. It highlights chaya's phytochemical profile, explores proposed anti-diabetic mechanisms, and summarizes evidence from in vivo, in vitro, and clinical studies. The results indicate that adding chaya leaf to the diet may help people with diabetes as a complementary therapy to conventional treatment; nonetheless, further clinical studies are required to comprehend the exact mechanisms and define specific usage instructions. Further investigation into the specific types of compounds present in chaya, their effective dosages, and their safety in human populations is essential to support its integration into medical practice.

Keywords: chaya leaf; diabetes; hypoglycemic effects; traditional medicine

1. Introduction

There is rising interest in investigating and recognizing sources like medicinal plants that have important phytochemicals and superior nutritional content compared to processed foods [1–3]. These sources could be used to create medications or food items that might aid in the prevention or management of transmissible chronic illnesses. Noncommunicable diseases (NCDs) are health conditions that develop from interactions among factors and external influences, like the environment and physiology, which need continuous attention and management and could result in disability or early mortality [4]. Key NCD categories encompass cancer, diabetes, heart diseases, and chronic respiratory disorders. NCD-related fatalities represented 71 percent of deaths and comprised 14 of the leading causes of death in the Americas in 2019 [4,5]. In the first half of 2021, in Mexico, over 1.5 million cases of non-communicable diseases were reported. There has been a rise in people using plants, which have been crucial in health for centuries, mostly to treat injuries or illnesses [6–9]. For a plant to be labeled "medicinal", it must show scientifically verified effects. Mexico boasts a variety of plants, totaling around 4500 species; however, only a small fraction of them, roughly 5%, have undergone pharmacological assessment [10]. One such plant that remains underexplored from this standpoint is chaya, which has been gaining attention for its health benefits, including blood sugar regulation [11,12]. Despite its properties, its application currently relies on empirical knowledge passed down through generations via oral communication, online publications, and recipe books. Knowledge about the bioactive compounds responsible for its health benefits, as well as whether there may be toxic or hazardous compounds in the plant, remains absent [13,14]. For this reason, the main aim of this review is to offer insights into the existing understanding of chaya's role in managing diabetes and to delve into future research avenues, as well to promote the incorporation of foods that have been ancestrally used as therapeutic alternatives. Mechanisms of action, involving bioactive substances, as well as in vivo and in vitro studies, are summarized. Most of the details regarding the use of chaya to treat diabetes were mainly gathered from the last five years. We also included relevant information from earlier years. To conduct this review on chaya, a comprehensive search was performed across several scientific databases, including PubMed, Scielo, Science Direct, Dialnet, Web of Science, and Google Scholar. Keywords used in the search included "chaya", "*Cnidoscolus chayamansa*", "chaya leaf", "diabetes", and "*Cnidoscolus aconitifolius*". First, Google Scholar was explored to determine whether the required information was available, where an initial number of 2310 articles were obtained. Then, the other databases were used. Articles were selected based on their relevance to the nutritional, pharmacological, and ethnobotanical aspects of chaya. Studies in English and Spanish were included. Duplicate, non-scientific, thesis, and popular articles were excluded. After screening the titles and abstracts, a total of 37 articles were selected for detailed review. The manuscripts were initially chosen based on their titles, before moving on to the abstracts and conducting an analysis of the text to confirm that they contained relevant information related to the subjects discussed in this review. The inclusion and exclusion of articles in this review focused on selecting studies that addressed key aspects of diabetes mellitus, as well as the implications of metabolites for the anti-diabetic effects of chaya. We performed the identification, screening, and selection according to the criteria stated previously.

2. Botanical and Ethnobotanical Information of *C. chayamansa*

The plant known as chaya is also recognized by the names *Cnidoscolus chayamansa* McVaugh and *Cnidoscolus aconitifolius* (Mill) [12,15]. It is also referred to as "tree spinach", or "quelite" [16]. It belongs to the *Euphorbiaceae* family and the genus *Cnidoscolus* spp. (Figure 1), which are distinguished by the number of lobes and the shape of their leaves. In the case of chaya, its leaves have three lobes connected by a petiole to the main stem. The plant can reach heights of 5 to 6 m based on the quality of the soil and its environment. It is native to the Yucatán Peninsula and is now grown in regions like Hidalgo and San Luis Potosí in Mexico. It is also being cultivated in Belize and Guatemala, as well as in the United States and Africa [12,15–17].

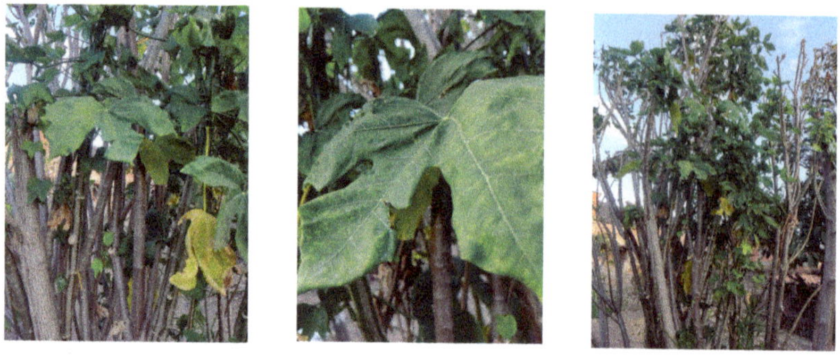

Figure 1. Chaya plant.

The chaya plant, or *Cnidoscolus chayamansa*, is commonly referred to as "chaya" or tree spinach, originating from the Maya regions in the Americas. It is a variety of the *Cnidoscolus aconitifolius* plant due to its lack of stinging hairs, which can cause skin irritation during harvesting. *C. chayamansa* is a cultivated, spineless (non-stinging) version of *C. aconitifolius*, selected for safer handling and easier consumption. It is not a separate species but a domesticated variant developed to be more suitable for human handling and food use. It is often grown in home gardens and used in cooking. When cooked as a vegetable dish for consumption purposes, chaya is rich in vitamin C content, along with beta carotene, proteins, calcium, phosphorus, iron, and vitamins, including riboflavin and niacin [12,15,18].

Throughout history, animals like livestock and horses have been given chaya as a food source. Historical records from the Maya civilization indicate that it was also consumed by humans due to its nutritional value [16]. Chaya stands out for its protein content exceeding 5%, containing seven of the nine essential amino acids (leucine, isoleucine, valine, lysine, methionine, phenylalanine, and threonine), and it has crude fiber content higher than 2% [12,19]. For this reason, people incorporate chaya leaves into their diets or consume them as an infusion. It is recommended to subject the leaves to heat treatment before consumption due to the presence of cyanogenic glycosides—compounds that are harmful to living beings but necessary for the plant's defense against predators [16,20]. Cyanogenic glycosides release cyanide when the plant is damaged. In chaya, the main cyanogenic compound is linamarin (as found in cassava), but this is reduced to a safe level when the plant is cooked. The nutritional value of the plant may vary according to environmental fluctuations, soil conditions, biotic factors, agricultural practices, and postharvest handling.

Preparing teas or infusions from the leaves is a common tradition in managing diabetes mellitus. In addition, the stems and roots can be utilized to brew infusions [12]. Some other customary applications encompass treating kidney stones, hemorrhoids, and eye ailments, as well as enhancing blood flow, lung decongestant effects promoting lactation, enhanced memory and brain function, and lowering cholesterol levels. In some laboratory experiments, chaya has demonstrated potential in terms of hypoglycemic and anti-diabetic properties. Doses and extraction methods vary from study to study, and most of the plants used are related to folk practices, since it is necessary to systematically explore extraction methods, concentrations, and doses. The present review identifies doses and extract concentrations.

Traditionally, chaya infusions were produced using water as a solvent. However, it was noted that some compounds were not fully extracted with water alone; therefore, other solvents, such as methanol and ethanol—and, in some cases, acetone—were used to improve the extraction efficiency. Studies have primarily examined the impacts of solvent extracts of chaya leaves, with findings showing that adding chaya leaves to the diets of rats had the effect of protecting the brain by reducing acetylcholinesterase levels, according to one study [21]. Furthermore, the capacity to lower blood sugar levels, as well as cholesterol and triglyceride levels, has been studied. Ethanolic extracts from chaya leaves have demonstrated promising results [22]. A recent study [19] revealed that ethanolic chaya extracts and ascorbate conferred protection against kidney and testicular damage induced by dimethylnitrosamine. Moreover, chaya shows antioxidant properties, along with inflammatory and cardioprotective effects, due to the presence of sterols, flavonoids, coumarins, and saponins [11].

Moreover, umami plays a role in developing food products by offering a rich and savory taste that improves overall food appeal. This characteristic flavor is primarily due to the presence of free amino acids, such as glutamic acid and aspartic acid, as well as 5′-nucleotides, such as 5′-AMP and 5′-GMP, along with 5′-inosine monophosphate. A research study has pinpointed acids, 5′-AMP, and short peptides as the umami components found in chaya leaves. Additionally, besides their umami flavor, chaya leaves are recognized for their medicinal properties, offering benefits for conditions such as diabetes and rheumatism, as well as gastrointestinal disorders and inflammation [23].

3. Phytochemistry of the Species *Cnidoscolus*

From a chemical perspective, the leaves and stems of this species have been identified to contain proteins and vitamins such as thiamine, niacin, riboflavin, retinol, beta-carotene, and ascorbic acid. It also contains minerals like calcium, iron, phosphorus, potassium, magnesium, sodium, manganese, zinc, and copper. Due to the presence of essential amino acids, the species is considered to have high nutritional value (the essential amino acids present in chaya are building blocks for protein synthesis in the body). Proteins are essential for the growth and repair of tissues, including muscles, skin, and organs [23].

The leaves contain essential oils and fatty acids like palmitic, oleic, stearic, myristic, arachidonic, and lauric acids, as well as flavones, including quercetin and kaempferol, among others like amentoflavone and astragalin (kaempferol-3-O-rutinoside). Moreover, coumarin, naringin, rutin, catechin, protocatechuic acid, and dihydromyricetin are also present in the leaves. Numerous harmful secondary substances have been identified, including glycosides like linamarin and compounds such as tannins, saponins, and lignin, which are typically removed through cooking and do not represent a safety concern [23].

Various investigations have explored the composition of *C. chayamansa* leaves through high-performance liquid chromatography (HPLC). It was discovered that the leaves harbored protocatechuic acid at a concentration of 0.242 mg/g and rutin at 2 mg/g by comparing them to known standards [24]. Chlorogenic acid in fresh leaves amounted to 1217.3 meq/kg, decreasing to 733.5 meq/kg in cooked leaves. Quercetin and kaempferol levels were measured at 44.7 μg/g and 22.4 μg/g, respectively, in raw leaves, and they decreased slightly in cooked leaves to 40.2 μg/g and 18.1 μg/g, respectively. Other identified compounds included kaempferol-3-O-rhamnosylglucoside, kaempferol-3-O-rhamnosylgalactoside-7-O-rhamnoside, and quercetin-3-O-rhamnoside in different concentrations [25].

Methanolic leaf extracts were analyzed for phenolic content using the Folin–Ciocalteu method. It was found that gallic acid (71.3 ± 1.7 mg/g), catechin (42.6 ± 3.7 mg/g), protocatechuic acid (0.24 mg/g), and rutin (2.0 mg/g) were present. Three organic extracts of the leaves were evaluated, identifying flavonoids and coumarins in the ethyl acetate extract; flavonoids, coumarins, and lignins in the ethanolic extract; and various fatty acids in the hexane extract, such as lauric acid (31.9%), myristic acid (11.7%), palmitic acid (28.3%), oleic acid (5%), and arachidonic acid (4.8%) [11,24]. The content of linamarin in the leaves and petioles of *Cnidoscolus chayamansa*, with evaluations of frozen and fresh samples, was higher in frozen samples (11.90 ± 1.8 μg/g in leaves and 14.79 ± 0.9 μg/g in petioles) than in fresh samples (2.89 ± 0.1 μg/g in leaves and 3.72 ± 1.5 μg/g in petioles). Similar results were obtained with UV–vis spectrometry, showing concentrations of 1.28 ± 0.4 μg/g in fresh leaves and 2.63 ± 0.4 μg/g in petioles, compared to 4.93 ± 2.3 μg/g in frozen leaves and 6.25 ± 0.2 μg/g in frozen petioles. The increase in linamarin in frozen plants is attributed to a physiological response to cold, which causes structural changes in lipid membranes and protein synthesis. Regarding hydrogen cyanide (HCN), the concentration in methanolic extracts determined by acid/base titration was 2.37 mg/100 g of dry extract by acid titration and 4.25 mg/100 g by alkaline titration. These levels are well below the FDA limit (20 mg HCN/100 g), indicating that chaya is safe for consumption after a five-minute cooking process. The HCN levels in chaya are considerably lower than those reported in broad beans and cassava, which range between 200 and 300 mg HCN/100 g [26]. Chaya, valued for its high content of proteins and polyphenols, was evaluated in its leaves and protein concentrates through SDS–gel electrophoresis, FTIR, and DSC. Amino acids, protein efficiency, and bioavailability were analyzed, finding protein purity of 63.52%. The identified polyphenols included anthocyanidins, hydroxycinnamic acids, hydroxybenzoic acids, and flavonols, suggesting that chaya may serve as a potential alternative source for functional foods [27].

In a study analyzing the chemical constituents of chaya leaves, samples were desiccated using both shade-drying and oven-drying techniques. Oven drying was found to be more efficient in minimizing residual moisture. The extraction of compounds was conducted through maceration using petroleum ether, ethanol, and distilled water. An examination of the constituents was executed via Soxhlet extraction processes, revealing the presence of flavonoids, alkaloids, tannins, and saponins. The moisture and total ash levels (10.7%) were within the established parameters, validating the quality of the plant [28].

4. Diabetes

Diabetes mellitus is a chronic condition caused by the body's resistance to insulin, which leads to disturbances in maintaining glucose balance and can result in blood sugar fluctuations and complications related to blood vessels. The prevalence of diabetes and metabolic diseases is rapidly increasing worldwide, becoming a significant health issue with associated personal, social, and economic burdens. Data from the International Diabetes Federation indicate that an estimated 463 million adults globally are affected by diabetes. If no measures are taken to address this pandemic, projections suggest that around 578 million individuals could be dealing with diabetes by the year 2030, and this number might increase even further to 700 million by 2045. The yearly worldwide healthcare spending related to diabetes has been approximated at USD 760 billion. Therefore, the projected direct costs associated with managing diabetes are expected to reach USD 825 billion (USD 2500 per person in the US) by the year 2030 and further rise to USD 845 billion (around USD 2600 per person in the US) by the year 2045 [29].

The widespread occurrence and diverse causes of diabetes emphasize the importance of finding treatments that can address its nature and associated complications effectively. Phytotherapeutic agents from natural sources, including chaya, are increasingly preferred over synthetic drugs because of their chemical diversity and lower incidence of adverse effects [30]. Assessments of plant-based sources have shown that certain natural substances directly enhance insulin secretion, prevent apoptosis in pancreatic beta cells, and modulate the differentiation and proliferation of pancreatic beta cells. Consequently, bioactive natural compounds offer significant potential as sources of new medications [31].

4.1. Utilization in Diabetes

4.1.1. Mechanisms of Action

The mechanisms of action of chaya against diabetes appear to be linked to compounds that influence the regulation of blood glucose levels. According to research findings, chaya extracts (especially methanolic and aqueous extracts) contain flavonoids like quercetin and rutin that could potentially lower blood sugar levels. The presence of antioxidants in chaya may aid in boosting insulin sensitivity for the management of blood sugar levels. Oxidative stress reduction by antioxidants could potentially enhance the performance of beta cells in the pancreas in terms of insulin production [24].

In diabetes, especially type 2 diabetes, cells undergo changes in how they process glucose, which may result in the production of oxygen species (ROS). These substances can harm cells by causing damage, including among beta cells that produce insulin, and can worsen insulin malfunction and resistance to it. Flavonoids are compounds found in chaya leaves and various plants, and they possess antioxidant qualities that enable them to counteract ROS' effects by reducing oxidative stress and safeguarding cells from harm. This is crucial for diabetic cells, as it helps to maintain cellular function and protects against diabetic complications. In diabetes, especially when poorly controlled, LDL levels may be elevated. Circulating LDL can undergo oxidation due to high ROS concentrations, becoming oxidized LDL (oxLDL), which is particularly harmful. oxLDL contributes to the development of atherosclerosis, a condition where the arteries harden and narrow due to cholesterol plaque buildup, increasing the risk of cardiovascular diseases. The consumption of flavonoids, such as those present in chaya leaves, can offer significant benefits for individuals with diabetes by reducing oxidative stress, improving cardiovascular health, and protecting cells from damage. These combined effects may aid in better diabetes management and reduce the risk of associated complications [24].

An increase in LDL levels in the bloodstream poses a risk of artery disease, especially when it comes to oxidized LDL cholesterol. The "oxidative hypothesis of atherogenesis" suggests that the development of atheroma begins with foam cells generated from macrophages absorbing oxidized LDL uncontrollably within the subendothelium. These lipoproteins are harmful to the endothelium since they attract macrophages and monocytes to accumulate in the layer of blood vessels. This accumulation contributes to diseases like artery disease and is closely linked to diabetes, significantly heightening the risk of such conditions [24].

Methanolic extracts from chaya have been found to boost the activity of beta cells and enhance insulin secretion, helping to regulate blood glucose levels in rats with diabetes induced by streptozotocin (STZ). However, the mechanism does not resemble insulin's action. Rather, it encourages efficient beta cell function. Oxidative stress is implicated in the pathogenesis of diabetes-related complications, including neuropathy, nephropathy, and retinopathy; nevertheless, the antioxidant compounds found in chaya may mitigate oxidative damage and thereby contribute to the prevention or delay of these complications [24].

The plant's effectiveness in lowering blood sugar levels through activity seems to depend on the concentration of the extract being used, according to studies conducted with different doses, which revealed similar outcomes to commonly prescribed medications like metformin and glibenclamide [32]. When tested on rats in lab settings, chaya methanolic extracts showed a decrease in blood glucose levels after glucose intake, which hints at its potential in managing post-meal blood sugar spikes [33]. The bioactive components found in the extract, including quercetin and rutin, are believed to be responsible for these properties. These substances could enhance the body's response to insulin and have antioxidant effects, offering properties that support the management of diabetes [26]. Figure **??** represents mechanism of action of quercetin.

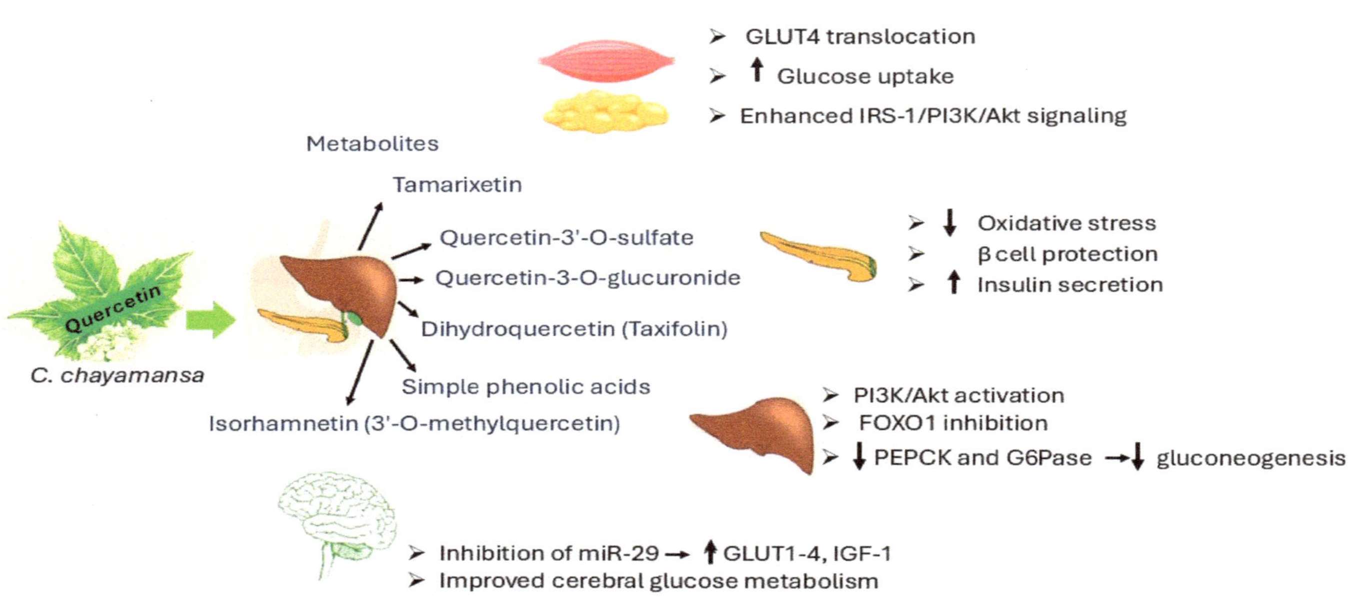

Figure 2. Mechanism of action of quercetin [34–39]. Akt = protein kinase B; FOXO1 = Forkhead box protein O1; G6Pase = glucose-6-phosphatase; GLUT1–4 = glucose transporter 1–4; GLUT 4 = glucose transporter type 4; IGF-1 = insulin-like growth factor-1; IRS-1 = insulin receptor substrate 1; miR-29 = microRNA-29; PEPCK = phosphoenolpyruvate carboxykinase; PI3K = phosphoinositide 3-kinase.

In addition to reducing glucose levels, chaya extracts have also been shown to reduce cholesterol and triglyceride levels in animal models, contributing to improved overall metabolic health in diabetic conditions. Type 2 diabetes often leads to inflammation and insulin resistance issues among affected individuals; the antioxidants and anti-inflammatory properties found in chaya may aid in reducing inflammation, according to research [32]. Overall, the anti-diabetic activity of chaya leaves is attributed to the combined action of its bioactive compounds, which enhance insulin secretion, reduce postprandial glucose, and have antioxidant and lipid profile improvement effects. These functions position chaya as a supplementary treatment choice for the management of diabetes.

4.1.2. In Vivo Studies

Several in vivo studies have explored how methanolic (MeOH) extracts of *Cnidoscolus chayamansa* affect blood sugar levels in Wistar rats with diabetes induced by streptozotocin (STZ). Wistar rats with streptozotocin (STZ)-induced diabetes were administered intraperitoneal doses of 10, 40, and 70 mg/kg, which were subsequently evaluated through postprandial glucose testing and fasting blood glucose measurements. It was discovered that only the 70 mg dose (twice the weight of a grain of rice) had an impact in lowering blood sugar levels when compared to the glibenclamide-treated group. There was a 1% decrease at 120 min (about 4 h) and an 18% decrease at 180 min (6 h). Nevertheless, this dosage did not exhibit a fasting effect, as seen with insulin [24,33].

Another study evaluated the effects of methanolic (MeOH) extracts in rats with alloxan-induced diabetes by administering doses of 0.5, 1.0, and 1.5 mg/kg. The outcomes revealed the levels of glucose, cholesterol, and triglycerides, with the reduction in glucose correlating to the dosage used. These results were comparable to the effects observed with standard anti-diabetic drugs such as metformin and glibenclamide [32].

Furthermore, experiments conducted in rats using water extracts from dried *Cnidoscolust chayamansa* leaves revealed a decrease in both body weight and blood sugar levels, which was linked to the presence of quercetin and rutin, suggesting the extract's potential efficacy and safety for consumption [26].

Recent studies have revealed that extracts from *C. chayamansa*, *E. prostrata*, and *J. dioica* contain ingredients known for their antioxidant properties. In this investigation, the amounts of these components were determined to be 6.34, 10.67, and 1.83 mg gallic acid equivalents/g of dry biomass (DB), respectively. Water-soluble antioxidants were measured using the ABTS method, yielding 5.89, 12.70, and 2.50 millimoles of Trolox equivalents/g of DB. After examining tissues under a microscope following the administration of these extracts during hyperglycemia induction, they showed changes that implied a beneficial effect [40].

Another study examined the impacts of aqueous extracts of chaya on glycemic control in streptozotocin-induced diabetic rat models. Chaya extracts from plants collected in Quintana Roo (Mayan region) and Durango (Northern Mexico) were compared, with metformin used as a reference drug for control purposes. The compositions of the extracts from both areas were examined using high-performance liquid chromatography coupled with tandem mass spectrometry (HPLC-MS/MS-QQQ). The researchers conducted this study on tissues to investigate the impacts of extracts on Langerhans islets. At two weeks of treatment, with both extracts, hypoglycemic effects were evidenced. There was partial recovery of Langerhans islets. This effect of the treatment was consistent despite the plants being grown 2350 km apart under varying conditions. The compounds found in the two extracts showed no differences [41].

In another research study performed on type 2 diabetic rats, it was examined how combining metformin with green tea and black tea derived from *Cnidoscolous aconitifolius* impacted the rats' health over a period of 28 days (around 4 weeks). The levels of phenols and flavonoids, as well as the antioxidant capacities of the teas, were analyzed. The study also explored blood sugar levels after fasting, as well as lipid profiles and markers related to liver and kidney function. Green tea exhibited the highest levels of phenols and flavonoids and demonstrated superior antioxidant properties. When combined with metformin, in a study group of participants who consumed both teas together with the medication, it showed improvements in health markers including fasting glucose levels and various blood lipid parameters, such as triglycerides and cholesterol levels (total and LDL). Additionally, a reduction in liver enzymes—alanine aminotransferase (ALT) and aspartate aminotransferase (AST)—as well as in creatinine and urea levels was observed, alongside an increase in serum protein levels. The combination of chaya tea infusions with metformin was more effective than metformin alone in regulating fasting glucose, with green tea being the most effective [42].

Another study focused on assessing the protective effects of chaya leaf on mitochondrial abnormalities and synaptic damage in the TallyHO (TH) mouse model of type 2 diabetes, which shares several characteristics with human diabetes. The results showed that diabetic TH mice had body weight and fasting glucose levels comparable to those of diabetic mice, but those fed chaya experienced notable reductions in both areas. This information suggests that chaya may provide a safeguard against mitochondrial and synaptic dysfunction in mice. This implies that chaya could be beneficial as a supplement for people at risk of or dealing with diabetes and metabolic disorders [43].

In a research study investigating the effects of methanolic leaf extracts of *Cnidoscolus aconitifolius* in alloxan-induced diabetic rats, GC-MS analysis was conducted as part of the experimental evaluation. The analysis revealed the presence of 37 compounds, including hydrocarbons, alcohols, phenols, and fatty acids, many of which possess biological activity. Different doses of the extract (100 mg/kg, 150 mg/kg, and 200 mg/kg) were administered to diabetic rats, resulting in a reduction in blood sugar levels, outperforming chlorpropamide, a known diabetes medication. These findings suggest that the plant may help in controlling blood sugar levels in people with diabetes [44].

Type 2 diabetes is a health concern that affects many people globally. While there are medications to manage blood sugar levels orally, some individuals opt for herbal remedies due to their proven benefits. However, limited research has been conducted to investigate the interactions between medications like metformin and herbal remedies. These interactions could potentially impact the effectiveness of each treatment. In a study, the combination of metformin and chaya (an extract of *Cnidoscolus aconitifolius*) was examined in Long Evans rats with diabetes induced by streptozotocin. Various combinations were tested, and blood glucose levels were measured in the rats. The compositions of the extracts were analyzed using HPLC-MS/MS. The results showed an antagonistic effect between the compounds, with high glucose levels maintained in three of the four treated groups. Certain identified elements present in chaya could explain this phenomenon. In conclusion, the findings suggest that the consistent consumption of chaya as a treatment might diminish the efficacy of metformin, as observed in part of the Mexican population. It is advisable to conduct investigations on pharmacodynamic interactions to better understand this behavior [45].

Patients diagnosed with type 2 diabetes commonly face inflammation caused by the production of pro-inflammatory proteins, like TNF alpha and ILS, due to NF-kB regulation and overexpression. A study aimed to explore the potential anti-inflammatory properties of specific fractions of chaya aqueous extracts that have been previously suggested to reduce inflammation levels in diabetic patients. The researchers examined the content of the sample fractions by employing solid-phase extraction and tracking them with HPLC-MS/MS analysis. The activation of NF-kB and the levels of the pro-inflammatory proteins TNF-alpha and IL-6 were evaluated in streptozotocin-induced diabetic rats. Two of the sample fractions exhibited notable anti-inflammatory properties in diabetic rats induced by streptozotocin. Two of the fractions demonstrated the most significant anti-inflammatory effects, even outperforming the crude extract, which contained the highest concentrations of compounds. The presence of ferulic acid in the chemical profile suggested that it may have played a key role in the observed anti-inflammatory effect. On the other hand, naringenin and apigenin, found exclusively in the extract, might have impeded this effect, accounting for the superior performance of these distinct fractions [46]. Table 1 summarizes chaya's biological activity, extract types, and dosages

4.1.3. In Vitro Studies

In a study performed to assess the antioxidant properties of a methanolic extract of *Cnidoscolus chayamansa* using a colorimetric method, when tested at a concentration of 5 mg/mL, the DPPH radical was inhibited by 45%. The ABTS radical showed an inhibition rate of 94%. At a concentration of 1 mg/mL, the inhibitory effects decreased to 13.75% for DPPH and 52.07% for the ABTS radical. The sample displayed antioxidant effectiveness (IC50 = 1693 μg/mL) in contrast to positive controls (gallic acid and Trolox), with IC50 values of 15.39 and 43.90 μg/mL, respectively [24].

Another assessment of the antioxidant properties through the oxygen absorbance capacity (ORAC) method found that uncooked leaves exhibited an ORAC value of 15.6 μeq Trolox/g. Meanwhile, cooked leaves showed a slightly lower value of 14.8 μeq Trolox/g. Furthermore, the total amount of phenolic compounds present was determined to be 1217.3 meq chlorogenic acid/kg in raw leaves and 733.5 meq/kg in cooked leaves. The decrease of 5% in ORAC and the 40% decrease in phenols in the leaves were attributed to the change in quercetin-3-O-rhamnoside content, which increased by 23% in the cooked leaves [25].

Moreover, when assessing the antioxidant capacity with the DPPH method across three leaf extracts, it was observed that the hexane extract saw a reduction of 10.58%, while that of the ethyl acetate extract decreased by 11.68%. The ethanol extract exhibited a decline of 10.66%. The ethanol extract displayed polyphenol content of 35.70 meq AG/g according to the Folin–Ciocalteu method. This was followed by the hexane extract at 22.35 meq AG/g and the acetic ether extract at 13.25 meq AG/g.

Another way to evaluate the antioxidant capacity in laboratory settings involves using the ferric reducing ability of plasma (FRAP) method. In this method, the hexane extract (Hex) showed an inhibition rate of 239.47 μmol Fe^{+2}/L, the ethyl acetate extract (AcOEt) showed an inhibition rate of 387 μmol Fe^{+2}/L, and the ethanolic extract (EtOH) showed an inhibition rate of 254 μmol Fe^{+2}/L [11]. According to [47], this method provides insights into the antioxidant properties. This study found that a 95% ethanolic extract of *C. chayamansa* showed antioxidant properties in tests using DPPH and FRAP micromethods. However, when tested using the macromethod approach, the antioxidant effect was minimal, leading to the conclusion that the EtOH extract may not exhibit antioxidant properties [47].

Non-communicable chronic diseases (NCDs) are the leading causes of death worldwide. They are associated with oxidative stress and inflammation. Researchers have found that certain natural compounds derived from plants like *Cnidoscolus aconitifolius* could play a role in preventing these diseases by helping to combat stress and inflammation. In another in vitro study, the antioxidant and anti-inflammatory activity of *C. aconitifolius* extracts were evaluated, highlighting their notable potential due to the presence of bioactive compounds. These findings hold implications for diseases like diabetes, a type of NCD, where oxidative stress and inflammation play roles in disease progression and management. Chaya extracts may have advantages in the treatment of diabetes by alleviating these detrimental processes [48].

A different research project focused on creating and assessing capsules containing dried *Cnidoscolus chayamansa* McVaugh extract through hot percolation extraction using a 70% *v/v* ethanol solution. Preformulation experiments were carried out to prepare three sets of capsules. Various properties, like the moisture level, drug content, and disintegration weight consistency, as well as the dissolution of the capsules, were analyzed. One formulation showed optimal drug release in in vitro tests and met the standards of the Pharmacopeia. It was concluded that these capsules are an effective means of administering *C. chayamansa* extracts for the management of diabetes mellitus [49].

Another study aimed to evaluate the antioxidant capacity of a water-based extract and a combined extract (methanol/acetone/water) derived from chaya leaves and their impacts on mitochondrial bioenergetics and fatty acid oxidation. The antioxidant properties of both extracts derived from chaya leaves were found to be similar to those of nopal, a plant commonly used in medicine. The results indicated that the liquid extract from chaya leaves improved the function of mitochondria and the oxidation of fatty acids in liver cells. This suggests that it could be a treatment for liver issues linked to metabolic disorders [50].

In addition, research conducted at the University of Querétaro in Mexico involved the cultivation of *Cnidoscolus aconitifolius* (chaya) from woody cuttings, initiated in 2014. During the summer of 2016, leaf samples were collected from all cultivated plants to analyze methanol–water and ethanol–water extracts (in 50:50 and 80:20 ratios) from both raw and boiled leaves. The objective was to evaluate the total phenolic content, total flavonoid content, and antioxidant capacity. Through RP-HPLC-DAD analysis, 11 phenolic compounds were identified and quantified, including gallic acid, vanillin, chlorogenic acid, and resveratrol. The findings revealed that boiling the leaves increased both the antioxidant capacity and phenolic compound content compared to raw leaves. The 80:20 ethanol extract showed the highest polyphenol concentration, suggesting that chaya leaves are a rich source of natural antioxidants [51].

A separate study was initially conducted on four atolls south of Tarawa in Kiribati and later extended to Tuvalu to investigate the mineral levels present in different types of local edible leafy plants. Variations in the ability of these plants to accumulate minerals in their leaves were analyzed, as well as their resistance to soils lacking essential nutrients. Farmers in the area grew plants in nurseries to then provide them to the rest of the farmers. Information leaflets highlighted the most suitable species among the 24 studied, including multiple examples of each. These included plants such as chaya, ofenga, hedgerow panax, and purslane, which have been shown in other studies to have beneficial effects against non-communicable diseases (NCDs) [18].

Chaya is a shrub known for its medicinal properties, used since the time of the Mayan culture in Southeastern Mexico, and has been studied to evaluate its effectiveness in reducing blood pressure and blood glucose levels through six different types of leaf extracts (aqueous and alcoholic). In a recent study, the leaves used were collected in Timucuy, Yucatan, Mexico as part of the process for this specific study. For the extraction,

48 h maceration was used, with the proportions consisting of one part of the sample for every ten parts of the solvent (weight/volume). The solvents used were the following: distilled water, a mixture of ethanol and acetone together with ethyl acetate, diethyl ether, and hexane. The tests carried out included enzymatic inhibition against ACE, and the inhibition effects on the alpha glucosidase and alpha amylase enzymes were also evaluated in tests under controlled conditions. The hypotensive impact, the glycemic response to oral glucose overload, and the hypoglycemic effects in rats induced with obesity, hypertension, and hyperglycemia were also analyzed. The extracts with the lowest 50% inhibition concentrations (IC50) for angiotensin-converting enzyme (ACE), alpha glucosidase, and alpha amylase were the following: acetone (12.61 μg/mL), ethyl acetate (22.97 μg/mL), and ethyl acetate (32 μg/mL). On the other hand, the aquaculture extract had a notable hypotensive effect, reducing systolic blood pressure by 15.5%. The highest percentage reduction in systolic blood pressure was observed in the methanol extract at a rate of 23%, while the hexane extract managed to reduce glucose levels by up to 22.88%. The findings revealed that all chaya extracts exhibited enzyme-inhibitory properties and hypotensive and hypoglycemic effects [52]. The use of different extracts is an advantage in studies, as it allows for the evaluation of various substances. However, the chemical profile of each extract should be determined to identify its composition and bioactive compounds. Since different articles present varying extraction methodologies, comparing their effects becomes difficult. Therefore, a study design that considers these variables is necessary to accurately assess the effects of chaya.

The study performed in [53] compared fried, roasted, boiled, and raw chaya in terms of the content of bioactives and nutrients, as well as antioxidant, anti-diabetic, and anti-thrombotic activity. It was concluded that chaya is a good option, finding that fried chaya increased the antioxidant activity and α-amylase inhibition (+30%) but that the boiled chaya decreased all parameters. Frying and roasting improved the sensory attributes while maintaining the plant's nutritional value and enhancing its functional properties, making chaya promising for dietary interventions in diabetes.

4.1.4. Clinical Studies

Proper nutrition is essential in maintaining good health; to achieve this, the diet should include vegetables such as quelites. Quelites are edible wild plants that may help to prevent diabetes due to their antioxidant and anti-inflammatory compounds. A study was conducted to determine the glycemic index (GI) and glycemic load (GL) of rice and a tamal prepared with and without two types of quelites: alache (*Anoda cristata*) and chaya (*Cnidoscolus aconitifolius*). The GI was measured in 10 healthy subjects, namely seven women and three men, with the following average metrics: age, 23 years; body weight, 61.3 kg; height, 1.65 m; body mass index, 22.7 kg/m^2; and fasting glucose, 77.4 mg/dL. Capillary blood samples were collected within 2 h after the meal. White rice (rice without quelites) had a GI of 75.35 ± 15.6 and a GL of 36.17 ± 7.8; rice with alache had a GI of 33.74 ± 5.85 and a GL of 33.74 ± 1.85. White tamal had a GI of 57.33 10.23 and a GL of 26.65 ± 5.12; tamal with chaya had a GI of 46.73 ± 22.1 and a GL of 23.36 ± 11. The GI and GL values recorded for the combinations of quelites with rice and tamal confirmed that quelites could be a beneficial alternative for healthy diets [54]. Based on in vitro studies, more clinical research is needed to establish the minimum and maximum effective doses. Until the appropriate dosing, the environmental influences on the metabolite profile of chaya, and its interaction with various drugs used in the treatment of diabetes are established, it will be difficult to position it as a suitable tool in diabetes management, and its effects will remain inconsistent. Table 2 summarizes limitations considered in researches performed in chaya.

Table 1. Summary of chaya's biological activity, extract types, and dosages.

Antioxidant	Anti-Inflammatory	Cardio-protective/Hypotensive	Renal Protection	Cognitive Function	Hypoglycemic	Anti-Mutagenic	Anti-Hypercholesterolemic	Anti-Hypertriglyceridemic	In Vitro	In Vivo	Model	Type of Extract	Clinica Assay	Extract	Dose	Drug Interactions	Toxicity	Reference
X	X	X							X	X	Male CD1 mice	Hex, EtOAc, and EtOH		135 g/ 5.68 g Hex, 5.27 g EtOAc, 9.44 g EtOH	2 mg, 500 mg/kg	-	LD50 > 5 g/kg EtOAC and EtOH, single dose	[11]
X									X			H_2O, EtOH		-	-	-	-	[17]
X			X							X	Wistar rats	EtOH		600 g to yield 12.78 g after evaporation to dryness	400 mg/kg	-	-	[19]
X					X				X	X	Wistar rats	H_2O		5 g/100 mL	5 mg/kg	-	LD50 1070.42 µg/mL	[20]
				X						X	Wistar Rats	Fine powder of dried leaves as meal		-	1%, 2.5%, 5%, and 10% supplemented diet	-	-	[21]

Table 1. *Cont.*

Antioxidant	Anti-Inflammatory	Cardio-protective/Hypotensive	Renal Protection	Cognitive Function	Hypoglycemic	Anti-Mutagenic	Anti-Hypercholesterolemic	Anti-Hypertriglyceridemic	In Vitro	In Vivo	Model	Type of Extract	Clinica Assay	Extract	Dose	Drug Interactions	Toxicity	Reference
					X		X	X		X	Mice	EtOH, Hex, MeOH, Chl		5000/2.5 L EtOH	250, 500, 1000, 2500, 3000, 3500, 4000, 4500, and 5000 mg/kg	-	EtOH LD50 of 4000 mg/kg, MeOH LD50 3500 mg/kg, Hex LD50 value of 2000 mg/kg, Chl LD50 2500 mg/kg	[22]
X					X	X			X	X	Wistar rats	MeOH		500 g/L	10, 40, and 70 mg/kg	-	-	[24]
X									X			H_2O		-	-	-	-	[25]
					X		X			X	Rats	MeOH		20 g of dried leaves in 250 mL 80% MeOH	0.5 and 1.5 g/kg	-	-	[32]
X					X				X	X	Wistar rats	H_2O		60 g/300 H_2O	-	-	-	[40]
					X					X	Wistar rats	H_2O		15 g of fresh leaf/L	-	-	-	[41]

Table 1. *Cont.*

Antioxidant	Anti-Inflammatory	Cardioprotective/Hypotensive	Renal Protection	Cognitive Function	Hypoglycemic	Anti-Mutagenic	Anti-Hypercholesterolemic	Anti-Hypertriglyceridemic	In Vitro	In Vivo	Model	Type of Extract	Clinica Assay	Extract	Dose	Drug Interactions	Toxicity	Reference
X					X		X		X	X	Wistar rats	H_2O		2 g of tea powder ("green" or "black") was infused (4 min) in 100 mL of boiling water	6 mL/kg	Metformin	-	[42]
X									X			EtOH		-	-	-	-	[47]
					X					X	Mice TallyHo/JngJ strain (TH) and mice SWR/J strain	Meal as powder		Diet with 25% ground chaya	-	-	-	[43]
					X					X	Wistar rats	MeOH		-	100, 150, and 200 mg/kg	-	-	[44]
					X					X	Rats	H_2O		7.5 mg of dry leaf in 1 L	25 to 100% extract	Metformin	.	[45]
	X				X					X	Long Evans rats	H_2O, EtOH, AcOEt		2.5 g/100 mL water	Ad libitum as drinking water	-	-	[46]

Table 1. *Cont.*

Antioxidant	Anti-Inflammatory	Cardioprotective/Hypotensive	Renal Protection	Cognitive Function	Hypoglycemic	Anti-Mutagenic	Anti-Hypercholesterolemic	Anti-Hypertriglyceridemic	In Vitro	In Vivo	Model	Type of Extract	Clinica Assay	Extract	Dose	Drug Interactions	Toxicity	Reference
X	X								X			H_2O, EtOH, Ace, AcOEt, Et2O, Hex		1:10 (*w*/*v*)	150, 300, 450, 600, 750, and 900 mg/mL; 10, 25, 50, 100, 250, and 500 mg/mL; 25, 50, and 100 mg/mL	-	-	[48]
X									X			EtOH-H_2O-MeOH-H_2O		1:10	-	-	-	[51]
		X			X				X	X	Wistar rats	H_2O, EtOH, Ace, AcOEt, Et2O, Hex		1:10	-	-	-	[52]
X		X			X				X			H_2O	X	5 g/100 mL	-	-	-	[53]

Abbreviations. H_2O, water; EtOH, ethanol; Ace, acetone; AcOEt, ethyl acetate; Et2O, ethyl ether; Hex, hexane. "—" indicates information not established. Dose: expressed in kg of body weight. "X" indicates a characteristic found in the study.

Table 2. Summary of the limitations considered in the studies.

Issue Assessed	Study Limitations
Experimental Lab/Animal Studies	• Mainly in vitro/in vivo studies; clinical applicability limited. Animal models only, lack of human or clinical trial support. • Food matrix interaction is not fully understood. • Limited dose standardization—no specific dosing guidelines or adverse effects discussed. • No long-term effects studied. • No correlation with human nutritional outcomes. • High heterogeneity in methods; limited clinical correlation. • Differences in animal models and impairment in sex distribution and variance because of species.
Ethnobotanical	• Mostly descriptive. • Biological validation of plant evaluated. • Does not link genetics and environmental changes to bioactivity.
Phytochemical/Nutritional Studies	• Lacks bioavailability and toxicity data; no in vivo relevance. • High heterogeneity in methods; limited clinical correlation.

5. Conclusions

In conclusion, scientific evidence supports the anti-diabetic properties of chaya leaf, highlighting its hypoglycemic and antioxidant properties. In vivo studies have demonstrated that the methanolic extract of *C. chayamansa* significantly reduces blood glucose levels in rats with streptozotocin- and alloxan-induced diabetes, favorably comparing with conventional medications such as metformin and glibenclamide [24,32,33]. Additionally, research has revealed that aqueous extracts of chaya not only decrease glucose levels but also improve lipid profiles and overall health in diabetes models, demonstrating its therapeutic potential [26,42].

Studies have also highlighted the role of the phenolic and antioxidant compounds present in chaya, such as quercetin and rutin, in reducing oxidative stress, a key factor in the pathogenesis of diabetes [40]. The combination of chaya extracts with standard treatments like metformin has shown promising results, although possible interactions have been observed, requiring further investigation to optimize their combined use [42,47].

In vitro research corroborates the antioxidant and anti-inflammatory capacity of chaya, suggesting that its consumption could mitigate the harmful effects of oxidative stress and inflammation in diabetes [48]. Additionally, the development of standardized formulations of chaya extracts, such as capsules, provides an effective means of administration that meets pharmaceutical standards, facilitating its use in diabetes management [49]; however, there is a need for evaluations to determine suitable formulations.

In summary, chaya leaf represents a valuable and safe option in complementary therapies for diabetes, underscoring the need for further clinical studies in humans to confirm and expand these findings. The integration of herbal remedies with conventional treatments could offer a more holistic and effective approach to managing this chronic disease, but it is necessary to systematically explore doses, extraction methods, concentrations, the effects of isolated compounds, and interactions with other drugs for diabetes treatment; without this information, this plant will remain in the domain of folk medicine.

Author Contributions: Conceptualization, F.I.G.R. and L.G.-M.; methodology, L.G.-M. and F.C.A.; investigation, S.N.J.-G.; writing—original draft preparation, F.I.G.R.; writing—review and editing, L.G.-M. and F.C.A. All authors have read and agreed to the published version of the manuscript.

Funding: This research received no external funding.

Data Availability Statement: The data presented in this study are available on request from the corresponding authors.

Conflicts of Interest: The authors declare no conflicts of interest.

References

1. Alvarez-Poblano, L.; Roman-Guerrero, A.; Vernon-Carter, E.J.; Alvarez-Ramirez, J. Exogenous Addition of Muicle (*Justicia spicigera* Schechtendal) Extract to White Maize Tortillas Affects the Antioxidant Activity, Texture, Color, and In Vitro Starch Digestibility. *LWT* **2020**, *133*, 110120. [CrossRef]
2. Pérez-Loredo, M.G.; Jesús, L.H.D.; Barragán-Huerta, B.E. Extracción de compuestos bioactivos de pitaya roja (*Stenocereus stellatus*) aplicando pretratamientos con microondas, ultrasonido y enzimáticos. *Agrociencia* **2017**, *51*, 135–151.
3. Wang, T.; Li, Q.; Bi, K. Bioactive flavonoids in medicinal plants: Structure, activity and biological fate. *Asian J. Pharm. Sci.* **2018**, *13*, 12–23. [CrossRef] [PubMed]
4. Organización Mundial de la Salud. Enfermedades no Transmisibles. Available online: https://www.paho.org/es/temas/enfermedades-no-transmisibles#:~:text=Las%20enfermedades%20no%20transmisibles%20(ENT)%20matan%20a%2041%20millones%20de,muertes%20por%20ENT%20cada%20a%C3%B1o (accessed on 12 July 2023).
5. Organización Panamericana de la Salud. Leading Causes of Death and Disability. Portal de Datos ENLACE. Available online: https://www.paho.org/en/enlace/leading-causes-death-and-disability (accessed on 12 July 2023).
6. Secretaría de Salud. Panorama Epidemiológico de las Enfermedades no Transmisibles en México, Cierre. 2021. Available online: https://www.gob.mx/cms/uploads/attachment/file/745354/PanoEpi_ENT_Cierre2021.pdf (accessed on 12 August 2023).
7. Acosta-Recalde, P.; Vera, G.Z.; Morinigo, M.; Maidana, G.M.; Samaniego, L. Uso de plantas medicinales y fito-terápicos en pacientes con Diabetes Mellitus tipo 2. *Mem. Inst. Investig. Cienc. Salud* **2018**, *16*, 6–11. [CrossRef]
8. Hernández, Y.V.V.; Munguía, A.R. Chaya: Fuente emergente de potencial nutraceútico y funcional. *Tlatemoani Rev. Acad. Investig.* **2022**, *13*, 140–151. [CrossRef]
9. Seetaloo, A.D.; Aumeeruddy, M.Z.; Rengasamy Kannan, R.R.; Mahomoodally, M.F. Potential of traditionally consumed medicinal herbs, spices, and food plants to inhibit key digestive enzymes geared towards diabetes mellitus management—A systematic review. *S. Afr. J. Bot.* **2019**, *120*, 3–24. [CrossRef]
10. Secretaría de Medio Ambiente y Recursos Naturales. Plantas Medicinales de México. Available online: https://www.gob.mx/semarnat/articulos/plantas-medicinales-de-mexico (accessed on 12 August 2023).
11. García-Rodríguez, R.V.; Gutiérrez-Rebolledo, G.A.; Méndez-Bolaina, E.; Sánchez-Medina, A.; Maldonado-Saavedra, O.; Domínguez-Ortiz, M.Á.; Vázquez-Hernández, M.; Muñoz-Muñiz, O.D.; Cruz-Sánchez, J.S. *Cnidoscolus chayamansa* Mc Vaugh, an important antioxidant, anti-inflammatory and cardioprotective plant used in Mexico. *J. Ethnopharmacol.* **2014**, *151*, 937–943. [CrossRef]
12. González Stuart, A. Chaya. Universidad de Texas. Available online: https://www.utep.edu/herbal-safety/hechos-herbarios/hojas-de-datos-a-base-de-hierbas/chaya.html (accessed on 13 August 2023).
13. Alonso-Castro, A.J.; Zapata-Morales, J.R.; Ruiz-Padilla, A.J.; Solorio-Alvarado, C.R.; Rangel-Velázquez, J.E.; Cruz-Jiménez, G.; Orozco-Castellanos, L.M.; Domínguez, F.; Maldonado-Miranda, J.J.; Carranza-Álvarez, C.; et al. Use of medicinal plants by health professionals in Mexico. *J. Ethnopharmacol.* **2017**, *198*, 81–86. [CrossRef]
14. Mazumder, M.E.H.; Rahman, S. Pharmacological Evaluation of Bangladeshi Medicinal Plants for Antioxidant Activity. *Pharm. Biol.* **2008**, *46*, 704–709. [CrossRef]
15. Chin-Chan, T.; Ortiz-García, M.M.; Ruiz-Gil, P.J.; Martínez-Castillo, J. Diversidad genética de la Chaya (*Cnidoscolus aconitifolius* (Mill.) I. M. Johnst. ssp. aconitifolius) en Yucatán, México, su posible centro de domesticación. *Polibotánica* **2021**, 185–201. [CrossRef]
16. Bendaña, G. La Chaya. Valor Nutritivo, Cultivo, Utilización. Available online: http://edn.link/qxyj3y (accessed on 12 August 2023).

17. Rodrigues, L.G.G.; Mazzutti, S.; Siddique, I.; da Silva, M.; Vitali, L.; Ferreira, S.R.S. Subcritical water extraction and microwave-assisted extraction applied for the recovery of bioactive components from Chaya (*Cnidoscolus aconitifolius* Mill.). *J. Supercrit. Fluids* **2020**, *165*, 104976. [CrossRef]
18. Lyons, G.; Dean, G.; Tongaiaba, R.; Halavatau, S.; Nakabuta, K.; Lonalona, M.; Susumu, G. Macro- and Micronutrients from Traditional Food Plants Could Improve Nutrition and Reduce Non-Communicable Diseases of Islanders on Atolls in the South Pacific. *Plants* **2020**, *9*, 942. [CrossRef]
19. Somade, O.T.; Ugbaja, R.N.; Idowu, M.A.; Akinloye, O.A. *Cnidoscolus aconitifolius* leaf extract and ascorbate confer amelioration and protection against dimethyl nitrosamine-induced renal toxicity and testicular abnormalities in rats. *Toxicol. Rep.* **2021**, *8*, 1098–1108. [CrossRef]
20. Valenzuela Soto, R.; Morales Rubio, M.E.; Verde Star, M.J.; Oranday Cárdenas, A.; Preciado-Rangel, P.; Antonio González, J.; Esparza-Rivera, J.R. *Cnidoscolus chayamansa* organic hydroponic and its hypoglycemic capacity, nutraceutical quality and toxicity. *Rev. Mex. Cienc. Agríc.* **2017**, *6*, 815–825.
21. Adebayo, O.G.; Ajayi, A.M.; Onasanwo, S.A. The Impact of *Cnidoscolus aconitifolius* (Linn)-Supplemented Diet on Cognitive Function, Oxidative Stress and Histological Changes in Wistar Rats. *IBRO Rep.* **2019**, *7*, 26–27. [CrossRef]
22. Achi, N.K.; Ohaeri, O.C.; Ijeh, I.I.; Eleazu, C. Modulation of the lipid profile and insulin levels of streptozotocin-induced diabetic rats by ethanol extract of *Cnidoscolus aconitifolius* leaves and some fractions: Effect on the oral glucose tolerance of normoglycemic rats. *Biomed. Pharmacother.* **2017**, *86*, 562–569. [CrossRef]
23. Hutasingh, N.; Tubtimrattana, A.; Pongpamorn, P.; Pewlong, P.; Paemanee, A.; Tansrisawad, N.; Siripatrawan, U.; Sirikantaramas, S. Unraveling the effects of drying techniques on chaya leaves: Metabolomics analysis of non-volatile and volatile metabolites, umami taste, and antioxidant capacity. *Food Chem.* **2024**, *446*, 138769. [CrossRef]
24. Loarca-Piña, G.; Mendoza, S.; Ramos, G.M.; Reynoso, R. Antioxidant, Antimutagenic and Antidiabetic Activities of Edible Leaves from *Cnidoscolus chayamansa* Mc. Vaugh. *J. Food Sci.* **2010**, *75*, 68–72. [CrossRef]
25. Kuti, J.O.; Konoru, H.B. Antioxidant capacity and phenolic content in leaf extracts of tree spinach (*Cnidoscolus* spp). *J. Agric. Food Chem.* **2004**, *52*, 117–121. [CrossRef] [PubMed]
26. González-Laredo, R.F.; Flores de la Hoya, M.E.; Quintero-Ramos, M.J.; Karchesy, J.J. Flavonoid and cyanogenic contents of chaya (Spinach Tree). *Plant Foods Hum. Nutr.* **2003**, *58*, 1–8. [CrossRef]
27. Ramírez Rodrigues, M.M.; Metri Ojeda, J.C.; González Díaz, M.; Baigts Allende, D.K. Use of Chaya (*Cnidoscolus chayamansa*) Leaves for Nutritional Compounds Production for Human Consumption. *J. Mex. Chem. Soc.* **2021**, *65*, 118–128. [CrossRef]
28. Mena Linares, Y.; González Mosquera, D.M.; Valido Díaz, A.; Pizarro Espín, A.; Castillo Alfonso, O.; Escobar Román, R. Estudio fitoquímico de extractos de hojas de *Cnidoscolus chayamansa* Mc Vaugh (Chaya). *Rev. Cubana Plantas Med.* **2016**, *21*, 1–13.
29. International Diabetes Federation. Diabetes Atlas. Available online: https://diabetesatlas.org/ (accessed on 10 February 2022).
30. Salehi, B.; Ata, A.V.; Anil Kumar, N.; Sharopov, F.; Ramírez-Alarcón, K.; Ruiz-Ortega, A.; Abdulmajid Ayatollahi, S.; Tsouh Fokou, P.V.; Kobarfard, F.; Amiruddin Zakaria, Z.; et al. Antidiabetic Potential of Medicinal Plants and Their Active Components. *Biomolecules* **2019**, *9*, 551. [CrossRef] [PubMed]
31. Oh, Y.S. Plant-Derived Compounds Targeting Pancreatic Beta Cells for the Treatment of Diabetes. *Evid.-Based Complement. Altern. Med.* **2015**, *2015*, 629863. [CrossRef]
32. Figueroa-Valverde, L.; Díaz-Cedillo, F.; Camacho-Luis, A.; López-Ramos, M. Efectos Inducidos por *Ruta graveolans* L., *Cnidoscolus chayamansa* Mc Vaugh y *Citrus aurantium* L. sobre los Niveles de Glucosa, Colesterol y Triacilglicéridos en un Modelo de Rata Diabética. *Rev. Bras. Farmacogn.* **2009**, *19*, 898–907. [CrossRef]
33. Kuti, J.O.; Torres, E.S. Potential Nutritional and Health Benefits of Tree Spinach. In *Progress in New Crops*; Janick, J., Ed.; ASHS Press: Arlington, VA, USA, 1996; pp. 516–520.
34. Yi, X.; Dong, M.; Guo, N.; Tian, J.; Lei, P.; Wang, S.; Yang, Y.; Shi, Y. Flavonoids Improve Type 2 Diabetes Mellitus and Its Complications: A Review. *Front. Nutr.* **2023**, *10*, 1192131. [CrossRef] [PubMed]
35. Ansari, P.; Choudhury, S.T.; Seidel, V.; Rahman, A.B.; Aziz, M.A.; Richi, A.E.; Rahman, A.; Jafrin, U.H.; Hannan, J.M.A.; Abdel-Wahab, Y.H.A. Therapeutic Potential of Quercetin in the Management of Type-2 Diabetes Mellitus. *Life* **2022**, *12*, 1146. [CrossRef]
36. Rahmani, A.H.; Alsahli, M.A.; Khan, A.A.; Almatroodi, S.A. Quercetin, a Plant Flavonol Attenuates Diabetic Complications, Renal Tissue Damage, Renal Oxidative Stress and Inflammation in Streptozotocin-Induced Diabetic Rats. *Metabolites* **2023**, *13*, 130. [CrossRef]
37. Mahmoud, M.F.; Hassan, N.A.; El Bassossy, H.M.; Fahmy, A. Quercetin Protects against Diabetes-Induced Exaggerated Vasoconstriction in Rats: Effect on Low Grade Inflammation. *PLoS ONE* **2013**, *8*, e63784. [CrossRef]
38. Dini, S.; Zakeri, M.; Ebrahimpour, S.; Dehghanian, F.; Esmaeili, A. Quercetin-Conjugated Superparamagnetic Iron Oxide Nanoparticles Modulate Glucose Metabolism-Related Genes and miR-29 Family in the Hippocampus of Diabetic Rats. *Sci. Rep.* **2021**, *11*, 8618. [CrossRef]

39. Wu, J.; Lv, T.; Liu, Y.; Liu, Y.; Han, Y.; Liu, X.; Cai, J. The Role of Quercetin in NLRP3-Associated Inflammation. *Inflammopharmacology* **2024**, *32*, 3585–3610. [CrossRef]
40. Valenzuela-Soto, R.; Jiménez-Villarreal, J.; García-Garza, R.; Betancourt-Martínez, N.D.; Lozoya-Martínez, R.; Almaráz-Celis, D.; Morán-Martínez, J. Evaluation of the Antioxidant Activity of *Cnidoscolus chayamansa* (Chaya), *Euphorbia prostrata* (Golondrina Herb), and *Jatropha dioica* (Dragon's Blood) in Wistar Rats Induced with Hyperglycemia. *Int. J. Morphol.* **2019**, *37*, 36–42. [CrossRef]
41. Guzmán, E.L.; González, J.C.C.; Flores, M.C.; Carrillo, A.S.; Pescador, M.G.N.; Cruz, F.J.M. Effect on Hyperglycemia and Pancreas Cells of Chaya Aqueous Extracts from Two Different Regions in Streptozotocin-Induced Diabetes Rats. *Braz. J. Pharm. Sci.* **2021**, *56*, e18782. [CrossRef]
42. Mahammad, A.; Tekou, F.A.; Woumbo, C.Y.; Kentsop, M.P.; Djuine, V.; Kuate, D. Simultaneous Consumption of Green and Black Tea Infusions from *Cnidoscolus aconitifolius* Leaves with Metformin Treatment Improves the Health Outcome in Type II Diabetic Rats. *CYTA J. Food* **2023**, *21*, 386–393. [CrossRef]
43. Ramasubramanian, B.; Griffith, C.; Hanson, M.; Bunquin, L.E.; Reddy, A.P.; Hegde, V.; Reddy, P.H. Protective Effects of Chaya against Mitochondrial and Synaptic Toxicities in the Type 2 Diabetes Mouse Model TallyHO. *Cells* **2022**, *11*, 744. [CrossRef] [PubMed]
44. Iheanacho, E.K.; Igwe, O.U.; Onyemachi, P.E.N. GC-MS Analysis and Hypoglycemic Properties of Methanolic Leaf Extract of *Cnidoscolus aconitifolius* on Alloxan-Induced Diabetic Wistar Rats. *Afr. Sci. Rep.* **2023**, *2*, 150. [CrossRef]
45. Guzmán, E.L.; Cruz, F.J.M.; Vidal, F.J.Q.; Rodríguez, D.Q.; Flores, M.C.; Pescador, M.G.N. Effects of the Combination of *Cnidoscolus aconitifolius* and Metformin on the Glycemia in Streptozotocin-Induced Diabetes Rats. *J. Diabetes Endocrinol.* **2019**, *10*, 30–35. [CrossRef]
46. Guzmán, E.L.; Godina, A.S.H.; Flores, M.C.; Pescador, M.G.N.; Mendiola, A.P.; Hernández, Á.A.V. Anti-Inflammatory Effect of Chaya Extracts Fractions. *J. Med. Plant Res.* **2023**, *17*, 218–224.
47. Cáceres, A.; Lange, K.; Cruz, S.M.; Velásquez, R.; Lima, S.; Menéndez, M.C.; Dardón, R.; Córdova, D.; González, J. Assessment of Antioxidant Activity of 24 Native Plants Used in Guatemala for Their Potential Application in Natural Product Industry. *Acta Hortic.* **2010**, *964*, 85–92. [CrossRef]
48. Us-Medina, U.; Millán-Linares, M.d.C.; Arana-Argaes, V.E.; Segura-Campos, M.R. Actividad Antioxidante y Anti-Inflamatoria In Vitro de Extractos de Chaya (*Cnidoscolus aconitifolius* (Mill.) I.M. Johnst). *Nutr. Hosp.* **2020**, *37*, 46–55.
49. Kumaraswamy, K.P.; Nallaperumal, N.; Karimulla, S.; Devarajan, S.; Jagannathan, P.; Thangavel, V.; Yusuff, I.; Boddu, B. Formulation and Evaluation of Capsule of Ethanolic Extract of Cnidoscolus chayamansa Mc Vaugh Leaves for the Treatment of Diabetes. *Ann. Phytomed.* **2022**, *11*, 339–343. [CrossRef]
50. Avila-Nava, A.; Acevedo-Carabantes, J.A.; Alamilla-Martinez, I.; Tobón-Cornejo, S.; Torre-Villalvazo, I.; Tovar, A.R.; Torres, N.; Noriega, L.G. Chaya (*Cnidoscolus aconitifolius* (Mill.) I.M. Johnst) Leaf Extracts Regulate Mitochondrial Bioenergetics and Fatty Acid Oxidation in C2C12 Myotubes and Primary Hepatocytes. *J. Ethnopharmacol.* **2023**, *312*, 116522. [CrossRef]
51. Godínez-Santillán, R.I.; Chávez-Servín, J.L.; García-Gasca, T.; Guzmán-Maldonado, S.H. Phenolic Characterization and Antioxidant Capacity of Alcoholic Extracts from Raw and Boiled Leaves of *Cnidoscolus aconitifolius* (Euphorbiaceae). *Acta Bot. Mex.* **2019**, e1493. [CrossRef]
52. Manzanilla Valdez, M.L.; Acevedo Fernández, J.J.; Segura Campos, M.R. Antidiabetic and Hypotensive Effect of *Cnidoscolus aconitifolius* (Mill) IM Johnst Leaves Extracts. *J. Food Meas. Charact.* **2021**, *15*, 5245–5255. [CrossRef]
53. Uuh Narvaez, J.J.; Huaroto Ramos, A.L.; Quintal Martinez, J.P.; Segura Campos, M.R. Traditional foods based on chaya (Cnidoscolus aconitifolius) cooked by different methods as a proposal for diabetes and thrombosis management. *J. Food Meas. Charact* **2025**, *19*, 3888–3899. [CrossRef]
54. Morales-Guerrero, J.C.; Rosas-Romero, R.; Mariscal-Gálvez, M.A.; Ayala-Alcántara, F.; Bourges-Rodríguez, H. Glycemic Index and Glycemic Load of Two Dishes Cooked with Alache (*Anoda cristata*) and Chaya (*Cnidoscolus aconitifolius*) Plants from the Traditional Mexican Diet. *J. Med. Food* **2023**, *26*, 416–421. [CrossRef] [PubMed]

pharmaceuticals

Review

Polyphenolic Compounds in Fabaceous Plants with Antidiabetic Potential

Lucia Guerrero-Becerra [1,2], Sumiko Morimoto [3], Estefania Arrellano-Ordoñez [1], Angélica Morales-Miranda [3], Ramón G. Guevara-Gonzalez [1], Ana Angélica Feregrino-Pérez [2,*] and Consuelo Lomas-Soria [3,*]

1 Center of Applied Research in Biosystems (CARB-CIAB), School of Engineering, Autonomous University of Querétaro-Campus Amazcala, Carr. Amazacala-Chichimequillas km 1.0, El Marqués, Querétaro 76265, Mexico; gubel28@gmail.com (L.G.-B.); eaordonez21@gmail.com (E.A.-O.); ramon.guevara@uaq.mx (R.G.G.-G.)
2 Research and Postgraduate Division, School of Engineering, Universidad Autónoma de Querétaro, Campus Amazcala, Carretera a Chichimequillas Km 1 s/n, Amazcala, El Marqués, Querétaro 76265, Mexico
3 Departamento de Biología de la Reproducción, Instituto Nacional de Ciencias Médicas y Nutrición Salvador Zubirán, Ciudad de México 14080, Mexico; sumiko.morimotom@incmnsz.mx (S.M.); angelica.moralesm@incmnsz.mx (A.M.-M.)
* Correspondence: feregrino.angge@hotmail.com (A.A.F.-P.); consuelo.lomass@incmnsz.mx (C.L.-S.)

Abstract: Diabetes mellitus (DM) is a chronic non-communicable disease with an increasing prevalence in Latin America and worldwide, impacting various social and economic areas. It causes numerous complications for those affected. Current treatments for diabetes include oral hypoglycemic drugs, which can lead to adverse effects and health complications. Other natural alternatives for DM treatment have been studied as adjunct therapies that could reduce or eliminate the need for antidiabetic medications. Several natural supplements may offer an alternative way to improve the quality of life for patients with DM, and they may have other nutraceutical applications. Due to their phenolic compound content, some leguminous substances have been proposed as these alternatives. Phenolic compounds, with their high antioxidant activity, have shown promising potential in insulin synthesis, secretion, and the functionality of the endocrine pancreas. This review provides valuable information on various leguminous plants with anti-diabetic properties, including antioxidant, hypoglycemic, anti-fat-induced damage, and anti-apoptotic properties in vitro and in vivo, attributed to the high content of phenolic compounds in their seeds. Natural products with antidiabetic and pharmacological treatment potential improve diabetes management by offering more effective and complementary alternatives. To integrate these herbal remedies into modern medicine, further research on phenolic compound type, doses, efficacy, and safety in the human population is needed.

Keywords: antioxidant; diabetes; legumes; secondary metabolites; phytochemicals

1. Introduction

Diabetes mellitus (DM) is a non-communicable disease characterized by high blood glucose levels (hyperglycemia), with disturbances in carbohydrate, fat, and protein metabolism. These metabolic disorders are caused by defects in insulin secretion and/or a lack of response to the action of this hormone in target organs. When DM is not controlled correctly, it can result in severe complications, including cardiovascular disease, renal failure, nerve damage, and blindness, as well as early death [1–3]. In treating DM, several therapeutic measures are fundamental for adequate metabolic control. These include some non-pharmacological measures, such as regular physical activity and a healthy diet,

https://doi.org/10.3390/ph18010069

and other pharmacological measures, including oral antidiabetic drugs [4]. In addition, therapeutic alternatives of natural origin, such as plants, have been sought out due to their containing of bioactive compounds with pharmacological properties that intervene in antioxidant action or their mechanisms of action that regulate glucose, among others properties [5,6]. Plants are considered important in traditional medicine and human nutrition, among which edible fabaceous plants (legumes) stand out, such as soybeans, beans, peas, broad beans, lentils, peanuts, and chickpeas. It has been suggested that these fabaceous plants can help prevent or reduce the complications of diabetes treatment and may even have similar effects to insulin [7]. Compounds such as alkaloids, phenolics, carotenoids, flavonoids, lectins, tannins, trypsin, glycosides, coumarins, and saponins have been identified in fabaceous plants as those responsible for some biological activities, i.e., phenolic acids, flavonoids, and isoflavonoids are classes of bioactive compounds found in plants that are known for their antioxidant, anti-inflammatory, and potential health-promoting effects [8,9].

Phenolic compounds are secondary metabolites that provide plants with essential properties such as color, flavor, and resistance to stress. Beyond their organoleptic properties, these compounds are critical to the human diet because they contain antioxidant properties which prevent cell damage [10,11], meaning they can help confront damage caused by free radicals in the body [12]. A comprehensive view of the benefits of polyphenols with antidiabetic effects present in common fabaceous plants can motivate clinical trials, attracting multiple disciplines for further investigation. Given the growing concern among individuals with DM about the potential side effects of synthetic pharmaceutical agents, the research community is increasingly looking for natural products as a safer alternative. This study aims to analyze and synthesize the most recent scientific evidence on the phenolic compounds present in commonly consumed fabaceous plants, evaluate their potential as antioxidants and in glucose modulation, understand their role in preventing and managing diabetes, and ways to incorporate fabaceous plants as dietary strategies for diabetes.

2. Diabetes Mellitus Generalities

According to the International Diabetes Federation, in 2021, the number of people living with diabetes worldwide was 537 million, of whom more than 95% had type 2 diabetes mellitus (T2DM) [1,13]. DM is diagnosed in patients who meet one of the following criteria: glycohemoglobin A1C ($\geq$48 mmol/mol), fasting plasma glucose (FPG) value ($\geq$126 mg/dL), 2 h glucose value ($\geq$200 mg/dL) during a 75 g oral glucose tolerance test (OGTT), or random glucose value ($\geq$200 mg/dL) [14].

Beta cells, one of the cells of the pancreatic islet, synthesize and secret insulin, regulating blood glucose levels [15]. After a meal, glucose is transported in the blood and enters the beta cell through the glucose transporter Glut2, glucose is then metabolized through glycolysis, increasing the intracellular ATP/ADP ratio, which in turn leads to the closure of the ATP-dependent potassium (KATP) channels in the plasma membrane. This causes membrane depolarization and opening of voltage-gated calcium channels, allowing Ca2+ to enter the cell, triggering insulin exocytosis, leading to the release of insulin into the bloodstream [16]. Impaired pancreatic beta cell function has been identified as a major factor contributing to the onset of T2DM. The mechanisms leading to beta cell failure in type 1 diabetes are classified into three categories: (a) reduction in beta cell number, (b) functional exhaustion of beta cells, and (c) loss of their cellular identity [17,18]. In type 2 diabetes, insulin resistance is the primary cause, while impaired insulin secretion results from inflammation and hyperglycemia. Hyperglycemia is a common trigger in both forms of diabetes as it causes oxidative stress [19], inflammation, cytokine secretion, cellular exhaustion, and apoptosis, contributing to beta cell damage and disease complications [20].

Based on the above information, antidiabetic agents target different steps in the signaling and functioning of insulin, such as the activation of insulin receptors (insulin analogs) and downstream signaling in multiple sensitive tissues [4], insulin sensitizers (sulfonylureas, biguadines) increasing glucose uptake in tissues of the whole body [21,22], the opening of voltage-dependent calcium channels (meglitinides) [23], and inhibitors of SGLT-2 [24]. Additionally, GLP-1 analogs represent a significant advancement in the treatment of type 2 diabetes by improving glycemic control, promoting weight loss, and having a low risk of hypoglycemia [25].

The treatment of diabetes mellitus is based on the diagnosis of the type of diabetes mellitus, the available treatment regimens, lifestyle changes (diet and exercise), oral hypoglycemic drugs, such as biguanides, sulfonylureas, meglitinides, thiazolidinediones, gliptins, α-glucosidase and sodium-glucose cotransporter inhibitors, and, finally, insulin. An alternative antidiabetic medication should, as much as possible, be capable of preventing the onset and progression of T2DM and should stop the loss of beta cells and/or promote the restoration of beta cell mass independently of reducing hyperglycemia and ameliorating glucotoxicity and oxidative stress in pancreatic islets. Plants and their fruit could be a good alternative with few or no adverse effects in the treatment of diabetes [26].

For centuries, plants have been used to treat diseases, being the precursors of modern medicine. The use of plants was intended to reduce the discomfort caused by diseases, ensuring that the plant worked through trial and error. Based on cultural beliefs and experiences transmitted from generation to generation, different parts of plants, such as the seeds, flowers, leaves, roots, bark, fruits, and stems, were used without knowing the active ingredient or mechanism [27,28]. Plant extracts are used as supplements for treating diseases, becoming a natural therapeutic alternative with almost no side effects because they come from commonly consumed plants such as fabaceous ones [29,30].

3. Importance of Secondary Metabolites in Fabaceous Plants

Fabaceae are part of a family of nitrogen-fixing plants comprising 770 genera and approximately 19,500 species, which help to grow other plants in infertile or nutrient-poor soils. The plants of these species are climbers (annuals), herbs, aquatic plants, woody lianas, trees, shrubs, and subshrubs [8]. This family includes the fabaceous plant, commonly known as legumes. They are characterized by producing pods containing seeds (one to twelve) that vary in color, size, and shape depending on the type of plant. Many fabaceous plants are used for human consumption and/or oil extraction, as well as for animal feed, the most common being soybeans, beans, peas, broad bean, lentils, peanuts, and chickpeas due to the quality of their nutrients (complex carbohydrates, unsaturated fats, proteins, amino acids, vitamins, and minerals) and their low cost [31,32]. Fabaceous plants also contain secondary metabolites (SM) that act in the plants as a chemical defense against insects or predators and attract pollinators; on the other hand, when they are consumed, they present biological activities with benefits to health [28,33–35].

Secondary metabolites are chemical compounds produced by plants, fungi, and other microorganisms which are essential for interacting with the environment; the SM has a molecular mass of <3000 kDa, and they are distributed throughout the plant [34,36]. The stress (biotic or abiotic) to which a plant is subjected influences the production of SM; this can be caused by herbivores, pathogens, salinity, solar radiation, extreme temperatures, drought, and lack of nutrients (Figure 1). The SM, being a response to stress, turn into defenders of the plant, thus achieving its adaptation to the environment and its survival [34,37]. Plants, through their SM, can attract pollinating insects, as well as nitrogen-fixing bacteria, forming nodules of different sizes and characteristics in their roots [38]. SM can be classified into four main groups: phenolic compounds, nitrogen compounds, sulfur compounds, and terpenes. Phenolic compounds are distinguished by their ability to defend plants, functioning as antimicrobials and herbivore repellents. They also contribute to the protection against oxidative damage [36].

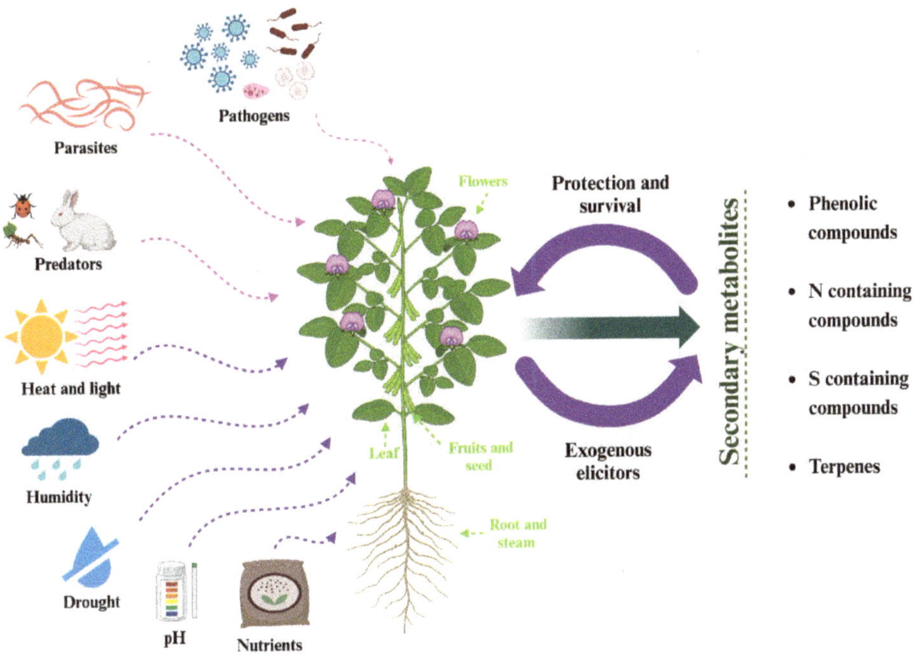

Figure 1. Secondary metabolite production in plants (N = nitrogen, S = sulfur) (created by BioRender).

4. Methodology

The search for information was performed following the PRISMA (Preferred Reporting Items for Systematic Review and Meta-Analysis) on Google Scholar, PubMed, Science Direct, and Scopus. Of all the articles found, those published within the previous 5 years were considered, with a maximum limit of 10 years for the plants with scarce information on them (less than five articles), ensuring the inclusion of recent and relevant advances, reflecting the area's current state. The keywords used for the search of articles were fabaceous (in general and for each of the species presented, it was also searched as legumes), "phenolic compounds", "antidiabetic phenolic compounds fabaceous", "extracts antidiabetic fabaceous", "antioxidant activity fabaceous", and each of the species names. From the selected articles, the general characteristics of fabaceous compounds, the phenolic compounds content, and the most outstanding compounds were considered, in addition to the results showing the hypoglycemic effect.

The inclusion and exclusion of articles in this review focused on selecting studies that addressed key aspects of diabetes mellitus, such as its description, development, and complications, as well as the production of secondary metabolites, especially phenolic compounds in fabaceous plants. Research that measured the antidiabetic potential of these phenolic compounds in commonly consumed species, such as soybeans, beans, peas, broad beans, lentils, and chickpeas, was included. However, articles that did not use the Fabaceae seed or its coating were excluded since these parts are the most relevant to studying the impact of phenolic compounds on diabetes management, ensuring that the review focused on the most pertinent and specific studies. Figure 2 shows the process of searching for information. First, we explored Google Scholar to determine whether the required information was available. Then, we used the most well-known databases and journals with a publication trend, precise information, and inclusion and exclusion criteria. In the record screening, a review of the titles and abstracts of the articles was carried out to evaluate their compliance with the established inclusion or exclusion criteria.

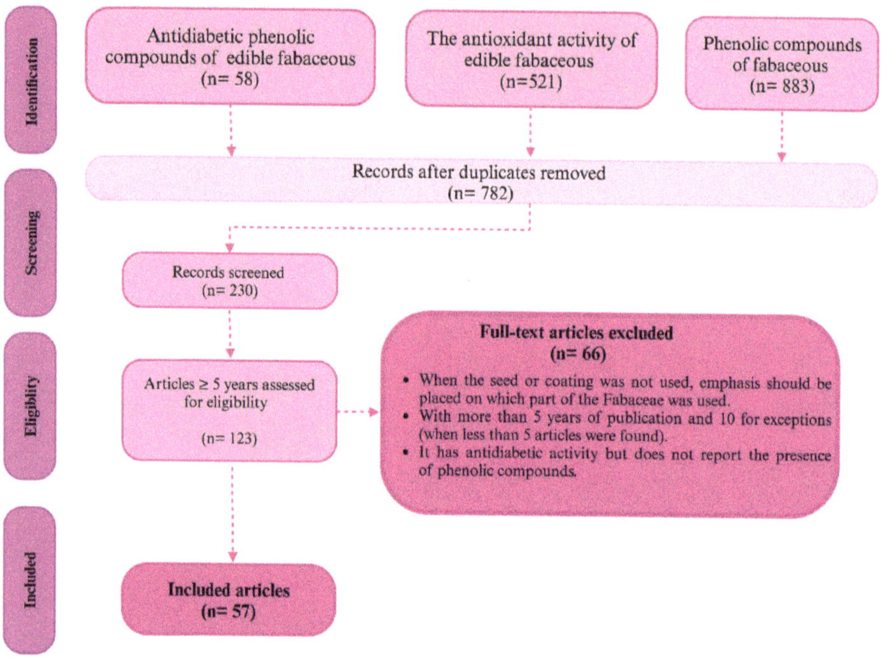

Figure 2. General diagram for the identification and selection of articles (created by BioRender).

5. Antioxidant Activity of Total Phenolic Compounds from Fabaceous Plants

The main characteristics of phenolic compounds are an aromatic ring and a hydroxyl group; within these, we can find catechol, derivatives of hydroxybenzoic acid, condensed tannins, flavonoids, stilbenes, and lignans. Phenolic compounds, being plant protectors, can function as toxins for herbivores or alter the growth or physiological processes of insects due to oxidation to toxic metabolites [34].

On the other hand, phenolic compounds also give color to the products extracted from red fruits (i.e., juices and wines), contributing to the aroma and enzymatic browning of the fruits [39]. Furthermore, phenolic compounds from vegetables and fruits, legumes, and grains included in the human diet are associated with health benefits [11,39].

Table 1 shows that the content of phenolic compounds in legumes varies significantly depending on the type of legume, the specific variety, and the region where they are grown. These differences show how factors such as the genetic variety of the legume and the growing conditions specific to each geographical region directly influence the accumulation of phenolic compounds, which are essential for their antioxidant properties and health benefits. For example, the highest concentration of these compounds in soybeans is reported in wild soybeans, 41.53 ± 1.25 mg GAE/g, compared to cultivated soybeans, whose concentration is lower (approximately 12.5 mg GAE/g). On the other hand, the color of the different varieties of bean seeds is also reflected in the values of phenolic compounds, such as in black, velvet, red, and white, where there is a range of 197–1328 mg GAE/g [40,41]. Something similar happens with pea varieties, although the concentration is lower than in beans, ranging from 0.12 to 2.66 mg GAE/g, a considerably wide range. The phenolic compound profile in the fabaceous plants of Table 1 is unique and presents an extensive range due to variety (genetic diversity), environment, stage of maturity, growing conditions, and cultivation methods [34].

Table 1. Phenolic compound content in fabaceous seed.

Fabaceous	Variety	Total Phenolic Content	Reference
Soybean	Black soybean	830.66 ± 5.46 mg GAE/kg	[42]
	Wild soybean	41.53 ± 1.25 mg GAE/g	[43]
	Cultivated soybean	12.5 mg GAE/g	
	Glycine max	2.04–6.10 mg GAE/g	[44]
	Local soy (China)	43.87± 3.22 mg GAE/100 g	[45]
Bean	*Different varieties*	0.57–10.34 mg de GAE/g	
	Black bean	197.23 ± 0.02 mg GAE/g	[40]
	Red kidney bean	1174.32 ± 103.11 mg GAE/g	[41]
	Velvet beans	12.19–37.30 mg GAE/g	[46]
	White kidney bean	1328.30 ± 156.63 mg GAE/g	[47]
	Vigna unguiculata	337.6 ± 14.6 mg GAE/100 g	
	Vigna mungo	547.2 ± 14.1 mg GAE/100 g	[48]
	Proteus vulgaris	440.2 ± 12.7 mg GAE/100 g	
Pea	Different varieties	12.6–128.6 mg GAE/100 g	[49]
	Different varieties	0.66–2.66 mg GAE/g	[50]
	Yellow pea	0.85–1.14 mg GAE/g	[51]
	Green pea	0.65–0.99 mg GAE/g	
Broad bean	Commercial (Tunisia)	115.21 mg GAE/g	[52]
	Commercial (Italy)	2.06 mg CAE/g	[53]
	Cultivated (Australian)	258–570 mg GAE/100 g	[54]
	Cultivated (Korea)	3.61 ± 0.11 mg GAE/g	[55]
	Cultivated (Tunisia)	1.122–1.225 mg GAE/g	[56]
Lentil	Commercial	26 mg GAE/100 g	[57]
	Different varieties	4.6–70 mg GAE/g	[58]
	Cultivated (Argelia)	49.65–59.12 mg GAE/g	[59]
	Black lentil	0.84 ± 0.03 mg GAE/g	[60]
	Green lentil	0.96 ± 0.07 mg GAE/g	
	Brown lentil	0.79 ± 0.02 mg GAE/g	
	Red lentil	0.81 ± 0.12 mg GAE/g	
Chickpea	Cicer reticulatum	8.02–10.84 mg GAE/g	[44]
	Different varieties	27.48–113.30 mg GAE/100 g	[61]

GAE: Gallic acid equivalent. CAE: Chlorogenic acid equivalents.

Moreover, the amount of phenolic compounds in fabaceous plants has been shown to correlate with antioxidant capacity and health benefits (Table 2). For example, in the case of soybeans, flavonoids predominate and have an associated relationship with biological activity, having a high antioxidant capacity of around 80% of the inhibition of free radicals through ABTS and DPPH reported [43]. In the case of beans, the presence of anthocyanins, which are responsible for giving red, blue, and purple colors, also influences the inhibitory activity of free radicals [47]. Although flavonoids are also reported in peas, they contain free phenolics that are more available to exert antioxidant activity. Fabaceous foods like beans and lentils have more phenolic compounds, influencing their antioxidant activity.

However, this activity does not reflect much variation based on the color of the seed but rather on the profile of the compounds (Table 2).

Table 2. Antioxidant activity of phenolic compounds from fabaceous plants.

Fabaceous Plant	Main Associated Compounds	ABTS	DPPH	Reference
Soybean (*Glycine max*) 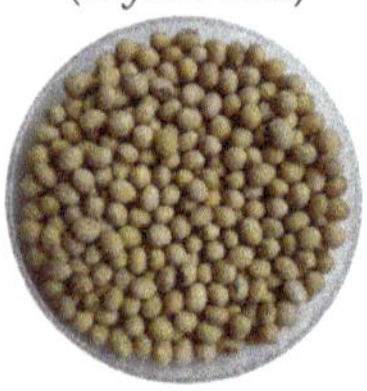	Flavonoids Anthocyanins Flavonoids (soybean; wild and cultivated) Flavonoids Flavonoids	92.74 ± 1.47 mmol eq. trolox/kg 84.28% inhibition 38.01% inhibition ----- EC_{50} 1.43 ± 0.12 mg/mL EC_{50} 1.64 ± 0.03 mg/mL	----- 82.58% inhibition 71.08% inhibition IC_{50} = 58.33 ± 0.26 µg/mL EC_{50} 1.33 ± 0.01 mg/mL EC_{50} 1.29 ± 0.02 mg/mL	[42] [43] [9] [62]
Bean (*Phaseolus vulgaris*) 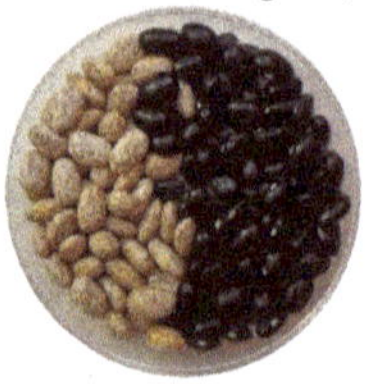	Phenolics (red and white *P. vulgaris*) Flavonoids Anthocyanins (*V. mungo*, *P. vulgaris*, and *V. angularis*) Flavonoids Phenolics	$1/EC_{50}$ 0.0061 ± 0.0008 mL/mg $1/EC_{50}$ 0.0035 ± 0.0005 mL/mg 56.4 ± 1.5 µmol eq. trolox/g 51.8 ± 1.0 µmol eq. trolox/g 84.1 ± 0.8 µmol eq. trolox/g ----- 1190.32 ± 42.77 mg eq. trolox/g	----- 52.1 ± 4.8 µmol eq. trolox/g 53.7 ± 3.6 µmol eq. trolox/g 98.7 ± 1.6 µmol eq. trolox/g IC_{50} 69.74 ± 0.08 µg/mL -----	[47] [48] [9] [63]
Pea (*Pisum sativum*) 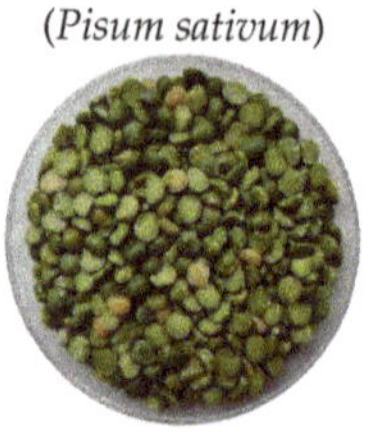	Flavonoids Flavonoids Free phenolic Bound phenolic Phenolics acids Flavonoids	----- ----- ----- 18.3 ± 1.2 mmol eq. trolox/kg	12.49 µmol eq. trolox/g IC_{50} 56.33 ± 0.13 µg/mL 2.3 µmol eq. trolox/g 0.5 µmol eq. trolox/g 13.7 ± 1.1 mmol eq. trolox/kg	[50] [9] [64] [65]
Broad bean (*Vicia faba*) 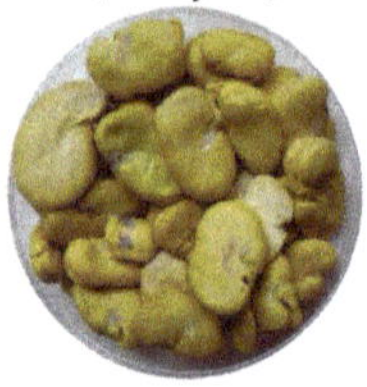	Flavonoid Condensed tannin Flavonoid Flavonoids	IC_{50} 610.61 ± 0.56 µg/mL ----- IC_{50} 2.35 ± 1.81 µg/mL	IC_{50} 157.94 ± 0.56 µg/mL IC_{50} 59.60 ± 0.24 µg/mL IC_{50} 74.71 ± 2.91 µg/mL	[52] [9] [53]

Table 2. *Cont.*

Fabaceous Plant	Main Associated Compounds	ABTS	DPPH	Reference
Lentil (*Lens culinaris*) 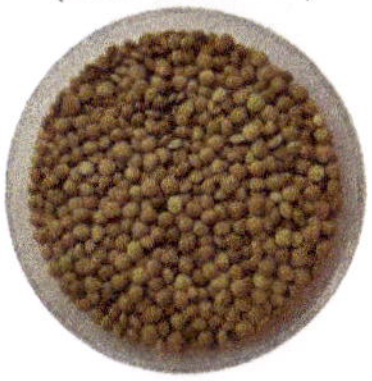	Flavonoids Condensed tannin Flavonoid Condensed tannin Proanthocyanin Anthocyanin (black, green, red, and brown) Flavonoids Phenolics acids Flavonoids (fermented seed; *A. oryzae* 24 h and *A. niger* 48 h)	EC_{50} 1.28 mg/mL 6.47 ± 0.81 mg eq. trolox/g 9.82 ± 0.71 mg eq. trolox/g 8.06 ± 0.47 mg eq. trolox/g 7.94 ± 0.12 mg eq. trolox/g ----- 6.81 μg eq. trolox/g 6.97 μg eq. trolox/g	EC_{50} 4.92 mg/mL 4.32 ± 0.08 mg eq. trolox/g 5.24 ± 0.02 mg eq. trolox/g 4.65 ± 0.02 mg eq. trolox/g 3.21 ± 0.08 mg eq. trolox/g IC_{50} 61.50 ± 0.16 μg/mL 7.48 μg eq. trolox/g 10.02 μg eq. trolox/g	[59] [60] [9] [66]
Chickpea (*Cicer arietinum*) 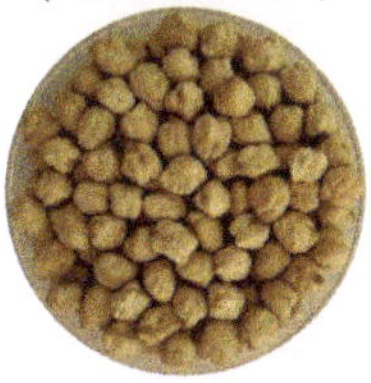	----- Flavonoids Isoflavonoids	25.06 mg/g de GAE 159–207 mmol eq. trolox/100 g	22.2 mg eq. trolox/g -----	[67] [68]

ABTS: 2,2′-azino-bis(3-ethylbenzothiazoline-6-sulfonic acid) and DPPH: 2,2-diphenyl-1-picrylhydrazyl; most used methods to evaluate antioxidant activity. Extracts or fractions of compounds with low IC_{50} and EC_{50} values are potent antioxidants. IC_{50}: concentration corresponding to 50% inhibition. EC_{50} is the sample concentration required for a 50% decrease in DPPH concentration.

Phenolic compound extraction and processing as phytotherapeutic practice has the potential to be effective therapeutic or preventative agents against different diseases [11,39], neutralizing free radicals and protecting cells from oxidative damage. This is known as antioxidant capacity, one of the most studied biological activities due to its relationship with chronic diseases. For example, in DM, an increase in free radicals affects the mechanism of insulin action, causing damage to pancreatic beta cells.

Phenolic compounds, as part of bioactive compounds, have been shown to significantly inhibit enzymes such as lipases, α-amylase, α-glucosidase, and β-glucosidase in vitro [69]. By inhibiting α-glucosidase, these compounds reduce glucose digestion and absorption in the intestine, which is crucial for managing type 2 diabetes as they help regulate blood sugar levels after meals. The activity of phenolic compounds underlines the importance of bioactive compounds in the diet, highlighting their potential to contribute to the prevention and control of metabolic diseases [69,70]. The bioactive compounds contained in fabaceous plants reduce the risk of suffering from T2DM [33,34]. In vitro antidiabetic studies of fabaceous plants have been evaluated through various methods, including glucose uptake assay and the inhibition of α-glucosidase, α-amylase, and DPP-IV (Dipeptidyl peptidase IV) [32].

6. In Vitro and In Vivo Antidiabetic Studies of Edible Fabaceous Plants

6.1. Soybean

Soybean (*Glycine max*) is one of the most edible fabaceous plants with the highest protein (40%) content; the wild soybean tends to have 10% more protein and 10% less oil than black soybean [71]. In addition to its nutritional composition, carbohydrates (33%), unsaturated fatty acids (20%), fiber, vitamins, minerals, and other bioactive compounds such as polyphenols, flavonoids, isoflavone, and glycosides are present [45,72,73]. The combination of phenolic compounds such as anthocyanins, proanthocyanidins, chlorophyll, and other pigments defines the characteristic color of their seed coat [42,74].

Identifying and analyzing the α-glucosidase enzyme inhibitors derived from black soybeans resulted in the bioactive compounds present in this fabaceous plant achieving inhibition of the enzyme; this lead to the regulation of glucose levels because the digestion of carbohydrates was reduced, which suggests a potential use for this inhibitor in the management of T2DM. Soy isoflavones (daidzin, glycitin, genistin, malonyldaidzin, malonylgenistin, genistein, and daidzein) inhibitors of α-glucosidase were identified, resulting in daidzein (IC_{50} 15.7 ± 0.3 μmol/L) and genistein (IC_{50} 3.2 ± 1.2 μmol/L) showing an inhibitory activity superior to that of acarbose (IC_{50} 632.5 ± 70.0 μmol/L). The structure–activity relationship indicated that isoflavone aglycones without glucosylation have higher inhibitory activity. Hydrophobic interactions and hydrogen bonds were the main forces involved in the interaction between isoflavones and α-glucosidase, suggesting that black soybean, through its isoflavones, has significant antidiabetic potential [72]. In another investigation conducted with the same animal model of T2DM, *Glycine max* fermented flour was used in a dose of 18.050 mg/kgBW, reducing blood glucose as the positive control group (administration of treatment). One of the hypoglycemic mechanisms is that isoflavone compounds can be transformed into aglycones (genistein, glycitein, and daidzein), which help reduce blood glucose. In addition, the fermentation process can transform the aglycone to produce compounds with greater biological activity, such as 6,7,4′ trihydroxy isoflavone, which has better antioxidant activity than daidzein and genistein. It also acts on free radicals caused by hyperglycemia. Isoflavones lower blood glucose by activating the peroxisome proliferator-activated receptor and protecting cells from cytokine pre-inflammation, fat-induced damage, and apoptosis [75].

Son et al. investigated the antidiabetic effects of *Glycine soja* extract in type 2 diabetic mice and insulin-resistant human hepatocytes for 6 weeks. Different concentrations were evaluated, with the group receiving the highest dose (300 mg/kg/day) achieving the lowest blood glucose levels (331.3 ± 78.6 mg/dL). Significant effects showed properties that improved insulin sensitivity by increasing adiponectin, and blood glucose and glycated hemoglobin levels were reduced, especially at doses higher than 150 mg/kg/day [71]. The hypoglycemic effect of fermented mulberry with soy has also been evaluated. This mixture for diabetic mice (type 2) reduced blood glucose levels, and improvements were observed in pancreatic function and insulin sensitivity. This indicates that the combination of mulberry and soy (1:5) enhances the beneficial effects at a concentration of 2.26 g/kg/day since the diabetic group reduced food consumption, improved glucose tolerance, and optimized the blood lipid profile, thanks to its antioxidant capacity [76].

6.2. Beans

Beans (*Phaseolus vulgaris*) are one of the most widely consumed fabaceous plant, with black beans being one of the main ones included in the diets of Latin America and Africa. This fabaceous plant stands out due to its rich nutritional composition of protein (17.9–31.1%), carbohydrates (25–60%), lipids (0.55–2.1%), fiber (4–20%), vitamins, and minerals. Despite being rich in carbohydrates, they have a low glycemic index, so they release their energy slowly, helping to keep blood sugar levels stable [77]. This fabaceous plant is rich in nutrients such as carbohydrates, proteins, fiber, and bioactive compounds (phenols, alkaloids, phytosterols, coumarins, and saponins). It has also been reported that they contain polysaccharides, peptides, and polyphenols. Bean seeds (*Phaseolus vulgaris*) are used as traditional medicine in some parts of China [78]. Polyphenol extracts in mung beans (a common compound in plants) have a hypoglycemic effect. By consuming foods with a low glycemic index and high dietary fiber content, the blood glucose is reduced, facilitating the elimination of glucose through the glucose transporter (GLUT4) [79,80].

A study evaluating the inhibitory effects of polyphenol-rich extracts (from six bean varieties) on α-amylase and α-glucosidase enzymes found that the *Sanghellato* variety had the highest amount of phenolic compounds. In carbohydrate digestion, polyphenolic extracts showed an inhibition of the α-amylase enzyme as well as inhibiting the α-glucosidase enzyme. The *Screziato Impalato* variety presented the best inhibition of α-amylase with an IC_{50} value of 69.02 μg/mL. For α-glucosidase, there was a more significant inhibition, presenting an IC_{50} of 90.40 μg/mL for the variety *Cannellino Rosso*. It is reported that tannins and proanthocyanidins (phenolic compounds) are related to the inhibition of both enzymes, suggesting a synergistic interaction between phenolic compounds and the inhibitory effect [81].

In a mouse model with T2DM, the hypoglycemic effect of beans was evaluated, where a significant reduction in blood glucose, cholesterol, and lipid levels was observed due to the influence on metabolic pathways related to insulin sensitivity and the regulation of lipid and carbohydrate metabolism [82]. The identified metabolites present significant potential for managing T2DM, related to the enrichment of soybean sprouts with γ-aminobutyric acid (GABA). This compound has been studied for its ability to improve metabolism and regulate blood glucose levels. It has been suggested that the enrichment of certain foods, such as soybean sprouts, with GABA could have beneficial effects on metabolic health and the control of type 2 diabetes. In addition, a decrease in urea and creatinine levels was observed, indicating that several metabolic parameters are improved in diabetic mice [82]. On the other hand, the effect of polyphenol extracts from germinated mung beans was evaluated in T2DM mice, obtaining significant improvements in blood glucose levels and the reduction in systemic inflammation associated with T2DM. Polyphenolic extracts reduce fasting glucose levels, improve glucose tolerance, and decrease insulin resistance, providing a better effect in the high concentration group (150 mg/kg) of the extract and improving lipid levels and liver enzymes. Along with these results, a balance was observed in the mice's intestinal microflora related to insulin sensitivity [83]. In another study, they evaluated the effect of bean-rice and rice-without-bean intake in adults with T2DM with consumption at different times; a significant difference was obtained in the groups that consumed bean-rice compared to those that did not. Three varieties of beans were evaluated; the groups that ingested pinto and black beans showed lower glycemic values than the red beans and the control (rice only). This study suggests that including beans in meals can reduce the glycemic response in patients with T2DM, offering a non-pharmacological dietary management alternative. In addition, promoting these traditional foods can improve dietary adherence and quality of life in minority and immigrant populations with diabetes [84]. Knowing the effect of the compounds present in beans is important, as few studies focus on the substances. Although the main phytonutrients studied as phytotherapeutics are secondary metabolites, the study of the various components of foods should be expanded.

6.3. *Pea*

The pea (*Pisum sativum*) is a bean of European origin [65] that is very adaptable to cultivation. Peas have a high nutritional value due to their composition of dietary fiber (11.34–16.13%), lipids (0.57–3.52%), and protein (19.75–26.48%), in addition to trace elements, phenolic compounds, and their glycemic index being less than 60 (considered medium or low). Flavonoids are the main polyphenols in peas so the content of their bioactive compounds can be used for functional foods or other products [50,85].

Di Stefano et al. investigated how bioprocessing (germination and fermentation) of fabaceous plants influences the inhibitory activities of DPP-IV and α-glucosidase. The findings indicated that bioprocessing facilitates the digestion and absorption of bioactive compounds, and that yellow pea extract can inhibit two critical enzymes in blood glucose regulation: DPP-IV and α-glucosidase. The inhibition of DPP-IV was approximately 55.1 ± 1.5 milliequivalents of Diprotin A, while the inhibition of α-glucosidase was 56.5 ± 5.2 milliequivalents of acarbose, suggesting that processed fabaceous plants could function as health supplements [85]. In another study, the inhibitory activity of the enzyme α-glucosidase from pea (*Cajanus cajan*) extract was tested. This extract containing saponins, flavonoids, phenolics, and tannins, among other compounds, caused a delay in the breakdown of carbohydrates, leading to a decrease in glucose absorption into the bloodstream and thus lowering postprandial hyperglycemia. The enzyme α-glucosidase results in an IC_{50} value of 69.67 ppm, a high level which indicates its potential as an antidiabetic drug [86]. The consumption of peas has presented advantages for potentially improving diseases associated with insulin resistance. Peas with a low glycemic index (22) can help maintain blood sugar levels, which can trigger an improvement in insulin sensitivity [51].

6.4. Broad Beans

Vicia faba, known as the broad beans, is a fabaceous plant rich in nutrients such as protein (present in high amounts; 29%), carbohydrates (56–68%), lipids (2.30–3.91%), fiber, vitamins, and phenolic compounds in the seed. Due to the root nodules, the bean plant has a greater capacity to fix nitrogen than other bean plants. The consumption of broad bean flowers benefits health due to their polyphenol content, which reduces the risk of cancer, cardiovascular diseases, and diabetes due to their ability to counteract free radicals [87,88]. The broad bean has a low glycemic index and little fat; this seed is a health promoter because it has anti-cancer, anti-diabetic, anti-obesity, and cardioprotective effects. The primary polyphenols in broad beans are tannins; broad bean seeds usually have many phenolic compounds, almost twice as many as other fabaceous plants [89]. Mejri et al. report different percentages in extracting broad bean's yield of phenolic compounds because different solvents were used to obtain them. Methanol presented the highest extraction with 25.8%, ethanol with 17.5%, butanol and ethyl acetate presented the lowest extraction percentage, at 11.3% and 0.81%, respectively. The methanolic extract also exhibited the highest total phenolic, flavonoid, and tannin content and showed antidiabetic effects in alloxan-induced diabetic mice. It was found that blood glucose concentration and deterioration of pancreatic β-cells produced by alloxan were reverted after the administration of BBP extract, apparently through its antioxidant properties [53]. Sharma and Giri reported an α-amylase inhibitory concentration IC_{50} of 264.69 μg/mL, thus providing data on the properties of natural antidiabetic agents of the broad bean; this result was better than the standard (acarbose IC_{50} of 52.76 μg/mL) [9]. When extracts are obtained with different solvents, there may be differences in the potential for inhibition of α-amylase, as shown in the study of the broad bean where the best concentration was 3-5 mg/mL with the acetone and methanol extracts having an IC_{50} value of 2.94 mg/mL, which could lead to a lower postprandial glucose level [90]. Broad beans are a rich source of polyphenolic compounds acting as antioxidants scavenging free radicals, helping in treating diabetes and, with the rejuvenation of beta cells of the pancreas, broad beans are ideal for consumption by diabetics as they inhibit α-glucosidase, thus delaying the absorption of carbohydrates [88].

6.5. Lentils

The lentil (*Lens culinaris*) contains many macro and micronutrients: carbohydrates (40–50%), protein (20–30%), fiber, vitamins, and minerals, highlighting that the green and gray seeds are preventative and, in many cases, have a health benefit [57,58,66]. Among the benefits of consuming lentils is their insoluble fiber content, as a source of prebiotics and prebiotic carbohydrates, stimulating the microbial flora, benefiting health, and preventing intestinal diseases. Lentils (sprouted) have been reported to improve blood glucose metabolism as well as decrease lipoproteins and lipids in diabetic patients. Compared to other fabaceous plants, lentils contain a high content of phenolic compounds, with a high concentration of phenolic acids, flavonoids, and condensed tannins. The polyphenols in lentils reduce the glycemic index, making them suitable for a healthy diet [57]. The consumption of lentils is recommended to prevent or control diabetes since it has been shown to improve the metabolism of lipids and lipoproteins, as well as help with blood glucose; the above is possible due to the fiber content, in addition to the flavonoids contained in them [58].

Magro et al. found phenolic compounds such as ferulic acid and quercetin in fermented lentils; vanillic acid and 3,4-dihydroxybenzoic acid were also detected (in fermented and non-fermented lentils). Lentils fermented with *Aspergillus niger* showed greater inhibition (91%; 48 h of fermentation) of α-glucosidase than those fermented with *Aspergillus oryzae* and non-fermented ones. For the inhibition of α-amylase, lentils were fermented with *A. oryzae* at different fermentation times (75%; 24 h, 73%; 48 h and 71%; 0 h); α-amylase is an enzyme that breaks down starches into simple sugars, and its activity may influence blood glucose control [66].

In an experimental study with diabetic male and female mice, methanolic extracts of fermented lentil seeds were administered for 6–8 weeks. Aqueous methanolic extracts of fermented lentils reduced blood glucose in diabetic mice; the reduction was significantly greater with the 400 mg/kg extract (169.92 $\pm$ 1.62 mg/dL) than with the 200 mg/kg extract (180.83 $\pm$ 2.858 mg/dL) and 100 mg/kg (190.83 $\pm$ 1.80 mg/dL). All three doses showed a statistically significant difference from the diabetic control group with blood glucose concentration (252.17 $\pm$ 3.84 mg/dL). The group treated with glibenclamide showed a hypoglycemic effect due to its direct impact on the mechanics of insulin release from beta cells and increasing glucose tolerance [91].

6.6. Chickpea

The chickpea is a fabaceous plant with a rich nutritional composition containing 17 to 22% of proteins, 18 to 22% of dietary fiber, and a higher lipid content of up to 7% [61]. Chickpea bioactive compounds, such as phenolics, help inhibit the hydrolysis of carbohydrates and some lipids, decreasing the risk of developing T2DM. Polyphenols also have a mechanism of action to inactivate the DPP-IV enzyme by 70-90% [92]. Seed chickpeas are other well-known and consumed fabaceous plants, but little research has been performed on their phenolic compounds with antidiabetic potential. Chickpea (*Cicer arietinum*) is characterized by its high protein content but also by the phenolic compounds it has, such as isoflavones (153 to 340 mg/100 g) [44].

Based on different experimental studies, the Table 3 summarizes the antidiabetic effects of various fabaceous, such as soybean, bean, pea, broad bean, lentil, and chickpea. Key mechanisms are highlighted, such as the inhibition of enzymes related to carbohydrate metabolism (α-glucosidase and DPP-IV), antioxidant activity, reduction in glucose, lipid, and glycosylated hemoglobin levels, as well as improvement in insulin sensitivity and decreased inflammation. This summary demonstrates fabaceous therapeutic potential in controlling and managing diabetes.

Table 3. Impact of fabaceous on diabetes control.

Fabaceous	Experimental Approach	Effect	Reference
Soybean	Isoflavones in vitro Isoflavones in vitro Polyphenolic in vivo Polyphenolic in vivo	α-glucosidase inhibition Antioxidant activity Reducing blood glucose Reducing blood glucose and glycated hemoglobin Insulin sensitivity	[72] [75] [71] [76]
Bean	Tannins and proanthocyanidins in vitro Polyphenolic in vivo Polyphenolic in vivo Clinical study	α-glucosidase and α-glucosidase enzyme inhibition Reducing blood glucose, cholesterol, and lipid levels Improves blood glucose levels and reduces inflammation Lower glycemic values	[81] [82] [83] [84]
Pea	Polyphenolic in vitro Flavonoids and tannins in vitro	Inhibitory activities of DPP-IV and α-glucosidase Inhibitory activity of the enzyme α-glucosidase	[85] [86]
Broad beans	Flavonoids and tannins in vivo Polyphenolic in vitro	Blood glucose concentration and pancreatic beta cell deterioration were reversed Inhibitory activity of the enzyme α-glucosidase	[53] [9,90]
Lentil	Polyphenolic in vitro Polyphenolic in vivo	α-glucosidase and α-glucosidase enzyme inhibition Reducing blood glucose	[66] [91]
Chickpea	Polyphenolic in vitro	Inactivate the DPP-IV enzyme	[92]

7. Perspectives

Natural products have been used as medicine throughout history and are still the basis for the development of drugs. Current research not only seeks new molecules but also focuses on the development of phytotherapeutics to prevent or treat diseases or find evidence to support the biological activity of plants. The design and development of phytotherapeutics must be standardized, and the chemical compounds associated with the medicinal properties present in plants must be identified. Phytotherapeutics or nutraceuticals can be formulated from bioactive compounds such as phenolics (Figure 3). Identifying phenolic compounds with antidiabetic potential can produce natural products in combination with pharmacological products that help prevent and/or treat diabetes mellitus, assisting patients with diabetes in the future. The analysis of bioactive molecules in plants drives the development of natural products, providing a new option for treating different diseases.

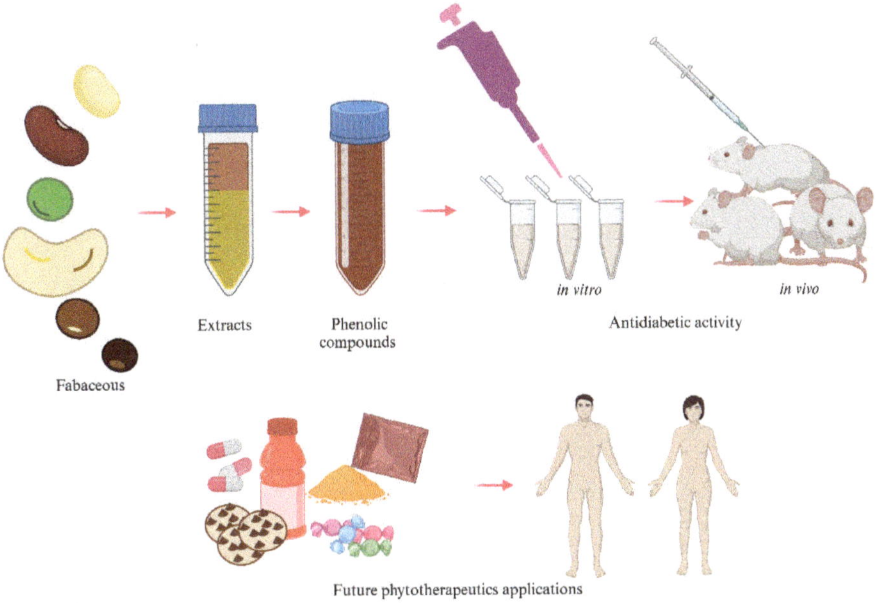

Figure 3. The process of obtaining and developing phytotherapeutics from fabaceous plants (created by BioRender).

Generally, plant consumption is assumed to be safe; however, it is important to consider that they contain chemical compounds that, in some cases, can cause oxidative damage in the body. Despite this, current evidence widely supports the safety of phytochemicals for treating DM. Improving the stability and bioavailability of phytotherapeutics is essential to ensure adequate absorption and maximize their efficacy as a treatment, offering an effective alternative with fewer side effects compared to conventional drugs used in the management of DM [93]. Phenolic compounds may have properties that can affect human health because they could act as endocrine disruptors, interfering with hormonal functions and influencing cellular processes such as energy production and generating reactive oxygen species [94].

Phenolic compounds exert their beneficial effects on health through a series of biochemical mechanisms that intervene at both the cellular and molecular level (Figure 4). These compounds, thanks to their chemical structure that includes a hydroxyl group (-OH), have the ability to donate electrons to free radicals or ROS species, neutralizing them and preventing cellular damage that can result from oxidative stress. This process protects cells from the damage that ROS can cause to key components, such as lipids, proteins and DNA. Regarding inflammation, phenolic compounds also modulate this response by reducing the release of proinflammatory cytokines such as TNF-α, IL-1β and IL-6, molecules that amplify and perpetuate inflammatory processes. In addition, many of these compounds have the ability to inhibit the activation of NF-κB (nuclear factor kappa B), a key protein in the regulation of chronic inflammation. Inhibition of NF-κB disrupts signals that promote persistent inflammation, which is crucial to preventing the development of various chronic diseases [93,95].

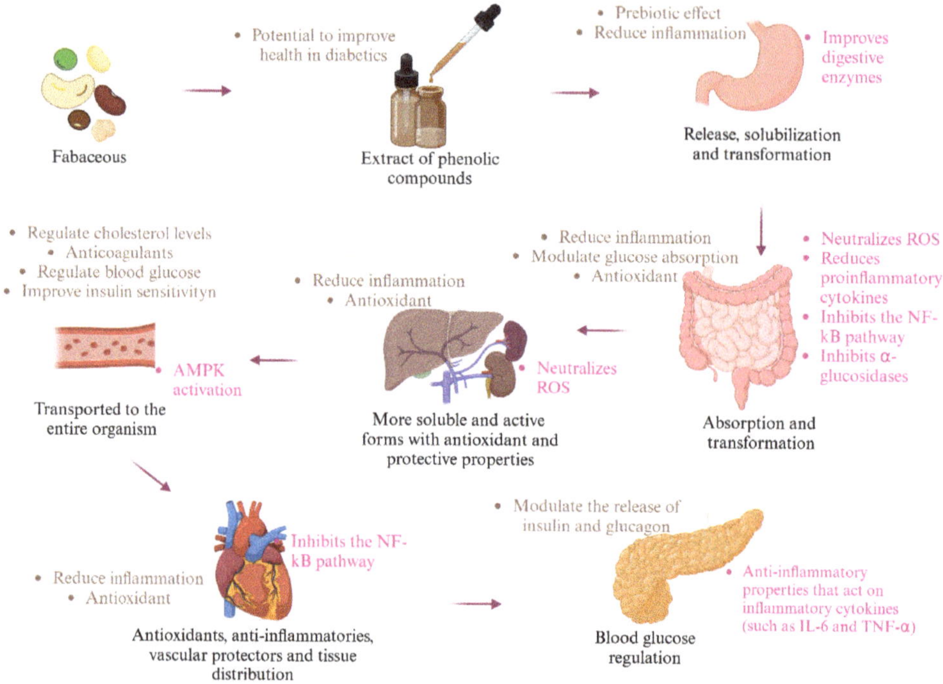

Figure 4. Potential mechanisms of action of phenolic compounds [93,95] (created by BioRender).

Although phenolic compounds may have certain adverse effects, they also have beneficial properties, such as their antioxidant capacity, which helps neutralize free radicals and protect cells from oxidative damage. In addition, some phenolic compounds are widely studied for their possible applications in the prevention of chronic diseases, such as cardiovascular diseases and certain types of cancer, thanks to their protective effects on the body when used in a controlled manner.

8. Conclusions

Fabaceous plants are accessible to virtually everyone and are essential for a healthy diet due to their nutritional profile. For some people, fabaceous plants are their primary source of protein as they avoid animal protein. The importance of fabaceous plants is highlighted by their bioactive compounds, such as phenols, which function as antioxidants and anti-inflammatory agents and play an essential role in health, stabilizing free radicals and preventing cell damage. Oxidative stress caused by free radicals in cells is associated with diabetes mellitus, which contributes to complications in different organs. The action of phenolic compounds helps mitigate damage and reduce risks due to their antioxidant and anti-inflammatory properties, benefiting patients with different pathologies.

Phenolic compounds have been evaluated in vitro and in vivo, where favorable results have been observed not only for their antioxidant capacity but also for their hypoglycemic effect, positively impacting the health of patients with diabetes mellitus; these characteristics make fabaceous plants of great interest with the potential to be used in future nutraceutical applications due to their efficacy.

The results of different studies summarized here support the role of fabaceous plants as adjuvants in the control of diabetes and show the importance of integrating the knowledge of traditional medicine with pharmacological medicine to improve the care of patients suffering from this condition. To integrate these herbal remedies into modern medicine, further research on phenolic compound type, doses, efficacy, and safety in humans is needed.

Author Contributions: Conceptualization L.G.-B.; Original draft preparation L.G.-B.; investigation L.G.-B., E.A.-O., S.M. and C.L.-S.; writing L.G.-B., E.A.-O., S.M., A.M.-M. and C.L.-S.; supervision L.G.-B., S.M., A.M.-M. and C.L.-S.; editor L.G.-B. S.M., C.L.-S.; R.G.G.-G. and A.A.F.-P. All authors have read and agreed to the published version of the manuscript.

Funding: This work was supported by CONAHCyT grant G-1176.

Institutional Review Board Statement: Not applicable.

Informed Consent Statement: Not applicable.

Data Availability Statement: Data sharing does not apply to this article.

Acknowledgments: The authors want to thank CONAHCyT for the PhD scholarship to the student L.G.-B. We would also like to thank L.G.-B. for creating the figures with BioRender.com.

Conflicts of Interest: The authors declare no conflicts of interest.

References

1. OMS. Diabetes. Available online: https://www.who.int/es (accessed on 25 April 2024).
2. Hu, K.; Huang, H.; Li, H.; Wei, Y.; Yao, C. Legume-Derived Bioactive Peptides in Type 2 Diabetes: Opportunities and Challenges. *Nutrients* **2023**, *15*, 1096. [CrossRef] [PubMed]
3. Yedjou, C.G.; Grigsby, J.; Mbemi, A.; Nelson, D.; Mildort, B.; Latinwo, L.; Tchounwou, P.B. The Management of Diabetes Mellitus Using Medicinal Plants and Vitamins. *Int. J. Mol. Sci.* **2023**, *24*, 9085. [CrossRef] [PubMed]
4. Rahman, M.S.; Hossain, K.S.; Das, S.; Kundu, S.; Adegoke, E.O.; Rahman, M.A.; Hannan, M.A.; Uddin, M.J.; Pang, M.G. Role of Insulin in Health and Disease: An Update. *Int. J. Mol. Sci.* **2021**, *22*, 6403. [CrossRef] [PubMed]
5. Sun, W.; Shahrajabian, M.H. Therapeutic Potential of Phenolic Compounds in Medicinal Plants—Natural Health Products for Human Health. *Molecules* **2023**, *28*, 1845. [CrossRef]
6. Kang, B.B.; Chiang, B.H. A Novel Phenolic Formulation for Treating Hepatic and Peripheral Insulin Resistance by Regulating GLUT4-Mediated Glucose Uptake. *J. Tradit. Complement. Med.* **2022**, *12*, 195–205. [CrossRef]
7. Przeor, M. Some Common Medicinal Plants with Antidiabetic Activity, Known and Available in Europe (A Mini-Review). *Pharmaceuticals* **2022**, *15*, 65. [CrossRef]
8. Maroyi, A. Medicinal Uses of the Fabaceae Family in Zimbabwe: A Review. *Plants* **2023**, *12*, 1255. [CrossRef]
9. Sharma, K.R.; Giri, G. Quantification of Phenolic and Flavonoid Content, Antioxidant Activity, and Proximate Composition of Some Legume Seeds Grown in Nepal. *Int. J. Food Sci.* **2022**, *2022*, 4629290. [CrossRef]
10. Alara, O.R.; Abdurahman, N.H.; Ukaegbu, C.I. Extraction of Phenolic Compounds: A Review. *Curr. Res. Food Sci.* **2021**, *4*, 200–214. [CrossRef]
11. Zhang, Y.; Cai, P.; Cheng, G.; Zhang, Y. A Brief Review of Phenolic Compounds Identified from Plants: Their Extraction, Analysis, and Biological Activity. *Nat. Prod. Commun.* **2022**, *17*, 1–14. [CrossRef]
12. Albergaria, E.T.; Oliveira, A.F.M.; Albuquerque, U.P. The Effect of Water Deficit Stress on the Composition of Phenolic Compounds in Medicinal Plants. *S. Afr. J. Bot.* **2020**, *131*, 12–17. [CrossRef]
13. International Diabetes Federation. Diabetes Atlas. Available online: https://www.diabetesatlas.org (accessed on 28 May 2024).
14. American Diabetes Association Professional Practice Committee. 2. Diagnosis and Classification of Diabetes: Standards of Care in Diabetes—2024. *Diabetes Care* **2024**, *47*, 20–42. [CrossRef] [PubMed]
15. Deepa-Maheshvare, M.; Raha, S.; König, M.; Pal, D. A Pathway Model of Glucose-Stimulated Insulin Secretion in the Pancreatic β-Cell. *Front. Endocrinol.* **2023**, *14*, 1185656. [CrossRef] [PubMed]
16. Galicia-Garcia, U.; Benito-Vicente, A.; Jebari, S.; Larrea-Sebal, A.; Siddiqi, H.; Uribe, K.B.; Ostolaza, H.; Martín, C. Pathophysiology of Type 2 Diabetes Mellitus. *Int. J. Mol. Sci.* **2020**, *21*, 6275. [CrossRef]
17. Wysham, C.; Shubrook, J. Beta-Cell Failure in Type 2 Diabetes: Mechanisms, Markers, and Clinical Implications. *Postgrad. Med.* **2020**, *132*, 676–686. [CrossRef]
18. Swisa, A.; Glaser, B.; Dor, Y. Metabolic Stress and Compromised Identity of Pancreatic Beta Cells. *Front. Genet.* **2017**, *8*, 21. [CrossRef]
19. González, P.; Lozano, P.; Ros, G.; Solano, F. Hyperglycemia and Oxidative Stress: An Integral, Updated and Critical Overview of Their Metabolic Interconnections. *Int. J. Mol. Sci.* **2023**, *24*, 9352. [CrossRef]

20. Volpe, C.M.O.; Villar-Delfino, P.H.; dos Anjos, P.M.F.; Nogueira-Machado, J.A. Cellular Death, Reactive Oxygen Species (ROS) and Diabetic Complications. *Cell Death Dis.* **2018**, *9*, 119. [CrossRef]
21. Mishra, V.; Nayak, P.; Sharma, M.; Albutti, A.; Alwashmi, A.S.S.; Aljasir, M.A.; Alsowayeh, N.; Tambuwala, M.M. Emerging Treatment Strategies for Diabetes Mellitus and Associated Complications: An Update. *Pharmaceutics* **2021**, *13*, 1568. [CrossRef]
22. Lamoia, T.E.; Shulman, G.I. Cellular and Molecular Mechanisms of Metformin Action. *Endocr. Rev.* **2021**, *42*, 77–96. [CrossRef]
23. Pakkir Maideen, N.M.; Manavalan, G.; Balasubramanian, K. Drug Interactions of Meglitinide Antidiabetics Involving CYP Enzymes and OATP1B1 Transporter. *Ther. Adv. Endocrinol. Metab.* **2018**, *9*, 259–268. [CrossRef] [PubMed]
24. Gilbert, M.P.; Pratley, R.E. GLP-1 Analogs and DPP-4 Inhibitors in Type 2 Diabetes Therapy: Review of Head-to-Head Clinical Trials. *Front. Endocrinol.* **2020**, *3*, 11. [CrossRef] [PubMed]
25. Kramer, C.K.; Zinman, B. Sodium–Glucose Cotransporter–2 (SGLT-2) Inhibitors and the Treatment of Type 2 Diabetes. *Annu. Rev. Med.* **2019**, *70*, 323–334. [CrossRef]
26. Chaudhury, A.; Duvoor, C.; Reddy Dendi, V.S.; Kraleti, S.; Chada, A.; Ravilla, R.; Marco, A.; Shekhawat, N.S.; Montales, M.T.; Kuriakose, K.; et al. Clinical Review of Antidiabetic Drugs: Implications for Type 2 Diabetes Mellitus Management. *Front. Endocrinol.* **2017**, *8*, 6. [CrossRef] [PubMed]
27. Salmerón-Manzano, E.; Garrido-Cardenas, J.A.; Manzano-Agugliaro, F. Worldwide Research Trends on Medicinal Plants. *Int. J. Environ. Res. Public Health* **2020**, *17*, 3376. [CrossRef]
28. Alqethami, A.; Aldhebiani, A.Y. Medicinal Plants Used in Jeddah, Saudi Arabia: Phytochemical Screening. *Saudi J. Biol. Sci.* **2021**, *28*, 805–812. [CrossRef]
29. Tang, F.; Yan, H.L.; Wang, L.X.; Xu, J.F.; Peng, C.; Ao, H.; Tan, Y.Z. Review of Natural Resources With Vasodilation: Traditional Medicinal Plants, Natural Products, and Their Mechanism and Clinical Efficacy. *Front. Pharmacol.* **2021**, *12*, 627458. [CrossRef]
30. Ullah, R.; Alqahtani, A.S.; Noman, O.M.A.; Alqahtani, A.M.; Ibenmoussa, S.; Bourhia, M. A Review on Ethno-Medicinal Plants Used in Traditional Medicine in the Kingdom of Saudi Arabia. *Saudi J. Biol. Sci.* **2020**, *27*, 2706–2718. [CrossRef]
31. Moreno-Valdespino, C.A.; Luna-Vital, D.; Camacho-Ruiz, R.M.; Mojica, L. Bioactive Proteins and Phytochemicals from Legumes: Mechanisms of Action Preventing Obesity and Type-2 Diabetes. *Food Res. Int.* **2020**, *130*, 108905. [CrossRef]
32. Looi, E.P.; Mohd, M.N. The Bioactivities of Legumes: A Review. *Food Res.* **2023**, *7*, 339–360. [CrossRef]
33. Ishaq, A.R.; El-Nashar, H.A.S.; Younis, T.; Mangat, M.A.; Shahzadi, M.; Ul Haq, A.S.; El-Shazly, M. Genus *Lupinus* (Fabaceae): A Review of Ethnobotanical, Phytochemical and Biological Studies. *J. Pharm. Pharmacol.* **2022**, *74*, 1700–1717. [CrossRef] [PubMed]
34. Divekar, P.A.; Narayana, S.; Divekar, B.A.; Kumar, R.; Gadratagi, B.G.; Ray, A.; Singh, A.K.; Rani, V.; Singh, V.; Singh, A.K.; et al. Plant Secondary Metabolites as Defense Tools against Herbivores for Sustainable Crop Protection. *Int. J. Mol. Sci.* **2022**, *23*, 2690. [CrossRef]
35. Hughes, J.; Pearson, E.; Grafenauer, S. Legumes—A Comprehensive Exploration of Global Food-Based Dietary Guidelines and Consumption. *Nutrients* **2022**, *14*, 3080. [CrossRef] [PubMed]
36. Twaij, B.M.; Hasan, M.N. Bioactive Secondary Metabolites from Plant Sources: Types, Synthesis, and Their Therapeutic Uses. *Int. J. Plant Biol.* **2022**, *13*, 4–14. [CrossRef]
37. Li, Y.; Kong, D.; Fu, Y.; Sussman, M.R.; Wu, H. The Effect of Developmental and Environmental Factors on Secondary Metabolites in Medicinal Plants. *Plant Physiol. Biochem.* **2020**, *148*, 80–89. [CrossRef]
38. Ku, Y.S.; Contador, C.A.; Ng, M.S.; Yu, J.; Chung, G.; Lam, H.M. The Effects of Domestication on Secondary Metabolite Composition in Legumes. *Front. Genet.* **2020**, *11*, 581357. [CrossRef]
39. Cheynier, V. Phenolic Compounds: From Plants to Foods. *Phytochem. Rev.* **2012**, *11*, 153–177. [CrossRef]
40. Nikolić, V.; Žilić, S.; Simić, M.; Perić, V. Black Soya Bean and Black Chia Seeds as a Source of Nutrients and Bioactive Compounds with Health Benefits. *Food Feed Res.* **2020**, *47*, 99–107. [CrossRef]
41. Chen, Q.; Wang, X.; Yuan, X.; Shi, J.; Zhang, C.; Yan, N.; Jing, C. Comparison of Phenolic and Flavonoid Compound Profiles and Antioxidant and α-Glucosidase Inhibition Properties of Cultivated Soybean (*Glycine max*) and Wild Soybean (*Glycine soja*). *Plants* **2021**, *10*, 813. [CrossRef]
42. De Camargo, A.C.; Favero, B.T.; Morzelle, M.C.; Franchin, M.; Alvarez-Parrilla, E.; De La Rosa, L.A.; Geraldi, M.V.; Maróstica, M.R.; Shahidi, F.; Schwember, A.R. Is Chickpea a Potential Substitute for Soybean? Phenolic Bioactives and Potential Health Benefits. *Int. J. Mol. Sci.* **2019**, *20*, 2644. [CrossRef]
43. Zhang, J.; Xia, N.; Teng, J.; Wei, B.; Huang, L. Effect of Lactic Acid Bacteria Fermentation on Extractable and Non-Extractable Polyphenols of Soybean Milk: Influence of β-Glucosidase and Okara. *Food Biosci.* **2023**, *56*, 2212–4292. [CrossRef]
44. Bhadkaria, A.; Srivastava, N.; Bhagyawant, S.S. A Prospective of Underutilized Legume Moth Bean (*Vigna aconitifolia* (Jacq.) Marechàl): Phytochemical Profiling, Bioactive Compounds and in Vitro Pharmacological Studies. *Food Biosci.* **2021**, *42*, 2212–4292. [CrossRef]
45. Mali, P.S.; Kumar, P. Optimization of Microwave Assisted Extraction of Bioactive Compounds from Black Bean Waste and Evaluation of Its Antioxidant and Antidiabetic Potential in Vitro. *Food Chem. Adv.* **2023**, *3*, 100543. [CrossRef]

46. Sowdhanya, D.; Singh, J.; Rasane, P.; Kaur, S.; Kaur, J.; Ercisli, S.; Verma, H. Nutritional Significance of Velvet Bean (*Mucuna pruriens*) and Opportunities for Its Processing into Value-Added Products. *J. Agric. Food Res.* **2024**, *15*, 100921. [CrossRef]
47. Thummajitsakul, S.; Piyaphan, P.; Khamthong, S.; Unkam, M.; Silprasit, K. Comparison of FTIR Fingerprint, Phenolic Content, Antioxidant and Anti-Glucosidase Activities among *Phaseolus vulgaris* L., *Arachis hypogaea* L. and *Plukenetia volubilis* L. *Electron. J. Biotechnol.* **2023**, *61*, 14–23. [CrossRef]
48. Tungmunnithum, D.; Drouet, S.; Lorenzo, J.M.; Hano, C. Effect of Traditional Cooking and in Vitro Gastrointestinal Digestion of the Ten Most Consumed Beans from the Fabaceae Family in Thailand on Their Phytochemicals, Antioxidant and Anti-Diabetic Potentials. *Plants* **2022**, *11*, 67. [CrossRef]
49. Wu, D.T.; Li, W.X.; Wan, J.J.; Hu, Y.C.; Gan, R.Y.; Zou, L. A Comprehensive Review of Pea (*Pisum sativum* L.): Chemical Composition, Processing, Health Benefits, and Food Applications. *Foods* **2023**, *12*, 2527. [CrossRef]
50. Chen, S.K.; Lin, H.F.; Wang, X.; Yuan, Y.; Yin, J.Y.; Song, X.X. Comprehensive Analysis in the Nutritional Composition, Phenolic Species and in Vitro Antioxidant Activities of Different Pea Cultivars. *Food Chem. X* **2023**, *17*, 100599. [CrossRef]
51. Kumari, T.; Deka, S.C. Potential Health Benefits of Garden Pea Seeds and Pods: A Review. *Legume Sci.* **2021**, *3*, 82. [CrossRef]
52. Mejri, F.; Selmi, S.; Martins, A.; Benkhoud, H.; Baati, T.; Chaabane, H.; Njim, L.; Serralheiro, M.L.M.; Rauter, A.P.; Hosni, K. Broad Bean (*Vicia faba* L.) Pods: A Rich Source of Bioactive Ingredients with Antimicrobial, Antioxidant, Enzyme Inhibitory, Anti-Diabetic and Health-Promoting Properties. *Food Funct.* **2018**, *9*, 2051–2069. [CrossRef]
53. Loizzo, M.R.; Bonesi, M.; Leporini, M.; Falco, T.; Sicari, V.; Tundis, R. Chemical Profile and In Vitro Bioactivity of *Vicia faba* Beans and Pods. *Proceedings* **2020**, *70*, 45. [CrossRef]
54. Johnson, J.B.; Skylas, D.J.; Mani, J.S.; Xiang, J.; Walsh, K.B.; Naiker, M. Phenolic Profiles of Ten Australian Faba Bean Varieties. *Molecules* **2021**, *26*, 4642. [CrossRef] [PubMed]
55. Duan, S.C.; Kwon, S.J.; Eom, S.H. Effect of Thermal Processing on Color, Phenolic Compounds, and Antioxidant Activity of Faba Bean (*Vicia faba* L.) Leaves and Seeds. *Antioxidants* **2021**, *10*, 1207. [CrossRef] [PubMed]
56. Rajhi, I.; Boulaaba, M.; Baccouri, B.; Rajhi, F.; Hammami, J.; Barhoumi, F.; Flamini, G.; Mhadhbi, H. Assessment of Dehulling Effect on Volatiles, Phenolic Compounds and Antioxidant Activities of Faba Bean Seeds and Flours. *S. Afr. J. Bot.* **2022**, *147*, 741–753. [CrossRef]
57. Ganesan, K.; Xu, B. Polyphenol-Rich Lentils and Their Health Promoting Effects. *Int. J. Mol. Sci.* **2017**, *18*, 2390. [CrossRef]
58. Mustafa, A.M.; Abouelenein, D.; Acquaticci, L.; Alessandroni, L.; Angeloni, S.; Borsetta, G.; Caprioli, G.; Nzekoue, F.K.; Sagradini, G.; Vittori, S. Polyphenols, Saponins and Phytosterols in Lentils and Their Health Benefits: An Overview. *Pharmaceuticals* **2022**, *15*, 1225. [CrossRef]
59. Attou, A.; Bouderoua, K.; Cheriguene, A. Effects of Roasting Process on Nutritional and Antinutritional Factors of Two Lentils Varieties (*Lens culinaris.* Medik) Cultivated in Algeria. *S. Asian J. Exp. Biol.* **2020**, *10*, 445–454. [CrossRef]
60. Xia, M.; Li, M.; de Souza, T.S.P.; Barrow, C.; Dunshea, F.R.; Suleria, H.A.R. LC-ESI-QTOF-MS^2 Characterization of Phenolic Compounds in Different Lentil (*Lens culinaris M.*) Samples and Their Antioxidant Capacity. *Front. Biosci.* **2023**, *28*, 44. [CrossRef]
61. Begum, N.; Khan, Q.U.; Liu, L.G.; Li, W.; Liu, D.; Haq, I.U. Nutritional Composition, Health Benefits and Bio-Active Compounds of Chickpea (*Cicer arietinum* L.). *Front. Nutr.* **2023**, *10*, 1218468. [CrossRef]
62. Lin, Y.; Wu, S. Vegetable Soybean (*Glycine max* (L.) Merr.) Leaf Extracts: Functional Components and Antioxidant and Anti-Inflammatory Activities. *J. Food Sci.* **2021**, *86*, 2468–2480. [CrossRef]
63. Charoensiddhi, S.; Chanput, W.P.; Sae-Tan, S. Gut Microbiota Modulation, Anti-Diabetic and Anti-Inflammatory Properties of Polyphenol Extract from Mung Bean Seed Coat (*Vigna radiata* L.). *Nutrients* **2022**, *14*, 2275. [CrossRef] [PubMed]
64. Liu, Y.; Ragaee, S.; Marcone, M.F.; Abdel-Aal, E.S.M. Composition of Phenolic Acids and Antioxidant Properties of Selected Pulses Cooked with Different Heating Conditions. *Foods* **2020**, *9*, 908. [CrossRef] [PubMed]
65. Castaldo, L.; Izzo, L.; Gaspari, A.; Lombardi, S.; Rodríguez-Carrasco, Y.; Narváez, A.; Grosso, M.; Ritieni, A. Chemical Composition of Green Pea (*Pisum sativum* L.) Pods Extracts and Their Potential Exploitation as Ingredients in Nutraceutical Formulations. *Antioxidants* **2022**, *11*, 105. [CrossRef]
66. Magro, A.E.A.; Silva, L.C.; Rasera, G.B.; de Castro, R.J.S. Solid-State Fermentation as an Efficient Strategy for the Biotransformation of Lentils: Enhancing Their Antioxidant and Antidiabetic Potentials. *Bioresour. Bioprocess* **2019**, *6*, 38. [CrossRef]
67. Bochenek, H.; Francis, N.; Santhakumar, A.B.; Blanchard, C.L.; Chinkwo, K.A. The antioxidant and anticancer properties of chickpea water and chickpea polyphenol extracts in vitro. *Cereal Chem.* **2023**, *100*, 895–903. [CrossRef]
68. Mekky, R.H.; Contreras, M.D.M.; El-Gindi, M.R.; Abdel-Monem, A.R.; Abdel-Sattar, E.; Segura-Carretero, A. Profiling of phenolic and other compounds from egyptian cultivars of chickpea (*Cicer arietinum* L.) and antioxidant activity: A comparative study. *RSC Adv.* **2015**, *5*, 17751–17767. [CrossRef]
69. Tan, Y.; Chang, S.K.C.; Zhang, Y. Comparison of α-Amylase, α-Glucosidase and Lipase Inhibitory Activity of the Phenolic Substances in Two Black Legumes of Different Genera. *Food Chem.* **2017**, *214*, 259–268. [CrossRef]

70. Zeb, A. Concept, Mechanism, and Applications of Phenolic Antioxidants in Foods. *J. Food Biochem.* **2020**, *44*, 13394. [CrossRef]
71. Son, E.; Jin Choi, H.; Kim, S.-H.; Jang, D.-G.; Cha, J.; June, J.; Ree Kim, M.; Kim, D.-S. Anti-Diabetic Effects of Wild Soybean *Glycine Soja* Seed 2 Extract on Type 2 Diabetic Mice and Human Hepatocytes Induced Insulin Resistance. *Preprints* **2020**, 2020080572. [CrossRef]
72. Zheng, Y.; Zhang, R.; Huang, F.; Cheng, L.H.; Xu, L.; Jia, X. α-Glucosidase Inhibitors Derived from Black Soybean and Their Inhibitory Mechanisms. *LWT* **2023**, *189*, 115502. [CrossRef]
73. Król-Grzymała, A.; Amarowicz, R. Phenolic Compounds of Soybean Seeds from Two European Countries and Their Antioxidant Properties. *Molecules* **2020**, *25*, 2075. [CrossRef] [PubMed]
74. Khosravi, A.; Razavi, S.H. Therapeutic Effects of Polyphenols in Fermented Soybean and Black Soybean Products. *J. Funct. Foods* **2021**, *81*, 104467. [CrossRef]
75. Laenggeng, A.H.; Hasanuddin, A.; Nuryanti, S. The Effect of Fermented Soybean Flour Towards Blood Glucose Level of Mice (*Mus musculus*). *World J. Adv. Res. Rev.* **2024**, *21*, 2356–2360. [CrossRef]
76. Long, X.S.; Liao, S.T.; Li, E.N.; Pang, D.R.; Li, Q.; Liu, S.C.; Hu, T.G.; Zou, Y.X. The Hypoglycemic Effect of Freeze-Dried Fermented Mulberry Mixed with Soybean on Type 2 Diabetes Mellitus. *Food Sci. Nutr.* **2021**, *9*, 3641–3654. [CrossRef]
77. Meenu, M.; Chen, P.; Mradula, M.; Chang, S.K.C.; Xu, B. New Insights into Chemical Compositions and Health-Promoting Effects of Black Beans (*Phaseolus vulgaris* L.). *Food Front.* **2023**, *4*, 1019–1038. [CrossRef]
78. Kabré, J.d.W.; Dah-Nouvlessounon, D.; Fatoumata, H.B.; Agonkoun, A.; Guinin, F.; Sina, H.; Kohonou, N.A.; Tchogou, P.; Senou, M.; Savadogo, A.; et al. Mung Bean (*Vigna radiata* (L.) R. Wilczek) from Burkina Faso Used as Antidiabetic, Antioxidant and Antimicrobial Agent. *Plants* **2022**, *11*, 3556. [CrossRef]
79. Moloto, M.R.; Phan, A.D.T.; Shai, J.L.; Sultanbawa, Y.; Sivakumar, D. Comparison of Phenolic Compounds, Carotenoids, Amino Acid Composition, in Vitro Antioxidant and Anti-Diabetic Activities in the Leaves of Seven Cowpea (*Vigna unguiculata*) Cultivars. *Foods* **2020**, *9*, 1285. [CrossRef]
80. Li, B.; Shen, X.; Shen, H.; Zhou, Y.; Yao, X. Effect of Optimized Germination Technology on Polyphenol Content and Hypoglycemic Activity of Mung Bean. *Front. Nutr.* **2023**, *10*, 1138739. [CrossRef]
81. Ombra, M.N.; d'Acierno, A.; Nazzaro, F.; Spigno, P.; Riccardi, R.; Zaccardelli, M.; Pane, C.; Coppola, R.; Fratianni, F. Alpha-Amylase, α-Glucosidase and Lipase Inhibiting Activities of Polyphenol-Rich Extracts from Six Common Bean Cultivars of Southern Italy, Before and After Cooking. *Int. J. Food Sci. Nutr.* **2018**, *69*, 824–834. [CrossRef]
82. Jiang, X.; Xu, Q.; Zhang, A.; Liu, Y.; Li, Z.; Tang, H.; Cao, D.; Zhang, D. Revealing the Hypoglycemic Effects and Mechanism of GABA-Rich Germinated Adzuki Beans on T2DM Mice by Untargeted Serum Metabolomics. *Front. Nutr.* **2021**, *8*, 791191. [CrossRef]
83. Shen, X.; Jiang, X.; Qian, L.; Zhang, A.; Zuo, F.; Zhang, D. Polyphenol Extracts From Germinated Mung Beans Can Improve Type 2 Diabetes in Mice by Regulating Intestinal Microflora and Inhibiting Inflammation. *Front. Nutr.* **2022**, *9*, 846409. [CrossRef] [PubMed]
84. Thompson, S.V.; Winham, D.M.; Hutchins, A.M. Bean and Rice Meals Reduce Postprandial Glycemic Response in Adults with Type 2 Diabetes: A Cross-Over Study. *Nutr. J.* **2012**, *11*, 23. [CrossRef] [PubMed]
85. Di Stefano, E.; Tsopmo, A.; Oliviero, T.; Fogliano, V.; Udenigwe, C.C. Bioprocessing of Common Pulses Changed Seed Microstructures, and Improved Dipeptidyl Peptidase-IV and α-Glucosidase Inhibitory Activities. *Sci. Rep.* **2019**, *9*, 15308. [CrossRef]
86. Ginaris, R.P.; Fauzah, N.R. The Effectiveness of Flavonoids in Pigeon Pea (*Cajanus cajan*) as Inhibitors of α-Glucosidase Enzyme in Anti-Diabetes. *J. Ilmiah Farmasi* **2023**, *13*, 139–145. [CrossRef]
87. Elessawy, F.M.; Hughes, J.; Khazaei, H.; Vandenberg, A.; El-Aneed, A.; Purves, R.W. A Comparative Metabolomics Investigation of Flavonoid Variation in Faba Bean Flowers. *Metabolomics* **2023**, *19*, 52. [CrossRef]
88. Kumar, R.; Duhan, A.; Sangwan, S.; Yadav, N. A Brief Overview of the Biological Activities of Faba Bean (*Vicia faba*). *Forage Res.* **2022**, *48*, 152–160. Available online: https://www.researchgate.net/publication/364814865 (accessed on 1 December 2024).
89. Rahate, K.A.; Madhumita, M.; Prabhakar, P.K. Nutritional Composition, Anti-Nutritional Factors, Pretreatments-Cum-Processing Impact and Food Formulation Potential of Faba Bean (*Vicia faba* L.): A Comprehensive Review. *LWT* **2021**, *138*, 110796. [CrossRef]
90. Choudhary, D.K.; Mishra, A. In Vitro and in Silico Interaction of Porcine α-Amylase with *Vicia faba* Crude Seed Extract and Evaluation of Antidiabetic Activity. *Bioengineered* **2017**, *8*, 393–403. [CrossRef]
91. Tefera, M.M.; Masresha Altaye, B.; Yimer, E.M.; Berhe, D.F.; Bekele, S.T. Antidiabetic Effect of Germinated *Lens culinaris* Medik Seed Extract in Streptozotocin-Induced Diabetic Mice. *J. Exp. Pharmacol.* **2020**, *12*, 39–45. [CrossRef]
92. Acevedo Martinez, K.A.; Yang, M.M.; Gonzalez de Mejia, E. Technological Properties of Chickpea (*Cicer arietinum*): Production of Snacks and Health Benefits Related to Type-2 Diabetes. *Compr. Rev. Food Sci. Food Saf.* **2021**, *20*, 3762–3787. [CrossRef]
93. Singh, S.; Bansal, A.; Singh, V.; Chopra, T.; Poddar, J. Flavonoids, alkaloids and terpenoids: A new hope for the treatment of diabetes mellitus. *J. Diabetes Metab. Disord.* **2022**, *21*, 941–950. [CrossRef] [PubMed]

94. Panigrahy, N.; Priyadarshini, A.; Sahoo, M.M.; Verma, A.K.; Daverey, A.; Sahoo, N.K. A comprehensive review on eco-toxicity and biodegradation of phenolics: Recent progress and future outlook. *Environ. Technol. Innov.* **2022**, *27*, 102423. [CrossRef]
95. Rahman, M.M.; Rahaman, M.S.; Islam, M.R.; Rahman, F.; Mithi, F.M.; Alqahtani, T.; Almikhlafi, M.A.; Alghamdi, S.Q.; Alruwaili, A.S.; Hossain, M.S.; et al. Role of Phenolic Compounds in Human Disease: Current Knowledge and Future Prospects. *Molecules* **2021**, *27*, 233. [CrossRef] [PubMed]

pharmaceuticals

MDPI

Review

The Potential Therapeutic Use of Agarwood for Diabetes: A Scoping Review

Mohammad Adi Mohammad Fadzil, Norhashimah Abu Seman and Aswir Abd Rashed *

Nutrition, Metabolism and Cardiovascular Research Centre (NMCRC), Institute for Medical Research (IMR), National Institutes of Health (NIH), Ministry of Health Malaysia (MOH), No. 1, Jalan Setia Murni U13/52, Seksyen U13 Setia Alam, Shah Alam 40170, Malaysia; adifadzil@moh.gov.my (M.A.M.F.); nor.hashimah@moh.gov.my (N.A.S.)

* Correspondence: aswir@moh.gov.my; Tel.: +603-33627841

Abstract: Introduction: In 2019, 9.3% (463 million) of adults worldwide had diabetes, according to the International Diabetes Federation (IDF). By 2030, the number will rise to 10.2% (578 million) and 10.9% (700 million) by 2045 if effective prevention methods are not implemented. Agarwood is a pathological product and valuable plant due to its numerous medicinal properties, and it is used as an essential ingredient in medicine. Therefore, we conducted this review to determine agarwood's potential health benefit effect on type 2 diabetes. Results and Discussion: Although no clinical trials were found, the evidence from in vitro and in vivo studies is promising. Agarwood has shown the ability to reduce the activity of α-glucosidase, α-amylase, and lipase, promote adiponectin secretion during adipogenesis, and reduce oxidative stress. Animal studies elucidated hypoglycaemic, antidyslipidemia, anti-obesity, and organ protective effects from agarwood. Materials and Methods: Original articles were searched in three databases (PubMed, Scopus, and Cochrane Library) using the medical subject heading (MeSH) term "diabetes" crossed with the term "agarwood" from 2008 to 2024. Synonyms and relevant search terms were also searched. Conclusions: This effect underscores the need for further research and the potential for groundbreaking discoveries in the field of diabetes treatment.

Keywords: agarwood; diabetic properties; phytochemicals; therapeutic potential

1. Introduction

Agarwood, also known as eaglewood, *oud*, *oudh*, aloeswood, *karas*, and *gaharu*, is a type of resinous, fragrant heartwood produced by the tree species of the family Thymelaeaceae. Typically, agarwood is obtained or harvested from the genera *Aquilaria* and *Gyrinops* [1]. Agarwood is a secondary metabolite produced as a defence mechanism by agarwood-producing species upon encountering injuries or infections. The dark and aromatic resin accumulates in the heartwood of the trees [1]. However, not all genus *Aquilaria* or *Gyrinops* trees can produce agarwood. There are only 17 recognised species around the world that have been recorded as being able to produce agarwood [2]. These species are commonly found in Southeast Asia, China, and India. *A. malaccensis*, *A. sinensis*, *A. rugosa*, *A. filaria*, *A. subintegra*, *A. crassna*, *A. agallocha*, and *A. beccariana* are the common species used for the harvesting of agarwood [3].

Due to its significant economic nontimber potential and limited availability, agarwood is highly sought after, especially in the Asia and Middle East markets. A recent review by the Convention of International Trade in Endangered Species of Wild Fauna and Flora (CITES) found that overharvesting has destroyed the agarwood-producing species' natural habitat. Thus, technological advancement has been made in producing artificial agarwood with physical and medicinal properties on par with natural agarwood [4]. The use of agarwood is deeply rooted in many traditions for various purposes, as its application is recorded in historical and religious scriptures such as those of the Sahih Muslims and the

Ayurveda [1]. Agarwood has been recorded in the literature as having various pharmacological benefits such as antibacterial, anticancer, anti-inflammation, antioxidant, analgesic, cough depressant, asthma reliever, anti-ageing, cardioprotective, and anti-depression effects [5–12]. The beneficial health properties are due to the various active compounds that have been identified through phytochemical studies, such as chromone derivatives, terpenoids, flavonoids, benzophenones, lignans, benzenoid derivatives, phenolic compounds, triterpenes, steroids, and other chemical compounds [1].

Diabetes mellitus is a complex metabolic disorder characterised by a chronic elevated sugar level in the bloodstream, a phenomenon commonly termed hyperglycaemia, which is the hallmark of the disease. Although there are more types of diabetes occurring, type 1 diabetes and type 2 diabetes are the two primary variants, making up 5% and 90% of diabetes cases worldwide [13].

The epidemiologic trend of diabetes is worrying, as the International Diabetes Federation reported that the global number of diabetes incidence is expected to increase from 537 million in the year 2021 to 783 million in the year 2045 [14]. In the year 2021 alone, 6.7 million mortalities of young adults and the elderly were caused by diabetes and its related diseases. The economic burden of diabetes is also worrisome, as the global cost of treating the disease is expected to reach 1.05 trillion USD by 2045 [14].

Diabetes is also known to be a polygenic disease caused by a multifactorial interaction of environmental factors and genetic variations. However, the common themes are that nutrition transition, rapid urbanisation, rising cases of obesity, and modern sedentary lifestyles lead to an increased risk of diabetes, especially type 2 diabetes [15]. Ultimately, the most preferred and effective therapeutic and management approaches to diabetes are lifestyle modifications involving diet changes, active lifestyles, and pharmacological interventions [16]. Interventions involving individualised precision and personalised strategy are becoming more popular nowadays, aiming to meet glycaemic goals.

Up to date, many oral conventional drugs are available to reduce glucose levels, such as sulfonylureas, meglitinides, biguanides, thiazolidinediones, α-glucosidase inhibitors, α-amylase inhibitors, dipeptidyl peptidase-4 (DPP-4) inhibitors, sodium-glucose cotransporter-2 (SGLT2) inhibitors, glucagon-like peptide-1 (GLP-1) agonist, and cycloset [16,17]. Among these conventional drugs, α-glucosidase and α-amylase inhibitors are designed to delay or prevent blood glucose spiking by inhibiting the hydrolysation of carbohydrates into glucose [18–20]. Examples include acarbose, miglitol, and voglibose, commonly prescribed for diabetes management. Other than that, it is well established that targeting and preventing obesity will result in a better prognosis and prevention of type 2 diabetes. Thus, lipase inhibitors are also commonly prescribed drugs aimed at disrupting fat absorption from food, resulting in reduced weight gain [21]. An example of a conventional drug is orlistat. However, these conventional drugs often come with side effects such as flatulence, oily stools, and gastrointestinal complications, leading to poor compliance and efficacy [18–20,22].

Due to their possible health advantages and minimal side effects, functional foods are becoming more popular for managing diabetes [23]. Compared to traditional diabetic treatments, functional foods are frequently more affordable and readily available, making them a viable choice for many people [24]. Agarwood can be potentially utilised as a functional food due to its high content of bioactive chemicals, providing an alternative to conventional diabetic treatments. Many studies have reported the anti-diabetic properties of agarwood. Therefore, this review will evaluate agarwood's potential as a supplementary or alternative agent for managing diabetes disease.

2. Materials and Methods

The study question was constructed based on the PICO framework [25]. The PICO framework stands for Population or subjects, Intervention or exposure, Comparison or control, and Outcome or benefits. The population/subjects investigated are individuals or animals with diabetes. The intervention is the application of agarwood. The comparison or control is the conventional diabetes treatment. The study aims to elucidate agarwood plants' potential use and mechanism in managing diabetes.

The inclusion criteria were as follows: (1) Primary studies that evaluated the efficacy of agarwood against diabetes. (2) Peer-reviewed studies with an available full text. (3) Studies published in the English language. (4) Included studies of any geographical origin from 2008–2024 (15 years). The exclusion criteria were as follows: (1) Duplicate publications. (2) Studies published in a non-English language. (3) Review articles, protocol papers, letters to editors, and short communications.

Original articles were comprehensively searched in three databases (PubMed, Scopus, and Cochrane Library) using the medical subject heading (MeSH) term "diabetes" crossed with the term "agarwood." Search terms also included synonyms and relevant keywords for diabetes and agarwood. The search terms were then connected using Boolean operators "OR" and "AND" before being subjected to database browsing. The search terms for each database are shown in the Supplementary Materials. The last search was carried out in February 2024. The decision to focus on studies published from 2008 onwards was based on the aim of capturing the most recent and relevant research developments in the field over the past 15 years. All database hits were subjected to automated duplicate screening using the citation manager EndNote X9 (Clarivate Analytics, Philadelphia, PA, USA). After that, the title and abstract of the records were screened manually for duplicates or illegibility. Finally, the remaining articles' full texts were assessed per the stated criteria. Mohammad Adi Mohammad Fadzil (MAMF) and Aswir Abd Rashed (AAR) were involved in the selection process following the eligibility criteria. Contradicting assessments were resolved through discussions. Flowcharts were constructed using the "Preferred Reporting Items for Systematic Reviews and Meta-Analyses" (PRISMA) [26]. The detailed process of the search strategy is elucidated using a flowchart in Figure 1.

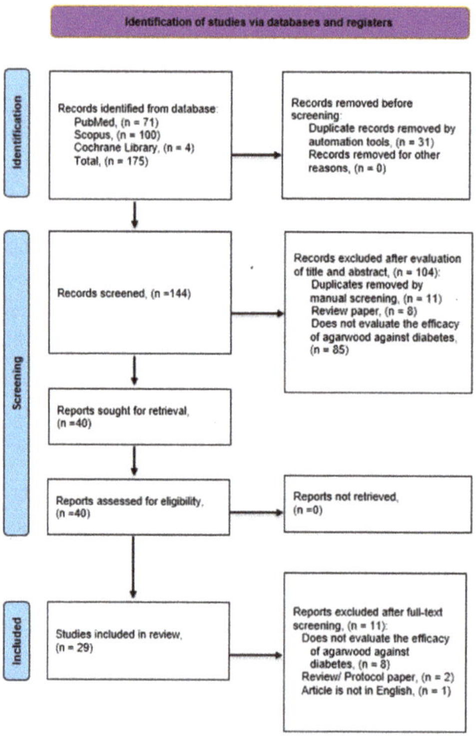

Figure 1. Flowchart of the Search Strategy.

3. Results

The search resulted in 175 articles produced with a refined search based on the availability of the full text, peer-reviewed articles, and library collection access. Upon further assessment, only 29 full-text articles were relevant and included for the final review (Tables 1 and 2). All the related articles were printed out for further evidence-based assessment to explore agarwood's effectiveness as a potential anti-diabetic agent. Overall, 22 studies were conducted in vitro [27–47] and 7 were in vivo studies [48–54]. Studies were conducted using agarwood plants obtained from various countries. Specimens from Thailand, Indonesia, Malaysia, Korea, Laos, Vietnam, India, Algeria, and China featured in most studies. Various agarwood-producing plant species were studied for their anti-diabetic potential. A total of 11 studies were conducted on *A. sinensis* [29,37,39–41,46–49,53,55], 7 studies on *A. malaccensis* [27,28,33,36,45,47,54], and 5 studies on *A. crassna* [32,38,39,44,50]. Other agarwood-producing plants studied are *A. filaria*, *A. subintegra*, *A. agallocha*, and *G. versteegii* [27,30,31,33,42,43,47,51,52], including two unspecified *Aquilaria* species [34,35]. Most studies were conducted on either the agarwood itself or the leaves; 14 studies were conducted using agarwood [28,30,31,34,35,37,39–45,51,52] whereas 13 studies were conducted using the leaves [27,29,31,33,36,38,46–50,53,55]. Other studies used different parts of the agarwood-producing plants, such as the stem bark, fruit bark, and branches. Three studies were conducted to investigate the potential synergistic effects of agarwood and other plants [36,52,54]. Ethanol was the most used extraction solvent, where it was used in 12 studies [36–44,46,47,53]. The second most used solvent was methanol extraction, used in nine studies [30–33,45,48,49,54,55] and the third was water extraction, used in seven studies [27,28,47,48,50–52]. Other extraction solvents used were hexane, ethyl ether, dichloromethane, and acetone [29,30,33–35,47].

Table 1. The effect of agarwood on diabetes in in vitro studies.

No.	References	Country	Plant Species	Plant Parts	Extraction Solvent	Key Findings
1	[40]	China	*A. sinensis*	Agarwood chips	95% Ethanol	• 2-(2-phenyl ethyl) chromone derivatives were isolated from *A. sinensis* and were subjected to an α-glucosidase inhibition assay. • Significant inhibitions were detected from three derivatives, namely, 6,7-dimethoxy-2-[2-(4-hydroxyphenyl) ethyl] chromone, 6,7-dihydroxy-2-[2-(4-methoxyphenyl) ethyl] chromone, and 6-hydroxy-2-[2-(3-methoxy-4-hydroxyphenyl) ethyl] chromone with IC_{50} values of 48.953, 15.655, and 16.318 μg/mL, respectively. Acarbose was used as the positive control (IC_{50} = 632.688 μg/mL).
2	[42]	Indonesia	*A. filaria*	Agarwood chips	95% ethanol	• 2-(2-phenyl ethyl) chromone derivatives were isolated from *A. filaria* and were subjected to an α-glucosidase inhibition assay. • The 21 compounds isolated reported α-glucosidase inhibition with IC_{50} values ranging from 2.256 ± 0.085 to 44.977 ± 0.984 μg/mL. Acarbose and genistein were used as controls, 479.939 ± 2.130 μg/mL and 2.243 ± 0.027 μg/mL, respectively. • 6,7-dihydroxy-2-(2-phenyl ethyl) chromone was the most potent α-glucosidase inhibitor with an IC_{50} value of 2.256 ± 0.085 μg/mL.

Table 1. *Cont.*

No.	References	Country	Plant Species	Plant Parts	Extraction Solvent	Key Findings
3	[45]	Laos	*A. malaccensis*	Agarwood chips	70% Methanol	• 2-(2-phenyl ethyl) chromone derivatives were isolated from *A. malaccensis* and investigated for their effects on adiponectin production. • 2-(2-phenyl ethyl) chromone derivatives promoted adiponectin production during adipogenesis in a bone marrow mesenchymal stem cell model. • The most potent enhancers of adiponectin production were identified as 6-methoxy-2-(2-phenyl ethyl) chromone and 7-methoxy-2-(2-phenyl ethyl) chromone.
4	[30]	Indonesia	*G. versteegii*	Agarwood chips	Methanol and Acetone	• Several wood extracts and extraction solvents of *G. versteegii* were tested for their α-glucosidase inhibitory activity and antioxidant potential. • Acetone extracts from infected wood of *G. versteegii* had the highest DPPH antioxidant activity with the IC_{50} value of 65.62 μg/mL. Quercetin was used as a control (8.59 ug/mL). • Acetone agarwood extracts had the highest α-glucosidase inhibitory activity with an IC_{50} value of 53.46 μg/mL. Quercetin was used as a control (5.34 ug/mL).
5	[46]	China	*A. sinensis*	Leaves	70% Ethanol	• Compounds were isolated from the ethanolic extracts of *A. sinensis* leaves and screened for α-glucosidase inhibitory activity. • Compounds were isolated using activity-directed fractionation and a purification process. • Mangiferin and iriflophenone 2-O-a-L-rhamnopyranoside, the significant components in the leaves of *A. sinensis*, showed potent inhibition with IC_{50} values of 126.5 ± 17.8 and 143.7 ± 10.6 ug/mL, respectively. Acarbose was used as a control (372.0 ± 37.8 ug/mL).
6	[39]	China	*A. sinensis* and *A. crassna*	Agarwood chips	95% Ethanol	• Artificial and wild agarwood extracts were investigated for their antioxidant potential and α-glucosidase inhibition. • Wild agarwood demonstrated more substantial antioxidant potential, followed by artificial *A. sinensis* agarwood. • IC_{50} values of the α-glucosidase inhibition for wild agarwood, artificial *A. sinensis*, and artificial *A. crassna* were reported at 156.400 ug/mL, 292.000 ug/mL, and 343.000 ug/mL, respectively.

Table 1. *Cont.*

No.	References	Country	Plant Species	Plant Parts	Extraction Solvent	Key Findings
7	[47]	Malaysia	*A. malaccensis*, *A. subintegra*, and *A. sinensis*	Leaves	100% Ethanol, 70% Ethanol, Water, and Hexane	• Several leaves of the *Aquilaria* spp. were extracted using various solvents and drying methods. The extracts were screened and compared for their α-glucosidase inhibition and DPPH radical scavenging activity. • Oven-dried *A. malaccensis* leaves extracted using 70% ethanol showed the highest inhibition of α-glucosidase and DPPH radicals with IC_{50} values of 0.13 ug/mL and 33.60 ug/mL, respectively. Acarbose was used as a control for the α-glucosidase inhibition test, whereas quercetin was used as the control for the DPPH radical scavenging test. The IC_{50} of the controls was 0.65 ug/mL and 20.75 ug/mL, respectively.
8	[33]	Malaysia	*A. subintegra* and *A. malaccensis*	Leaves and Barks	Hexane, Dichloromethane, and Methanol	• Using several extraction solvents, 12 extracts from the leaves and barks of *A. subintegra* and *A. malaccensis* were screened for anti-lipase activity. • At 100 ug/mL, *A. malaccensis* bark extracted using dichloromethane showed the most potent lipase inhibition with 91% inhibition.
9	[44]	Laos	*A. crassna*	Agarwood chips	95% Ethanol	• Four new derivatives of bi-2-(2-phenyl ethyl) chromone were isolated from the *A. crassna* extracts, which were named crassin A, crassin B, crassin C, and crassin D. • α-glucosidase inhibition screening was conducted. None of the derivatives showed significant α-glucosidase inhibition activity.
10	[41]	China	*A. sinensis*	Agarwood chips	95% Ethanol	• Four new derivatives of bi-phenyl ethyl chromones were isolated from the *A. sinensis* extracts, which were (5S,6R,7S,8R)-2-[2-(4-Methoxyphenyl)ethyl]-5,6,7-trihydroxy-5,6,7,8-tetrahydro-8-{6-methoxy-2-[2-(3‴-methoxy-4‴-hydroxyphenyl)ethyl]chromonyl-7-oxy}chromone, (5S,6R,7S,8R)-2-[2-(4-Methoxyphenyl)ethyl]-5,6,7-trihydroxy-5,6,7,8-tetrahydro-8-{2-[2-(4‴-methoxyphenyl)ethyl]chromonyl-6-oxy}chromone, 5S,6R,7S,8R)-2-(2-Phenylethyl)-5,6,7-trihydroxy-5,6,7,8-tetrahydro-8-[2-(2-phenyl ethyl)chromonyl-6-oxy]chromone, and (5R,6R,7R,8S)-2-(2-Phenylethyl)-5,6,7-trihydroxy-5,6,7,8-tetrahydro-8-[2-(2-phenyl ethyl)chromonyl-6-oxy]chromone. • α-glucosidase inhibition screening was conducted. None of the derivatives showed significant α-glucosidase inhibition activity.

Table 1. *Cont.*

No.	References	Country	Plant Species	Plant Parts	Extraction Solvent	Key Findings
11	[43]	Indonesia	*A. filaria*	Agarwood chips	95% Ethanol	• Six 8,12-epoxyguaiane sesquiterpenes were isolated from *A. filaria* agarwood extracts. The extracts were then screened for α-glucosidase inhibitory activity. • The most potent α-glucosidase inhibitor was reported from guaianolide with an IC_{50} value of 53.332 ± 2.273 μg/mL. Acarbose was used as a control (IC_{50} = 479.939 ± 2.130 μg/mL).
12	[38]	Thailand	*A. crassna*	Leaves	95% Ethanol	• Mangiferin was determined as the active metabolite of *A. crassna* leaf extracts. Mangiferin and crude extracts of *A. crassna* leaves were screened for α-glucosidase inhibition and antioxidant activity. • α-glucosidase inhibition of *A. crassna* extracts and mangiferin were reported with IC_{50} values of 184.000 ± 3.200 μg/mL and 571.400 ± 4.400 μg/mL, respectively. Acarbose was used as a control (IC_{50} = 17,394.700 ± 18.9 μg/mL). • A DPPH radical scavenging assay, nitric oxide scavenging assay, and superoxide scavenging assay showed that *A. crassna* extracts and mangiferin were significantly antioxidant. Mangiferin reported higher antioxidant potential than the crude extracts, suggesting its role as the active compound.
13	[27]	Malaysia	*A. malaccensis* and *A. subintegra*	Leaves	Water	• Various particle sizes of *A. subintegra* and *A. malaccensis* leaves were extracted and screened for lipase inhibition. • Highest inhibition was reported using the extracts obtained from the smallest particle size, 250 μm, with *A. subintegra* leaves being the most potent at 82% lipase inhibition. • Kinetic study revealed the mode of lipase inhibition from *A. subintegra* and *A. malaccensis* leaves was determined as mixed inhibition that mimics noncompetitive binding.
14	[35]	Thailand	*Aquilaria* spp.	Agarwood chips	Ethyl ether	• Sesquiterpenoid derivatives were isolated from unspecified *Aquilaria* spp. and were subjected to an α-glucosidase inhibition assay. • Aquilarene D and Aquilarene E reported significant inhibition against α-glucosidase with IC_{50} values of 57.460 and 522.104 μg/mL. Acarbose was used as a control (IC_{50} = 781.176 μg/mL).

Table 1. *Cont.*

No.	References	Country	Plant Species	Plant Parts	Extraction Solvent	Key Findings
15	[31]	Indonesia	*G. versteegii*	Fruit bark, Stem bark, and Leaves	Methanol	• Extracts obtained from various parts of *G. versteegii* were tested for their α-glucosidase inhibitory activity and antioxidant potential. • Leaf extracts of *G. versteegii* had the highest potency against α-glucosidase activity with an IC_{50} value of 55.01 ± 2.4 ug/mL. Quercetin was used as a control (IC_{50} = 5.34 ± 0.2 ug/mL). • Leaf extracts of *G. versteegii* showed the highest antioxidant potential using a DPPH radical scavenging assay with an IC_{50} value of 32.89 ± 2.7 ug/mL. Quercetin was used as a control (IC_{50} = 8.59 ± 0.3 ug/mL).
16	[34]	Thailand	*Aquilaria* spp.	Agarwood chips	Ethyl ether	• Sesquiterpenoids derivatives were isolated from unspecified *Aquilaria* spp. and were subjected to an α-glucosidase inhibition assay. • Significant α-glucosidase inhibition was reported from agarozizanol E, jinkohol I, jinkohol II, and isokhusenol, with IC_{50} values ranging from 27.308 μg/mL to 109.274 μg/mL. Acarbose was used as a control (IC_{50} = 479.939 μg/mL). • A kinetic study reported an uncompetitive mode of inhibition against α-glucosidase activity.
17	[29]	China	*A. sinensis*	Leaves	Not stated	• Several benzophenone O-glycosides were synthesised from *A. sinensis* leaf extracts and screened for their potential to inhibit α-glucosidase activity. • Significant α-glucosidase inhibition was reported using 4,4′,6-O-Trihydroxylbenzophenone 2-O-a-D-mannopyranosyl-(1-4)-a-L-rhamnoside and 2,4′,6-O-Trihydroxylbenzophenone 4-O-a-D-mannopyranosyl-(1-4)-a-L-rhamnoside, they reported IC_{50} values of 93.713 ± 7.721 μg/mL and 116.710 ± 13.276 μg/mL, respectively. Acarbose was used as a control (IC_{50} = 367.540 ± 32.086 μg/mL).
18	[32]	Vietnam	*A. crassna*	Branches	Methanol	• Several polyphenols, namely, iriflophenone 3,5-C-β-D-diglucoside, iriflophenone 3-C-β-D-glucoside, mangiferin, iriflophenone 2-O-α-rhamnoside, genkwanin 5-O-β-primeveroside, genkwanin 4′-methyl ether 5-O-β-primeveroside, and genkwanin, were isolated from *A. crassna* branches and screened for their potential to inhibit α-glucosidase activity. • Genkwanin was found to have the highest inhibition of α-glucosidase activity with an IC_{50} value of 6.822 ug/mL. Acarbose was used as a control (IC_{50} = 50.05 ug/mL).

Table 1. *Cont.*

No.	References	Country	Plant Species	Plant Parts	Extraction Solvent	Key Findings
19	[28]	India	*A. malaccensis*	Agarwood chips	Water	• Essential oil extracted from *A. malaccensis* agarwood was screened for its α-amylase inhibitory and antioxidant activity. • The IC_{50} value for the α-amylase inhibitory assay was reported at 30.78 ± 0.0018 μL/mL. Acarbose was used as a control (IC_{50} = 44.77 ± 0.0006 μL/mL). • DPPH, 2,2′-Azino-bis (3-ethylbenzothiazoline-6-sulfonic acid) (ABTS) radical scavenging and metal chelating assays were conducted to determine its antioxidant activity. The IC_{50} values reported were 40.14 ± 0.0192, 76.95 ± 0.0090, and 26.96 ± 0.0244 μL/mL, respectively. α-tocopherol was used as a control for the DPPH and ABTS assays, with IC_{50} values of 18.53 ± 0.0141 and 61.93 ± 0.0018 μL/mL, respectively. Ethylenediaminetetraacetic acid (EDTA) was used as a control for the metal chelating assay with an IC_{50} value of 19.52 ± 0.0192 μL/mL.
20	[37]	China	*A. sinensis*	Agarwood chips	Ethanol	• Artificial and wild agarwood extracts were investigated for their antioxidant potential and α-glucosidase inhibition. • Showing a similar trend from 2021, IC_{50} values of the α-glucosidase inhibition for wild agarwood were higher compared to artificial *A. sinensis* with IC_{50} values of 0.147 ug/mL and 0.212 ug/mL, respectively. • Wild agarwood reported higher antioxidant capacity than artificial agarwood via DPPH and ABTS assays. However, the differences were not statistically significant ($p > 0.05$).
21	[36]	Indonesia	*A. malaccensis*	Leaves	Ethanol	• The synergistic effect of *A. malaccensis* leaves and *Cinnamomum burmannii* bark extracts on α-glucosidase and α-amylase was investigated. • 750:250 ug/mL *C. burmannii* and *A. malaccensis* extracts reported increased inhibition of α-glucosidase and α-amylase compared to using the extracts individually.
22	[55]	China	*A. sinensis*	Leaves	Methanol	• *A. sinensis* leaf extracts were isolated using different elution solvents, starting with water, 30% ethanol, 50% ethanol, 75% ethanol, and 95% ethanol. The eluates were tested for α-glucosidase inhibitory and antioxidant potential. • 75% ethanol eluates reported the highest α-glucosidase inhibition with EC_{50} value 844 ug/mL. Acarbose was used as a control (EC_{50} = 183 ug/mL). • 30% ethanol eluates reported the highest antioxidant capacity through ABTS and ferric reducing antioxidant power (FRAP) radical scavenging assays. IC_{50} values were 366 ug/mL and 833 ug/mL, respectively.

Table 2. The effect of agarwood on diabetes in in vivo studies.

No.	References	Country	Plant Species	Part of Plant	Extraction Solvent	Experimental Model	Main Outcomes
1	[48]	Thailand	*A. sinensis*	Leaves	Water and Methanol	Model: male Sprague–Dawley rats. Induction of disease: streptozotocin. Treatment: 1 g/kg of extracts. Control: 4 U/kg/day of insulin. Treatment duration: 7 days.	• *A. sinensis* extracts reduced fasting blood glucose up to 54%, comparable to insulin control at 73%. • *A. sinensis* extracts enhanced glucose uptake by adipocytes by up to 176%, comparable to insulin control at 166%.
2	[53]	China	*A. sinensis*	Leaves	95% Ethanol	Model: db/db mice. Induction of disease: genetically diabetic mice. Treatment: 300–600 mg/kg of extracts. Control: 5 mg/kg of rosiglitazone. Treatment duration: 1 month.	• *A. sinensis* extracts reduced hyperglycaemia in oral glucose tolerance tests and glycosylated haemoglobin (HbA1C) levels, implying that the treatment managed to reduce insulin resistance. • *A. sinensis* extracts also attenuated weight gain, which is a side effect of thiazolidinediones. • Western blot analysis revealed that the mechanism of the hypoglycaemic effect by *A. sinensis* may be related to the activation of AMP-activated protein kinase (AMPK).
3	[49]	Thailand	*A. sinensis*	Leaves	Methanol	Model: imprinting control region mice. Induction of disease: streptozotocin. Treatment: 0.1–1 g of extracts or 0.047–0.47 g of iriflophenone 3-C-β-glucoside. Control: 8 U/kg/day of insulin. Treatment duration: 3 weeks.	• Iriflophenone 3-C-β-glucoside was identified as the main constituent in *A. sinensis* extracts at 3.17%. • *A. sinensis* extracts and iriflophenone 3-C-β-glucoside reduced blood glucose levels by 40.3% and 46.4%, respectively. • *A. sinensis* extracts and iriflophenone 3-C-β-glucoside enhanced glucose uptake by adipocytes up to 152% and 153%, respectively. • Iriflophenone 3-C-β-glucoside was suggested as the main active compound for the hypoglycaemic effect in *A. sinensis* extracts.

Table 2. *Cont.*

No.	References	Country	Plant Species	Part of Plant	Extraction Solvent	Experimental Model	Main Outcomes
4	[51]	Korea	*A. lignum (A. agallocha)*	Agarwood	Water	Model: female Specific Pathogen-Free/Virus Antibody Free Crj: CD-1 (SPF/VAF CrljOri:CD1) Imprinting Control Region (ICR) mice. Induction of disease: high-fat diet. Treatment: 100–400 mg/kg of agarwood-fermented green tea or 400 mg/kg of green tea. Control: 250 mg/kg of metformin or 10 mg/kg of simvastatin. Treatment duration: 84 days.	• Agarwood-fermented green tea improves the anti-diabetic potential of normal green tea by enhancing its antihyperglycemic, antidyslipidemia, antioxidant, hepatoprotective, and kidney protective effects. • Agarwood-fermented green tea attenuated the decrease in glucokinase and the increase in glucose-6-phosphatase and phosphoenolpyruvate carboxykinase, which are liver enzymes related to glucose homeostasis.
5	[52]	Korea	*A. lignum (A. agallocha)*	Agarwood	Water	Model: female C57BL/6NCrljOri mice and db/db mice. Induction of disease: genetically diabetic mice. Treatment: 100–400 mg/kg of agarwood-fermented green tea or 400 mg/kg of green tea. Control: 250 mg/kg of metformin. Treatment duration: 84 days.	• Synergistic effects of agarwood and green tea were reported by enhanced anti-obesity, hypoglycaemic, hypolipidemic, anti-hepatopathy, anti-nephropathy, and antioxidant effects.
6	[50]	Thailand	*A. crassna*	Leaves	Water	Model: Male ddY mice. Induction of disease: streptozotocin and nicotinamide. Treatment: 5–1000 mg/kg of extracts. Control: 5 mg/kg of glibenclamide. Treatment duration: 28 days.	• *A. crassna* extracts treatment managed to attenuate blood glucose spiking significantly and promoted a hypoglycaemic effect of up to 86% compared to the control ($p < 0.01$). • *A. crassna* extracts also presented anti-α-glucosidase effects with an IC_{50} value of 36.3 ug/mL and an antioxidative effect with an IC_{50} value of DPPH inhibition determined at 34.6 ug/mL. • Enzyme-kinetic analysis revealed the uncompetitive inhibition of α-glucosidase by *A. crassna* extracts.

Table 2. *Cont.*

No.	References	Country	Plant Species	Part of Plant	Extraction Solvent	Experimental Model	Main Outcomes
7	[54]	Algeria	*A. malaccensis*	Stem barks	70% Methanol	Model: Female albino rats. Induction of disease: high-fructose, high-fat diet. Treatment: 200 mg/kg of agarwood extracts or 400 mg/kg of *P. oleracea* extracts or both. Control: 300 mg/kg of metformin. Treatment duration: 1 month.	• *A. malaccensis* extracts significantly attenuated the effect of insulin resistance induced by a high-fructose, high-fat diet in mice • Hypoglycaemic and anti-dyslipidaemia were reported by reduced blood glucose and serum lipid profile. • *A. malaccensis* reduced liver and kidney damage caused by insulin resistance by improving kidney and liver function markers. • *A. malaccensis* showed antioxidant potential by significantly reducing the lipid peroxidation marker malondialdehyde. • However, no synergistic effect was found between *A. malaccensis* and *P. oleracea*.

4. Discussion

4.1. In Vitro Anti-Diabetic Findings of Agarwood

In vitro studies on the anti-diabetic mechanisms of agarwood are mainly characterised by the plant's potent efficacy in inhibiting enzymes associated with carbohydrate metabolism, exhibiting lipase inhibitory activity, and increasing the production of adiponectin as well as oxidative stress. Figure 2 shows the overview of the in vitro anti-diabetic mechanism of agarwood on carbohydrates and dietary fats in the intestine.

4.1.1. α-Glucosidase Inhibition

α-glucosidase is an enzyme involved in the breaking down of oligosaccharides and disaccharides into glucose [56]. Excess glucose rapidly absorbed and retained in the bloodstream, especially after meals, is commonly described as postprandial hyperglycaemia [57]. The conventional drugs prescribed are α-glucosidase inhibitors, such as acarbose and miglitol; they are associated with side effects, such as gastrointestinal discomfort and long-term tolerance [58,59]. Therefore, alternative and complementary natural products with minimal side effects are needed to inhibit α-glucosidase to manage type 2 diabetes.

Several studies have reported promising α-glucosidase inhibitors in various compounds extracted from agarwood, particularly polyphenols, sesquiterpenes, chromones, and benzophenone O-glycosides. One of the most studied compounds is the 2-(2-phenylmethyl) chromone due to its strong α-glucosidase inhibition. In a study using *A. filaria* agarwood from Indonesia, 6,7-dihydroxy-2-(2-phenyl ethyl) chromone was identified as the most potent chromone derivative to inhibit the α-glucosidase activity with an IC_{50} value of 2.256 ± 0.085 μg/mL, surpassing the potency of the conventional drug, acarbose, and comparable to genistein with IC_{50} values of 479.939 ± 2.130 μg/mL and 2.243 ± 0.027 μg/mL, respectively [42]. Another study conducted using *A. sinensis* agarwood from China reported 6,7-dihydroxy-2-[2-(4-methoxyphenyl) ethyl] chromone as the most potent derivative from that agarwood species with an IC_{50} value of 15.655 μg/mL [40]. Besides chromones, sesquiterpenoid derivatives are among the primary compounds isolated from agarwood for their bioactive potential. In a study of sesquiterpenoid derivatives isolated from agarwood obtained from Thailand, the most potent inhibitor of α-glucosidase was identified as Aquilarene D with an IC_{50} value of 57.460 μg/mL, also surpassing the potency of the conventional drug acarbose with an IC_{50} value of 781.176 μg/mL [35]. For *A. filaria* agarwood, the most potent sesquiterpenes against α-glucosidase activity were determined as guaianolide, with an IC50 value of 53.332 ± 2.273 μg/mL [43]. Also in 2019, screening for new sesquiterpenoids from agarwood found a newly discovered zizaane-type sesquiterpenoid named agarozizanol E with an IC_{50} value of 27.308 μg/mL, and it was found to act as an uncompetitive inhibitor due to the compound's ability to modify the active site of the α-glucosidase enzyme. The authors emphasised that uncompetitive inhibitors are preferred in drug discovery due to their high efficacy in living models [34].

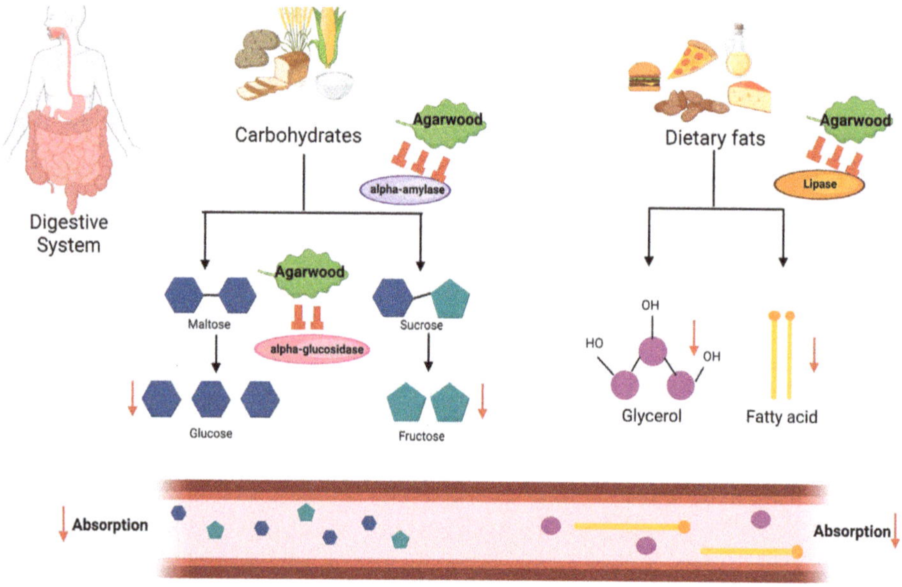

Figure 2. Overview of in vitro studies on the anti-diabetic mechanisms of agarwood.

Other than these types of compounds, benzophenone O-glycosides are also commonly studied in agarwood for their α-glucosidase inhibition potential. 4,4′,6-O-trihydroxylbenzophenone 2-O-α-D-mannopyranosyl-(1-4)-α-L-rhamnoside, isolated from the leaves of *A. sinensis*, showed notable inhibitory activity with an IC_{50} value of 93.713 ± 7.721 μg/mL, adding to the diverse array of bioactive compounds found in agarwood [29]. Mangiferin is a significant polyphenolic commonly identified as the active compound responsible for the anti-α-glucosidase properties of agarwood. Mangiferin content was determined to make up 2.1130% of the dried leaf powder [38]. Mangiferin isolated from the leaves of *A. sinensis* and *A. crassna* showed IC_{50} inhibition of α-glucosidase at 126.5 ± 17.8 ug/mL and 571.4 ± 4.4 ug/mL, respectively [38,46]. However, a study conducted using *A. crassna* leaves from Vietnam revealed genkwanin, another polyphenol, to be the most potent α-glucosidase inhibitor with an IC_{50} value of 6.822 ug/mL [32].

Studies have also focused on comparing the α-glucosidase inhibition between wild and artificially induced agarwood. Artificial technology aims at a faster and more sustainable production of agarwood. For instance, wild agarwood demonstrated an IC_{50} value of 156.4 μg/mL, compared to 292.0 μg/mL for artificially produced agarwood [39]. A more recent study in 2023 reported similar trends, with wild agarwood showing an IC_{50} value of 147.2 μg/mL, compared to 211.9 μg/mL for the artificially induced variant [37]. These studies elucidated that although wild agarwood is still superior in terms of α-glucosidase inhibition, this signals that artificially produced agarwood technology is improving and approaching the efficacy of natural agarwood.

Much research has been carried out involving the optimisation of using different solvents, drying methods, and parts of the plant to achieve the highest α-glucosidase inhibition. For instance, acetone is the preferred extraction solvent for *Gyrinops versteegii* from Indonesia, showing the highest potency against α-glucosidase compared to other solvents [30]. Also, the leaf extracts of *Gyrinops* versteegii performed better than the fruits and barks of the plant [31]. On the other hand, an ethanolic extract of *A. crassna* leaves from Thailand reported an IC_{50} value of 184.0 ± 3.2 ug/mL against α-glucosidase [38]. Interestingly, another study reported a much higher potency from *A. crassna* leaves extracted using boiling water with an IC_{50} value of 36.3 ± 2.3 μg/mL [50]. In a Malaysian study, leaves from *A. malaccensis*, *A. subintegra*, and *A. sinensis* were compared for their α-glucosidase inhibition using different drying methods and solvents. The study found that 70% ethanol extraction from oven-dried *A. malaccensis* leaves resulted in the highest potency, with an IC_{50} value of 0.13 μg/mL, almost five times more potent than the acarbose control [47]. These various studies prove that extraction parameters significantly influence the potency of the bioactive compounds from agarwood against α-glucosidase.

Interestingly, a synergistic effect between C. *burmannii* bark and *A. malaccensis* leaves on α-glucosidase inhibition was reported [36]. A 750:250 μg/mL *C. burmannii* and *A. malaccensis* extract combination showed higher inhibition at 96.368 ± 0.00870% compared to a pure 1000 μg/mL *A. malaccensis* extract at 83.133 ± 0.00870% inhibition. In the same study, in silico molecular docking revealed that palustrol, a secondary metabolite from A. malaccensis, was able to bind strongly to the receptor-ligand of the human maltase-glucoamylase receptor. The binding affinity of palustrol was −10.2 kcal/mol, whereas the acarbose control was −8.1 kcal/mol [36]. These findings highlight the potential of agarwood and its active compounds in the discovery and development of effective α-glucosidase inhibitors for diabetes management.

4.1.2. Lipase Inhibition

Lipase is one of the enzymes involved in the function of the gastrointestinal tract. Lipase breaks down into triacylglycerides, monoacylglycerols, and free fatty acids [60]. Inhibiting lipase is a strategy to manage obesity and type 2 diabetes, as it reduces lipid levels and relieves stress on pancreatic β-cells, improving insulin regulation. However, synthetic inhibitors like orlistat can cause side effects, making the search for natural alternatives important in managing these conditions [61].

In a study conducted in Malaysia, two *Aquilaria* spp. were collected to investigate their potential to inhibit lipase activity [33]. The leaves and bark of *A. subintegra* and *A. malaccensis* were collected, dried, and grided for homogenisation. Then, the leaves and bark of *A. subintegra* and *A. malaccensis* were individually extracted using macerations for 72 h using three different solvents—hexane, dichloromethane, and methanol. In total, there were 12 crude extracts of the *Aquilaria* spp. The anti-lipase activity was measured by employing a colorimetric assay using porcine pancreatic lipase and olive oil as the natural substrate. The positive control used was lipase enzyme and substrate without the crude extracts. Lipase activity in the positive control was measured at 0.753 U/mL ± 0.037. Then, 100 μg/mL of the crude extracts were screened for inhibitory potential. Among the 12 crude extracts, *A. malaccensis* bark extracted using dichloromethane showed the highest inhibitory activity at 91% inhibition, $p < 0.01$ (0.065 U/mL ± 0.147). As for *A. subintegra*, the highest inhibition was observed from its leaves extracted using hexane at 54% inhibition, $p < 0.01$ (0.348 U/mL ± 0.077). Phytochemical screening was conducted, and all extracts were found to have flavonoids, steroids, and terpenoids. The authors concluded that anti-lipase activity may be attributed to the polyphenol activity [33]. This study proves that different parts and extraction solvents play an important role in determining the inhibition of lipase activity using agarwood.

In another study from Malaysia, the roles of particle size and the kinetic behaviour of lipase inhibition using *A. subintegra* and *A. malaccensis* were studied [27]. *A. subintegra* and *A. malaccensis* leaves were collected, dried, milled, and sieved into five separate particle sizes ranging from 250 μm to 1000 μm. The powdered leaves were macerated using distilled water for 24 h before being sonicated for 30 min at 60 °C. The crude extracts were obtained using hydrodistillation. After that, the total polyphenols and total flavonoids were determined, and a kinetic study of lipase inhibition was carried out. The study found that crude extracts extracted using the smallest particle size (250 μm) contained the highest concentration of the gallic acid equivalent of the total polyphenols and quercetin equivalent of the total flavonoids. The gallic acid equivalent concentrations for A. *subintegra* and *A. malaccensis* using a 250 μm particle size are 101,273.0 μg/mL and 89,991.0 μg/mL, respectively. The quercetin equivalent concentrations for *A. subintegra* and *A. malaccensis* using a 250 μm particle size are 37.0 μg/mL and 29.0 μg/mL, respectively. Also worth noting is that the gallic acid and quercetin equivalents were 10% and 20% higher in *A. subintegra* compared to *A. malaccensis*. Similarly, the highest percentage inhibition of lipase activity was recorded at 82% using 1 mL of *A. subintegra* crude extracts from a 250 μm particle size powder. These findings support that a higher surface area of powder allows for the better extraction of polyphenols and flavonoids, leading to a higher lipase inhibition potential. Using Lineweaver–Burk plots, the mode of inhibition exhibited by *A. malaccensis* and *A. subintegra* leaf crude extract was described as a mixed inhibition that closely mimics noncompetitive binding. The authors described the possibility of an allosteric binding site on the lipase enzyme. This reaction allows the *Aquilaria* spp. extracts to bind to free lipase enzymes and to the lipase–fat complex. The study concluded that both the lipase–*Aquilaria* spp. complex and the lipase–*Aquilaria* spp.–fat complex prevent the formation of fatty acid products [27].

4.1.3. α-Amylase Inhibition

α-amylase breaks down digestive starches into simpler sugars to be absorbed into the bloodstream, causing blood glucose levels to increase [62]. Thus, it is a therapeutic strategy to lower complex sugar breakdown by inhibiting α-amylase activity to aid in the gradual release of glucose into the blood [63]. Therefore, screening for anti-α-amylase properties is common in testing natural products' anti-diabetic potential.

In India, *A. malaccensis* resinous agarwood was obtained by naturally infesting the tree with insects. The produced resinous agarwood was tested for α-amylase inhibitory activity. Tiny chips of the resinous agarwood were subjected to extraction using the Clevenger apparatus to obtain agarwood essential oils. At 60 μL/mL, the essential oil showed 85.90 ± 0.0018% inhibition, better than the conventional drug control, acarbose, at 68.42 ± 0.0080%. Following this, the IC_{50} was determined for the agarwood essential oil at 30.78 ± 0.0018 μL/mL, whereas the IC_{50} for acarbose was determined at 44.77 ± 0.0006 μL/mL [28]. These promising results unequivocally demonstrate the potential use of agarwood essential oil as an alternative strategy to inhibit α-amylase activity, marking a significant advancement in the field of pharmacology and herbal medicine.

Next, the α-amylase inhibition potential of *A. malaccensis* leaves and *Cinnamomum burmannii* barks was investigated [36]. The plant's materials were obtained from Indonesia. Ethanolic extraction was employed using the maceration technique. A sample of 0.25 mL of 1000 μg/mL of the *A. malaccensis* leaf extract showed 77.098 ± 0.521% inhibition towards α-amylase, whereas 1000 μg/mL *Cinnamomum burmannii* barks showed 79.397 ± 0.099% inhibition. The results are comparable to the acarbose control at 78.143 ± 0.099% inhibition. It is worth noting that both plants showed synergistic effects in inhibiting α-amylase. A combination of 75% *Cinnamomum burmannii* and 25% *A. malaccensis* showed the highest inhibition at 86.366 ± 0.451% [36]. These results support the polyherbal use of agarwood and other herbal products for synergistic effects.

4.1.4. Adiponectin Production

Adiponectin is a hormone produced by white adipose that has been linked to anti-obesity, anti-diabetes, and anti-cardiovascular diseases [45]. Studies have shown that adiponectin activates the Peroxisome Proliferator-Activated Receptor Alpha (PPAR-α) and AMPK pathways, which enhance insulin sensitivity and fat metabolism and reduce serum glucose and triglyceride levels. However, long-term use of synthetic PPARγ agonists, like thiazolidinediones, can cause side effects, emphasising the need for safer alternatives [64–69]. This underscores the urgent need for research to discover alternatives that can minimise the risk of the side effects of synthetic PPARγ modulators.

In a study by Ahn et al. (2019), the bioactive compounds of phenyethylchromone were isolated from agarwood chips of *A. malaccensis* [45]. The extracts, obtained by reflux in 70% methanol, were further fractionated using multiple solvents—water, diethyl ether, ethyl acetate, and n-butanol. Later, the respective chromone compounds were isolated using a chromatographic technique. Using a human bone marrow mesenchymal stem cell model, each of the obtained chromone compounds was tested for their effects on adiponectin production during adipogenesis. The compounds 6-methoxy-2-(2-phenylethyl) chromone and 7-methoxy-2-(2-phenylethyl) chromone were identified as the most potent promoters of adiponectin production, with EC_{50} values at 4.541 µg/mL, and 5.690 µg/mL, respectively, ensuring the reliability of the results. Further investigation found that the increased adiponectin was due to the activation of the PPARγ. Thus, Ahn et al. (2019) reported that *A. malaccensis* contains bioactive phenyethylchromone that exhibited PPARγ partial agonism, causing increased adiponectin production [45]. This discovery holds significant promise for diabetic patients, as increased adiponectin levels promote insulin sensitivity and decreased inflammation in diabetic patients.

4.1.5. Antioxidant Potential

Various studies have investigated the antioxidant capacity of agarwood extracts and essential oils using different assays such as DPPH, ABTS, and FRAP radical scavenging activities. First, methanol, methanol-water, and acetone of inoculated *G. versteegii* wood were tested using a DPPH radical scavenging assay. Results showed that all the extracts contained a promising antioxidant value, with the best antioxidant value being acetone extract with an IC_{50} value of 65.62 µg/mL [30].

Ma et al. (2021) conducted a comparative study on the antioxidant potential of various agarwoods [39]. The study found that the most potent IC_{50} values of DPPH and ABTS free radicals were reported in wild *A. sinensis* at 307.0 µg/mL and 236.8 µg/mL, respectively. An 18-month inoculated *A. sinensis* was reported as the best antioxidant artificial agarwood with the IC_{50} values of the DPPH and ABTS free radicals at 390.2 µg/mL and 447.2 µg/mL, respectively. Similar studies were conducted in 2023 by Ma et al. to compare the antioxidant potential of artificial and wild agarwood [37]. As a result, the IC_{50} values for DPPH free radical scavenging by artificial and wild agarwood were 187.3 µg/mL and 151.5 µg/mL, respectively. Furthermore, the IC_{50} values for the ABTS free radical scavenging assays for artificial agarwood and wild agarwood were 60.2 µg/mL and 56.3 µg/mL, respectively. Statistical analysis showed that the difference between artificial and wild agarwood is not significant ($p > 0.05$) [37]. Thus, regarding antioxidant potential, artificial technology in producing agarwood is improving and approaching naturally produced agarwood.

A study in Malaysia investigated the DPPH activity of *A. malaccensis*, *A. subintegra*, and *A. sinensis* leaf extracts using various extraction solvents and drying techniques [47]. The DPPH activity assay revealed that oven-dried *A. malaccensis* leaves extracted using 70% ethanol have the most potent antioxidant capacities with an IC_{50} value of 33.60 ug/mL. Correlation studies showed a positive correlation between the total polyphenols content and DPPH activity ($r = 0.796$, $p < 0.05$) [47]. This correlation might signal that the antioxidant capacity of agarwood leaf extracts is due to the rich polyphenol content.

A. crassna leaf crude extracts and mangiferin isolated from the extracts were tested for antioxidant activity [38]. A DPPH scavenging assay using *A. crassna* leaf extracts and mangiferin reported IC_{50} values of 21.54 ± 0.17 ug/mL and 0.64 ± 0.005 ug/mL, respectively. The DPPH activity of mangiferin isolated from *A. crassna* proved to be more potent than quercetin with an IC_{50} value of 3.46 ± 0.09 ug/mL. The IC_{50} values for a nitric oxide radical scavenging assay using *A. crassna* leaf extracts and mangiferin were recorded at 79.13 ± 0.74 ug/mL and 40.55 ± 0.17 ug/mL, respectively. Next, the IC_{50} values for a superoxide radical scavenging assay using *A. crassna* leaf extracts and mangiferin were recorded at 278.12 ± 4.29 ug/mL and 105.49 ± 1.28 ug/mL, respectively. Thus, this study demonstrates that *A. crassna* leaf extracts exhibit potent antioxidant activity. Mangiferin is suggested as the active compound contributing to the antioxidant potential, outperforming the crude leaf extracts in various radical scavenging assays and quercetin in the DPPH scavenging assays [38].

A study compared the antioxidant DPPH radical scavenging potential of fruit bark, stem bark, and the leaves of an agarwood-producing plant, *G. versteegii* [31]. The study also compared the antioxidant potential between healthy and inoculated *G. versteegii*. As a result, the inoculated specimens reported higher DPPH radical scavenging potential, with the most potent being the inoculated leaves of *G. versteegii* extracts with an IC_{50} value of 32.89 ± 2.7 ug/mL. Thus, this study showed that *G. versteegii* leaves possess the most potent antioxidant potential compared to other parts of the plant, with enhanced bioactivity due to inoculation [31]. Gogoi et al. (2023) determined the antioxidant potential of *A. malaccensis* using its essential oil [28]. The *A. malaccensis* essential oil reported an IC_{50} value of 40.14 ± 0.0192 μL/mL using the DPPH free radical scavenging assay. An ABTS scavenging assay of the agarwood essential oil reported an IC_{50} value of 76.95 ± 0.0090 μL/mL, whereas the IC_{50} value for a metal chelating assay was reported at 26.96 ± 0.0244 μL/mL [28]. These findings further emphasised the antioxidant potential of the essential oil extracted from *A. malaccensis* agarwood.

In the most recent study of the antioxidant potential of agarwood, the methanolic extract of an *A. sinensis* leaf was subjected to chromatographic isolation using different elution solvents, starting with water and then increasing the concentration of ethanol [55]. Later, the elutions were tested for their antioxidant potential using ABTS and FRAP radical scavenging assays. As a result, the highest antioxidant potential was determined from the 30% ethanol elution with EC_{50} values for the ABTS and FRAP assays of 366.0 ug/mL and 833.0 ug/mL, respectively. The crude total extracts reported EC_{50} values for the ABTS and FRAP assays of 542.0 ug/mL and 899.0 ug/mL, respectively. Further analysis using tandem mass spectrometry revealed that the 30% ethanol elution fraction is high in antioxidant molecules, particularly mangiferin [55]. These findings further support mangiferin as the main bioactive compound in the antioxidant properties of agarwood leaf extracts.

Strong antioxidant activity was reported, particularly from the ethanol and acetone extractions of *A. malaccensis*, *A. sinensis*, and *G. versteegii* leaves. Mangiferin was found to be the main active compound for antioxidant potential. The antioxidant potential of artificial agarwood is approaching the level of natural agarwood. In conclusion, these studies reviewed and demonstrated significant antioxidant capacities using different parts, compounds, and species of agarwood.

4.2. In Vivo Anti-Diabetic Findings of Agarwood

Several in vivo studies have explored the antidiabetic potential of agarwood and agarwood-producing plants. This research explored the potential of pure extracts as well as synergistic effects with different plant products. Figure 3 summarises the overview of the in vivo anti-diabetic mechanism of agarwood with multiple pathways involved.

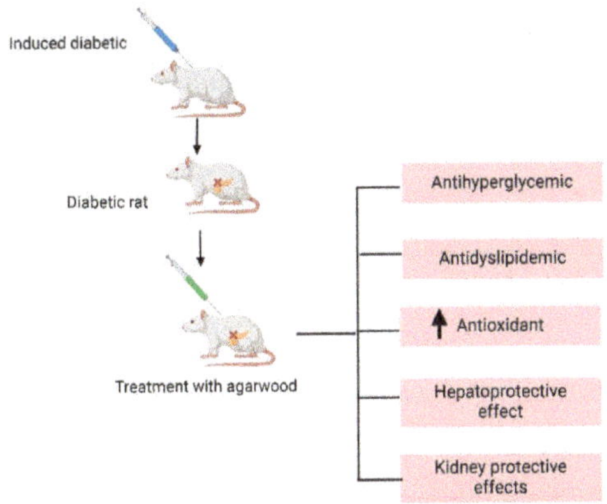

Figure 3. Overview of the in vivo anti-diabetic mechanisms of agarwood.

First, Pranakhon et al. (2011) demonstrated the hypoglycaemic effect of *A. sinensis* leaf extracts using streptozotocin-induced diabetic rats [48]. Hyperglycaemia was induced by an intraperitoneal injection of 45 mg/kg bodyweight of STZ. After seven days, treatment was given daily for one week by subcutaneous injections of 4 U/kg/day of insulin or the oral administration of 1 g/kg bodyweight/day of 0.15 g/mL of *A. sinensis* leaf extracts. A reduced fasting blood glucose was reported in the methanol and water extract rats of 54% and 40%, respectively. The insulin control group reported a 73% fasting blood glucose reduction. Further analysis also showed that the methanol and water extracts increased glucose uptake by the rat adipocytes by 172% and 176%, similar to the effect of a 1.5 nM insulin treatment. These results showed that agarwood leaves have a hypoglycaemic effect in diabetic rats by increasing glucose uptake from the blood into the adipocytes [48].

In 2015, Pranakhon et al. continued to analyse further the hypoglycaemic effects of *A. sinensis* leaf extracts [49]. Chromatographic isolation revealed iriflophenone 3-C-β-glucoside as the main compound isolated from the *A. sinensis* leaf extracts. Streptozotocin was used to induce diabetes in mice models. The diabetic mice models then received a daily oral administration of 1 g/kg of *A. sinensis* extracts or 0.47 g/kg of iriflophenone 3-C-β-glucoside. The treatment continued for 3 weeks. The iriflophenone 3-C-β-glucoside lowered the glucose level by 46.4%, whereas the crude *A. sinensis* leaf extracts lowered the glucose level by 40.3%. Glucose analysis using rat adipocytes also showed that iriflophenone 3-C-β-glucoside increased glucose uptake by 153%, whereas the crude *A. sinensis* leaf extracts increased glucose uptake by 152%. These findings suggest that iriflophenone 3-C-β-glucoside is the active compound contributing to the hypoglycaemic effect of *A. sinensis* leaves [49].

A study in 2011 further investigated the mechanisms and hypoglycaemic effects of *A. sinensis* leaves using genetically diabetic db/db mice models [53]. The mice received an oral administration of 300 mg/kg of *A. sinensis* extracts in the low-dose group or 600 mg/kg in the high-dose group. After 1 month of treatment, the high-dose group recorded a significant reduction in fasting blood glucose and HbA1c levels. Western blot analysis revealed that the high-dose and rosiglitazone control groups had a higher ratio of phosphorylated AMPK to total AMPK in comparison to the negative control groups. This finding signals the possibility that the hypoglycaemic property effects of *A. sinensis* leaf extracts are due to the activation of AMPK. The study also ran an oral glucose tolerance test (OGTT), which revealed that the extracts protected the mice from sugar spikes by increasing insulin sensitivity. Weight analysis also showed that the extracts did not cause weight gain, unlike the side effects caused by the conventional drug type of thiazolidinediones [53]. These findings further emphasised the potentials and mechanisms of the hypoglycaemic properties of *A. sinensis* leaf extracts.

Two studies were conducted to investigate the synergistic therapeutic effect of *A. lignum* fermented with green tea against diabetes [51,52]. High-fat-fed mice and genetically type 2 diabetes db/db mice were used as diabetic animal models. *A. lignum* was described as the stem of an agarwood plant, *A. agallocha*. The process of producing agarwood-fermented green tea was started by mixing dried green leaves and *A. lignum* powder using a ratio of 49:1. The mixtures were then subjected to several steps of fermentation. In both studies, the mice were administered up to 400 mg/kg of agarwood-fermented green tea orally. The findings reported that in both the high-fat-fed mice and db/db mice, there were significantly stronger hypoglycaemic effects in the agarwood-fermented green tea group than in the conventional green tea group. Histopathological studies reported that agarwood-fermented green tea treatment attenuated the hypertrophy or hyperplasia of pancreatic islet cells by normalising the ratio of insulin-producing pancreatic cells and glucagon-producing cells. Further analysis reported that agarwood-fermented green tea significantly reduced the effect of high-fructose, high-fat diets on the levels of key enzymes involved in glucose metabolism, such as glucokinase, glucose-6-phosphatase, and phosphoenolpyruvate carboxykinase, which may explain the mechanism of hypoglycaemic effects. Other than that, agarwood-fermented green tea also attenuated the increase in lipids and weight gain in both obese and diabetic mice. Agarwood-fermented green tea groups reported a marked decrease in lipid profiles, serum leptin, and faecal lipid content, as well as attenuated adipose accumulation. Further analysis also showed that agarwood-fermented green tea reduced the levels of pancreatic digestive enzymes in the mice and reduced the number of pancreatic zymogen granules. The authors presumed the product's ability to inhibit the release and activity of pancreatic lipid-digesting enzymes may be the mechanism explaining the anti-dyslipidaemia effects. Histopathological analysis, along with kidney and liver serum profiles, showed that agarwood-fermented green tea had stronger hepatoprotective and nephroprotective effects against diabetic hepatopathy and nephropathy. Both studies also reported stronger anti-radicals and antioxidant potential in agarwood-fermented green tea groups [51,52]. These findings summarise the synergistic effect of agarwood and green tea against diabetes due to its hypoglycaemic, anti-obesity, anti-dyslipidaemia, kidney protective, liver protective, and antioxidant effects.

Another study used streptozotocin-nicotinamide-induced type 2 diabetic mice to illustrate the hypoglycaemic effect of *A. crassna* leaf extracts. The mouse models were induced with 150 mg/kg of streptozotocin and 120 mg/kg of nicotinamide. After 1 month of intragastric intervention with 1000 mg/kg *A. crassna*, blood glucose levels were reduced by 86%. Thus, this study showed the hypoglycaemic potential of *A. crassna* leaf extracts in diabetic mouse models [50].

The most recent in vivo study investigated the synergistic anti-diabetic effect of *Portulaca oleracea* and *A. malaccensis* leaf extracts using high-fructose, high-fat diet rats [54]. The rats were fed a diet containing 60% fructose and fat calories for 70 days to induce insulin resistance. The treatment group received an oral administration of 400 mg/kg/day of *P. oleracea* or 200 mg/kg/day of *A. malaccensis*, or both. The treatment continued for 1 month. The treatment groups showed attenuated weight gain, decreased blood glucose levels, and lipid peroxidation markers. The treatment also reported improvement in lipid, renal, and liver profiles. However, no synergistic effects were reported from the combination of the *P. oleracea* and *A. malaccensis* groups [54].

The findings from these studies elucidated the antidiabetic potentials of various *Aquilaria* extracts, including *A. sinensis*, *A. crassna*, and *A. malaccensis*, as well as the bark of *A. agallocha*, also called *A. lignum*. Considering the results from these studies, the agarwood dosage range of 200–1000 mg/kg appears to be effective for achieving significant hypoglycaemic effects and improving insulin sensitivity in mice models. Future researchers may start with a low dose of 200 mg/kg to assess the initial effects and safety, a medium dose of 400 mg/kg, and a high dosage of 1000 mg/kg to determine if further benefits can be achieved without adverse effects. This dosage range balances efficacy and safety, as seen in the studies, and allows for a comprehensive evaluation of agarwood's therapeutic potential in diabetes mice models. The antidiabetic effects of agarwood and agarwood-producing plants are demonstrated in the in vivo studies by lowering blood glucose levels, improving insulin sensitivity, and providing antioxidant benefits. Therefore, future research should focus on clinical studies to confirm the efficacy of these products.

5. Limitations of the Study

This review paper has certain limitations. Some information could not be fully retrieved from the original articles. The use of various substances, such as ethanol or methanol in extraction, essential oils, and emulsions, makes it challenging to draw precise conclusions. Additionally, different studies utilised various parts of the agarwood tree, such as the fruit bark, stem bark, or leaves, complicating the assessment of its effectiveness against diabetes-related enzymes. Since agarwood is native to specific regions, the species studied may vary by country, making direct comparisons difficult. Furthermore, the limited number of the selected studies restricts the ability to fully determine agarwood's effectiveness.

6. Future Research

The current review presents the potential of agarwood as an anti-diabetic agent. With the advancement in technology, it makes it possible for us to identify the active compound of agarwood. The improvement of agarwood's isolation and bioactive characterisation is essential for a better understanding of the mechanisms of anti-diabetic action, including insulin sensitivity, glucose uptake, and lipid metabolism. From the bioactive compound, researchers could explore developing functional food products incorporating agarwood extracts, focusing on palatability and bioavailability. The nutritional profile of these functional foods could be analysed to further study the anti-diabetic properties of agarwood-infused foods. We also suggest investigating the effects of anti-diabetic properties when combining agarwood with other herbal remedies that have been known for anti-diabetic properties to evaluate their synergistic effects.

This review has shown the anti-diabetic properties of agarwood using an animal model. Future research could conduct long-term animal studies to assess the impact of prolonged agarwood supplementation on blood glucose levels and insulin sensitivity. The impact of agarwood on diabetes complications such as neuropathy, retinopathy, and nephropathy could be further investigated using a diabetic animal model.

Further research is needed to elucidate its mechanisms, efficacy, and safety in clinical settings. From our scoping, no clinical trials have been conducted using agarwood to study its anti-diabetic effect. In the future, researchers could conduct a small-scale pilot study to assess the safety and efficacy of agarwood in diabetic patients. Later, randomised controlled trials (RCTs) could be designed to evaluate the efficacy of agarwood in lowering blood glucose levels compared to the standard glucose-lowering agents in diabetic patients. It is interesting to study how genetic, dietary, and lifestyle factors affect the efficacy of the anti-diabetic properties in agarwood in different populations. By addressing existing research gaps, exploring holistic approaches, and considering their use in functional foods, future research can contribute significantly to diabetes management strategies complementary to the current diabetes management.

7. Conclusions

Agarwood-producing plants, particularly agarwood and leaf extracts, possess promising potential as alternative or supplementary treatments for diabetes. The crude extracts, as well as isolated bioactive compounds such as polyphenols, phenylethyl chromone, and sesquiterpenoids, have demonstrated significant α-glucosidase, lipase, and α-amylase inhibition, and strong antioxidant capacity. Overall, *A. malaccensis* shows great promise for inhibiting α-glucosidase and α-amylase and promoting antioxidant activity, as well as stimulating adiponectin production, highlighting its potential therapeutic applications in diabetes management. The main bioactive compounds identified include phenylethylchromone and polyphenols such as genkwanin and mangiferin. Diabetic animal models treated with agarwood plants showed significant hypoglycaemic, anti-obesity, anti-dyslipidaemia, and organ protection effects. However, from our scoping and literature search, no clinical trials on agarwood in relation to diabetes have been performed. Although these findings suggest that agarwood and agarwood-producing plants could act as valuable agents in managing diabetes, further clinical trials are warranted.

Supplementary Materials: The following supporting information can be downloaded at: https://www.mdpi.com/article/10.3390/ph17111548/s1.

Author Contributions: Conceptualisation, M.A.M.F., N.A.S. and A.A.R.; literature review: M.A.M.F., N.A.S. and A.A.R.; tables: M.A.M.F., N.A.S. and A.A.R.; writing and review: M.A.M.F., N.A.S. and A.A.R.; editing: M.A.M.F., N.A.S. and A.A.R.; revisions and final editing: M.A.M.F. All authors have read and agreed to the published version of the manuscript.

Funding: This research received no external funding.

Acknowledgments: The authors thank the Director General of Health Malaysia and the Director of the Institute for Medical Research (IMR), Malaysia, for permitting them to publish this article. We also thank the staff of the Nutrition, Metabolism and Cardiovascular Centre, Institute for Medical Research, NIH, for their continuous support.

Conflicts of Interest: The authors declare no conflicts of interest.

Abbreviations

ABTS	2,2′-Azino-bis (3-ethylbenzothiazoline-6-sulfonic acid)
AMPK	AMP-activated protein kinase
CITES	Convention of International Trade in Endangered Species of Wild Fauna and Flora
db/db mice	Diabetic and obese mice
DPP-4	Dipeptidyl Peptidase-4
DPPH	2,2-Diphenyl-1-picrylhydrazyl
EC50	Half maximal effective concentration
EDTA	Ethylenediaminetetraacetic acid
FBG	Fasting Blood Glucose
FRAP	Ferric Reducing Antioxidant Power
GLP-1	Glucagon-Like Peptide-1
HbA1c	Glycosylated Haemoglobin
IC50	Half maximal inhibitory concentration
ICR mice	Imprinting Control Region mice
IDF	International Diabetes Federation
IR	Insulin Resistance
MeSH	Medical Subject Heading
PICO	Population, Intervention, Comparison, Outcome
PPAR	Peroxisome Proliferator-Activated Receptor
PRISMA	Preferred Reporting Items for Systematic reviews and Meta-Analyses
RCT	Randomised clinical trials
SGLT2	Sodium-Glucose Cotransporter-2
SPF/VAF CrljOri ICR mice	Specific Pathogen-Free/Virus Antibody Free Crj: CD-1 ICR mice

References

1. Shivanand, P.; Arbie, N.F.; Krishnamoorthy, S.; Ahmad, N. Agarwood-The Fragrant Molecules of a Wounded Tree. *Molecules* **2022**, *27*, 3386. [CrossRef]
2. Wang, Y.; Hussain, M.; Jiang, Z.; Wang, Z.; Gao, J.; Ye, F.; Mao, R.; Li, H. Aquilaria Species (Thymelaeaceae) Distribution, Volatile and Non-Volatile Phytochemicals, Pharmacological Uses, Agarwood Grading System, and Induction Methods. *Molecules* **2021**, *26*, 7708. [CrossRef]
3. Alamil, J.M.R.; Paudel, K.R.; Chan, Y.; Xenaki, D.; Panneerselvam, J.; Singh, S.K.; Gulati, M.; Jha, N.K.; Kumar, D.; Prasher, P.; et al. Rediscovering the Therapeutic Potential of Agarwood in the Management of Chronic Inflammatory Diseases. *Molecules* **2022**, *27*, 3038. [CrossRef]

4. Wyn, L.T.; Anak, N.A. *Wood for the Trees: A Review of the Agarwood (Gaharu) Trade in Malaysia*; TRAFFIC Southeast Asia: Kuala Lumpur, Malaysia, 2010.
5. Dahham, S.S.; Tabana, Y.M.; Iqbal, M.A.; Ahamed, M.B.K.; Ezzat, M.O.; Majid, A.S.A.; Majid, A.M.S.A. The anticancer, antioxidant and antimicrobial properties of the sesquiterpene β-caryophyllene from the essential oil of *Aquilaria crassna*. *Molecules* **2015**, *20*, 11808–11829. [CrossRef]
6. Li, W.; Cai, C.-H.; Dong, W.-H.; Guo, Z.-K.; Wang, H.; Mei, W.-L.; Dai, H.-F. 2-(2-Phenylethyl)chromone derivatives from Chinese agarwood induced by artificial holing. *Fitoterapia* **2014**, *98*, 117–123. [CrossRef]
7. Suzuki, A.; Miyake, K.; Saito, Y.; Rasyid, F.A.; Tokuda, H.; Takeuchi, M.; Suzuki, N.; Ichiishi, E.; Fujie, T.; Goto, M.; et al. Phenylethylchromones with in vitro antitumor promoting activity from *Aquilaria filaria*. *Planta Med.* **2017**, *83*, 300–305. [CrossRef]
8. Wang, S.; Zhou, Y.; MA, F.; Zhang, Q.; Liu, Y.; Gong, B.; Guo, P.; Wei, J. Effect of agarwood produced by whole-tree agarwood-inducing technique on hypnotic and spontaneous activity inhibition of mice. *J. Int. Pharm. Res.* **2016**, *43*, 1082–1087.
9. Wu, G.L. A brief discussion on the clinical effect of anesthetic medicine Ba Wei Chen Xiang in the treatment of bronchial asthma. *Latest Med. Inf. Abs* **2017**, *17*, 142–144.
10. Wang, S.; Yu, Z.; Wang, C.; Wu, C.; Guo, P.; Wei, J. Chemical constituents and pharmacological activity of agarwood and Aquilaria plants. *Molecules* **2018**, *23*, 342. [CrossRef]
11. Lin, F.H.; Peng, Y.H.; Ke, F.F.; Deng, Y.L. Experimental study on the content, antioxidant activity in vitro, and delaying aging effect of tannins from the leaf of *Aquilaria sinensis* (Lour.) Gilg. *J. Guangdong Pharm. Univer* **2012**, *3*, 259–262.
12. Yang, M.; Li, Y.F.; Ma, Q.S.; Ge, R.L. Effect of 50% ethanol-extract from Bawei Chenxiang Powder on hemodynamics in myocardial ischemia rats. *Chin. J. Trad. Chin. Med.* **2011**, *11*, 2740–2742.
13. Mekala, K.C.; Bertoni, A.G. Epidemiology of diabetes mellitus. In *eBooks*; Elsevier: Amsterdam, The Netherlands, 2020; pp. 49–58.
14. Magliano, D.J.; Boyko, E.J. *IDF Diabetes Atlas*, 10th ed.; IDF DIABETES ATLAS: Brussels, Belgium, 2021.
15. Hossain, M.J.; Al-Mamun, M.; Islam, M.R. Diabetes mellitus, the fastest growing global public health concern: Early detection should be focused. *Health Sci. Rep.* **2024**, *7*, e2004. [CrossRef]
16. Ganesan, K.; Rana, M.B.M.; Sultan, S. *Oral Hypoglycaemic Medications*; StatPearls Publishing: Treasure Island, FL, USA, 2023. Available online: https://www.ncbi.nlm.nih.gov/books/NBK482386/ (accessed on 1 September 2024).
17. Mohamed, W.; Jamil, A.; Huri, H.; Zuhdi, A. The effects of SGLT-2 inhibitor on epicardial adipose tissue (EAT) thickness in general cardiology admission patient. *Int. J. Cardiol.* **2023**, *393*, 131519. [CrossRef]
18. Tiwari, A.K.; Rao, J.M. Diabetes mellitus and multiple therapeutic approaches of phytochemicals: Present status and future prospects. *Curr. Sci.* **2002**, *83*, 30–38.
19. Hanefeld, M. Cardiovascular benefits and safety profile of acarbose therapy in prediabetes and established type 2 diabetes. *Cardiovasc. Diabetol.* **2007**, *6*, 20. [CrossRef]
20. Laar, F.A.V.D. Alpha-glucosidase inhibitors in the early treatment of type 2 diabetes. *Vasc. Health Risk Manag.* **2008**, *4*, 1189–1195. [CrossRef]
21. Wang, T.Y.; Liu, M.; Portincasa, P.; Wang, D.Q.H. New insights into the molecular mechanism of intestinal fatty acid absorption. *Eur. J. Clin. Investig.* **2013**, *43*, 1203–1223. [CrossRef]
22. Ballinger, A. Orlistat in the treatment of obesity. *Expert. Opin. Pharmacother.* **2000**, *1*, 841–847. [CrossRef]
23. Mezouara, M.; Hbyaj, K.; Soufiani, A.; Mouniane, Y.; Chriqui, A.; Ramdane, K.B.; Ouhammou, I.; Mabrouki, J.; Hmouni, D. Potential of Functional Foods in Diabetes Management: A Review of Coriandrum sativum, Ficus carica, Camellia sinensis. In *Advancements in Climate and Smart Environment Technology*; Mabrouki, J., Azrour, M., Eds.; IGI Global: Hershey, PA, USA, 2024; pp. 88–99.
24. Keservani, R.K.; Ahire, E.D. *Applications of Functional Foods in Disease Prevention*, 1st ed.; CRC Press: Boca Raton, FL, USA, 2024.
25. Eriksen, M.B.; Frandsen, T.F. The impact of patient, intervention, comparison, outcome (Pico) as a search strategy tool on literature search quality: A systematic review. *J. Med. Libr. Assoc.* **2018**, *106*, 420–431. [CrossRef]
26. Page, M.J.; McKenzie, J.E.; Bossuyt, P.M.; Boutron, I.; Hoffmann, T.C.; Mulrow, C.D.; Shamseer, L.; Tetzlaff, J.M.; Akl, E.A.; Brennan, S.E.; et al. The PRISMA 2020 statement: An updated guideline for reporting systematic reviews. *BMJ* **2021**, *372*, n71. [CrossRef]
27. Rodhi, M.N.M.; Hamzah, F.; Hamid, K.H.K. Kinetic behaviour of pancreatic lipase inhibition by Ultrasonicated A. malaccensis and A. subintegra leaves of different particle sizes. *Bull. Chem. React. Eng. Catal.* **2020**, *15*, 818–828. [CrossRef]
28. Gogoi, R.; Sarma, N.; Begum, T.; Chanda, S.K.; Lekhak, H.; Sastry, G.N.; Lal, M. Agarwood (*Aquilaria malaccensis* L.) a quality fragrant and medicinally significant plant based essential oil with pharmacological potentials and genotoxicity. *Ind. Crops. Prod.* **2023**, *197*, 116535. [CrossRef]
29. Liu, Q.; Guo, T.; Li, W.; Li, D.; Feng, Z. Synthesis and evaluation of benzophenone O-glycosides as α-glucosidase inhibitors. *Arch. Pharm.* **2012**, *345*, 771–783. [CrossRef]
30. Sukito, A.; Darmawan, S.; Turjaman, M. Anti-oxidant and anti-diabetes activities of agarwood extracts from Gyrinops versteegii (Gilg.) Domke and their cytotoxicity. *Earth Environ. Sci.* **2020**, *415*, 012001.
31. Sukito, A.; Darmawan, S.; Prihantini, A.I. Screening of antioxidant and antidiabetic activity from fruit bark, stem bark and leaves of *Gyrinops versteegii* (Gilg.) Domke. In *IOP Conference Series: Materials Science and Engineering*, 1st ed.; IOP Publishing Ltd.: Bristol, UK, 2020. [CrossRef]

32. Nguyen, T.N.T.; Le, T.D.; Nguyen, P.L.; Nguyen, D.H.; Nguyen, H.V.T.; Nguyen, T.K.; Tran, M.H.; Van Le, T.H. α-Glucosidase Inhibitory Activity and Quantitative Contribution of Phenolic Compounds from Vietnamese Aquilaria crassna Leaves. *Nat. Prod. Commun.* **2022**, *17*, 1934578X221080326. [CrossRef]
33. Ibrahim, M.; Azziz, S.S.S.A.; Wong, C.F.; Din, W.N.I.W.M.; Mahamod, W.R.W.; Bakri, Y.M.; Ahmad, M.S.; Yahaya, R.; Hadiani, N. Evaluation of anti-lipase activity of leaf and bark extracts from *Aquilaria subintegra* and *A. malaccensis*. *Marmara Pharm. J.* **2018**, *22*, 91–95.
34. Yang, L.; Yang, Y.L.; Dong, W.H.; Li, W.; Wang, P.; Cao, X.; Yuan, J.Z.; Chen, H.Q.; Mei, W.L.; Dai, H.F. Sesquiterpenoids and 2-(2-phenylethyl) chromones respectively acting as α-glucosidase and tyrosinase inhibitors from agarwood of an Aquilaria plant. *J. Enzym. Inhib. Med. Chem.* **2019**, *34*, 853–862. [CrossRef]
35. Yang, Y.-L.; Li, W.; Wang, H.; Yang, L.; Yuan, J.-Z.; Cai, C.-H.; Chen, H.-Q.; Dong, W.-H.; Ding, X.-P.; Jiang, B.; et al. New tricyclic prezizaane sesquiterpenoids from agarwood. *Fitoterapia* **2019**, *138*, 104301. [CrossRef]
36. Bahtiarsyah, A.A.; Hidayati, L.; Wijayanti, N.; Nuringtyas, T.R. Synergistic Activity of Cinnamomum burmannii (Nees & T. Nees) Blume and *Aquilaria malaccensis* Lamk. Extracts for Antidiabetic Study. *Indones. Biomed. J.* **2023**, *15*, 132–140. [CrossRef]
37. Ma, S.; Huang, M.; Fu, Y.; Qiao, M.; Li, Y. How Closely Does Induced Agarwood's Biological Activity Resemble that of Wild Agarwood? *Molecules* **2023**, *28*, 2922. [CrossRef]
38. Thitikornpong, W.; Palanuvej, C.; Ruangrungsi, N. In vitro antidiabetic, antioxidation and cytotoxicity activities of ethanolic extract of aquilaria crassna leaves and its active compound; mangiferin. *Indian J. Tradit. Knowl.* **2019**, *18*, 144–150. Available online: https://www.scopus.com/inward/record.uri?eid=2-s2.0-85060180022&partnerID=40&md5=93953b4873bf8fc6f7498252bb10d216 (accessed on 1 September 2024).
39. Ma, S.; Qiao, M.; Fu, Y.; Wei, P.; Li, Y.; Liu, Z. Comparative analysis of biological activity of artificial and wild agarwood. *Forests* **2021**, *12*, 1532. [CrossRef]
40. Liao, G.; Mei, W.L.; Dong, W.H.; Li, W.; Wang, P.; Kong, F.D.; Gai, C.J.; Song, X.Q.; Dai, H.F. 2-(2-Phenylethyl)chromone derivatives in artificial agarwood from *Aquilaria sinensis*. *Fitoterapia* **2016**, *110*, 38–43. [CrossRef] [PubMed]
41. Xiang, P.; Mei, W.; Chen, H.; Kong, F.; Wang, H.; Liao, G.; Zhou, L.; Dai, H. Four new bi-phenylethylchromones from artificial agarwood. *Fitoterapia* **2017**, *120*, 61–66. [CrossRef]
42. Mi, C.-N.; Yuan, J.-Z.; Zhu, M.-M.; Yang, L.; Wei, Y.-M.; Wang, H.; Long, W.-X.; Mei, W.-L.; Dai, H.-F. 2-(2-Phenylethyl)chromone derivatives: Promising α-glucosidase inhibitors in agarwood from *Aquilaria filaria*. *Phytochemistry* **2021**, *181*, 112578. [CrossRef]
43. Mi, C.-N.; Mei, W.-L.; Wang, H.; Yang, L.; Dong, W.-H.; Gai, C.-J.; Yuan, J.-Z.; Long, W.-X.; Dai, H.-F. Four new guaiane sesquiterpenoids from agarwood of *Aquilaria filaria*. *Fitoterapia* **2019**, *135*, 79–84. [CrossRef]
44. Yang, Y.; Mei, W.-L.; Kong, F.-D.; Chen, H.-Q.; Li, W.; Chen, Z.-B.; Dai, H.-F. Four new bi-2-(2-phenylethyl)chromone derivatives of agarwood from *Aquilaria crassna*. *Fitoterapia* **2017**, *119*, 20–25. [CrossRef]
45. Ahn, S.; Ma, C.T.; Choi, J.M.; An, S.; Lee, M.; Le, T.H.V.; Pyo, J.J.; Lee, J.; Choi, M.S.; Kwon, S.W.; et al. Adiponectin-secretion-promoting phenylethylchromones from the agarwood of *Aquilaria malaccensis*. *J. Nat. Prod.* **2019**, *82*, 259–264. [CrossRef]
46. Feng, J.; Yang, X.W.; Wang, R.F. Bio-assay guided isolation and identification of a-glucosidase inhibitors from the leaves of *Aquilaria sinensis*. *Phytochemistry* **2011**, *72*, 242–247. [CrossRef]
47. Wan-Nadilah, W.A.; Ghani, D.A.; Jalil, M.S.A.; Ali, A.M.; Mamat, W.N.A.W.; Mahmod, N.H. Effects of drying methods and solvents on phenolic and flavonoids content, dpph radical scavenging and α-glucosidase activities of aquilaria leaves extract. *Malays. Appl. Biol.* **2020**, *49*, 201–205. [CrossRef]
48. Pranakhon, R.; Pannangpetch, P.; Aromdee, C. Antihyperglycemic activity of agarwood leaf extracts in STZ-induced diabetic rats and glucose uptake enhancement activity in rat adipocytes. *Songklanakarin J. Sci. Technol.* **2011**, *33*, 405–410.
49. Pranakhon, R.; Aromdee, C.; Pannangpetch, P. Effects of iriflophenone 3-C-β-glucoside on fasting blood glucose level and glucose uptake. *Pharmacogn. Mag.* **2015**, *11*, 82–89. Available online: https://www.scopus.com/inward/record.uri?eid=2-s2.0-84961310035&doi=10.4103/0973-1296.149711&partnerID=40&md5=f711a19ce653edd51d18da02592700b4 (accessed on 1 September 2024). [PubMed]
50. Manoka, S.; Sungthong, B.; Sato, H.; Sugiyama, E.; Sato, V.H. Hypoglycaemic and Antioxidant Activities of the Water Extract of Aquilaria crassna Leaves in Streptozotocin-Nicotinamide-Induced Type-2 Diabetic Mice. *Nat. Prod. Commun.* **2016**, *11*, 757–761. [PubMed]
51. Lee, J.E.; Kang, S.J.; Choi, S.H.; Song, C.H.; Lee, Y.J.; Ku, S.K. Fermentation of Green Tea with 2% Aquilariae lignum Increases the Anti-Diabetic Activity of Green Tea Aqueous Extracts in the High Fat-Fed Mouse. *Nutrients* **2015**, *7*, 9046–9078. [CrossRef]
52. Kang, S.J.; Lee, J.E.; Lee, E.K.; Jung, D.H.; Song, C.H.; Park, S.J.; Choi, S.H.; Han, C.H.; Ku, S.K.; Lee, Y.J. Fermentation with Aquilariae Lignum enhances the anti-diabetic activity of green tea in type II diabetic db/db mouse. *Nutrients* **2014**, *6*, 3536–3571. [CrossRef]
53. Jiang, S.; Jiang, Y.; Guan, Y.F.; Tu, P.F.; Wang, K.Y.; Chen, J.M. Effects of 95% ethanol extract of Aquilaria sinensis leaves on hyperglycemia in diabetic db/db mice. *J. Chin. Pharm. Sci.* **2011**, *20*, 609–614. [CrossRef]
54. Derouiche, S.; Degachi, O.; Gharbi, K. The Effect of Purslane and Aquilaria Malaccensis on Insulin-Resistance and Lipid Peroxidation in High-Fructose Diet Rats. *Rom. J. Diabetes Nutr. Metab. Dis.* **2020**, *27*, 357–365. Available online: https://www.rjdnmd.org/index.php/RJDNMD/article/view/784 (accessed on 1 September 2024).

55. Yang, Y.L.; Sun, H.D.; Yang, J.; Liu, C.Z.; Kang, C.Z.; Liu, J.; Guo, L.P. Tandem mass spectrometry (MS/MS) molecular networking guided profiling of small molecules from *Aquilaria sinensis* (Lour.) Gilg leaves and their bioactivity evaluation. *Phytochem. Anal.* **2024**, *35*, 135–145. [CrossRef]
56. Kashtoh, H.; Baek, K.H. Recent Updates on Phytoconstituent Alpha-Glucosidase Inhibitors: An Approach towards the Treatment of Type Two Diabetes. *Plants* **2022**, *11*, 2722. [CrossRef]
57. Kumar, S.; Narwal, S.; Kumar, V.; Prakash, O. α-glucosidase inhibitors from plants: A natural approach to treat diabetes. *Pharmacogn. Rev.* **2011**, *5*, 19–29. [CrossRef]
58. Ojah, E.O.; Moronkola, D.O.; Akintunde, A. α-amylase and α-glucosidase antidiabetic potential of ten essential oils from *Calophyllum inophyllum* Linn. *Iberoam. J. Med.* **2020**, *2*, 253–260. [CrossRef]
59. Dirir, A.M.; Daou, M.; Yousef, A.F.; Yousef, L.F. A review of alpha-glucosidase inhibitors from plants as potential candidates for the treatment of type-2 diabetes. *Phytochem. Rev.* **2022**, *21*, 1049–1079. [CrossRef] [PubMed]
60. Zhu, G.; Fang, Q.; Zhu, F.; Huang, D.; Yang, C. Structure and Function of Pancreatic Lipase-Related Protein 2 and Its Relationship with Pathological States. *Front. Genet.* **2021**, *12*, 693538. [CrossRef] [PubMed]
61. Duarte, A.M.; Guarino, M.P.; Barroso, S.; Gil, M.M. Phytopharmacological Strategies in the Management of Type 2 Diabetes Mellitus. *Foods* **2020**, *9*, 271. [CrossRef] [PubMed]
62. Quazi, A.; Patwekar, M.; Patwekar, F.; Alghamdi, S.; Rajab, B.S.; Babalghith, A.O.; Islam, F. In vitro Alpha-Amylase Enzyme Assay of Hydroalcoholic Polyherbal Extract: Proof of Concept for the Development of Polyherbal Teabag Formulation for the Treatment of Diabetes. *Evid. Based Complement. Alternat Med.* **2022**, *2022*, 1577957. [CrossRef]
63. Kashtoh, H.; Baek, K.H. New Insights into the Latest Advancement in α-Amylase Inhibitors of Plant Origin with Anti-Diabetic Effects. *Plants* **2023**, *12*, 2944. [CrossRef]
64. Choi, H.M.; Doss, H.M.; Kim, K.S. Multifaceted Physiological Roles of Adiponectin in Inflammation and Diseases. *Int. J. Mol. Sci.* **2020**, *21*, 1219. [CrossRef]
65. Khoramipour, K.; Chamari, K.; Hekmatikar, A.A.; Ziyaiyan, A.; Taherkhani, S.; Elguindy, N.M.; Bragazzi, N.L. Adiponectin: Structure, Physiological Functions, Role in Diseases, and Effects of Nutrition. *Nutrients* **2021**, *13*, 1180. [CrossRef]
66. Nguyen, T.M.D. Adiponectin: Role in Physiology and Pathophysiology. *Int. J. Prev. Med.* **2020**, *11*, 136. [CrossRef]
67. Dubuisson, O.; Dhurandhar, E.J.; Krishnapuram, R.; Kirk-Ballard, H.; Gupta, A.K.; Hegde, V.; Floyd, E.; Gimble, J.M.; Dhurandhar, N.V. PPARgamma-independent increase in glucose uptake and adiponectin abundance in fat cells. *Endocrinology* **2011**, *152*, 3648–3660. [CrossRef]
68. Guo, M.; Li, C.; Lei, Y.; Xu, S.; Zhao, D.; Lu, X.Y. Role of the adipose PPARγ-adiponectin axis in susceptibility to stress and depression/anxiety-related behaviors. *Mol. Psychiatry* **2017**, *22*, 1056–1068. [CrossRef]
69. Maeda, N.; Takahashi, M.; Funahashi, T.; Kihara, S.; Nishizawa, H.; Kishida, K.; Nagaretani, H.; Matsuda, M.; Komuro, R.; Ouchi, N.; et al. PPARgamma ligands increase expression and plasma concentrations of adiponectin, an adipose-derived protein. *Diabetes* **2001**, *50*, 2094–2099. [CrossRef]

pharmaceuticals

Review

Updated Progress on Polysaccharides with Anti-Diabetic Effects through the Regulation of Gut Microbiota: Sources, Mechanisms, and Structure–Activity Relationships

Xiaoyu Zhang [1], Jia Wang [1], Tingting Zhang [1], Shuqin Li [1], Junyu Liu [1], Mingyue Li [1], Jingyang Lu [1], Min Zhang [2,3] and Haixia Chen [1,*]

1 Tianjin Key Laboratory for Modern Drug Delivery and High-Efficiency, School of Pharmaceutical Science and Technology, Faculty of Medicine, Tianjin University, Tianjin 300072, China; 15153501767@163.com (X.Z.); jiawangcongcong@163.com (J.W.); 17622636510@163.com (T.Z.); lisq2013@sina.com (S.L.); junyuliu@tju.edu.cn (J.L.); lmy15357831056@163.com (M.L.); jyl10192022@163.com (J.L.)

2 China-Russia Agricultural Processing Joint Laboratory, Tianjin Agricultural University, Tianjin 300384, China; zhangmin@tjau.edu.cn

3 State Key Laboratory of Nutrition and Safety, Tianjin University of Science & Technology, Tianjin 300457, China

* Correspondence: chenhx@tju.edu.cn

Abstract: Diabetes mellitus (DM) is a common chronic metabolic disease worldwide. The disturbance of the gut microbiota has a complex influence on the development of DM. Polysaccharides are one type of the most important natural components with anti-diabetic effects. Gut microbiota can participate in the fermentation of polysaccharides, and through this, polysaccharides regulate the gut microbiota and improve DM. This review begins by a summary of the sources, anti-diabetic effects and the gut microbiota regulation functions of natural polysaccharides. Then, the mechanisms of polysaccharides in regulating the gut microbiota to exert anti-diabetic effects and the structure–activity relationship are summarized. It is found that polysaccharides from plants, fungi, and marine organisms show great hypoglycemic activities and the gut microbiota regulation functions. The mechanisms mainly include repairing the gut burrier, reshaping gut microbiota composition, changing the metabolites, regulating anti-inflammatory activity and immune function, and regulating the signal pathways. Structural characteristics of polysaccharides, such as monosaccharide composition, molecular weight, and type of glycosidic linkage, show great influence on the anti-diabetic activity of polysaccharides. This review provides a reference for the exploration and development of the anti-diabetic effects of polysaccharides.

Keywords: polysaccharides; anti-diabetic effects; the gut microbiota; mechanism; structure–activity relationship

1. Introduction

Diabetes mellitus (DM) is a metabolic disease characterized by hyperglycemia, which is a typical and complex chronic metabolic disease worldwide. Generally, it is classified into type 1 DM (T1DM), type 2 DM (T2DM), gestational DM and specific types of diabetes due to other causes like monogenic diabetes syndromes [1]. T1DM is an autoimmune illness caused by the destruction of β cells, which typically results in a lack of insulin, accounting for 5–10% of the prevalence of DM [2]. About 90% of DM cases are T2DM, which is caused by a gradual decrease in β-cell insulin secretion [3].

The incidence of DM is rising as a result of the changing of lifestyles and living circumstances. DM is considered a global disease and more and more people suffer from it. According to a prediction of the International Diabetes Federation (IDF), there may be up to 700 million people living with DM by 2045. Persistent hyperglycemia can cause chronic damage to and dysfunction of numerous organs and tissues, such as eyes, kidneys, heart, blood vessels, and nerves [4,5]. For example, abnormal blood glucose metabolism is usually accompanied by blood lipid metabolism disorder [6]. Additionally, patients with DM have a notable increase in microvascular risk, which can lead to the development of hypertension [7]. What is more, DM may predispose toward Parkinson-like pathology [8,9]. These complications seriously endanger human health. Nowadays, the prevention and treatment of DM mainly focus on improvement in lifestyle and control of blood sugar by drugs. Although there are many drugs on the market that can be used to treat DM, like biguanides, acarbose, sulfonylureas and thiazolidinediones, these drugs have some limitations that cannot be ignored, such as side effects or high cost [10,11]. The development of lower-toxicity and more effective drugs is necessary.

Polysaccharides are carbohydrate macromolecules composed of at least more than 10 monosaccharides linked to each other by glycosidic bonds, and can be mainly found in plants, fungi, and marine organisms in nature. Numerous functions, including hypoglycemic, anti-inflammatory, immunomodulatory, neuromodulatory, and anticancer activities, have been demonstrated by studies on polysaccharides [12–16]. In addition, there are many advantages of polysaccharides, including good biodegradability and biocompatibility and few side effects [17,18]. Polysaccharides are utilized extensively in the food and pharmaceutical industries as emulsifiers, adjuvants for vaccines, and materials to treat oral diseases [19–21]. Therefore, polysaccharides can be regarded as a promising strategy for the prevention and treatment of DM.

The human gut is a crucial organ that is directly connected to the outside environment. The human the gut microbiota comprises trillions of microorganisms, including archaea, eukaryotes, viruses and bacteria at the domain level [22]. At the phylum level, it mainly consists of Firmicutes, Bacteroidetes, Actinobacteria, Proteobacteria, Verrucomicrobia and Fusobacteria [23–25]. They participate in nutrient metabolism, immune regulation and chemical modifications of dietary components, and the health of the host is closely related to the diversity and stability of the gut microbiota [26–28]. In normal conditions, the gut microbiota and its metabolites are maintained in a reasonably steady ecological balance with the host, but many factors can affect the composition and function of the gut microbiota such as dietary habits and hereditary and environmental factors [29]. The destruction of the gut microbiota may lead to many diseases, such as osteoporosis, obesity, T2DM, non-alcoholic fatty liver, and hypertension [30]. Research has found that a reduction in gut microbiota biodiversity and gut-associated metabolites contributes to heart failure [31]. The dysbiosis state of the gut microbiota and disruption in the energy metabolism contribute to the pathogenic mechanisms of neurodegeneration [32]. The modulation of gut microbiota biodiversity and gut-associated metabolites is associated with anti-diabetic activities [33–36].

The host cannot digest and absorb the majority of polysaccharides. In the human body, polysaccharides can interact with the gut microbiota and ferment into absorbable substances, mainly short-chain fatty acids (SCFAs) in the colon [37,38]. SCFAs consist of free fatty acids with two to five carbons, such as acetic acid, propanoic acid, and butyric acid, participating in signal transmission, nutrition provision and many other healthy protection functions in human body [39]. During these processes, polysaccharides are involved in the balance of the gut microbiota and host as a kind of prebiotic [40]. In turn, the gut microbiota can influence the host digestive efficiency by altering the bioavailability of polysaccharides [41].

In our earlier research, we discovered that mulberry leaf polysaccharides (MLPs) had a substantial negative link with the risk of obesity and might considerably lower the Firmicutes/Bacteroidetes (F/B) ratio, which may result in diminished energy absorption in mice [42]. Additionally, we discovered that *Lentinula edodes* soluble dietary fibers (LESDF) promoted Bacteroides production, indicating that LESDF was one of the dietary elements with an impact on the composition and relative abundance of the gut microbial community in vitro [43].

Nowadays, polysaccharides are highly valued by researchers in the field of medicine and health food and more and more polysaccharides have been discovered to prevent and treat DM. In addition, the gut microbiota is a hot topic in the management of DM. Although there are some reviews about the anti-diabetic effects and gut microbiota regulation function of polysaccharides, there is no comprehensive review about how polysaccharides exert anti-diabetic effects through the regulation of the gut microbiota and the related mechanisms. This article gives a summary of the relationship between polysaccharides and the gut microbiota in the prevention and treatment of DM, which may provide a reference for developing more effective anti-diabetic strategies.

2. Sources of Polysaccharides and Their Anti-Diabetic Effects

In the 21st century, scientific researchers paid more attention to natural products. Polysaccharides, natural compounds with low toxicity and multiple functions, can be regarded as lead compounds to be screened for developing new drugs and health foods [44]. Researchers discovered that the gut microbiota were linked to the onset of DM and played an important role in the maintenance of good health [23]. Although the human digestive system is capable of breaking down and absorbing certain polysaccharides like starch, there are polysaccharides that cannot be digested by the host because of high molecular weight and low bioavailability. They can enter the colon and interact with the gut microbiota, exerting dietary or medicinal effects [45,46]. For example, researchers found that polysaccharides from *Dendrobium officinale* were fermented and degraded into SCFAs in the large intestine and modulated bioactivities associated with the gut microbiota in rats [47].

The sources of polysaccharides and the structure of some examples are shown in Figure 1. The anti-diabetic effects of polysaccharides from different sources and their regulation effects on the gut microbiota are summarized in the following.

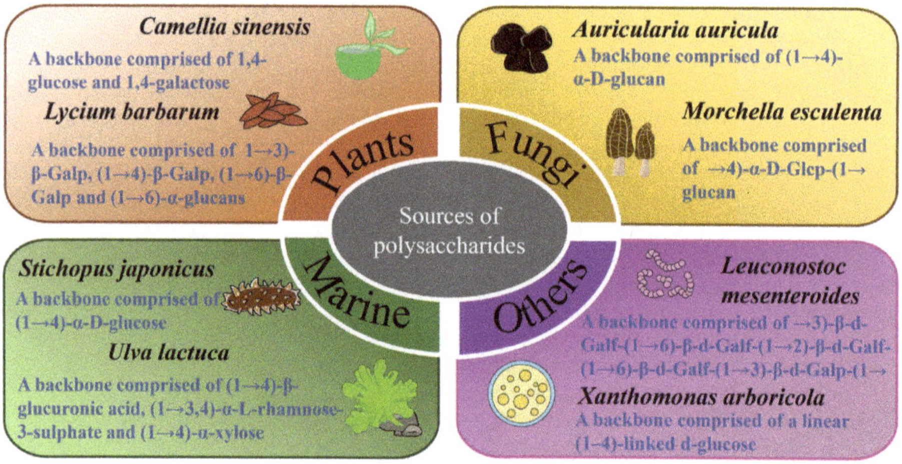

Figure 1. Sources of polysaccharides and the structures of some examples [48–55].

2.1. *Polysaccharides Extracted from Plants*

Plants are one of the main sources of polysaccharides. Polysaccharides can be extracted from different kinds of plants like herbs, woody plants, and shrubs [56]. For example, *Camellia sinensis*, which is commonly called a tea tree, is a kind of shrub and the source of tea polysaccharides with famous anticancer and anti-diabetic effects in vitro or in vivo [57,58]. Various plant parts, including the leaves, stems, roots, and flowers, can also be used to extract polysaccharides. Polysaccharides extracted from the leaves and fruits of baobab (*Adansonia digitata* L.) have different molecular weights, solution viscosity-enhancing properties and other characteristics [59]. In our previous study, we found that polysaccharides from plants showed good anti-diabetic effects. Polysaccharides from *Camellia sinensis* showed α-glucosidase inhibitory capacity and hypoglycemic effect on L6 cells by promoting glucose uptake [60]. MLP treatment considerably improved metabolic diseases by lowering the Firmicutes/Bacteroidetes (F/B) ratio and increasing the amounts of Bifidobacterium, Lactobacillus, and Akkermansia, which were linked to the generation of butyric acid and/or propionic acid in mice [42].

Many other polysaccharides from various plants also showed anti-diabetic effects and the gut microbiota regulation function. The sources, structures, anti-diabetic effects and the gut microbiota regulation function of polysaccharides from plants are shown in Table 1.

Polysaccharides from plants show different gut microbiota regulation function. On the one hand, polysaccharides increase the diversity of probiotics in gut. Probiotics in the gut show positive effects on DM, such as decreasing lipid accumulation, ameliorating oxidative stress and inflammation, and increasing SCFAs in the gut [61]. Lactobacillus and Bifidobacterium are two main probiotics at the genus level and can even be used commercially [62,63]. Lactobacillus participates in glycolipid metabolism and produces SCFAs like lactic acid and acetic acid [64]. One study found that Lactobacillus could also reduce hepatic insulin resistance and liver deterioration in diabetic mice [65]. Bifidobacterium has great saccharolytic capability, plays an anti-inflammatory role, manages obesity, protects mucosal barrier integrity, and participates in the production of SCFAs in the gut [66,67].

Polysaccharides from kiwifruit (*Actinidia chinensis*), ginseng, and soy hull increase the abundance of Lactobacillus in mice or rats [68–70]. Polysaccharides from the tuberous root of *Ophiopogon japonicus* significantly enrich Bifidobacterium in mice [71,72]. On the other hand, polysaccharides regulate the gut microbiota by decreasing pathogenic bacteria. For example, the in vitro fermentation of human fecal microbiota showed that polysaccharides from *Polygonatum kingianum* decrease the abundance of Proteobacteria, which was positively correlated with dysbiosis of the gut microbiota and the occurrence of DM. It exhibited similar effects in diabetic rats [73,74].

2.2. *Polysaccharides Extracted from Fungi*

Fungi have been widely eaten and used by humans all over the world for thousands of years. Polysaccharides from fungi can be extracted from different parts like fruiting body, mycelium, or fermentation broth, and β-glucan accounts for the main structure of fungi polysaccharides [75,76]. Fungi polysaccharides possess many health-enhancing activities, such as immune modulation, fatigue relief, anti-aging and hypolipidemic activities in vivo or in vitro [77–81]. For example, researches revealed that oral β-1,3/1,6 glucan per day prevented the occurrence or reduced the severity of upper respiratory tract infection in older individuals [82]. High-purity yeast β-glucan induced innate immune regulation in gut mucosa, protecting against T1DM in mice [83]. *Grifola frondose* polysaccharides improved the disorder in lipid metabolism in high-fat diet (HFD)- and STZ-induced mice by increasing hepatic Acox1 expression and reducing the hepatic free fatty acid levels [84].

Polysaccharides from fungi can play an anti-diabetic role through modulation of the gut microbiota. The sources, structures, anti-diabetic effects and gut microbiota regulation function of polysaccharides from fungi are shown in Table 2.

Polysaccharides from fungi have anti-diabetic and the gut microbiota regulation functions in different respects. For example, *Grifola frondosa* polysaccharides improved the diversity and composition of the gut microbiota in HFD-induced diabetic mice [85]. Polysaccharides from *Agaricus bisporus* promoted the growth of beneficial bacteria, including Prevotella, Megamonas, and Bacteroides during the in vitro fermentation process [86]. *Hirsutella sinensis* mycelium (HSM) polysaccharides showed protective effects on gut integrity by selectively promoting the growth of a commensal bacterium, Parabacteroides goldsteinii, whose level was reduced in HFD-induced mice. HSM polysaccharides reduced inflammation associated with metabolic disorders, relieved insulin resistance, and improved lipid metabolism to treat obesity and T2DM [87].

Table 1. Interactions between plant polysaccharides and the gut microbiota in diabetic mellitus.

Polysaccharide Source	Mw (kDa)	Monosaccharide Composition	Research Model	Anti-Diabetic Activity	Gut Microbiota Modulation	Reference
Apocynum venetum leaves	289.2	Man, Rha, GluA, GalA, Glu, Gal, and Ara with a ratio of 2.90:28.06:1.92 :21.72:10.47:26.69:8.42;	HFD and STZ induced C57BL/6J male mice	↓ liquid intake; liver and heart indexes; insulin resistance; GSP; TG; LDL-C; NEFA; ALT; AST; ↑ liver glycogen; glucose tolerance; β-cell function; CAT, SOD; GSH; SCFAs (acetate; butyrate); relieve the histopathological injuries of liver and pancreas	↓ Firmicutes to Bacteroidetes ratio (P); Proteobacteria (P); Enterococcus (G); Klebsiella (G); Aerocuccus (G); ↑ Odoribacter (G); Anaeroplasma (G); Muribaculum (G); Parasutterella (G);	[10]
Astragalus membranaceus	161.15	Ara, Gal, Glu, Xyl, Man, GalA, and GluA with a ratio of 13.60:7.20:63.73: 0.25:0.13:14.73:0.37	HFD and STZ induced C57BL/6J male mice	↓ body weight loss; food and water intake; FBG; GSP; FINs; TC; TG; LDL-C; LPS; TNF-α; IL-6; MDA; ALT; AST; hepatic lipid accumulation and steatosis; epididymal adipose; DAO; D-LA; ↑ glucose tolerance; HDL-C; IL-10; CAT; SOD; GSH; hepatic glycogen; relieve the histopathological injuries of pancreas and colon	↓ Helicobacter (G); Cupriavidus (G); Halomonas (G); Bacteroides (G); Odoribacter (G); Erysipelotrichaceae_Clostridium (G); Enterococcus (G); Shigella (G); Akkermansia (G); Anaeroplasma (G); AF12 (G); [Prevotella] (G); Streptococcus (G); ↑ Allobaculum (G); Lactobacillus (G);	[88]
Berberis dasystachya	102	Man, Ara, Glu, Gal, Xyl, and Fru with a ratio of 113.59:89.07:69.46:59.55: 7.48:2.33	HFD and STZ induced Sprague Dawley male rats	↓ food and water intake; weight loss; organ index (pancreas, liver, kidneys, and heart); FBG; insulin resistance; GSP; HbAlc; MDA; NO; NOS; ↑ glucose tolerance; insulin sensitivity index; GSH-Px; SOD; SCFAs (acetic, propionic, butyric, isobutyric, valeric, and isovaleric acids); relieve the histopathological injuries of pancreas, colon tissues	↓ Bacteroidetes (P); Klebsiella (G); Ruminococcus torques group (G); Skermanella (G); Odoribacter (G); ↑ Firmicutes (P); Lactobacillus (G); Ruminococcaceae UCG-005 (G); Prevotellaceae NK3B31 group (G); Blautia (G); Ruminococcaceae NK4A214 group (G); Ruminococcus 2 (G); Eubacterium coprostanoligenes_group (G); Romboutsia (G);	[89]
Brasenia schreberi	50–100	-	HFD and STZ induced C57BL/6 male mice	↓ FBG; insulin resistance; TC; LDL-C; ↑ glycogen level; regulate PI3K/Akt signal pathway	↓ Firmicutes to Bacteroidetes ratio (P); Romboutsia; Desulfovibrio; ↑ Allopravotella; Lactobacillus (G); Bacteroides (G)	[90]

Table 1. *Cont.*

Polysaccharide Source	Mw (kDa)	Monosaccharide Composition	Research Model	Anti-Diabetic Activity	Gut Microbiota Modulation	Reference
Camellia sinensis	289.734	Rha, Rib, Ara, Man, Glu, and Gal with a ratio of 1.26:3.18:4.08:1.00: 1.52:3.92	HFD and STZ induced male Wistar male rats	↓ FBG; insulin resistance; TC; TG; LDL-C; FFA; Bax protein; colonic pH value; ↑ glucose tolerance; ADP; GLP-1; HDL-C; Bcl-2 protein; SCFAs (acetic acid; propionic acid; n-butyric acid; i-butyric acid and n-valeric acid); relieve the histopathological injury of pancreas	↓ Bacteroidetes (P); ↑ Proteobacteria (P); Fluviicola (G); Roseburia (G); Victivallis (G); Lachnospira (G);	[91]
Coix seed	13.285	Fuc, Rha, Ara, Gal, Glu, Xyl, Man, Fru, Rib, GalA, GulA, GluA, and ManA with a ratio of 0.25:1.05: 2.79:3.86:79.64:2.75: 3.54:0.31:0.08:4.26:0.31: 0.81:0.18	HFD and STZ induced C57BL/6J male mice	↓ FBG; body weight loss; food intake; insulin resistance; TC; TG; LDL-C; ↑ glucose tolerance; HDL-C; SCFAs; ZO-1 expression; relieve the histopathological injury of colon; regulate IGF1/PI3K/AKT signaling pathway	↓ Firmicutes (P); Helicobacter; ↑ Bacteroidetes (P); Lactobacillus (G), Akkermansia (G), Bacteroides (G); Bifidobacterium (G);	[92]
Lycium barbarum	98.0	Rha, Ara, Xyl, Man, Glu, Gal, GluA, and GalA with a ratio of 0.23:1.90:0.26: 0.20:1.0:1.26:0.44:1.49	HFD and STZ induced C57BL/6 male mice	↓ body weight loss; food and water intake; FBG; insulin resistance; HbA1c; GSP; insulin; TC; TG; LDL-C; ALT; AST; MDA; IL-6; IL-1b; TNF-α; LPS; ↑ glucose tolerance; insulin sensitivity; GLP-1; PYY; TBA; HDL-C; CAT; SOD; GSH-Px; TAOC; β cell function; glycogen; SCFAs (acetate, propionate, butyrate, isobutyrate, valerate, iso-valerate, and isovalerate); relieve the histopathological injuries of pancreas, liver, and skeletal muscle	↓ Firmicutes (P); Allobaculum (G); Dubosiella (G); Romboutsia (G); ↑ Bacteroidetes (P); Bacteroides (G); Ruminococcaceae_UCG-014 (G); Mucispirillum (G); Intestinimonas (G); Ruminococcaceae_UCG-009 (G);	[93]

Table 1. *Cont.*

Polysaccharide Source	Mw (kDa)	Monosaccharide Composition	Research Model	Anti-Diabetic Activity	Gut Microbiota Modulation	Reference
Cyclocarya paliuru	2.584	Glu, Ara, Gal, Man, Xyl, Rha, GalA, GluA, Fuc, and Rib in a ratio of 27.90:9.68:7.67:1.93:1.67: 1.26:0.72:0.66:0.17:0.16	HFD and STZ induced Sprague-Dawley male rats	↓ FBG; insulin resistance; TC; TG; LDL-C; ↑ glucose intolerance; HDL-C; GLP-1; PYY; CAZyme subtypes; SCFAs (malonic acid, propionic acid, isobutyric acid; glutaric acid); SCFAs derivates (D-3-hydroxybutyricacid; D (-)-beta-hydroxy butyric acid and 3-hydroxycapric acid)	↓ Spirochaetes (P); Proteobacteria (P); Enterococcus_faecium (S) ↑ Firmicutes(P); Ruminococcaceae (F); Eubacteriaceae (F); Lachnospiraceae (F); Ruminococcus_bromii (S); Anaerotruncus_colihominis (S); Clostridium_methylpentosum (S); Roseburia_intestinalis (S); Roseburia_hominis (S); Clostridium_asparagiforme (S); Pseudoflavonifractor_capillosus (S); Intestinimonas_butyriciproducens (S); Intestinimonas_sp._GD2 (S); Oscillibacter_valericigenes (S); Oscillibacter_ruminantium (S)	[22]
Nigella sativa seed	-	-	HFD and STZ induced Kunming male mice	↓ FBG; GSP; body weight loss; TC; TG; LDL-C; MDA; IL-6; TNF-α; IL-1β; ↑ insulin; HDL-C; T-AOC; SOD; CAT; p-AKT; GLUT4; SCFAs (↑propionic acid; ↓acetic acid); relieve the histopathological injuries of liver and pancreas	↓ Firmicutes (P); Lachnospiraceae_NK4A136_group (G); f_Lachnospiraceae_Unclassified (G); ↑ Bacteroidetes (P); Bacteroides (G); f_Muribaculaceae_Unclassified (G); Lactobacillus (G);	[94]
Moutan Cortex	164	Glu and Ara with a ratio of 3.31:2.25	high-fat and high-sugar diet, and STZ induced SD male rats	↓ HbA1c; insulin resistance; renal function index (UP/24 h, Scr, BUN, UACR); IL-6; isovaleric acid; ↑ GLP-1; expression of tight junction proteins (ZO-1, Claudin-1, Occludin); IL-10; SCFAs (acetic acid, propionic acid, butyric acid); relieve the histopathological injuries of kidney, ileum, colon	↑ Verrucomicrobia (P); Mollicutes (G), Bacteroidia (G); Lactobacillus (G); Akkermansia (G); Ruminococcaceae_UCG-014 (G); Muribaculaceae_unclassified (G)	[95]

Table 1. *Cont.*

Polysaccharide Source	Mw (kDa)	Monosaccharide Composition	Research Model	Anti-Diabetic Activity	Gut Microbiota Modulation	Reference
Setaria italica	-	Man, Rha, Gal, Xyl, and Ara in a ratio of 0.72:0.59:76.26:1.03:0.83	HFD and STZ induced Kunming male rats	↓ body weight loss; FBG; TC; TG; LDL-C; MDA ↑ glucose tolerance; HDL-C; CAT; SOD; GSH-Px; SCFAs (acetic acid, propionic acid, butyric acid); relieve the histopathological injuries of liver and pancreas	↓ Firmicutes (P); Verrucomicrobiota (P); Peptostreptococcales-Tissierellales (O); Lachnospirales (O); Romboutsia (O); Bacteroides (O); ↑ Proteobacteria (P); Pseudomonadales (O); Pseudomonas (G); Alloprevotella (G); Akkermansia (G); Alistipes (G)	[11]

P: phylum; O: order; F: family; G: genus; S: species.

Table 2. Interactions between fungi polysaccharides and gut microbiota in diabetic mellitus.

Polysaccharide Source	Mw (kDa)	Monosaccharide Composition	Research Model	Anti-Diabetic Activity	Gut Microbiota Modulation	Reference
Auricularia auricula-judae	-	Man, Glu, Gal, Rha, Xyl, and Fru in a ratio of 62:12.6:4:1.31:4: 3.8	HFD and STZ induced C57BL/6 male mice	↓ relative epididymal fat weight; FBG; insulin resistance; TC; TG; LDL-C; lipid accumulation; ALT; AST; TNF-α; IL-6; ↑ glucose tolerance; GLP-1; HDL-C; relieve the histopathological injuries of liver and pancreas; regulate the AKT/AMPK signaling pathways; enrich KEGG pathways	↓ Firmicutes to Bacteroidetes ratio (P); Proteobacteria (P); Alistipes; Allobaculum; unidentified_Lachnospiraceae; Clostridium; ↑ Lactobacillus; Oscillospira; Rikenella; Bacteroides; Lactococcus; Odoribacter; Ruminococcus; Anaerotruncus;	[96]
Ganoderma lucidum	11.079	Ara, Gal, Glu, Xyl, Man, Rib, and Rha in a ratio of 5.32:5.47:57.63:0.84:25.41: 1.95:3.38	HFD and STZ induced Kunming male mice	↓ body weight loss; liver and kidney weight; FBG; insulin resistance; LDL-C; TC; TG; ALT; AST; MDA; fat accumulation; ↑ HDL-C; GSH-Px; SOD; liver glycogen; relieve the histopathological injuries of liver and pancreas	↓ Firmicutes (P); Proteobacteria (P); Desulfovibrionaceae (F); Bacteroidaceae (F); Lachnospiraceae (F); Lactobacillaceae (F); _f__Desulfovibrionaceae (G); Acetatifactor (G); Lactobacillus (G); ↑ Bacteroidetes (P); Epsilonbacteraeota (P); Muribaculaceae (F); Helicobacteraceae (F); Peptococcaceae (F); Lactobacillaceae (F); Ruminococcaceae (F); Prevotellaceae(F); Alloprevotella (G); Ruminiclostridium_5 (G); f__Peptococcaceae (G); Tyzzerella (G);	[97]

Table 2. *Cont.*

Polysaccharide Source	Mw (kDa)	Monosaccharide Composition	Research Model	Anti-Diabetic Activity	Gut Microbiota Modulation	Reference
Cordyceps militaris	87.8	Man, Gal, and Glu in a ratio of 2.2:15.1:1	HFD and STZ induced C57BL/6 male mice	↓ food and water intake; FBG; insulin resistance; LEP; TC; TG; ALT; AST; BUN; Cr; LPS; TNF-α; IL-1β; IL-6; ↑ glucose tolerance; GLP-1; ADP; colon tight junction proteins (Claudin1, Occludin, and ZO-1); relieve the histopathological injuries of liver, kidney, pancreas and colon; inhibit TLR4/NF-κB pathway	↓ Firmicutes/Bacteroidetes ratio (P); Verrucomicrobiota (P); Proteobacteria (P); Desulfobacterota (F); Escherichia-Shigella (G); Enterococcus (G); ↑ Bacteroidota (P); Campilobacterota (F); Actinobacteriota (F); norank_f_Muribaculaceae (G); Lachnospiraceae_NK4A136_group (G); norank_o__Clostridia_UCG-014 (G); Alistipes (G), Helicobacter (G); Eubacterium_xylanophilum_group (G)	[98]
Grifola frondosa	12,600	Ara, Man and Glu in a ratio of 3.79:1.00:49.70.	high-fat, high-sugar diet and STZ induced ICR male mice	↓ FBG; HbA1c; expression of JNK1/2; ↑ glucose tolerance; β-cells function; expression of IRS1and PI3K; GLUT4; relieve the histopathological injuries of liver and kidney	↓ Firmicutes (P); Proteobacteria (P); ↑ Bacteroidetes (P); Porphyromonas gingivalis (S); Akkermansia muciniphila (S); Lactobacillus acidophilus (S); Tannerella forsythia (S); Bacteroides acidifaciens (S); Roseburia intestinalis (S)	[99]
Morchella esculenta	-	Man, Rib, Rha, GluA, GalA, Glu, Gal, Ara, and Fuc in a ratio of 5.77: 0.263:0.018:0.036:0.006: 81.35:3.543:8.99:0.016	HFD and STZ induced BALB/c male mice	↓ body weight loss; FBG; insulin resistance; IL-6; IL-1β; TNF-α; LPS; ↑ glucose tolerance; colon tight junction proteins (ZO-1, occludin, and claudin-1); MUC2 protein; relieve the histopathological injuries of colon; regulate the KEGG pathways	↓ Firmicutes (P); Corynebacterium (G); Facklamia (G); Corynebacteriaceae (F); Actinomyceletes (C); Staphylococcaceae (S); ↑ Actinobacteria (P); Lactobacillus (G); Lactobacillaceae (F); Lachnospiraceae (F); Enterobacteriaceae (F); Lactobacilliaceae (S)	[100]

P: phylum; F: family; G: genus; S: species.

In a recent study, we discovered that soluble dietary fiber from *Lentinula edodes* byproducts combined with Lactobacillus plantarum LP90 repaired intestinal epithelial injury in dextran sulfate sodium-induced colitis mice. Additionally, the synbiotic therapy enhanced the production of butyric acid and upregulated the expression of tight junction proteins [101].

2.3. Polysaccharides Extracted from Marine Organisms

Marine organisms are a huge source of material for drug development. Many marine organisms are used as food ingredients and supplements due to their great taste and nutrition. Researchers are paying more attention to marine active ingredients because of the unique environmental characteristics like the high salt, high pressure and the lack of light. For example, *Ishige okamurae* extract showed multiple activities such as anti-obesity, anti-diabetic, anti-inflammatory and antioxidant activities in vitro or in mice [102–105]. As one of the major components of the active ingredients from marine organisms, polysaccharides play various activities. Two polysaccharides (laminaran SdL, fucoidan SdF) extracted from brown alga *Sargassum duplicatum* had different structures and fucoidan SdF showed anticancer effect in vitro on colon cancer cells [106]. *Undaria pinnatifida* polysaccharides exhibited α-glucosidase inhibitory activity in vitro and alleviated HFD/STZ-induced hyperglycemia by increasing glucose tolerance, relieving insulin resistance and the histopathological injuries of pancreas and liver [107]. They also showed anti-inflammatory activity by inhibiting IFN-γ expression in mice [108]. In addition to the examples above, the sources, structures, anti-diabetic effects and gut microbiota regulation function of polysaccharides from marine organisms are shown in Table 3.

An in vitro digestion experiment showed that polysaccharides from *Gracilaria lemaneiformis* were mostly degraded in the fermentation process, promoting the production of SCFAs and inhibiting the growth of the Firmicutes community [109]. Another in vitro experiment illustrated that fermentation of fucosylated chondroitin sulfate from *Stichopus chloronotus* contributed to Bacteroidetes and Fusobacteria and benefited host health by lowering the F/B ratio in turn [110].

Experiments in vivo showed similar results. For instance, the seaweed polysaccharides laminaran and ulvan were slowly fermented by Bifidobacterium as well as stimulated the growth of Bifidobacterium and promoted the production of acetate, propionate and lactate [111]. The mixture of algal polysaccharides ulvan and astaxanthin increased the level of Bacteroidia, Bacilli, Clostridia, and Verrucomicrobia [112]. Sulfated sea cucumber *Stichopus japonicus* significantly enriched the relative abundance of Parabacteroides and Akkermansia, as well as reduced the level of Proteobacteria [113,114]. *Sargassum fusiforme* polysaccharides decreased the relative abundance of Bacteroidetes and increased that of Oscillospira, Mucispirillum, and Clostridiales [115]. *Laminaria japonica* polysaccharides upregulated Turicibacter, which produced SCFAs, especially lactic acid [116].

Table 3. Interactions between marine polysaccharides and gut microbiota in diabetic mellitus.

Polysaccharide Source	Mw (kDa)	Monosaccharide Composition	Research Model	Anti-Diabetic Activity	Gut Microbiota Modulation	Reference
Dictyopteris divaricata	63.06	Man, Rib, Rha, GluA, Glu, Gal, Xyl, Ara, and Fuc in a ratio of 15.02: 9.90:1.28:17.54:1.86:17.19: 4.54:0.55	high sugar diet and STZ induced Balb/c male mice	↓ body weight loss; food and water intake; FBG; PBG-2h; insulin resistance; TC; TG; LDL-C; IL-1β; IL-2; IL-6, TNF-α; IFN-γ; MDA; ↑ glucose tolerance; β cell function; HDL-C; SOD; MUC-2; ZO-1; tight junction proteins (Occludin; Claudin-1); IRS-1; relieve histopathological injury of colon	↓ Bacteroidetes (P); Proteobacteria (P); Actinobacteria (P); S24-7 (F); Paraprevotellaceae (F); Odoribacteraceae (F); Corynebacteriaceae (F); Bacteroides (G); Corynebacterium (G); Ruminococcus (G); Parabacteroides (G); ↑ Firmicutes (P); Lactobacillus (G); Prevotella (G); Oscillospira (G); Lactobacillaceae (F); Ruminococaceae (F); Lachnospiraceae (F); Rikenellaceae (F)	[117]
Holothuria leucospilota	52.8	Rha, Fuc, Glua, galactose, Glu, and Xyl in a ratio of 39.1:35.7: 10.7:8.4:4.2:1.8	GK male rats and age-matched Wistar rats	↓ FBG; TC; TG; LDL-C; insulin; LEP; CD36; Bax; ↑ glucose tolerance; HDL-C; adiponectin; GLP-1; PI3K; AKT; PPAR-α; GLUT4; Bcl-2; SCFAs (acetic, butyric acid, pentanoic acid); relieve histopathological injuries of pancreas, colon	↓ Firmicutes (P); Proteobacteria (P); Spirochaetes (P); Actinobacteria (P); Bilophila (G); Bifidobacterium (G); Mucispirillum (G); Colinsella (G); Gemella (G); Treponema (G); Anaerobiospirillum (G); Aggregatibacter (G); Facklamia (G); Lactobacillus (G); ↑ Bacteroidetes (P); TM7 (P); Cyanobacteria (P); Tenericutes (P); Ruminococcus (G); Holdemania (G); Clostridium (G); Helicobacter (G); Turicibacter (G); Paraprevotella (G); Bacteroides (G); Faecalibacterium (G)	[118]
Ulva lactuca	224	Rha, GluA, Gal, and Xyl in a ratio of 32.75:22.83: 1.07:6.46	high-fat high sugar diet and STZ induced ICR male mice	↓ FBG; body weight loss; MDA; ↑ glucose tolerance; CAT; SOD; GSH-PX; relieve the histopathological injury of liver; regulate JAK/STAT3 pathway	↓ Firmicutes (P); ↑ Bacteroidetes (P); Actinobacteria (P); s_weissella_cibaria (G); g_Candidatus_Saccharimonas (G); f_Saccharimonadaceae (G); c_Saccharimonadia (G); o_Saccharimonadales (G)	[119]

Table 3. *Cont.*

Polysaccharide Source	Mw (kDa)	Monosaccharide Composition	Research Model	Anti-Diabetic Activity	Gut Microbiota Modulation	Reference
Macrocystis pyrifera	342.1	Gal, Fuc, Man, and GluA in ratio of 29.29:27.59: 21.24: 16.99	high-fat, high-sugar and STZ induced Sprague Dawley male rats	↓ body weight loss; glucose; HbA1c; insulin resistance; TG; TC; LDL-C; AST; ALT; BUN; Cr; TNF-α; IL-6; MDA ↑ glucose tolerance; GSH-Px;	↓ Escherichia–Shigella (G); ↑ Muribaculaceae_norank (G); Akkermansia (G); Bifidobacterium (G); Lactobacillus (G); Olsenella (G); Lachnospiraceae_NK4A136_group (G); Ruminococcaceae_UCG-014 (G); Ruminococcus_1 (G); Eubacterium_coprostanoligenes_group (G)	[120]
Onchidium struma	8–14	Ara, Man and Glu in a ratio of 3.79:1.00:49.70.	high-sucrose high-fat diet and STZ induced Kungming male mice	↓ body weight loss; FBG; blood glucose; FIN level; HOMA-IRI; TC; TG; LDL-C; GSP; IL-6; LPS; TNF-α; GSK-3β; ↑ daily intake; glucose tolerance; FER value; HOMA-ISI; HOMA-β; HDL-C; IL-10; mRNA expression (PI3K, AKT-1, mTOR, GLUT-2); SCFAs (acetate, propionate, isobutyrate, butyrate, isovalerate, valerate); relieve the histopathological injury of liver	↓ Firmicutes to Bacteroidetes (P); Lachnoclostridium; Parabacteroides; ↑ Alipipes; Lactobacillus	[121]

P: phylum; F: family; G: genus.

3. Mechanism of the Anti-Diabetic Effects of Polysaccharides through Regulating Gut Microbiota

The gut microbiota is closely related to human health maintenance. Research has shown that there is an important relationship between the gut microbiota and DM [122]. The gut microbiota forms a network regulating the gut barrier, the production and utilization of metabolites, and the immune function of the gut [123]. It also influences the use of glucose and the conversion of glycogen, and its composition is related to the progression of insulin resistance in T2DM as well as the development of complications of DM [124,125]. Below, the anti-diabetic mechanisms of polysaccharides through regulating the gut microbiota are summarized and are shown in Figure 2.

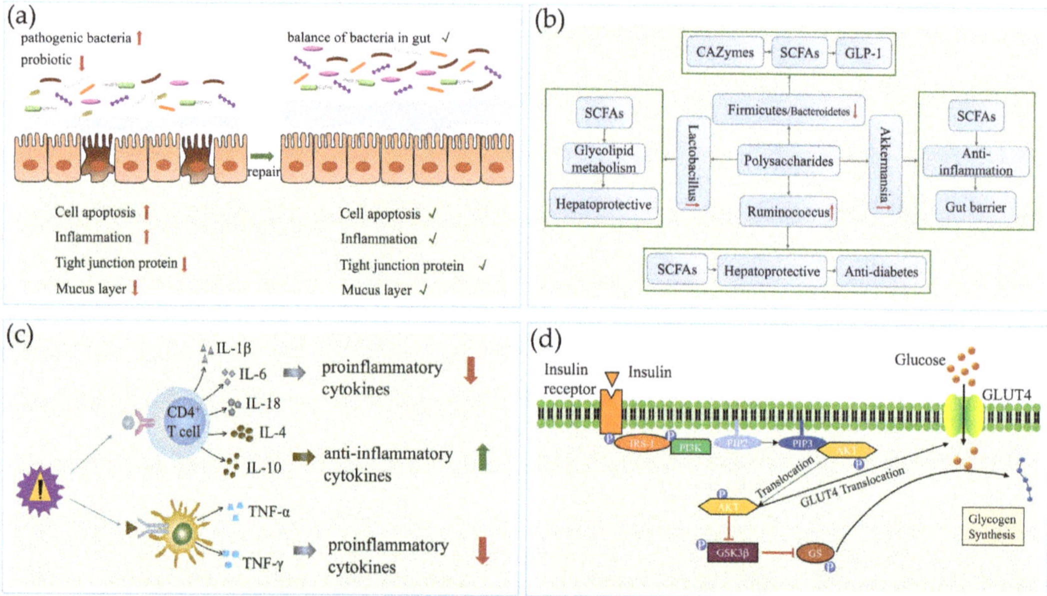

Figure 2. Mechanisms of polysaccharides: (**a**) repairing gut barrier, (**b**) changing gut microbiota composition and metabolites, (**c**) regulating anti-inflammatory activity and immune function, and (**d**) regulating signal pathways. The up-pointing or right-pointing arrow (red or green) means increase, and the down-pointing arrow (red) means decrease. √ means improvement.

3.1. Repairing the Gut Barrier

The mucus layer and the intestinal apical junctional protein complex make up the complex gut barrier, which protects host health from many acute and chronic illnesses [126]. Inflammatory bowel disease (IBD), colon cancer, and many other illnesses were related to damage to the gut barrier [127]. In diabetic mice, the destruction of the gut barrier was shown in a reduction in the number of goblet cells, shorter and irregular villi, a reduction in mucosal space, an influx of inflammatory cells, and weakened epithelial cells [121,128,129]. When the gut barrier was damaged, its function was decreased or even disturbed. Many studies have shown that polysaccharides showed great protective effects on gut barrier integrity. For example, *Pleurotus eryngii* polysaccharide interacted with intestinal mucus layer after in vitro fermentation by the gut microbiota [130]. *Ganoderma atrum* polysaccharides maintained the intestinal barrier and its permeability in rats [131]. The mixture of hawthorn flavonoids and two kinds of polysaccharides from *Auricularia auricula* and *Tremella* improved injuries to the intestinal barrier and epithelial cells in rats [132]. Dandelion polysaccharides repaired the intestinal barrier and improved the structure of the gut microbiota in mice [133].

Polysaccharides can also relieve the injury of the gut barrier through improving tight junction proteins. Cultured *Cordyceps sinensis* polysaccharides, *Dictyopteris divaricate* polysaccharides, and *Phellinus linteus* polysaccharides upregulated tight junction proteins such as occludin, claudin-1, and ZO-1 in intestinal barrier injury in mice, maintaining the gut structure and barrier permeability in mice or rats [47,121,134]. Mucin-2 protein (MUC2) is a kind of heavily glycosylated mucin proteins secreted by intestinal cells protecting the human gut from potentially harmful bacteria and substances [135]. Polysaccharides from the fruit of *Lycium barbarum* increased the mRNA expression of MUC2 in mouse colon [136]. Quinoa seed polysaccharides increased the production of intestinal mucus in rats, protecting host from infection [137].

3.2. Changing Gut Microbiota Composition and Metabolites

Research found that the production of bacteria-derived metabolite damaging to human health was strongly associated with gut dysbiosis reversal [89]. Polysaccharides, regarded as a kind of prebiotics, were found to promote the growth and/or activity of beneficial bacteria and to suppress pathogenic bacteria in rat gut [47]. Polysaccharides also influenced the metabolism of SCFAs and other metabolites indirectly by changing the composition and diversity of the gut microbiota in rats [138]. The metabolites of the gut microbiota influenced the gut and system function by circulation or acting as ligands for cell receptors [139]. For example, increased expression of GPCR 41/43 in the intestinal L cells caused by higher SCFAs may cause the production of GLP-1 [140].

At the phylum level, the Gram-positive Firmicutes and Gram-negative Bacteroidetes were two dominant bacteria in the gut microbiota, comprising more than 90% of total 16S rRNA-targeted sequences from bacteria [141]. Firmicutes and Bacteroidetes had many carbohydrate metabolism pathways, which promoted the expression of CAZymes to degrade most polysaccharides to produce SCFAs, participating in the regulation of glycol metabolism [142,143]. One study found that the F/B ratio was related to metabolic disorders, and compared with a normal group, the F/B ratio was considerably increased in diabetic model mice [68]. Regulation of the F/B ratio is one important way for polysaccharides to modulate the composition of the gut microbiota and improve the gut metabolites.

Dendrobium officinale leaf polysaccharides change gut microbiota composition and derived microbial compounds. They decrease the F/B ratio and upregulate butyrate production to repair the intestinal microenvironment in mice [128]. The treatment of polysaccharide from *Cyclocarya paliurus* leaves attenuated the decrease in the F/B ratio induced by diabetes, while in nondiabetic rats, polysaccharide administration did mot have the same effect [144]. *Astragalus membranaceus* polysaccharide treatment decreased the F/B ratio and promoted the production of acetic acid, butyric acid, and propanoic acid in feces from db/db mice. Konjac glucomannans (KGMs) increased Bacteroidetes and decreased Firmicutes abundance in diabetic mice. KGMs increased the abundance of Muribaculaceae, part of Bacteroidetes, and produced SCFAs to improve pancreatic β-cell function and reduce the release of proinflammatory cytokines [145].

It was also found that Akkermansia is closely related to human health and some DM related indices and is a potential probiotic for the treatment of diabetes [146]. Akkermansia is a kind of representative bacterium in the mucus layer of the intestine that participates in the degradation process of mucin, thereby protecting the intestinal mucosal barrier and reducing protein deposition [147]. Metformin therapy enhances the relative abundance of Akkermansia in mice [148]. Polysaccharides from pumpkin, gougunao tea, and *Gastrodia elata* increased Akkermansia in T2DM mice [149–151].

Ruminococcus, which is abundant and common in the mammalian gut environment, can degrade polysaccharides to produce SCFAs and is a predominant acetogen producing acetic acid and propionate [152]. It was reported that Ruminococcaceae UCG-005 is a key genus for protecting against diabetes [144]. One study found that Ruminococcus was negatively connected with FBG and positively related to body weight [74]. Ruminococcaceae UCG-014 and UCG-005 genera were negatively correlated with indices including liver weight, AST and ALT levels, hepatic steatosis and inflammation degree, which revealed their hepatoprotective effect [153]. *Grifola frondosa, Ganoderma atrum* and *Cordyceps militaris* polysaccharide supplementation enriched the relative abundance of Ruminococcus in HFD rats [154].

Furthermore, a number of studies have shown that reducing the amount of Alistipes in the gut may decrease the generation of antimicrobial peptides, which in turn promotes the colonization of harmful microbes on the gut barrier and results in liver illnesses. For example, Alistipes play a crucial part in the prevention of dextran sulfate sodium-induced colitis in mice [155]. Polysaccharides from *Grifola frondose* and *Lentinula edodes* significantly increased the abundance of Alistipes in mice [156,157]. *Auricularia auricula* polysaccharides markedly increased the level of Bifidobacterium animalis, Morchella esculenta, and *Inonotus obliquus* polysaccharides enhanced the level of Lactobacillus in mice [77,158,159].

SCFAs belong to beneficial metabolites, positively correlated with the health of the body. *Phellinus linteus* polysaccharides increased the abundance of Roseburia, Lachnospiraceae-NK4A136, Lachnospiraceae-UCG-006, and Prevotella9 that decomposed fiber polysaccharides and produced SCFAs in STZ-induced male Sprague Dawley rats [134]. Similarly, *Ganoderma lucidum* and *Poria cocos* polysaccharides increased SCFA-producing bacteria like Prevotella and Paraprevotella clara, and *Poria cocos* polysaccharides greatly increased Bacteroides xylanolyticus, a xylan-degrading bacterium in mice [160].

3.3. Regulating Anti-Inflammatory Activity and Immune Function

Inflammation and disorder of the immune system in the host, e.g., IBD, systemic lupus erythematosus, asthma, arthritis, and many other diseases, are impacted by changes in the normal gut microbiota [161,162]. A low-grade inflammatory and autoimmune condition that is closely linked to T2DM may be caused directly by changes in the gut microbiota's composition. According to the results of Pearson analysis, the relative abundance of some of the gut microbiota was closely correlated with indices of immunological organs like the spleen and thymus and immunoglobulins like IgG and IgM, and $CD4^+$ T cells [163]. Investigation of the connection between the gut microbiota and biochemical profiles showed Bifidobacterium was involved in inflammation and Fusobacterium modulated host immune responses [93,164]. Similarly, relevant studies showed that members of the Lachnospira family in the human gut express two "superantigens" that stimulate the IgA response and are crucial for intestinal homeostasis [165]. Another study found that an increase in Proteobacteria resulted in immune dysregulation in the host [166]. *Agaricus blazei* Murill polysaccharides decreased Proteobacteria and increased Lachnospiraceae and Lactobacillaceae, suppressing the inflammation response in mice [167].

The intervention of polysaccharides can improve the inflammatory and immune response. For example, water extract of *Berberis kansuensis* reduced inflammatory factors such as TNF-α, IL-1β and IL-6 in diabetic mice [168]. *Lycium berry* polysaccharides downregulated proinflammatory cytokines including IL-1β and IL-18 and M1 macrophage markers and increased anti-inflammatory cytokines like IL-4 and IL-10 and M2 macrophage markers to facilitate the shifting of the epithelial immunity from the pro- to the anti-inflammatory microenvironment in mice [169]. *Nigella sativa* seed polysaccharides decreased the levels of cytokines, including IL-6, IL-1β and TNF-α [94]. *Dictyopteris divaricate* polysaccharides downregulated the expression of IL-1β, IL-2, IL-6, TNF-α and IFN-γ in T1DM mice [121].

3.4. Regulating the Signal Pathway

Many signal pathways have been found to be related to glucose metabolism as well as DM. For example, the mTOR signal pathway regulates energy intake and is related to metabolic disorders like T2DM [170]. The PI3K/Akt pathway is a key signaling pathway and regulates insulin signal and glucose metabolism [171,172]. Inactivation of the PI3K/Akt signaling pathway in liver reduces the synthesis of liver glycogen, resulting in insulin resistance, a typical symptom of T2DM [173]. The phosphorylation of ISR1, PI3K and Akt in succession activates GLUT4/GLUT2, leading to glucose uptake of cells [174]. Many polysaccharides relieve the symptoms of DM by regulating the PI3K/Akt signal pathway. For examples, azuki bean (*Vigna angularis*) polysaccharides control glucose metabolism and oxidative stress by considerably upregulating the expression of INSR, IRS-1, PI3K, Akt, and GLUT2 in this signal pathway [175]. *Brasenia schreberi* polysaccharides increase the expression of PI3K and Akt in T2DM mice [90]. Oligosaccharides from seaweed *Sargassum confusum* significantly upregulate the expression of IRS1 and PI3K genes and downregulate the expression of JNKs,h contributing to DM in high-fat/high-sucrose-fed hamsters [176].

Besides the signal pathways in the liver and muscle for glucose uptake, the signal pathways in the gut and other organs are also affected. Coix seed polysaccharides increase the expression of insulin-like growth factor 1 (IGF1) and insulin-like growth factor 1 receptor (IGF1R), which participates in the secretion of insulin [92]. Dietary inulin and *Lycium barbarum* polysaccharides improve the expression of Toll-like receptor 2 (TLR2) on the surface of $\gamma\delta$ T cells, which can be recognized by the metabolites of the gut microbiota and increase the integrity of the gut microbiota in rats [177]. At the same time, a Scutellaria–Coptis herb couple downregulated the expression of Toll-like receptor 4 (TLR4) and MyD88 protein in the colon, decreasing the secretion of proinflammatory factors in mice [178]. It has been reported that polysaccharides can interact with enteroendocrine L cells directly and enhance the production of glucagon-like peptide-1 (GLP-1) through the cAMP signaling pathway and Ca^{2+}/calmodulin/calmodulin-dependent protein kinase 2 signaling pathway [136]. *Cyclocarya paliuru* polysaccharides can increase the mRNA expression of G-protein-coupled receptors (GPRs) like GPR41, GPR43 and GPR109a, which are receptors of SCFAs in colon tissue in T2DM mice [118].

3.5. Action on Related Tissue and Organs

The gut microbiota is closely related to other tissue and organs, and the mostly studied include muscle, liver, kidney and pancreas. The relationship of the gut microbiota and to these organs is shown in Figure 3.

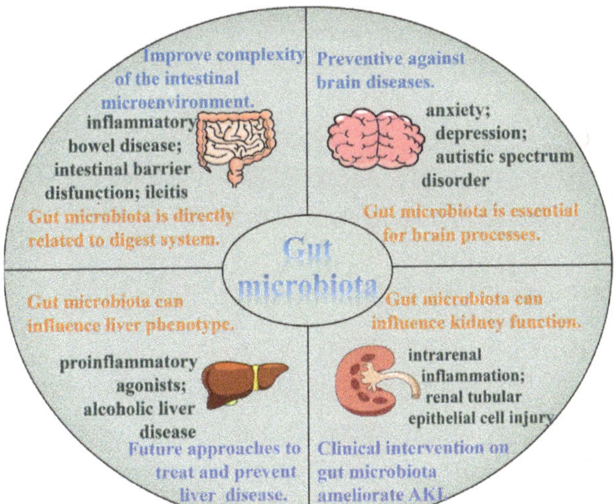

Figure 3. Gut microbiota and related organs.

The metabolites of the gut microbiota enter the blood and interact with receptors on muscle, liver, pancreas, and other organs, influencing their functions [179]. The microbiota–liver axis, microbiota–brain axis, microbiota–kidney, microbiota–lung, and other microbiota–organ axes have been studies [180–184]. For example, one study found that hepatic markers were associated with Ruminococcaceae family [153]. The regulation effects and communication with other tissue and organs of the gut microbiota has aroused researchers' interest.

Polysaccharides can play protective roles by regulating intestinal flora. For instance, water extracts of *Plukenetia volubilis* leaves restored pancreas injury, including the improvement in injured pancreas islets and pancreatic β-cells in T1DM mice [185]. Polysaccharides from red kidney bean also showed pancreas-protective effects in T2DM mice [186]. Mulberry fruit polysaccharides healed damage to the liver, kidneys and pancreas of obese diabetic mice [187].

4. Structure–Activity Relationship of the Anti-Diabetic Effects of Polysaccharides through Regulating Gut Microbiota

As a kind of biological macromolecule, polysaccharides have complex structures. The differences in the structure of polysaccharides, such as monosaccharide composition, molecular weight, types of glycosidic linkages and other intrinsic physicochemical characteristics, can profoundly influence their anti-diabetic effects [188]. Their structural characteristics are closely related to the fermentability of polysaccharides by the gut microbiota [189]. The structure–activity relationship of the anti-diabetic effects of polysaccharides through regulating the gut microbiota is summarized in the following section.

4.1. Monosaccharide Composition

Monosaccharide composition is an essential factor influencing the anti-diabetic effects of polysaccharides. In general, the hypoglycemic activity of polysaccharides increases with the complexity of monosaccharide composition [190]. For example, polysaccharides from four legume species—mung bean, azuki bean, pea and cowpea—with different monosaccharide composition show different hypoglycemic activity. Azuki bean polysaccharides with more complex monosaccharide types, including arabinose, galactose, glucose, xylose, mannose, and galacturonic acid (unique monosaccharide among the four polysaccharides), exhibit the best hypoglycemic effects in STZ-induced diabetic mice. What is more, polysaccharides from mung bean and cowpea with the same monosaccharide type but in different proportions had different hypoglycemic activity, indicating that galactose and glucose might be two important monosaccharides in the anti-diabetic process [175]. Similarly, polysaccharides from four *Gastrodia elata* plants with the same monosaccharide type but in different proportions showed different hypoglycemic activity. *G. elata Bl. f. elata* polysaccharides possessed the highest hypoglycemic activity with the lowest glucose content and highest xylose content, which indicated that xylose was also an important kind of monosaccharide participating in the anti-diabetic process [191].

4.2. Molecular Weight

Molecular weight significantly influences the anti-diabetic and gut microbiota regulation activity of polysaccharides [192]. Typically, polysaccharides have stronger anti-diabetic activity when their molecular weight is lower [76]. For example, blackberry polysaccharides with lower molecular weight were more easily broken down and consumed by the gut microbiota and exhibited better prebiotic effects [193]. Pectin from artichoke and citrus promoted the growth of Bifidobacterium and Lactobacillus, and the enzymatically modified pectin with lower molecular weight showed higher activity [194]. Rhamnogalacturonan-I (RG-I)-enriched pectin (WRP) from citrus and its depolymerized fraction (DWRP) with lower molecular weight showed different gut microbiota regulation function. WRP increased the abundance of Ruminococcaceae, while the abundance of prebiotics like Bifidobacterium and Lactobacillus were significantly by DWRP [195].

There are also some polysaccharides with higher or medium molecular weight showing higher hypoglycemic activity. For instance, Chinese yam polysaccharides HSY-I (>50 kDa) and HSY-II (10 to 50 kDa) exhibited hypoglycemic activity by digestion resistance or β-insulin cell repair. HSY-III (<10 kDa) had no hypoglycemic effect [196]. Peach gum polysaccharides (PGPs) promoted the growth of Bacteroides and Parabacteroides. PGPs with high molecular weight played the most significant role in the production of SCFAs [197]. Konjac glucomannan with medium molecular weight displayed higher hypoglycemic effects and regulated the gut microbiota by modulating gut microbiota composition and improving gut microbiota-related metabolites [145].

Laminaria japonica polysaccharides with higher (HLJP) and lower (LLJP) molecular weight showed different gut microbiota and metabolite regulation function. The function of HLJP focused more on the regulation of SCFAs and metabolites, while that of LLJP focused more on the proliferation probiotic of gut microbiota like Akkermansiaceae [198].

Numerous polysaccharide characteristics, such as viscosity and advanced structure, are correlated with molecular weight. More research is needed to determine the relationship between polysaccharide molecular weight and anti-diabetic activity.

4.3. Types of Glycosidic Linkage

The orientation and position of glycosidic bonds affect the anti-diabetic activity of polysaccharides. For example, fucoidan from Ascophyllum nodosum with alternating (1→3) and (1→4)-α-l-fucose showed better α-glucosidase inhibitory activity than that with repeated (1→3)-α-l-fucose from Fucus vesiculosus, while the inhibitory effect on α-amylase was opposite to α-glucosidase [199]. The glycosidic linkage also influenced the production of SCFAs. The fermentation of polysaccharides with diglucose α-(1→1) structure is positively related to the production of butyrate and negatively related to the production of acetate. Fermentation of polysaccharides with diglucose β-(1→4) structure produces more butyrate, propionate and butyrate than diglucose β-(1→4) structure [200]. As for gut regulation, fucogalactan sulfate from Laminaria japonica, with more branched sugar residues like (1→2, 3, 4)-linked β-D-ManpA and sulfate ester groups, showed better effects in terms of the proliferation of beneficial bacteria and production of SCFAs and other metabolites than mannogluconic acid [201].

5. Conclusions and Prospects

The gut microbiota is closely related to DM and is becoming a new target in the treatment of DM. In this paper, we discussed the anti-diabetic effects of polysaccharides through regulation of the gut microbiota. Most polysaccharides cannot be digested by the human body directly, but are fermented by the gut microbiota to produce SCFAs and other metabolites. The interaction between polysaccharides and the gut microbiota can result in the formation of different metabolites and remodeling of the microbiota. The proposal of the gut–organ axis also provides a model for the understanding and treatment of human diseases. However, due to the complexity of the gut microbiota and the uncertainty of polysaccharide structure, the exact interaction between polysaccharides and the gut microbiota still needs further study. It is necessary to give a more detailed description of polysaccharide structure so that we can gain a clearer picture of how polysaccharides influence the gut microbiota and improve DM. The regulatory functions of the gut microbiota, including the metabolism process and the metabolites themselves and their interactions with other organs or tissue types, also need further study.

Author Contributions: Conceptualization, X.Z. and H.C.; investigation, J.W. and T.Z.; writing—original draft preparation, X.Z. and J.L. (Junyu Liu).; writing—review and editing, S.L., M.L. and J.L. (Jingyang Lu).; figure visualization, X.Z. and J.W.; visualization, T.Z. and S.L.; supervision, M.Z. and H.C.; project administration, M.Z. and H.C.; funding acquisition, H.C. All authors have read and agreed to the published version of the manuscript.

Funding: This research was funded by the National Key Research and Development Program of China (grant 2021YFE0110000), the National Natural Science Foundation of China (grant 32372245), and the Tianjin Municipal Science and Technology Foundation (grant 22JCYBJC00160).

Institutional Review Board Statement: Not applicable.

Informed Consent Statement: Not applicable.

Data Availability Statement: Data sharing is applicable.

Conflicts of Interest: The authors declare no conflicts of interest.

Abbreviations

STZ (streptozotocin); IFN-γ (interferon γ); GPCR 41/43 (G-protein-coupled receptor 41/43); FBG (fasting blood glucose); GSP (glycosylated serum protein); TG (triglyceride); LDL-C (low-density-lipoprotein cholesterol); NEFA (non-esterified fatty acid); ALT (glutamic pyruvic transaminase); AST (glutamic oxaloacetic transaminase); CAT (catalase); SOD (superoxide dismutase); GSH (glutathione); FINS (fasting insulin); TC (total cholesterol); LPS (lipopolysaccharide); TNF-α (tumor necrosis factor α); IL-2/4/6/8/10/18/1β/1b (interleukin-2/4/6/8/10/18/1β/1b); MDA (malondialdehyde); DAO (diamine oxidase); D-LA (D-lactic acid); HDL-C (high-density-lipoprotein cholesterol); HbAlc (glycosylated hemoglobin, type A1C); NO (nitric oxide); NOS (nitric oxide synthase); GSH-Px (glutathione peroxidase); FFA (free fatty acid); Bax (Bcl2-associated X); ADP (adenosine diphosphate); Bcl-2 (B-cell lymphoma 2); ZO-1 (zonula occludens 1); PYY (peptide YY); TBA (total bile acid); TAOC (total antioxidant capacity); UP (urine protein); Scr (serum creatinine); BUN (blood urea nitrogen); UACR (urine microalbumin:creatinine ratio); LEP (leptin); Cr (creatinine); LPS (lipase); JNK (c-Jun N-terminal kinase); PBG (postprandial blood glucose); CD36 (cluster of differentiation 36); PPAR-α (peroxisome proliferator-activated receptor α); HOMA-IRI (HOMA insulin resistance index); FER (food efficiency rate); IgA/M (immunoglobulin A/M).

References

1. ElSayed, N.A.; Aleppo, G.; Aroda, V.R.; Bannuru, R.R.; Brown, F.M.; Bruemmer, D.; Collins, B.S.; Hilliard, M.E.; Isaacs, D.; Johnson, E.L.; et al. 2. Classification and Diagnosis of Diabetes: Standards of Care in Diabetes-2023. *Diabetes Care* **2023**, *46*, S19–S40. [CrossRef] [PubMed]
2. Craciun, C.I.; Neag, M.A.; Catinean, A.; Mitre, A.O.; Rusu, A.; Bala, C.; Roman, G.; Buzoianu, A.D.; Muntean, D.M.; Craciun, A.E. The Relationships between Gut Microbiota and Diabetes Mellitus, and Treatments for Diabetes Mellitus. *Biomedicines* **2022**, *10*, 308. [CrossRef]
3. Giovannini, P.; Howes, M.J.R.; Edwards, S.E. Medicinal plants used in the traditional management of diabetes and its sequelae in Central America: A review. *J. Ethnopharmacol.* **2016**, *184*, 58–71. [CrossRef]
4. Baek, S.M.; Kim, K.; Kim, S.; Son, Y.; Hong, H.S.; Yu, S.Y. SP prevents T2DM complications by immunomodulation. *Sci. Rep.* **2020**, *10*, 16753. [CrossRef]
5. Yi, X.R.; Dong, M.S.; Guo, N.F.; Tian, J.L.; Lei, P.; Wang, S.; Yang, Y.F.; Shi, Y. Flavonoids improve type 2 diabetes mellitus and its complications: A review. *Front. Nutr.* **2023**, *10*, 1192131. [CrossRef] [PubMed]
6. Wu, Z.; Zeng, W.Z.; Zhang, X.; Yang, J.F. Characterization of Acidic Tea Polysaccharides from Yellow Leaves of Wuyi Rock Tea and Their Hypoglycemic Activity via Intestinal Flora Regulation in Rats. *Foods* **2022**, *11*, 617. [CrossRef]
7. Perreault, L.; Pan, Q.; Aroda, V.R.; Barrett-Connor, E.; Dabelea, D.; Dagogo-Jack, S.; Hamman, R.F.; Kahn, S.E.; Mather, K.J.; Knowler, W.C.; et al. Exploring residual risk for diabetes and microvascular disease in the Diabetes Prevention Program Outcomes Study (DPPOS). *Diabet. Med.* **2017**, *34*, 1747–1755. [CrossRef]
8. Pagano, G.; Polychronis, S.; Wilson, H.; Giordano, B.; Ferrara, N.; Niccolini, F.; Politis, M. Diabetes mellitus and Parkinson disease. *Neurology* **2018**, *90*, e1654–e1662. [CrossRef] [PubMed]
9. Schmidt, A.M. Diabetes Mellitus and Cardiovascular Disease Emerging Therapeutic Approaches. *Arter. Throm. Vas.* **2019**, *39*, 558–568. [CrossRef]
10. Yuan, Y.; Zhou, J.; Zheng, Y.; Xu, Z.; Li, Y.; Zhou, S.; Zhang, C. Beneficial effects of polysaccharide-rich extracts from Apocynum venetum leaves on hypoglycemic and gut microbiota in type 2 diabetic mice. *Biomed. Pharmacother.* **2020**, *127*, 110182. [CrossRef]
11. Zhang, J.H.; Wang, W.J.; Guo, D.Y.; Bai, B.Q.; Bo, T.; Fan, S.H. Antidiabetic Effect of Millet Bran Polysaccharides Partially Mediated via Changes in Gut Microbiome. *Foods* **2022**, *11*, 3406. [CrossRef] [PubMed]
12. Cui, J.F.; Ye, H.; Zhu, Y.J.; Li, Y.P.; Wang, J.F.; Wang, P. Characterization and Hypoglycemic Activity of a Rhamnan-Type Sulfated Polysaccharide Derivative. *Mar. Drugs* **2019**, *17*, 21. [CrossRef] [PubMed]
13. Kholiya, F.; Chatterjee, S.; Bhojani, G.; Sen, S.; Barkume, M.; Kasinathan, N.K.; Kode, J.; Meena, R. Seaweed polysaccharide derived bioaldehyde nanocomposite: Potential application in anticancer therapeutics. *Carbohydr. Polym.* **2020**, *240*, 116282. [CrossRef] [PubMed]
14. Roszczyk, A.; Turlo, J.; Zagozdzon, R.; Kaleta, B. Immunomodulatory Properties of Polysaccharides from Lentinula edodes. *Int. J. Mol. Sci.* **2022**, *23*, 8980. [CrossRef] [PubMed]
15. Wei, H.; Shi, Y.Q.; Yuan, Z.X.; Huang, Z.N.; Cai, F.H.; Zhu, J.F.; Zhang, W.W.; Li, J.; Xiong, Q.P.; Wang, Y.P.; et al. Isolation, Identification, and Anti-Inflammatory Activity of Polysaccharides of Typha angustifolia. *Biomacromolecules* **2021**, *22*, 2451–2459. [CrossRef] [PubMed]
16. Zhao, Z.K.; Yu, H.L.; Liu, B.; Wang, H.; Luo, Q.; Ding, X.G. Antioxidative mechanism of Lycium barbarum polysaccharides promotes repair and regeneration following cavernous nerve injury. *Neural Regen. Res.* **2016**, *11*, 1312–1321. [PubMed]

17. Fan, Y.M.; Zhou, X.F.; Huang, G.L. Preparation, structure, and properties of tea polysaccharide. *Chem. Biol. Drug Des.* **2022**, *99*, 75–82. [CrossRef] [PubMed]
18. Ullah, S.; Khalil, A.A.; Shaukat, F.; Song, Y.D. Sources, Extraction and Biomedical Properties of Polysaccharides. *Foods* **2019**, *8*, 304. [CrossRef] [PubMed]
19. Alba, K.; Dimopoulou, M.; Kontogiorgos, V. Baobab polysaccharides as emulsifiers. *LWT* **2021**, *144*, 111235. [CrossRef]
20. Sun, B.N.; Yu, S.; Zhao, D.Y.; Guo, S.H.; Wang, X.H.; Zhao, K. Polysaccharides as vaccine adjuvants. *Vaccine* **2018**, *36*, 5226–5234. [CrossRef]
21. Yang, Z.J.; Liu, W.W.; Liu, H.M.; Li, R.; Chang, L.; Kan, S.N.; Hao, M.; Wang, D.X. The applications of polysaccharides in dentistry. *Front. Bioeng. Biotech.* **2022**, *10*, 970041. [CrossRef] [PubMed]
22. Yao, Y.; Yan, L.J.; Chen, H.; Wu, N.; Wang, W.B.; Wang, D.S. Cyclocarya paliurus polysaccharides alleviate type 2 diabetic symptoms by modulating gut microbiota and short-chain fatty acids. *Phytomedicine* **2020**, *77*, 153268. [CrossRef] [PubMed]
23. Blandino, G.; Inturri, R.; Lazzara, F.; Di Rosa, M.; Malaguarnera, L. Impact of gut microbiota on diabetes mellitus. *Diabetes Metab.* **2016**, *42*, 303–315. [CrossRef] [PubMed]
24. Hermann-Bank, M.L.; Skovgaard, K.; Stockmarr, A.; Larsen, N.; Molbak, L. The Gut Microbiotassay: A high-throughput qPCR approach combinable with next generation sequencing to study gut microbial diversity. *BMC Genom.* **2013**, *14*, 788. [CrossRef] [PubMed]
25. Tan, X.J.; Wang, Y.Z.; Gong, T. The interplay between oral microbiota, gut microbiota and systematic diseases. *J. Oral. Microbiol.* **2023**, *15*, 2213112. [CrossRef] [PubMed]
26. Huttenhower, C.; Gevers, D.; Knight, R.; Abubucker, S.; Badger, J.H.; Chinwalla, A.T.; Creasy, H.H.; Earl, A.M.; FitzGerald, M.G.; Fulton, R.S.; et al. Structure, function and diversity of the healthy human microbiome. *Nature* **2012**, *486*, 207–214.
27. Sonnenburg, E.D.; Smits, S.A.; Tikhonov, M.; Higginbottom, S.K.; Wingreen, N.S.; Sonnenburg, J.L. Diet-induced extinctions in the gut microbiota compound over generations. *Nature* **2016**, *529*, 212–215. [CrossRef]
28. Zhang, Y.J.; Li, S.; Gan, R.Y.; Zhou, T.; Xu, D.P.; Li, H.B. Impacts of Gut Bacteria on Human Health and Diseases. *Int. J. Mol. Sci.* **2015**, *16*, 7493–7519. [CrossRef]
29. Fan, H.X.; Liu, X.C.; Ren, Z.Y.; Fei, X.N.; Luo, J.; Yang, X.Y.; Xue, Y.Y.; Zhang, F.F.; Liang, B. Gut microbiota and cardiac arrhythmia. *Front. Cell Infect. Microbiol.* **2023**, *13*, 1147687. [CrossRef] [PubMed]
30. Shi, Q.W.; Dai, L.L.; Zhao, Q.; Zhang, X. A review on the effect of gut microbiota on metabolic diseases. *Arch. Microbiol.* **2022**, *204*, 192. [CrossRef]
31. Masenga, S.K.; Kirabo, A. Salt and Gut Microbiota in Heart Failure. *Curr. Hypertens. Rep.* **2023**, *25*, 173–184. [CrossRef] [PubMed]
32. Mulak, A.; Bonaz, B. Brain-gut-microbiota axis in Parkinson's disease. *World J. Gastroenterol.* **2015**, *21*, 10609–10620. [CrossRef] [PubMed]
33. AL-Ishaq, R.K.; Samuel, S.M.; Büsselberg, D. The Influence of Gut Microbial Species on Diabetes Mellitus. *Int. J. Mol. Sci.* **2023**, *24*, 8118. [CrossRef]
34. Bajinka, O.; Tan, Y.R.; Darboe, A.; Ighaede-Edwards, I.G.; Abdelhalim, K.A. The gut microbiota pathway mechanisms of diabetes. *Amb. Express* **2023**, *13*, 16. [CrossRef] [PubMed]
35. Gong, P.; Xiao, X.Y.; Wang, S.; Shi, F.X.; Liu, N.; Chen, X.F.; Yang, W.J.; Wang, L.; Chen, F.X. Hypoglycemic effect of astragaloside IV via modulating gut microbiota and regulating AMPK/SIRT1 and PI3K/AKT pathway. *J. Ethnopharmacol.* **2021**, *281*, 114558. [CrossRef] [PubMed]
36. Ma, S.T.; Tian, S.H.; Sun, J.; Pang, X.Y.; Hu, Q.B.; Li, X.F.; Lu, Y.J. Broccoli microgreens have hypoglycemic effect by improving blood lipid and inflammatory factors while modulating gut microbiota in mice with type 2 diabetes. *J. Food Biochem.* **2022**, *46*, e14145. [CrossRef] [PubMed]
37. Wang, X.L.; Wang, X.; Jiang, H.; Cai, C.; Li, G.Y.; Hao, J.J.; Yu, G.L. Marine polysaccharides attenuate metabolic syndrome by fermentation products and altering gut microbiota: An overview. *Carbohydr. Polym.* **2018**, *195*, 601–612. [CrossRef]
38. Xie, G.X.; Zhong, W.; Zheng, X.J.; Li, Q.; Qiu, Y.P.; Li, H.K.; Chen, H.Y.; Zhou, Z.X.; Jia, W. Chronic Ethanol Consumption Alters Mammalian Gastrointestinal Content Metabolites. *J. Proteome Res.* **2013**, *12*, 3297–3306. [CrossRef] [PubMed]
39. Sam, Q.H.; Ling, H.; Yew, W.S.; Tan, Z.H.; Ravikumar, S.; Chang, M.W.; Chai, L.Y.A. The Divergent Immunomodulatory Effects of Short Chain Fatty Acids and Medium Chain Fatty Acids. *Int. J. Mol. Sci.* **2021**, *22*, 6453. [CrossRef]
40. Alvarez-Mercado, A.I.; Plaza-Diaz, J. Dietary Polysaccharides and Gut Microbiota Ecosystem. *Nutrients* **2022**, *14*, 4285. [CrossRef]
41. Riedl, R.A.; Atkinson, S.N.; Burnett, C.M.L.; Grobe, J.L.; Kirby, J.R. The Gut Microbiome, Energy Homeostasis, and Implications for Hypertension. *Curr. Hypertens. Rep.* **2017**, *19*, 1–7. [CrossRef] [PubMed]
42. Li, R.L.; Xue, Z.H.; Li, S.Q.; Zhou, J.N.; Liu, J.Y.; Zhang, M.; Panichayupakaranant, P.; Chen, H.X. Mulberry leaf polysaccharides ameliorate obesity through activation of brown adipose tissue and modulation of the gut microbiota in high-fat diet fed mice. *Food Funct.* **2022**, *13*, 561–573. [CrossRef] [PubMed]
43. Xue, Z.H.; Ma, Q.Q.; Chen, Y.; Lu, Y.P.; Wang, Y.J.; Jia, Y.N.; Zhang, M.; Chen, H.X. Structure characterization of soluble dietary fiber fractions from mushroom Lentinula edodes (Berk.) Pegler and the effects on fermentation and human gut microbiota in vitro. *Food Res. Int.* **2020**, *129*, 108870. [CrossRef] [PubMed]
44. Jiao, R.; Liu, Y.X.; Gao, H.; Xiao, J.; So, K.F. The Anti-Oxidant and Antitumor Properties of Plant Polysaccharides. *Am. J. Chin. Med.* **2016**, *44*, 463–488. [CrossRef]

45. Ge, Y.Z.; Ahmed, S.; Yao, W.Z.; You, L.J.; Zheng, J.X.; Hileuskaya, K. Regulation effects of indigestible dietary polysaccharides on intestinal microflora: An overview. *J. Food Biochem.* **2021**, *45*, e13564. [CrossRef]
46. Xu, X.F.; Xu, P.P.; Ma, C.W.; Tang, J.; Zhang, X.W. Gut microbiota, host health, and polysaccharides. *Biotechnol. Adv.* **2013**, *31*, 318–337. [CrossRef] [PubMed]
47. Cai, Y.; Liu, W.; Lin, Y.X.; Zhang, S.B.; Zou, B.R.; Xiao, D.; Lin, L.; Zhong, Y.P.; Zheng, H.H.; Liao, Q.F.; et al. Compound polysaccharides ameliorate experimental colitis by modulating gut microbiota composition and function. *J. Gastroenterol. Hepatol.* **2019**, *34*, 1554–1562. [CrossRef] [PubMed]
48. Bo, R.; Liu, Z.; Zhang, J.; Gu, P.; Ou, N.; Sun, Y.; Hu, Y.; Liu, J.; Wang, D. Mechanism of Lycium barbarum polysaccharides liposomes on activating murine dendritic cells. *Carbohydr. Polym.* **2019**, *205*, 540–549. [CrossRef]
49. Chen, N.; Zhang, H.; Zong, X.; Li, S.; Wang, J.; Wang, Y.; Jin, M. Polysaccharides from Auricularia auricula: Preparation, structural features and biological activities. *Carbohydr. Polym.* **2020**, *247*, 116750. [CrossRef]
50. Gong, P.X.; Wu, Y.C.; Liu, Y.; Lv, S.Z.; You, Y.; Zhou, Z.L.; Chen, X.; Li, H.J. Structure and hypoglycemic effect of a neutral polysaccharide isolated from sea cucumber Stichopus japonicus. *Int. J. Biol. Macromol.* **2022**, *216*, 14–23. [CrossRef]
51. Guidara, M.; Yaich, H.; Amor, I.B.; Fakhfakh, J.; Gargouri, J.; Lassoued, S.; Blecker, C.; Richel, A.; Attia, H.; Garna, H. Effect of extraction procedures on the chemical structure, antitumor and anticoagulant properties of ulvan from Ulva lactuca of Tunisia coast. *Carbohydr. Polym.* **2021**, *253*, 117283. [CrossRef] [PubMed]
52. Kumar, A.; Rao, K.M.; Han, S.S. Application of xanthan gum as polysaccharide in tissue engineering: A review. *Carbohydr. Polym.* **2018**, *180*, 128–144. [CrossRef] [PubMed]
53. Svensson, M.V.; Zhang, X.; Huttunen, E.; Widmalm, G. Structural studies of the capsular polysaccharide produced by Leuconostoc mesenteroides ssp. cremoris PIA2. *Biomacromolecules* **2011**, *12*, 2496–2501. [CrossRef] [PubMed]
54. Teng, S.; Zhang, Y.; Jin, X.; Zhu, Y.; Li, L.; Huang, X.; Wang, D.; Lin, Z. Structure and hepatoprotective activity of Usp10/NF-kappaB/Nrf2 pathway-related Morchella esculenta polysaccharide. *Carbohydr. Polym.* **2023**, *303*, 120453. [CrossRef] [PubMed]
55. Yuan, Q.H.; Xie, F.; Tan, J.; Yuan, Y.; Mei, H.; Zheng, Y.; Sheng, R. Extraction, structure and pharmacological effects of the polysaccharides from Cordyceps sinensis: A review. *J. Funct. Foods* **2022**, *89*, 104909. [CrossRef]
56. Zhou, Y.; Chen, X.X.; Chen, T.T.; Chen, X.Q. A review of the antibacterial activity and mechanisms of plant polysaccharides. *Trends Food Sci. Tech.* **2022**, *123*, 264–280. [CrossRef]
57. Zhou, J.N.; Li, R.L.; Jia, Y.A.; Wang, Y.J.; Liu, J.Y.; Panichayupakaranant, P.; Chen, H.X. Recent Progress in Natural Anticancer Agents Discovery from Tea (Camellia sinensis): A Review. *Recent. Pat. Anti-Cancer* **2022**, *17*, 343–357. [CrossRef] [PubMed]
58. Zhu, J.X.; Chen, Z.Y.; Zhou, H.; Yu, C.; Han, Z.; Shao, S.R.; Hu, X.C.; Wei, X.L.; Wang, Y.F. Effects of extraction methods on physicochemical properties and hypoglycemic activities of polysaccharides from coarse green tea. *Glycoconj. J.* **2020**, *37*, 241–250. [CrossRef] [PubMed]
59. Alba, K.; Offiah, V.; Laws, A.P.; Falade, K.O.; Kontogiorgos, V. Baobab polysaccharides from fruits and leaves. *Food Hydrocoll.* **2020**, *106*, 105874. [CrossRef]
60. Xu, L.L.; Chen, Y.; Chen, Z.Q.; Gao, X.D.; Wang, C.L.; Panichayupakaranant, P.; Chen, H.X. Ultrafiltration isolation, physicochemical characterization, and antidiabetic activities analysis of polysaccharides from green tea, oolong tea, and black tea. *J. Food Sci.* **2020**, *85*, 4025–4032. [CrossRef]
61. Guilbaud, A.; Howsam, M.; Niquet-Léridon, C.; Delguste, F.; Fremont, M.; Lestavel, S.; Maboudou, P.; Garat, A.; Schraen, S.; Onraed, B.; et al. The Effect of Lactobacillus fermentum ME-3 Treatment on Glycation and Diabetes Complications. *Mol. Nutr. Food Res.* **2020**, *64*, e1901018. [CrossRef] [PubMed]
62. Bao, Y.; Zhang, Y.C.; Zhang, Y.; Liu, Y.; Wang, S.Q.; Dong, X.M.; Wang, Y.Y.; Zhang, H.P. Screening of potential probiotic properties of Lactobacillus fermentum isolated from traditional dairy products. *Food Control* **2010**, *21*, 695–701. [CrossRef]
63. Saavedra, J.M.; Bauman, N.A.; Perman, J.A.; Yolken, R.H.; Saavedra, J.M.; Bauman, N.A.; Oung, I. Feeding of Bifidobacterium bifidum and Streptococcus thermophilus to infants in hospital for prevention of diarrhoea and shedding of rotavirus. *Lancet* **1994**, *344*, 1046–1049. [CrossRef] [PubMed]
64. Makras, L.; Triantafyllou, V.; Fayol-Messaoudi, D.; Adriany, T.; Zoumpopoulou, G.; Tsakalidou, E.; Servin, A.; De Vuyst, L. Kinetic analysis of the antibacterial activity of probiotic lactobacilli towards Salmonella enterica serovar Typhimurium reveals a role for lactic acid and other inhibitory compounds. *Res. Microbiol.* **2006**, *157*, 241–247. [CrossRef] [PubMed]
65. Chen, X.Y.; Tan, F.; Yi, R.K.; Mu, J.F.; Zhao, X.; Yang, Z.N. Effects of Lactobacillus on Mice with Diabetes Induced by High-Fat Diet with Streptozotocin (STZ). *Appl. Sci.* **2018**, *8*, 1249. [CrossRef]
66. Din, A.U.; Hassan, A.; Zhu, Y.; Zhang, K.; Wang, Y.; Li, T.; Wang, Y.; Wang, G. Inhibitory effect of Bifidobacterium bifidum ATCC 29521 on colitis and its mechanism. *J. Nutr. Biochem.* **2020**, *79*, 108353. [CrossRef] [PubMed]
67. Fernando, W.M.A.D.B.; Flint, S.H.; Ranaweera, K.K.D.S.; Bamunuarachchi, A.; Johnson, S.K.; Brennan, C.S. The potential synergistic behaviour of inter- and intra-genus probiotic combinations in the pattern and rate of short chain fatty acids formation during fibre fermentation. *Int. J. Food Sci. Nutr.* **2018**, *69*, 144–154. [CrossRef] [PubMed]
68. Chen, M.; Xiao, D.; Liu, W.; Song, Y.; Zou, B.; Li, L.; Li, P.; Cai, Y.; Liu, D.; Liao, Q.; et al. Intake of Ganoderma lucidum polysaccharides reverses the disturbed gut microbiota and metabolism in type 2 diabetic rats. *Int. J. Biol. Macromol.* **2020**, *155*, 890–902. [CrossRef]
69. Li, S.; Qi, Y.; Chen, L.; Qu, D.; Li, Z.; Gao, K.; Chen, J.; Sun, Y. Effects of Panax ginseng polysaccharides on the gut microbiota in mice with antibiotic-associated diarrhea. *Int. J. Biol. Macromol.* **2019**, *124*, 931–937. [CrossRef]

70. Yang, L.N.; Huang, J.H.; Wu, X.H.; Li, L.; Cai, W.Q.; Zhu, L.J.; Wang, S.N.; Song, H.; Zhu, D.S.; Ma, T.; et al. Interactions between gut microbiota and soy hull polysaccharides regulate the air-liquid interfacial activity. *Food Hydrocoll.* **2021**, *119*, 106704. [CrossRef]
71. Turroni, F.; Milani, C.; Duranti, S.; Mahony, J.; van Sinderen, D.; Ventura, M. Glycan Utilization and Cross-Feeding Activities by Bifidobacteria. *Trends Microbiol.* **2018**, *26*, 339–350. [CrossRef] [PubMed]
72. Wang, H.Y.; Guo, L.X.; Hu, W.H.; Peng, Z.T.; Wang, C.; Chen, Z.C.; Liu, E.Y.L.; Dong, T.T.X.; Wang, T.J.; Tsim, K.W.K. Polysaccharide from tuberous roots of Ophiopogon japonicus regulates gut microbiota and its metabolites during alleviation of high-fat diet-induced type-2 diabetes in mice. *J. Funct. Foods* **2019**, *63*, 103593. [CrossRef]
73. Li, J.; Pang, B.; Yan, X.; Shang, X.; Hu, X.; Shi, J. Prebiotic properties of different polysaccharide fractions from Artemisia sphaerocephala Krasch seeds evaluated by simulated digestion and in vitro fermentation by human fecal microbiota. *Int. J. Biol. Macromol.* **2020**, *162*, 414–424. [CrossRef] [PubMed]
74. Yan, H.L.; Lu, J.M.; Wang, Y.F.; Gu, W.; Yang, X.X.; Yu, J. Intake of total saponins and polysaccharides from Polygonatum kingianum affects the gut microbiota in diabetic rats. *Phytomedicine* **2017**, *26*, 45–54. [CrossRef] [PubMed]
75. Liang, J.J.; Zhang, M.N.; Wang, X.N.; Ren, Y.C.; Yue, T.L.; Wang, Z.L.; Gao, Z.P. Edible fungal polysaccharides, the gut microbiota, and host health. *Carbohydr. Polym.* **2021**, *273*, 118558. [CrossRef] [PubMed]
76. Yang, L.A.; Li, L.; Wu, X.H.; Cai, W.Q.; Lin, Q.; Zhu, D.S. The Effect of Natural Soluble Polysaccharides on the Type 2 Diabetes through Modulating Gut Microbiota: A Review. *Curr. Med. Chem.* **2021**, *28*, 5368–5385. [CrossRef] [PubMed]
77. Rehman, A.U.; Khan, A.I.; Xin, Y.; Liang, W. Morchella esculenta polysaccharide attenuate obesity, inflammation and modulate gut microbiota. *Amb. Express* **2022**, *12*, 114. [CrossRef] [PubMed]
78. Ren, F.; Meng, C.; Chen, W.J.; Chen, H.M.; Chen, W.X. Ganoderma amboinense polysaccharide prevents obesity by regulating gut microbiota in high-fat-diet mice. *Food Biosci.* **2021**, *42*, 101107. [CrossRef]
79. Su, A.X.; Ma, G.X.; Ma, N.; Pei, F.; Yang, W.J.; Hu, Q.H. Effects of Flammulina velutipes polysaccharides on gut microbiota composition and metabolism in vitro fermentation. *Food Sci. Biotechnol.* **2023**, *32*, 361–369. [CrossRef]
80. Zhong, L.; Ma, N.; Zheng, H.H.; Ma, G.X.; Zhao, L.Y.; Hu, Q.H. Tuber indicum polysaccharide relieves fatigue by regulating gut microbiota in mice. *J. Funct. Foods* **2019**, *63*, 103580. [CrossRef]
81. Yu, R.X.; Luo, J.M.; Liu, L.; Peng, X.C.; Gan, R.Y.; Wu, D.T.; Hu, Y.C. Hypoglycemic Effect of Edible Fungi Polysaccharides Depends on Their Metabolites from the Fermentation of Human Fecal Microbiota. *Foods* **2024**, *13*, 103580. [CrossRef]
82. Fuller, R.; Moore, M.V.; Lewith, G.; Stuart, B.L.; Ormiston, R.V.; Fisk, H.L.; Noakes, P.S.; Calder, P.C. Yeast-derived β-1,3/1,6 glucan, upper respiratory tract infection and innate immunity in older adults. *Nutrition* **2017**, *39–40*, 30–35. [CrossRef]
83. Gudi, R.; Perez, N.; Johnson, B.M.; Sofi, M.H.; Brown, R.; Quan, S.; Karumuthil-Melethil, S.; Vasu, C. Complex dietary polysaccharide modulates gut immune function and microbiota, and promotes protection from autoimmune diabetes. *Immunology* **2019**, *157*, 70–85. [CrossRef] [PubMed]
84. Guo, W.L.; Deng, J.C.; Pan, Y.Y.; Xu, J.X.; Hong, J.L.; Shi, F.F.; Liu, G.L.; Qian, M.; Bai, W.D.; Zhang, W.; et al. Hypoglycemic and hypolipidemic activities of Grifola frondosa polysaccharides and their relationships with the modulation of intestinal microflora in diabetic mice induced by high-fat diet and streptozotocin. *Int. J. Biol. Macromol.* **2020**, *153*, 1231–1240. [CrossRef]
85. Ouyang, Y.Z.; Nie, J.P.; Gao, X.X.; Zhao, C. Grifola Frondosa Polysaccharide Ameliorates Hyperglycemia and Gut Microbiota in Type 2 Diabetic Mice. *Free Radic. Biol. Med.* **2022**, *180*, s65. [CrossRef]
86. Fu, C.J.; Ye, K.; Ma, S.; Du, H.J.; Chen, S.G.; Liu, D.H.; Ma, G.X.; Xiao, H. Simulated gastrointestinal digestion and gut microbiota fermentation of polysaccharides from Agaricus bisporus. *Food Chem.* **2023**, *418*, 135849. [CrossRef]
87. Tsung-Ru, W.; Chuan-Sheng, L.; Chih-Jung, C.; Tzu-Lung, L.; Jan, M.; Yun-Fei, K.; David, M.O.; Chia-Chen, L.; John, D.Y.; Hsin-Chih, L. Gut commensal Parabacteroides goldsteiniiplays plays a predominant role in the anti-obesity effects of polysaccharides isolated from Hirsutella sinensis. *Gut* **2019**, *68*, 248.
88. Chen, X.X.; Chen, C.; Fu, X. Hypoglycemic effect of the polysaccharides from Astragalus membranaceus on type 2 diabetic mice based on the "gut microbiota-mucosal barrier". *Food Funct.* **2022**, *13*, 10121–10133. [CrossRef] [PubMed]
89. Zhou, W.; Han, L.J.; Raza, S.H.A.; Yue, Q.M.; Sun, S.N.; Zhao, Y.X.; Lv, L.F.; Deng, Y.R.; Yuan, Z.Z.; Alsharif, I.; et al. Polysaccharides in Berberis dasystachya improve intestinal flora depending on the molecular weight and ameliorate type 2 diabetes in rats. *J. Funct. Foods* **2023**, *100*, 105381. [CrossRef]
90. Liu, G.D.; Feng, S.M.; Yan, J.D.; Luan, D.; Sun, P.L.; Shao, P. Antidiabetic potential of polysaccharides from Brasenia schreberi regulating insulin signaling pathway and gut microbiota in type 2 diabetic mice. *Curr. Res. Food Sci.* **2022**, *5*, 1465–1474. [CrossRef]
91. Li, H.S.; Fang, Q.Y.; Nie, Q.X.; Hu, J.L.; Yang, C.; Huang, T.; Li, H.; Nie, S.P. Hypoglycemic and Hypolipidemic Mechanism of Tea Polysaccharides on Type 2 Diabetic Rats via Gut Microbiota and Metabolism Alteration. *J. Agric. Food Chem.* **2020**, *68*, 10015–10028. [CrossRef] [PubMed]
92. Xia, T.; Liu, C.S.; Hu, Y.N.; Luo, Z.Y.; Chen, F.L.; Yuan, L.X.; Tan, X.M. Coix seed polysaccharides alleviate type 2 diabetes mellitus via gut microbiota-derived short-chain fatty acids activation of IGF1/PI3K/ AKT signaling. *Food Res. Int.* **2021**, *150*, 110717. [CrossRef] [PubMed]
93. Ma, Q.Y.; Zhai, R.H.; Xie, X.Q.; Chen, T.; Zhang, Z.Q.; Liu, H.C.; Nie, C.X.; Yuan, X.J.; Tu, A.B.; Tian, B.M.; et al. Hypoglycemic Effects of Lycium barbarum Polysaccharide in Type 2 Diabetes Mellitus Mice Modulating Gut Microbiota. *Front. Nutr.* **2022**, *9*, 916271. [CrossRef] [PubMed]

94. Dong, J.; Liang, Q.X.; Niu, Y.; Jiang, S.J.; Zhou, L.; Wang, J.M.; Ma, C.Y.; Kang, W.Y. Effects of Nigella sativa seed polysaccharides on type 2 diabetic mice and gut microbiota. *Int. J. Biol. Macromol.* **2020**, *159*, 725–738. [CrossRef] [PubMed]
95. Zhang, M.; Yang, L.C.; Zhu, M.M.; Yang, B.; Yang, Y.J.; Jia, X.B.; Feng, L. Moutan Cortex polysaccharide ameliorates diabetic kidney disease via modulating gut microbiota dynamically in rats. *Int. J. Biol. Macromol.* **2022**, *206*, 849–860. [CrossRef]
96. Xu, N.; Zhou, Y.J.; Lu, X.Y.; Chang, Y.N. Auricularia auricula-judae (Bull.) polysaccharides improve type 2 diabetes in HFD/STZ-induced mice by regulating the AKT/AMPK signaling pathways and the gut microbiota. *J. Food Sci.* **2021**, *86*, 5479–5494. [CrossRef]
97. Shao, W.M.; Xiao, C.; Yong, T.Q.; Zhang, Y.F.; Hu, H.P.; Xie, T.; Liu, R.J.; Huang, L.H.; Li, X.M.; Xie, Y.Z.; et al. A polysaccharide isolated from Ganoderma lucidum ameliorates hyperglycemia through modulating gut microbiota in type 2 diabetic mice. *Int. J. Biol. Macromol.* **2022**, *197*, 23–38. [CrossRef] [PubMed]
98. Zhao, H.; Li, M.; Liu, L.; Li, D.; Zhao, L.; Wu, Z.; Zhou, M.; Jia, L.; Yang, F. Cordyceps militaris polysaccharide alleviates diabetic symptoms by regulating gut microbiota against TLR4/NF-κB pathway. *Int. J. Biol. Macromol.* **2023**, *230*, 123241. [CrossRef]
99. Chen, Y.Q.; Liu, D.; Wang, D.Y.; Lai, S.S.; Zhong, R.T.; Liu, Y.Y.; Yang, C.F.; Liu, B.; Sarker, M.R.; Zhao, C. Hypoglycemic activity and gut microbiota regulation of a novel polysaccharide from Grifola frondosa in type 2 diabetic mice. *Food Chem. Toxicol.* **2019**, *126*, 295–302. [CrossRef]
100. Rehman, A.U.; Siddiqui, N.Z.; Farooqui, N.A.; Alam, G.; Gul, A.; Ahmad, B.; Asim, M.; Khan, A.I.; Xin, Y.; Zexu, W.; et al. Morchella esculenta mushroom polysaccharide attenuates diabetes and modulates intestinal permeability and gut microbiota in a type 2 diabetic mice model. *Front. Nutr.* **2022**, *9*, 984695. [CrossRef]
101. Xue, Z.H.; Li, R.L.; Liu, J.Y.; Zhou, J.N.; Zhang, X.Y.; Zhang, T.T.; Zhang, M.; Yang, Y.; Chen, H.X. Preventive and synbiotic effects of the soluble dietary fiber obtained from Lentinula edodes byproducts and Lactobacillus plantarum against dextran sulfate sodium-induced colitis in mice. *J. Sci. Food Agric.* **2023**, *103*, 616–626. [CrossRef] [PubMed]
102. Kang, N.; Oh, S.; Kim, S.Y.; Ahn, H.; Son, M.; Heo, S.J.; Byun, K.; Jeon, Y.J. Anti-obesity effects of Ishophloroglucin A from the brown seaweed Ishige okamurae (Yendo) regulation of leptin signal in ob/ob mice. *Algal Res.* **2022**, *61*, 102533. [CrossRef]
103. Lee, S.H.; Kim, M.; Park, M.H. Diphlorethohydroxycamalol isolated from Ishige okamurae prevents H2O2-induced oxidative damage via BMP2/Runx2 signaling in osteoblastic MC3T3-E1 cells. *Fitoterapia* **2021**, *152*, 104921. [CrossRef]
104. Xiao, Z.B.; Yang, S.T.; Liu, Y.; Zhou, C.X.; Hong, P.Z.; Sun, S.L.; Qian, Z.J. A novel glyceroglycolipid from brown algae Ishige okamurae improve photoaging and counteract inflammation in UVB-induced HaCaT cells. *Chem.-Biol. Interact.* **2022**, *351*, 109737. [CrossRef]
105. Yang, H.W.; Fernando, K.H.N.; Oh, J.Y.; Li, X.; Jeon, Y.J.; Ryu, B. Anti-Obesity and Anti-Diabetic Effects of Ishige okamurae. *Mar. Drugs* **2019**, *17*, 202. [CrossRef] [PubMed]
106. Usoltseva, R.V.; Anastyuk, S.D.; Shevchenko, N.M.; Surits, V.V.; Silchenko, A.S.; Isakov, V.V.; Zvyagintseva, T.N.; Thinh, P.D.; Ermakova, S.P. Polysaccharides from brown algae Sargassum duplicatum: The structure and anticancer activity. *Carbohydr. Polym.* **2017**, *175*, 547–556. [CrossRef] [PubMed]
107. Zhong, Q.W.; Zhou, T.S.; Qiu, W.H.; Wang, Y.K.; Xu, Q.L.; Ke, S.Z.; Wang, S.J.; Jin, W.H.; Chen, J.W.; Zhang, H.W.; et al. Characterization and hypoglycemic effects of sulfated polysaccharides derived from brown seaweed. *Food Chem.* **2021**, *341*, 128148. [CrossRef] [PubMed]
108. Park, J.; Cha, J.D.; Choi, K.M.; Lee, K.Y.; Han, K.M.; Jang, Y.S. Fucoidan inhibits LPS-induced inflammation in vitro and during the acute response in vivo. *Int. Immunopharmacol.* **2017**, *43*, 91–98. [CrossRef] [PubMed]
109. Han, R.; Pang, D.R.; Wen, L.R.; You, L.J.; Huang, R.M.; Kulikouskaya, V. In vitro digestibility and prebiotic activities of a sulfated polysaccharide from Gracilaria Lemaneiformis. *J. Funct. Foods* **2020**, *64*, 103652. [CrossRef]
110. Mou, J.J.; Li, Q.; Shi, W.W.; Qi, X.H.; Song, W.G.; Yang, J. Chain conformation, physicochemical properties of fucosylated chondroitin sulfate from sea cucumber Stichopus chloronotus and its in vitro fermentation by human gut microbiota. *Carbohydr. Polym.* **2020**, *228*, 115359. [CrossRef]
111. Seong, H.; Bae, J.H.; Seo, J.S.; Kim, S.A.; Kim, T.J.; Han, N.S. Comparative analysis of prebiotic effects of seaweed polysaccharides laminaran, porphyran, and ulvan using in vitro human fecal fermentation. *J. Funct. Foods* **2019**, *57*, 408–416. [CrossRef]
112. Pratap, K.; Majzoub, M.E.; Taki, A.C.; Hernandez, S.M.; Magnusson, M.; Glasson, C.R.K.; de Nys, R.; Thomas, T.; Lopata, A.L.; Kamath, S.D. The Algal Polysaccharide Ulvan and Carotenoid Astaxanthin Both Positively Modulate Gut Microbiota in Mice. *Foods* **2022**, *11*, 565. [CrossRef]
113. Liu, Z.Q.; Yan, C.H.; Lin, X.P.; Ai, C.Q.; Dong, X.P.; Shao, L.; Wang, S.T.; Song, S.; Zhu, B.W. Responses of the gut microbiota and metabolite profiles to sulfated polysaccharides from sea cucumber in humanized microbiota mice. *Food Funct.* **2022**, *13*, 4171–4183. [CrossRef]
114. Zhu, Z.J.; Zhu, B.W.; Sun, Y.J.; Ai, C.Q.; Wang, L.L.; Wen, C.R.; Yang, J.F.; Song, S.; Liu, X.L. Sulfated Polysaccharide from Sea Cucumber and its Depolymerized Derivative Prevent Obesity in Association with Modification of Gut Microbiota in High-Fat Diet-Fed Mice. *Mol. Nutr. Food Res.* **2018**, *62*, e1800446. [CrossRef]
115. Wei, B.; Zhong, Q.-W.; Ke, S.-Z.; Zhou, T.-S.; Xu, Q.-L.; Wang, S.-J.; Chen, J.-W.; Zhang, H.-W.; Jin, W.-H.; Wang, H. Sargassum fusiforme Polysaccharides Prevent High-Fat Diet-Induced Early Fasting Hypoglycemia and Regulate the Gut Microbiota Composition. *Mar. Drugs* **2020**, *18*, 444. [CrossRef]
116. Lin, H.T.; Zhang, J.W.; Li, S.Y.; Zheng, B.D.; Hu, J.M. Polysaccharides isolated from Laminaria japonica attenuates gestational diabetes mellitus by regulating the gut microbiota in mice. *Food Front.* **2021**, *2*, 208–217. [CrossRef]

117. Siddiqui, N.Z.; Rehman, A.U.; Yousuf, W.; Khan, A.I.; Farooqui, N.A.; Zang, S.Z.; Xin, Y.; Wang, L. Effect of crude polysaccharide from seaweed, Dictyopteris divaricata (CDDP) on gut microbiota restoration and anti-diabetic activity in streptozotocin (STZ)-induced T1DM mice. *Gut Pathog.* **2022**, *14*, 39. [CrossRef]
118. Zhao, F.Q.; Liu, Q.B.; Cao, J.; Xu, Y.S.; Pei, Z.S.; Fan, H.F.; Yuan, Y.Q.; Shen, X.R.; Li, C. A sea cucumber (Holothuria leucospilota) polysaccharide improves the gut microbiome to alleviate the symptoms of type 2 diabetes mellitus in Goto-Kakizaki rats. *Food Chem. Toxicol.* **2020**, *135*, 110886. [CrossRef]
119. Ruan, Q.L.; Chen, Y.H.; Wen, J.H.; Qiu, Y.H.; Huang, Y.J.; Zhang, Y.; Farag, M.A.; Zhao, C. Regulatory mechanisms of the edible alga Ulva lactuca polysaccharide via modulation of gut microbiota in diabetic mice. *Food Chem.* **2023**, *409*, 135287. [CrossRef]
120. Jia, R.B.; Li, Z.R.; Lin, L.Z.; Luo, D.H.; Chen, C.; Zhao, M.M. The potential mechanisms of Macrocystis pyrifera polysaccharides mitigating type 2 diabetes in rats. *Food Funct.* **2022**, *13*, 7918–7929. [CrossRef]
121. Zhao, Y.F.; Song, P.L.; Yin, S.; Fan, T.Y.; Li, F.W.; Ge, X.D.; Liu, T.T.; Xu, W.; Xu, S.; Chen, L.G. Onchidium struma polysaccharides exhibit hypoglycemic activity and modulate the gut microbiota in mice with type 2 diabetes mellitus. *Food Funct.* **2023**, *14*, 1937–1951. [CrossRef]
122. Zhao, L.P.; Zhang, F.; Ding, X.Y.; Wu, G.J.; Lam, Y.Y.; Wang, X.J.; Fu, H.Q.; Xue, X.H.; Lu, C.H.; Ma, J.L.; et al. Gut bacteria selectively promoted by dietary fibers alleviate type 2 diabetes. *Science* **2018**, *359*, 1151–1156. [CrossRef]
123. Sun, Z.Y.; Yu, S.; Tian, Y.; Han, B.Q.; Zhao, Y.; Li, Y.Q.; Wang, Y.; Sun, Y.J.; Shen, W. Chestnut polysaccharides restore impaired spermatogenesis by adjusting gut microbiota and the intestinal structure. *Food Funct.* **2022**, *13*, 425–436. [CrossRef]
124. Martínez-López, Y.E.; Esquivel-Hernández, D.A.; Sánchez-Castañeda, J.P.; Neri-Rosario, D.; Guardado-Mendoza, R.; Resendis-Antonio, O. Type 2 diabetes, gut microbiome, and systems biology: A novel perspective for a new era. *Gut Microbes* **2022**, *14*, 2111952. [CrossRef]
125. Yang, J.P.; Summanen, P.H.; Henning, S.M.; Hsu, M.; Lam, H.; Huang, J.J.; Tseng, C.H.; Dowd, S.E.; Finegold, S.M.; Heber, D.; et al. Xylooligosaccharide supplementation alters gut bacteria in both healthy and prediabetic adults: A pilot study. *Front. Physiol.* **2015**, *6*, 216. [CrossRef]
126. Santilli, A.; Stefanopoulos, S.; Cresci, G.A.M. The gut barrier and chronic diseases. *Curr. Opin. Clin. Nutr.* **2022**, *25*, 178–185. [CrossRef]
127. Wang, Y.J.; Chen, Y.; Zhang, X.Y.; Lu, Y.P.; Chen, H.X. New insights in intestinal oxidative stress damage and the health intervention effects of nutrients: A review. *J. Funct. Foods* **2020**, *75*, 104248. [CrossRef]
128. Fang, J.Y.; Lin, Y.; Xie, H.L.; Farag, M.A.; Feng, S.M.; Li, J.J.; Shao, P. Dendrobium officinale leaf polysaccharides ameliorated hyperglycemia and promoted gut bacterial associated SCFAs to alleviate type 2 diabetes in adult mice. *Food Chem. X* **2022**, *13*, 100207. [CrossRef]
129. Macho-González, A.; Garcimartín, A.; Redondo, N.; Cofrades, S.; Bastida, S.; Nova, E.; Benedí, J.; Sánchez-Muniz, F.J.; Marcos, A.; López-Oliva, M.E. Carob fruit extract-enriched meat, as preventive and curative treatments, improves gut microbiota and colonic barrier integrity in a late-stage T2DM model. *Food Res. Int.* **2021**, *141*, 110124. [CrossRef]
130. Ma, G.X.; Ma, S.; Du, H.J.; Li, X.Y.; Tao, Q.; Hu, Q.H.; Xiao, H. Interactions between intestinal microbial fermentation products of Pleurotus eryngii polysaccharide with gut mucus. *Food Funct.* **2024**, *15*, 1476–1488. [CrossRef]
131. Jiang, G.Y.; Lei, A.T.; Chen, Y.; Yu, Q.; Xie, J.H.; Yang, Y.; Yuan, T.J.; Su, D. The protective effects of the Ganoderma atrum polysaccharide against acrylamide-induced inflammation and oxidative damage in rats. *Food Funct.* **2021**, *12*, 397–407. [CrossRef]
132. Bai, Y.F.; Yue, Z.L.; Wang, Y.N.; Li, Y.D.; Li, C.; Liu, X.T.; Shi, R.H.; Huo, N.N.; Li, D.D.; Gao, S.; et al. Synergistic effect of polysaccharides and flavonoids on lipid and gut microbiota in hyperlipidemic rats. *Food Funct.* **2023**, *14*, 921–933. [CrossRef]
133. Li, Z.; Li, X.Y.; Shi, P.P.; Li, P.P.; Fu, Y.; Tan, G.F.; Zhou, J.J.; Zeng, J.G.; Huang, P. Modulation of Acute Intestinal Inflammation by Dandelion Polysaccharides: An In-Depth Analysis of Antioxidative, Anti-Inflammatory Effects and Gut Microbiota Regulation. *Int. J. Mol. Sci.* **2024**, *25*, 1429. [CrossRef]
134. Liu, Y.Y.; Wang, C.R.; Li, J.S.; Li, T.T.; Zhang, Y.; Liang, Y.X.; Mei, Y.X. Phellinus linteus polysaccharide extract improves insulin resistance by regulating gut microbiota composition. *FASEB J.* **2020**, *34*, 1065–1078. [CrossRef]
135. van Muijlwijk, G.H.; van Mierlo, G.; Jansen, P.W.T.C.; Vermeulen, M.; Bleumink-Pluym, N.M.C.; Palm, N.W.; van Putten, J.P.M.; de Zoete, M.R. Identification of Allobaculum mucolyticum as a novel human intestinal mucin degrader. *Gut Microbes* **2021**, *13*, 1966278. [CrossRef]
136. Zhou, W.T.; Yang, T.T.; Xu, W.Q.; Huang, Y.J.; Ran, L.W.; Yan, Y.M.; Mi, J.; Lu, L.; Sun, Y.; Zeng, X.X.; et al. The polysaccharides from the fruits of Lycium barbarum L. confer anti-diabetic effect by regulating gut microbiota and intestinal barrier. *Carbohydr. Polym.* **2022**, *291*, 119626. [CrossRef]
137. Cordeiro, L.M.C.; Reinhardt, V.D.; Baggio, C.H.; Werner, M.F.D.; Burci, L.M.; Sassaki, G.L.; Iacomini, M. Arabinan and arabinan-rich pectic polysaccharides from quinoa (Chenopodium quinoa) seeds: Structure and gastroprotective activity. *Food Chem.* **2012**, *130*, 937–944. [CrossRef]
138. Wang, M.X.; Chen, Y.X.; Wang, Y.Y.; Li, Y.; Zheng, H.H.; Ma, F.L.; Ma, C.W.; Zhang, X.J.; Lu, B.Y.; Xie, Z.Y.; et al. The effect of probiotics and polysaccharides on the gut microbiota composition and function of weaned rats. *Food Funct.* **2018**, *9*, 1864–1877. [CrossRef]
139. Guo, C.L.; Zhang, S.H.; Wang, Y.Q.; Li, M.X.; Ding, K. Isolation and structure characterization of a polysaccharide from Crataegus pinnatifida and its bioactivity on gut microbiota. *Int. J. Biol. Macromol.* **2020**, *154*, 82–91. [CrossRef]

140. Song, Q.B.; Cheng, S.W.; Li, D.; Cheng, H.Y.; Lai, Y.S.; Han, Q.B.; Wu, H.Y.; Shaw, P.C.; Zuo, Z. Gut microbiota mediated hypoglycemic effect of Astragalus membranaceus polysaccharides in db/db mice. *Front. Pharmacol.* **2022**, *13*, 1043527. [CrossRef]
141. Granado-Serrano, A.B.; Martín-Garí, M.; Sánchez, V.; Solans, M.R.; Berdún, R.; Ludwig, I.A.; Rubió, L.; Vilaprinyó, E.; Portero-Otín, M.; Serrano, J.C.E. Faecal bacterial and short-chain fatty acids signature in hypercholesterolemia. *Sci. Rep.* **2019**, *9*, 1772. [CrossRef]
142. Huang, Y.Z.; Chen, H.; Zhang, K.F.; Lu, Y.M.; Wu, Q.Z.; Chen, J.L.; Li, Y.; Wu, Q.X.; Chen, Y. Extraction, purification, structural characterization, and gut microbiota relationship of polysaccharides: A review. *Int. J. Biol. Macromol.* **2022**, *213*, 967–986. [CrossRef]
143. Soverini, M.; Turroni, S.; Biagi, E.; Quercia, S.; Brigidi, P.; Candela, M.; Rampelli, S. Variation of Carbohydrate-Active Enzyme Patterns in the Gut Microbiota of Italian Healthy Subjects and Type 2 Diabetes Patients. *Front. Microbiol.* **2017**, *8*, 299497. [CrossRef]
144. Li, Q.; Hu, J.; Nie, Q.; Chang, X.; Fang, Q.; Xie, J.; Li, H.; Nie, S. Hypoglycemic mechanism of polysaccharide from Cyclocarya paliurus leaves in type 2 diabetic rats by gut microbiota and host metabolism alteration. *Sci. China Life Sci.* **2021**, *64*, 117–132. [CrossRef]
145. Deng, J.; Zhong, J.; Long, J.; Zou, X.Y.; Wang, D.; Song, Y.; Zhou, K.; Liang, Y.X.; Huang, R.M.; Wei, X.Q.; et al. Hypoglycemic effects and mechanism of different molecular weights of konjac glucomannans in type 2 diabetic rats. *Int. J. Biol. Macromol.* **2020**, *165*, 2231–2243. [CrossRef]
146. Zhong, L.; Peng, X.J.; Wu, C.T.; Li, Q.; Chen, Y.F.; Wang, M.; Li, Y.T.; He, K.Y.; Shi, Y.; Bie, C.Q.; et al. Polysaccharides and flavonoids from cyclocarya paliurus modulate gut microbiota and attenuate hepatic steatosis, hyperglycemia, and hyperlipidemia in nonalcoholic fatty liver disease rats with type 2 diabetes mellitus. *Int. J. Diabetes Dev. Ctries.* **2023**, *43*, 317–327. [CrossRef]
147. Collado, M.C.; Derrien, M.; Isolauri, E. Intestinal integrity and Akkermansia muciniphila, a mucin-degrading member of the intestinal microbiota present in infants, adults, and the elderly. *Appl. Environ. Microb.* **2007**, *73*, 7767–7770. [CrossRef]
148. Shin, N.R.; Lee, J.C.; Lee, H.Y.; Kim, M.S.; Whon, T.W.; Lee, M.S.; Bae, J.W. An increase in the Akkermansia spp. population induced by metformin treatment improves glucose homeostasis in diet-induced obese mice. *Gut* **2014**, *63*, 727–735. [CrossRef]
149. Deng, Q.H.; Wang, W.J.; Zhang, L.Y.; Chen, L.L.; Zhang, Q.F.; Zhang, Y.; He, S.C.; Li, J.E. Gougunao tea polysaccharides ameliorate high-fat diet-induced hyperlipidemia and modulate gut microbiota. *Food Funct.* **2023**, *14*, 703–719. [CrossRef]
150. Huo, J.Y.; Lei, M.; Li, F.F.; Hou, J.J.; Zhang, Z.J.; Long, H.L.; Zhong, X.C.; Liu, Y.M.; Xie, C.; Wu, W.Y. Structural Characterization of a Polysaccharide from Gastrodia elata and Its Bioactivity on Gut Microbiota. *Molecules* **2021**, *26*, 4443. [CrossRef]
151. Wu, H.Q.; Ma, Z.L.; Zhang, D.X.; Wu, P.; Guo, Y.H.; Yang, F.; Li, D.Y. Sequential Extraction, Characterization, and Analysis of Pumpkin Polysaccharides for Their Hypoglycemic Activities and Effects on Gut Microbiota in Mice. *Front. Nutr.* **2021**, *8*, 769181. [CrossRef]
152. Fu, Z.F.; Han, L.F.; Zhang, P.; Mao, H.P.; Zhang, H.; Wang, Y.F.; Gao, X.M.; Liu, E.W. Cistanche polysaccharides enhance echinacoside absorption in vivo and affect the gut microbiota. *Int. J. Biol. Macromol.* **2020**, *149*, 732–740. [CrossRef]
153. Milton-Laskibar, I.; Cuevas-Sierra, A.; Portillo, M.P.; Martínez, J.A. Effects of Resveratrol Administration in Liver Injury Prevention as Induced by an Obesogenic Diet: Role of Ruminococcaceae. *Biomedicines* **2022**, *10*, 1797. [CrossRef]
154. Li, L.; Guo, W.L.; Zhang, W.; Xu, J.X.; Qian, M.; Bai, W.D.; Zhang, Y.Y.; Rao, P.F.; Ni, L.; Lv, X.C. Grifola frondosa polysaccharides ameliorate lipid metabolic disorders and gut microbiota dysbiosis in high-fat diet fed rats. *Food Funct.* **2019**, *10*, 2560–2572. [CrossRef]
155. Dziarski, R.; Park, S.Y.; Kashyap, D.R.; Dowd, S.E.; Gupta, D. Pglyrp-Regulated Gut Microflora Prevotella falsenii, Parabacteroides distasonis and Bacteroides eggerthii Enhance and Attenuates Colitis in Mice. *PLoS ONE* **2016**, *11*, e0146162. [CrossRef]
156. Gao, X.X.; Liu, D.; Gao, L.Y.; Ouyang, Y.Z.; Wen, Y.X.; Ai, C.; Chen, Y.Q.; Zhao, C. Health benefits of Grifola frondosa polysaccharide on intestinal microbiota in type 2 diabetic mice. *Food Sci. Hum. Well* **2022**, *11*, 68–73. [CrossRef]
157. Xu, X.F.; Zhang, X.W. Lentinula edodes-Derived Polysaccharide Alters the Spatial Structure of Gut Microbiota in Mice. *PLoS ONE* **2015**, *10*, e0115037. [CrossRef]
158. Liu, Q.; An, X.; Chen, Y.; Deng, Y.X.; Niu, H.L.; Ma, R.S.; Zhao, H.A.; Cao, W.; Wang, X.R.; Wang, M. Effects of Auricularia auricula Polysaccharides on Gut Microbiota and Metabolic Phenotype in Mice. *Foods* **2022**, *11*, 2700. [CrossRef]
159. Su, L.; Xin, C.X.; Yang, J.T.; Dong, L.R.; Mei, H.R.B.; Dai, X.J.; Wang, Q. A polysaccharide from Inonotus obliquus ameliorates intestinal barrier dysfunction in mice with type 2 diabetes mellitus. *Int. J. Biol. Macromol.* **2022**, *214*, 312–323. [CrossRef] [PubMed]
160. Khan, I.; Huang, G.X.; Li, X.A.; Leong, W.; Xia, W.R.; Hsiao, W.L.W. Mushroom polysaccharides from Ganoderma lucidum and Poria cocos reveal prebiotic functions. *J. Funct. Foods* **2018**, *41*, 191–201. [CrossRef]
161. Christovich, A.; Luo, X.M. Gut Microbiota, Leaky Gut, and Autoimmune Diseases. *Front. Immunol.* **2022**, *13*, 946248. [CrossRef] [PubMed]
162. Richards, J.L.; Yap, Y.A.; McLeod, K.H.; Mackay, C.R.; Mariño, E. Dietary metabolites and the gut microbiota: An alternative approach to control inflammatory and autoimmune diseases. *Clin. Transl. Immunol.* **2016**, *5*, e82. [CrossRef] [PubMed]
163. Wang, Y.; Sun, M.Y.; Jin, H.Y.; Yang, J.B.; Kang, S.; Liu, Y.; Yang, S.; Ma, S.C.; Ni, J. Effects of Lycium barbarum Polysaccharides on Immunity and the Gut Microbiota in Cyclophosphamide-Induced Immunosuppressed Mice. *Front. Microbiol.* **2021**, *12*, 701566. [CrossRef] [PubMed]

164. Tan, T.G.; Sefik, E.; Geva-Zatorsky, N.; Kua, L.; Naskar, D.; Teng, F.; Pasman, L.; Ortiz-Lopez, A.; Jupp, R.; Wu, H.J.J.; et al. Identifying species of symbiont bacteria from the human gut that, alone, can induce intestinal Th17 cells in mice. *Proc. Natl. Acad. Sci. USA* **2016**, *113*, E8141–E8150. [CrossRef] [PubMed]
165. Bunker, J.J.; Drees, C.; Watson, A.R.; Plunkett, C.H.; Nagler, C.R.; Schneewind, O.; Eren, A.M.; Bendelac, A. B cell superantigens in the human intestinal microbiota. *Sci. Transl. Med.* **2019**, *11*, eaau9356. [CrossRef] [PubMed]
166. Shin, N.R.; Whon, T.W.; Bae, J.W. Proteobacteria: Microbial signature of dysbiosis in gut microbiota. *Trends Biotechnol.* **2015**, *33*, 496–503. [CrossRef]
167. Zhao, M.Q.; Tang, F.; Huang, X.Y.; Ma, J.J.; Wang, F.M.; Zhang, P. Polysaccharide Isolated from Agaricus blazei Murill Alleviates Intestinal Ischemia/Reperfusion Injury through Regulating Gut Microbiota and Mitigating Inflammation in Mice. *J. Agric. Food Chem.* **2024**, *72*, 2202–2213. [CrossRef] [PubMed]
168. Xu, T.; Ge, Y.M.; Du, H.; Li, Q.; Xu, X.M.; Yi, H.; Wu, X.Y.; Kuang, T.T.; Fan, G.; Zhang, Y. Berberis kansuensis extract alleviates type 2 diabetes in rats by regulating gut microbiota composition. *J. Ethnopharmacol.* **2021**, *273*, 113995. [CrossRef]
169. Xia, W.; Li, X.; Su, L.; Khan, I.; Leong, W.K.; Yin, L.; Bian, X.; Su, J.; Huang, G.; Hsiao, W.L.W. Corrigendum to "Lycium Berry Polysaccharides Strengthen Gut Microenvironment and Modulate Gut Microbiota of the Mice". *Evid. Based Complement. Altern. Med.* **2020**, *2020*, 4840656. [CrossRef]
170. Zhang, F.H.; Wang, M.; Yang, J.J.; Xu, Q.; Liang, C.; Chen, B.; Zhang, J.M.; Yang, Y.; Wang, H.L.; Shang, Y.F.; et al. Response of gut microbiota in type 2 diabetes to hypoglycemic agents. *Endocrine* **2019**, *66*, 485–493. [CrossRef]
171. Liu, X.; Zhang, J.J.; Li, Y.M.; Sun, L.Y.; Xiao, Y.; Gao, W.G.; Zhang, Z.S. Mogroside derivatives exert hypoglycemics effects by decreasing blood glucose level in HepG2 cells and alleviates insulin resistance in T2DM rats. *J. Funct. Foods* **2019**, *63*, 103566. [CrossRef]
172. Jiang, Q.H.; Chen, L.; Wang, R.; Chen, Y.; Deng, S.G.; Shen, G.X.; Liu, S.L.; Xiang, X.W. Hypoglycemic mechanism of Tegillarca granosa polysaccharides on type 2 diabetic mice by altering gut microbiota and regulating the PI3K-akt signaling pathway. *Food Sci. Hum. Well* **2024**, *13*, 842–855. [CrossRef]
173. Zhong, R.T.; Chen, L.B.; Liu, Y.Y.; Xie, S.X.; Li, S.M.; Liu, B.; Zhao, C. Anti-diabetic effect of aloin via JNK-IRS1/PI3K pathways and regulation of gut microbiota. *Food Sci. Hum. Well* **2022**, *11*, 189–198. [CrossRef]
174. Li, D.; Feng, G.L.; Li, Y.; Pan, H.; Luo, P.; Liu, B.; Ding, T.; Wang, X.; Xu, H.B.; Zhao, Y.F.; et al. Benefits of Huang Lian mediated by gut microbiota on HFD/STZ-induced type 2 diabetes mellitus in mice. *Front. Endocrinol.* **2023**, *14*, 1120221. [CrossRef] [PubMed]
175. Wu, G.J.; Bai, Z.Y.; Wan, Y.J.; Shi, H.F.; Huang, X.J.; Nie, S.P. Antidiabetic effects of polysaccharide from azuki bean (Vigna angularis) in type 2 diabetic rats via insulin/PI3K/AKT signaling pathway. *Food Hydrocoll.* **2020**, *101*, 105456. [CrossRef]
176. Yang, C.F.; Lai, S.S.; Chen, Y.H.; Liu, D.; Liu, B.; Ai, C.; Wan, X.Z.; Gao, L.Y.; Chen, X.H.; Zhao, C. Anti-diabetic effect of oligosaccharides from seaweed Sargassum confusum via JNK-IRS1/PI3K signalling pathways and regulation of gut microbiota. *Food Chem. Toxicol.* **2019**, *131*, 110562. [CrossRef] [PubMed]
177. Lu, H.; Liu, P.; Zhang, X.; Bao, T.; Wang, T.; Guo, L.; Li, Y.; Dong, X.; Li, X.; Dong, Y.; et al. Inulin and Lycium barbarum polysaccharides ameliorate diabetes by enhancing gut barrier via modulating gut microbiota and activating gut mucosal TLR2+ intraepithelial $\gamma\delta$ T cells in rats. *J. Funct. Foods* **2021**, *79*, 104407. [CrossRef]
178. Zhang, C.H.; Sheng, J.Q.; Sarsaiya, S.; Shu, F.X.; Liu, T.T.; Tu, X.Y.; Ma, G.Q.; Xu, G.L.; Zheng, H.X.; Zhou, L.F. The anti-diabetic activities, gut microbiota composition, the anti-inflammatory effects of Scutellaria-coptis herb couple against insulin resistance-model of diabetes involving the toll-like receptor 4 signaling pathway. *J. Ethnopharmacol.* **2019**, *237*, 202–214. [CrossRef] [PubMed]
179. Fernandez-Quintela, A.; Macarulla, M.T.; Gómez-Zorita, S.; González, M.; Milton-Laskibar, I.; Portillo, M.P. Relationship between changes in microbiota induced by resveratrol and its anti-diabetic effect on type 2 diabetes. *Front. Nutr.* **2023**, *9*, 1084702. [CrossRef]
180. Chassaing, B.; Etienne-Mesmin, L.; Gewirtz, A.T. Microbiota-Liver Axis in Hepatic Disease. *Hepatology* **2014**, *59*, 328–339. [CrossRef]
181. de Clercq, N.C.; Frissen, M.N.; Groen, A.K.; Nieuwdorp, M. Gut Microbiota and the Gut-Brain Axis: New Insights in the Pathophysiology of Metabolic Syndrome. *Psychosom. Med.* **2017**, *79*, 874–879. [CrossRef]
182. Dumas, A.; Bernard, L.; Poquet, Y.; Lugo-Villarino, G.; Neyrolles, O. The role of the lung microbiota and the gut-lung axis in respiratory infectious diseases. *Cell Microbiol.* **2018**, *20*, e12966. [CrossRef] [PubMed]
183. Huang, Y.H.; Xin, W.; Xiong, J.C.; Yao, M.Y.; Zhang, B.; Zhao, J.H. The Intestinal Microbiota and Metabolites in the Gut-Kidney-Heart Axis of Chronic Kidney Disease. *Front. Pharmacol.* **2022**, *13*, 837500. [CrossRef] [PubMed]
184. Tong, A.J.; Li, Z.Q.; Liu, X.Y.; Ge, X.D.; Zhao, R.F.; Liu, B.; Zhao, L.A.; Zhao, C. Laminaria japonica polysaccharide alleviates type 2 diabetes by regulating the microbiota-gut-liver axis: A multi-omics mechanistic analysis. *Int. J. Biol. Macromol.* **2024**, *258*, 128853. [CrossRef] [PubMed]
185. Lin, J.M.; Wen, J.M.; Xiao, N.; Cai, Y.T.; Xiao, J.; Dai, W.H.; Chen, J.P.; Zeng, K.W.; Liu, F.S.; Du, B.; et al. Anti-diabetic and gut microbiota modulation effects of sacha inchi (*Plukenetia volubilis* L.) leaf extract in streptozotocin-induced type 1 diabetic mice. *J. Sci. Food Agric.* **2022**, *102*, 4304–4312. [CrossRef] [PubMed]
186. Bai, Z.Y.; Huang, X.J.; Wu, G.J.; Ye, H.; Huang, W.Q.; Nie, Q.X.; Chen, H.H.; Yin, J.Y.; Chen, Y.; Nie, S.P. Polysaccharides from red kidney bean alleviating hyperglycemia and hyperlipidemia in type 2 diabetic rats via gut microbiota and lipid metabolic modulation. *Food Chem.* **2023**, *404*, 134598. [CrossRef]

187. Chen, C.; You, L.J.; Huang, Q.; Fu, X.; Zhang, B.; Liu, R.H.; Li, C. Modulation of gut microbiota by mulberry fruit polysaccharide treatment of obese diabetic db/db mice. *Food Funct.* **2018**, *9*, 3732–3742. [CrossRef]
188. Ding, W.; Wang, Y.N.; Zhou, J.F.; Shi, B. Effect of structure features of polysaccharides on properties of dialdehyde polysaccharide tanning agent. *Carbohydr. Polym.* **2018**, *201*, 549–556. [CrossRef]
189. Silva, I.M.V.; Machado, F.; Moreno, M.J.; Nunes, C.; Coimbra, M.A.; Coreta-Gomes, F. Polysaccharide Structures and Their Hypocholesterolemic Potential. *Molecules* **2021**, *26*, 4559. [CrossRef]
190. Ji, X.L.; Guo, J.H.; Cao, T.Z.; Zhang, T.T.; Liu, Y.Q.; Yan, Y.Z. Review on mechanisms and structure-activity relationship of hypoglycemic effects of polysaccharides from natural resources. *Food Sci. Hum. Well* **2023**, *12*, 1969–1980. [CrossRef]
191. Ji, N.; Liu, P.; Zhang, N.; Yang, S.Y.; Zhang, M.S. Comparison on Bioactivities and Characteristics of Polysaccharides from Four Varieties of Gastrodia elata Blume. *Front. Chem.* **2022**, *10*, 956724. [CrossRef] [PubMed]
192. Wang, H.T.; Li, H.L.; Hou, Y.T.; Zhang, P.J.; Tan, M.Q. Plant polysaccharides: Sources, structures, and antidiabetic effects. *Curr. Opin. Food Sci.* **2023**, *51*, 101013. [CrossRef]
193. Dou, Z.M.; Chen, C.; Fu, X. Digestive Property and Bioactivity of Blackberry Polysaccharides with Different Molecular Weights. *J. Agric. Food Chem.* **2019**, *67*, 12428–12440. [CrossRef] [PubMed]
194. Ferreira-Lazarte, A.; Kachrimanidou, V.; Villamiel, M.; Rastall, R.A.; Moreno, F.J. In vitro fermentation properties of pectins and enzymatic-modified pectins obtained from different renewable bioresources. *Carbohydr. Polym.* **2018**, *199*, 482–491. [CrossRef] [PubMed]
195. Mao, G.Z.; Li, S.; Orfila, C.; Shen, X.M.; Zhou, S.Y.; Linhardt, R.J.; Ye, X.Q.; Chen, S.G. Depolymerized RG-I-enriched pectin from citrus segment membranes modulates gut microbiota, increases SCFA production, and promotes the growth of Bifidobacterium spp., Lactobacillus spp. and Faecalibaculum spp. *Food Funct.* **2019**, *10*, 7828–7843. [CrossRef] [PubMed]
196. Li, Q.; Li, W.Z.; Gao, Q.Y.; Zou, Y.X. Hypoglycemic Effect of Chinese Yam (Dioscorea opposita rhizoma) Polysaccharide in Different Structure and Molecular Weight. *J. Food Sci.* **2017**, *82*, 2487–2494. [CrossRef] [PubMed]
197. Wei, C.Y.; Yao, L.; Zhang, L.; Zhang, Y.; Luo, Q.; Qiu, S.Y.; Zeng, X.Y.; Chen, S.G.; Ye, X.Q. In Vitro Digestion and Fecal Fermentation of Peach Gum Polysaccharides with Different Molecular Weights and Their Impacts on Gut Microbiota. *Foods* **2022**, *11*, 3970. [CrossRef] [PubMed]
198. Lu, X.Y.; Xu, H.T.; Fang, F.; Liu, J.C.; Wu, K.Z.; Zhang, Y.W.; Wu, J.H.; Gao, J. In vitro effects of two polysaccharide fractions from Laminaria japonica on gut microbiota and metabolome. *Food Funct.* **2023**, *14*, 3379–3390. [CrossRef]
199. Kim, K.T.; Rioux, L.E.; Turgeon, S.L. Alpha-amylase and alpha-glucosidase inhibition is differentially modulated by fucoidan obtained from Fucus vesiculosus and Ascophyllum nodosum. *Phytochemistry* **2014**, *98*, 27–33. [CrossRef]
200. Harris, H.C.; Edwards, C.A.; Morrison, D.J. Impact of Glycosidic Bond Configuration on Short Chain Fatty Acid Production from Model Fermentable Carbohydrates by the Human Gut Microbiota. *Nutrients* **2017**, *9*, 26. [CrossRef]
201. Fang, F.; Xiao, C.Q.; Wan, C.; Li, Y.Q.; Lu, X.Y.; Lin, Y.; Gao, J. Two Laminaria japonica polysaccharides with distinct structure characterization affect gut microbiota and metabolites in hyperlipidemic mice differently. *Food Res. Int.* **2022**, *159*, 111615. [CrossRef] [PubMed]

MDPI AG
Grosspeteranlage 5
4052 Basel
Switzerland
Tel.: +41 61 683 77 34

Pharmaceuticals Editorial Office
E-mail: pharmaceuticals@mdpi.com
www.mdpi.com/journal/pharmaceuticals

www.ingramcontent.com/pod-product-compliance
Lightning Source LLC
Chambersburg PA
CBHW041944260926
51850CB00018B/781
9783725865888